**This book is to be returned on or before
the last date stamped below.**

BENIGN PROSTATIC HYPERPLASIA

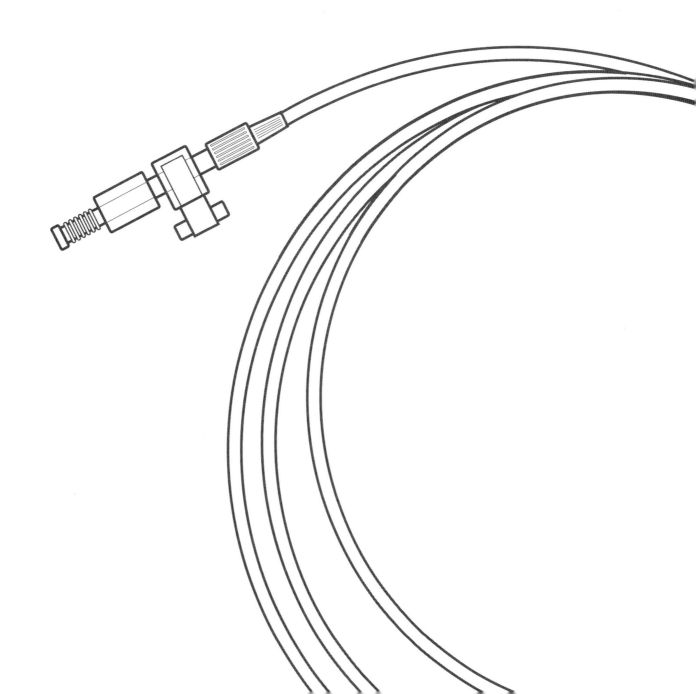

Commissioning Editor	Sue Hodgson
Project Development Manager	Tim Kimber
Project Manager	Rolla Couchman
Production Manager	Helen Sofio
Design and Cover Design	Deborah Gyan

BENIGN PROSTATIC HYPERPLASIA

Perinchery Narayan MD

Professor and Chief of Urology
Division of Urology
College of Medicine
University of Florida
Florida, USA

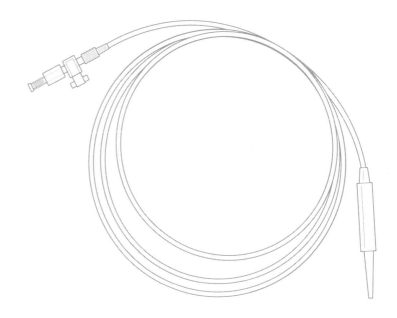

CHURCHILL
LIVINGSTONE London • Edinburgh • New York • Philadelphia • St Louis • Sydney • Toronto 2000

CHURCHILL LIVINGSTONE
An imprint of Harcourt Publishers Limited

First published 2000

ISBN 0 443 05637 4

Cataloguing in Publication Data:
Catalogue records for this book are available from the British Library and
the US Library of Congress.

Note
Medical knowledge is constantly changing. As new information becomes
available, changes in treatment, procedures, equipment and the use of
drugs become necessary. The editors, authors, contributors and the
publishers have, as far as possible, taken care to ensure that the
information given in this text is accurate and up to date. However,
readers are strongly advised to confirm that the information, especially
with regard to drug usage, complies with the latest legislation and
standards of practice.

Printed in Spain by Grafos SA

PREFACE

Unprecedented advances are occurring rapidly in the field of lower urinary tract dysfunction. Traditional definitions of what constitutes Benign Prostatic Hyperplasia (BPH) or enlarged prostate are changing. The field of prostatism is rapidly becoming indistinguishable from the fields of bladder dysfunction, sphincteric dysfunction, and urethral problems. These conditions are often collectively referred to as lower urinary tract symptoms or LUTS. There is now a plethora of traditional and alternative therapies for many of these common symptoms.

This textbook of BPH provides a state-of-the-art compilation of data and commentary from the world's leading experts in this field. Considerable effort and time were spent on covering all aspects of the subject, from molecular biology to alternative therapies. The materials covered in this book are unique since they bring together both the European and American perspectives on the subject.

A major emphasis throughout the book has been the cost-effectiveness of newer treatments (both medical and minimally invasive) and how they compare to standard therapy. With the increased emphasis throughout the world on cost-effective medical practice these considerations are paramount. All of the experts who have contributed have also strived to provide rational explanations for the use of various modalities.

Another valuable feature of this textbook is the Overview section before each set of related chapters and the Commentary sections that follow each chapter. These summaries are designed to provide a succinct overview of each section and chapter for the busy clinician in practice. The authors and the Editor realize the time constraints faced by clinicians 'in the trenches', who need factual, peer-reviewed data quickly and accurately so as to form their own opinion about various aspects of BPH therapy.

It is anticipated that this book will be useful to a broad spectrum of health care providers, including primary care physicians, who are rapidly becoming the gatekeepers and initial contacts for patients, as well as practicing urologists and academic researchers.

Dr Perinchery Narayan
1999

Dedication

Dedicated to my wife and two children, whose continuous support allowed for completion of this book, and to my mentors, students and patients whose teachings and contributions made this book possible.

Acknowledgement

We would like to thank Monika Depalo for her editorial assistance and Pete Betancourt for providing original material for the medical illustrations

CONTENTS

Contents

CONTRIBUTORS

Gopal H Badlani MD, FACS
Associate Chairman
Department of Urology
Long Island Jewish Medical Center
also: Professor of Urology at Albert Einstein College of
Medicine
New York, New York, USA

Michael J Barry MD
Director, Medical Practices Evaluation Center
Medical Practices Evaluation Center
Massachusetts General Hospital
Boston, Massachusetts, USA

John P Blandy CBE, DM, MCH, FRCS, FRCSI, FACS
Emeritus Professor of Urology
Royal London Hospital
London, United Kingdom

Reginald C Bruskewitz MD
Professor of Surgery
Division of Urology
Department of Surgery
University of Wisconsin Hospital and Clinics
Madison, Wisconsin, USA

Carl Cascione MD
Assistant Clinical Professor and Chief
Urology Section
Gainesville VA Medical Center
University of Florida
Gainesville, Florida, USA

R Duane Cespedes MD
Director, Female Urology and Urodynamics
Wilford Hall Medical Center
Lackland Air Force Base
San Antonio, Texas, USA

Toby C Chai MD
Dornier Research Scholar
American Foundation for Urologic Disease
Division of Urology
University of Maryland
Baltimore, Maryland, USA

Marlene Corujo MD
Physician-in-Charge of Voiding Dysfunction and Female
Urology
Phillips Ambulatory Care Center
Beth Israel Medical Center
New York, New York, USA

Louis Denis MD
Director, Oncology Center Antwerp
Antwerp, Belgium

Mark R Feneley MB BChir, MA, BA, MD, FRCS
Senior Registrar
St Bartholomew's Hospital
London, United Kingdom

John M Fitzpatrick MCH, FRCSI, FRCS
Professor of Surgery and Consultant Urologist
Department of Urology
Mater Misericordiae Hospital
University College Dublin
Dublin, Ireland

Jaimie Furman MD
Assistant Professor
Division of Pathology
College of Medicine
University of Florida
Gainesville, Florida, USA

John Hines MB ChB, FRCS (England), FRCS (Edinburgh)
Senior Urological Registrar
Department of Urology
Lister Hospital
Stevenage, United Kingdom

H Logan Holtgrewe MD
Associate Professor of Urology
Department of Urology
School of Medicine
The Johns Hopkins Hospital
Johns Hopkins University
Baltimore, Maryland, USA

Muta M Issa MD, FACS
Assistant Professor of Urology
Emory University School of Medicine
Chief of Urology
Atlanta Veterans Affairs Medical Center
Atlanta, Georgia, USA

Günter Janetschek MD
Assistant Professor of Urology
Department of Urology
University of Vienna,
Vienna, Austria

Steven A Kaplan MD
Vice Chairman and Professor of Urology
Columbia University
College of Physicians and Surgeons
New York, New York, USA

Roger S Kirby MB BChir, MD, FRCS (Urology),
FRCS (England)
Consultant Urologist
St George's Hospital
London, United Kingdom

Gerald M Lennon MCh, FRCSI (Urol)
Consultant Urologist
Department of Urology
Altnagelvin Hospital
Londonderry, Northern Ireland

Stephan Madersbacher MD, F.E.B.U.
Associate Professor of Urology
Department of Urology
University of Vienna
Vienna, Austria

Rajesh Makkenchery MB BS, MD
Surgical Resident
Department of Surgery
Lincoln Medical Center
Bronx, New York, USA

Michael Marberger MD
Professor and Chairman
Department of Urology
University of Vienna
Vienna, Austria

Edward J McGuire MD
Professor of Surgery
Department of Urology
University of Michigan Health Systems
Ann Arbor, Michigan, USA

Tom A McNicholas MB BS, FRCS
Consultant Urological Surgeon
Department of Urology
Lister Hospital
Stevenage, United Kingdom

Douglas F Milam
Professor
Departments of Biomedical Engineering and Urologic
Surgery
Vanderbilt University
Nashville, Tennessee, USA

Perinchery Narayan MD
Professor and Chief of Urology
Division of Urology
College of Medicine
University of Florida
Gainesville, Florida, USA

William H Nau MD
Assistant Professor
Departments of Biomedical Engineering and Urologic
Surgery
Vanderbilt University
Nashville, Tennessee, USA

Michael P O'Leary MD
Associate Professor
Department of Surgery
Division of Urology
Harvard Medical School
Brigham & Women's Hospital
Boston, Massachusetts, USA

Joseph E Oesterling MD
Former Professor and Chief
Division of Urology
The Michigan Medical Center
Ann Arbor, Michegan, USA

Manoj Patel MD
Research Fellow
Division of Urology and Pathology
College of Medicine
University of Florida
Gainesville, Florida, USA

Lori Rice MD
Research Scientist
Division of Urology and Pathology
College of Medicine
University of Florida
Gainesville, Florida, USA

Claus G Roehrborn MD
Associate Professor
Department of Urology
Southwestern Medical School
The University of Texas
Dallas, Texas, USA

Robert J Roselli PhD
Professor of Biomedical Engineering
Departments of Biomedical Engineering and Urologic
Surgery
Vanderbilt University
Nashville, Tennessee, USA

Ghazi Sakr MD
Associate
Department of Surgery
American University of Beirut
Medical Center
Beirut, Lebanon

Mogens Sall MD
Research Fellow
Department of Surgery
Division of Urology
University of Wisconsin Hospital and Clinics
Madison, Wisconsin, USA

Katsuto Shinohara MD
Assistant Professor
Department of Urology
School of Medicine
University of California
San Francisco, California, USA

Joseph A Smith MD
Professor and Chair
Departments of Biomedical Engineering and Urologic
Surgery
Vanderbilt University
Nashville, Tennessee, USA

Bo Standaert MD
Senior Epidemiologist
Oncology Center Antwerp
Antwerp, Belgium

William D Steers MD
Chairman
Jay Y Gillenwater Professor of Urology
Department of Urology
University of Virginia Health Sciences Center
Charlottesville, Virginia, USA

Barry S Stein MD
Professor and Chief of Urology
Division of Urology
Brown University School of Medicine
Providence, Rhode Island, USA

Mitchell S Steiner MD
Professor
Department of Urology
College of Medicine
University of Tennessee
Memphis, Tennessee, USA

Nikolas P Symbas MD
Assistant Professor
Department of Urology
Emory University School of Medicine and
Atlanta Veterans Affairs Medical Center
Atlanta, Georgia, USA

Alexis E Te MD
Assistant Professor of Urology
College of Physicians and Surgeons
Columbia University
New York, New York, USA

Ashutosh Tewari MD
Josephine Ford Scholar
Department of Urology
Josephine Ford Cancer Center
Detroit, Michigan, USA

Graham Watson MB BChir, MD, FRCS (Urology),
FRCS (England)
Consultant Urologist
Eastbourne District General Hospital
Eastbourne, United Kingdom

Section I

INTRODUCTION, SOCIOECONOMICS, QUALITY OF LIFE

Anatomy, Biochemistry, and Endocrinology: Molecular Biology, Endocrinology, and Physiology of the Prostate and Male Accessory Sex Glands

1

P. Narayan, M. Patel, L. Rice, and J. Furman

INTRODUCTION

The human prostate is a complex organ composed of four glandular zones that differ in their histology and biology. The organ is the target of three common clinical conditions of benign prostatic hyperplasia (BPH), prostatitis, and carcinoma of the prostate. The basic anatomy, physiology, and biochemistry of the prostate is reasonably clear. However, insights into its molecular biology and homeostatic regulation are still evolving.

ANATOMY AND EMBRYOGENESIS OF THE PROSTATE

The prostate is the largest accessory gland in the male reproductive system. Anatomically, it is the shape of an inverted pyramid, where the base (the vesicular surface) is the superior surface adjacent to the bladder, while the apex is inferior. The normal prostate weighs about 20 g. The prostate measures between 3 and 4 cm at its widest portion; it is 4–6 cm long, and 2–3 cm thick. The prostate is partly glandular (50–70%) and partly fibromuscular (30–50%), lying in the true pelvis below the inferior border of the symphysis pubis in front of the ampulla of the rectum (Figure 1.1). Structurally, the fibromuscular component is present mostly anteriorly, while the glandular element is mostly in the posterior and lateral aspects of the gland. The upper end of the prostate is continuous with the neck of the bladder, and its apex rests on the superior fascia of the urogenital diaphragm, the medial margins of the levator ani muscles, and the sphincter urethra muscle. The prostate is the size of a walnut and surrounds the prostatic urethra, which runs through the prostate from base to apex, making an anterior 35° angulation at the proximal part of the verumontanum (colliculus seminalis). This angulation divides the urethra into proximal and distal portions, each approximately 15 mm long.

The prostate gland is enveloped in a thin, dense, fibrous capsule (called the true capsule), which is enclosed within a loose sheath, derived from the pelvic fascia, called the prostatic sheath (also known as the false capsule). The prostatic venous plexus lies between this fibrous capsule and the prostatic sheath. The fibrous capsule is composed of collagen, elastin, and smooth muscle. The capsule condenses to form the puboprostatic ligaments, attaching the prostate to the symphysis pubis.

The puboprostatic ligaments support the prostate anterioinferiorly to the pubic bone and inferolaterally to the pubococcygeal segment of the levator ani muscle (Figures 1.1 and 1.2). It is further supported posteriorly by the rectovesical fascia, which separates the posterior surface of the prostate from the lower rectum. Even though the prostate seems to be well anchored to the surrounding bony structures, it is not the case. According to several studies,[1–5] there is a variation in the position of the prostate relative to the bony anatomy. It has been shown that the prostate's position is influenced by the movement of the bony anatomy (i.e. leg rotation), by filling of the rectum, and by filling of the urinary bladder. The prostate is least mobile in the lateral direction and most mobile in the craniocaudal and ventrodorsal directions. The significance of this variability is evident when attempting to position a patient (with prostate cancer) accurately for administration of radiotherapy. However, other studies[6] have shown that the higher the stage of carcinoma, the less mobile the prostate gland; possibly as a result of tumor infiltration into adjacent tissues.

The prostate is perforated posteriorly by the ejaculatory ducts (formed by the seminal vesicles and the ampulla of vas deferens), which pass obliquely through the gland for approximately 2 cm to empty into the verumontanum on the floor of the prostatic urethra just proximal to the striated external urinary sphincter (Figure 1.3A and B).

The posterior surface of the prostate is triangular and flattened transversely. It faces posteriorly and slightly interiorly toward the urogenital diaphragm. It rests on the ampulla of the rectum, and it is this surface that can be palpated by digital rectal exam (DRE) (Figure 1.4). Because the posterior surface is in contact with the anterior wall of the rectum, the layers of Denonvilliers' fascia, the pouch of Douglas, and the rectovesical septum are the only structures separating the examiner's gloved digit from the prostate. Rectal palpation of the prostate provides information about its size and consistency. A normal prostate has a soft, non-tender, elastic texture; whereas, a malignant (cancerous) prostate feels hard and nodular, and an inflamed prostate (prostatitis) results in an enlarged (>2 cm), tender "hot" gland. Upon rectal exam, the position of the prostate depends on the fullness of the bladder; a full bladder will displace the gland inferiorly, so it is more readily palpable.

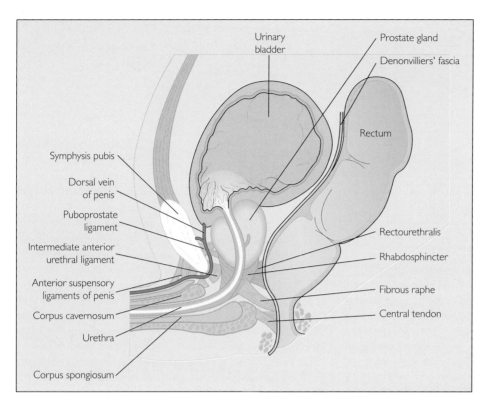

Figure 1.1 Sagittal view of the true pelvis. Note the relationship of the prostate gland to the rhabdosphincter and urinary bladder

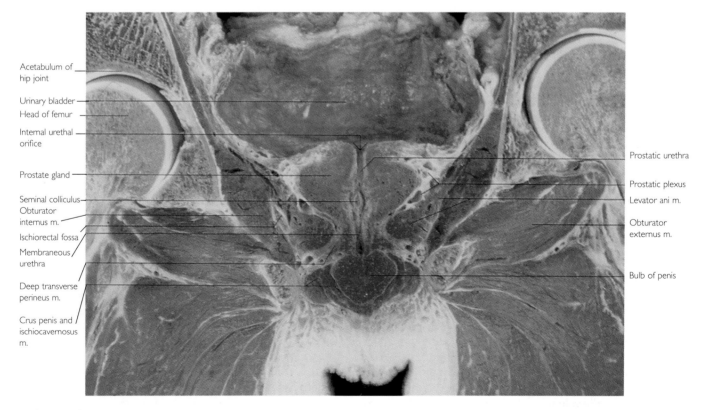

Figure 1.2 Coronal section anatomy of the prostate and supporting muscular structures

Source: Reproduced with permission from *Colour Atlas of Anatomy*, 3rd edn. Rohen and Yokochi. New York: Igaku-Shoin, 1992

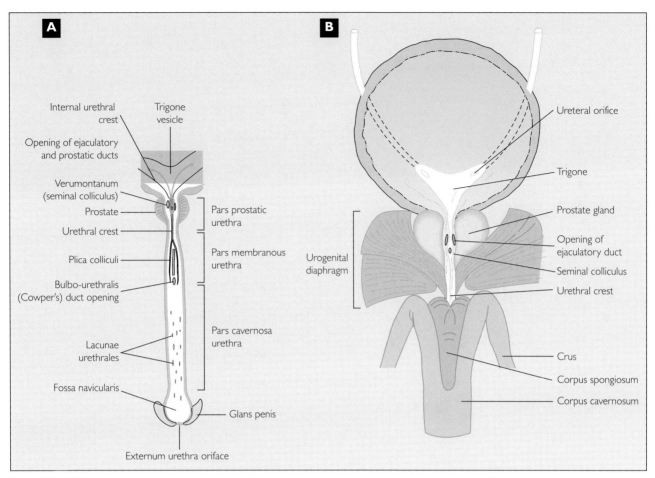

Figure 1.3 (A) Transverse section of the urethra; (B) section of the prostatic urethra showing relationships of the urogenital diaphragm, bladder, and penis

The posterior surface also has a shallow median groove demarcating the lateral lobes. However, because the lateral lobes are often fused, urologists sometimes refer to them as the posterior lobe. Superior to this on the posterior surface, there is a shallow groove where the ejaculatory ducts enter the prostate gland. This area has a slight indentation and indicates the area of the median lobe. When hypertrophied, the median lobe can act like a valve, causing obstructive urinary symptoms.

The anterior surface of the prostate is transversely narrow and convex. The inferolateral surfaces of the prostate meet anteriorly with the convex anterior surface and rest on the fascia covering the levator ani muscles. The 20–30 prostatic ducts open chiefly into the prostatic sinuses on each side of the urethral crest on the posterior wall of the prostatic urethra. This arrangement is present because most glandular tissue is located posterior and lateral to the prostatic urethra. This glandular tissue is responsible for the secretion of a thin, milky fluid upon contraction of the smooth muscles in the prostate. Prostatic fluid provides about 20% of the volume of the semen or seminal fluid. The seminal vesicles lie in a coronal plane with an axis at a 20–30° angle, lateral to the prostate gland.

THE "RHABDOSPHINCTER"

The distal part of the urethra is surrounded by a sphincter of striated muscle fibers (known as the rhabdosphincter), which is a proximal extension of the external sphincter located distal to the prostate apex. This sphincter and the associated membranous urethra that it covers must be dissected during radical prostatectomy. The anatomic relations between this muscle, the levator ani muscle, the membranous urethra, and the pudendal nerves play a crucial role in radical prostatectomy, particularly with regard to postoperative urinary incontinence.

With regard to anatomy, two concepts of the striated external sphincter anatomy have existed. Most investigators have described the sphincter as part of the "urogenital diaphram" caudal to the prostate;[7–10] others, however, define it as a striated muscle, which extends from the base of the bladder to the region of the "urogenital diaphragm".[11,12] Traditionally, the shape of this muscle was considered to be circular and completely enclosing the membranous urethra;[11–14] but this concept has been questioned in the last few years.[15–17] Data from anatomic studies reveal that the striated muscle fibers run in a cranial direction from the bulb

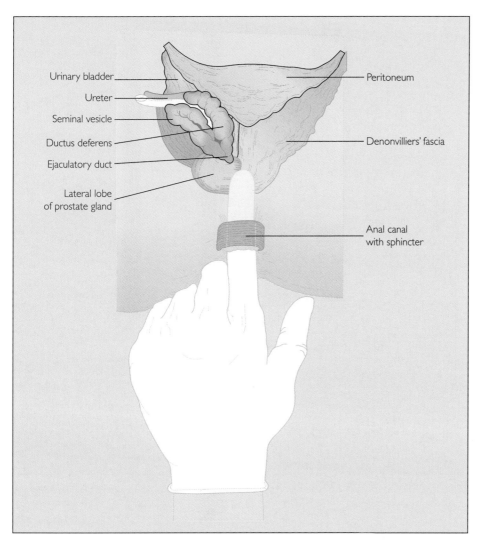

Urinary bladder

Ureter

Seminal vesicle

Ductus deferens

Ejaculatory duct

Lateral lobe
of prostate gland

Peritoneum

Denonvilliers' fascia

Anal canal
with sphincter

Figure 1.4 Note the structures that can be palpated upon DRE. The Denonvilliers' fascia is not shown on the left side, in order to reveal the underlying structures

of the penis to the base of the bladder along the anterolateral aspects of the prostate and the membranous urethra[11,12,14] (Figures 1.5A and B). The fibers of this vertically oriented muscle were arranged in a loop-shaped fashion on the ventral and lateral aspects of the urethra. It has also been noted that the rhabdosphincter does not form a complete collar around the membranous urethra. In the past some authors have depicted the rhabdosphincter as fully encircling the urethra. Although variations in muscular development may cause this to happen occasionally (Figure 1.5B) this is not the norm in most patients; rather, it is muscular "collar" ventral and lateral to the membranous urethra and prostate, the core of which is an omega-shaped (Ω) loop around the urethra.[16,17] Both ends of the omega-shaped sphincter insert at the perineal body (Figure 1.5A and B). The rhabdosphincter is also separated from the ventral portion of the levator ani muscle by a sheet of connective tissue; thus, contrary to previous understanding, the rhabdosphincter is an independent muscle unit that is not in direct contact with the fibers of the levator ani muscle.[18]

The innervation of this sphincter muscle is also a subject of controversy. Some authors[19,20] believe that it is under the

control of the sacral plexus (which runs on the pelvic surface of the levator ani) or possibly fibers from the cavernous nerves.[21-23] However, Narayan and associates[18] found that the rhabdosphincter is innervated by small branches of the pudendal nerve after leaving the pudendal canal[18] (Figures 1.7A–C, 1.8, and 1.9A and B). Regardless of which nerve innervates it, the sacral plexus, the pudendal nerve branches and the rhabdosphincter muscle all have to be preserved during radical prostatectomy in order to obtain good urinary continence results. It is Narayan's hypothesis that the wide variation in sphincteric strength between individuals occurs in large part owing to the variable growth of the prostate between the bladder neck and the external sphincter. In the prepubertal male, the urethral sphincter is a 4–5-cm-long segment extending continuously from the bladder neck and ending at the striated sphincter. At puberty, the prostate literally grows through this tissue between the bladder neck and distal external sphincter, disrupting it variably. The resultant remnants of muscle at the bladder neck and external sphincter are variable and, depending on its residual length, a radical prostatectomy can cause near total removal or preservation of a significant portion of it. Much of this is

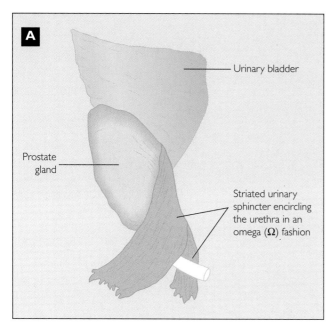

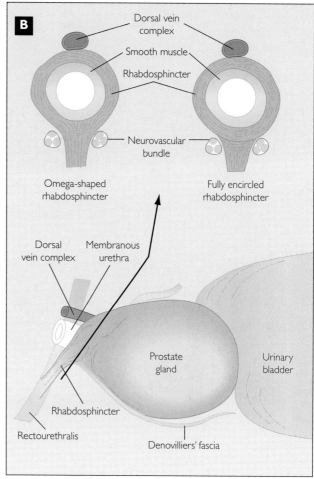

Figure 1.5 (A) Orientation of the rhabdosphincter in relation to the prostate gland and membranous urethra. In some patients, the muscle has circular fibers completing this omega shape (see Figure 1.5B). (B) Note the two variations of the rhabdosphincter encircling the urethra

not under the control of the surgeon, since the prostate length, shape, and apical extension into the distal sphincter are widely variable.

The degree of urinary incontinence is dependent to some extent on the anatomical condition of the striated external sphincter after radical prostatectomy. In healthy adult males, the rhabdosphincter, during contraction, pulls the membranous urethra interiorly towards the perineal body to compress the urethra. Gosling and associates[27] demonstrated that the rhabdosphincter consists of fibers that are functionally capable of maintaining tone over prolonged time periods without developing fatigue; the combination of the ability for chronic tonic contracture and its strategic location suggest that the rhabdosphincter is a core part of the sphincteric mechanism that maintains incontinence after radical prostatectomy. Additional data from Helweg et al., who conducted a transurethral sonographic evaluation of the rhabdosphincter, also suggest that injuries to this muscle inevitably will lead to urinary incontinence.[24]

Data from a study of both fetal anatomy and adult reveals that the proportions of striated and smooth muscle fibers in the rhabdosphincter change during life. In the fetus, the number of striated fibers of the rhabdosphincter is comparatively high. In the adult male, on the contrary, the content of the sphincter is gradually replaced by smooth muscle and connective tissue. The replacement of muscle tissue by fibrous tissue with advancing age is the reason for increased incidence of postoperative urinary incontinence in men more than 70 years old.[11,25]

BLOOD AND LYMPHATIC SUPPLY TO THE PROSTATE

The prostate is a highly vascular gland with extensive collateral circulation. The arterial blood supply to the prostate enters on either side at the base close to the bladder neck. The anterior division of the internal iliac artery is the major blood supplier to the prostate gland also giving rise to three branches. The main arterial branch to the prostate is the inferior vesical artery, but the middle rectal (hemorrhoidal) artery and the internal pudendal artery also provide some anastomosing circulation to the prostate (Figures 1.10 and 1.11). The inferior vesical artery divides into a prostatic and vesical branch; the prostatic artery then divides into the urethral and capsular arteries.

The first main branch off the prostatic artery is the urethral artery, which penetrates the prostate gland at the prostaticovesical junction in a posterolateral fashion at the 5 o'clock and 7 o'clock positions. It enters the gland, perpendicular to the urethra; then it turns caudally to run parallel

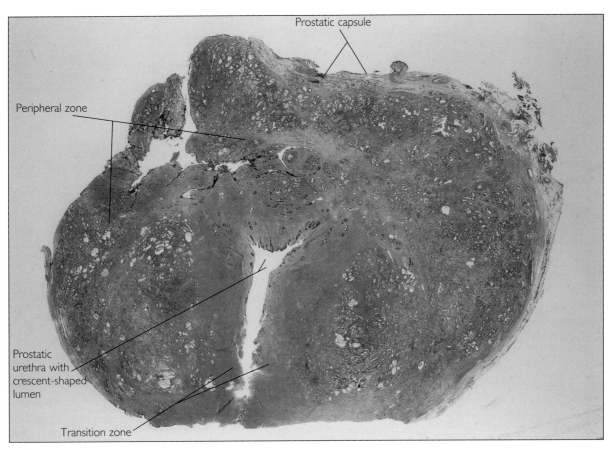

Figure 1.6 Low-power view of a whole mount of the prostate gland. Note the transition zone, peripheral zone, urethra, and prostatic capsule

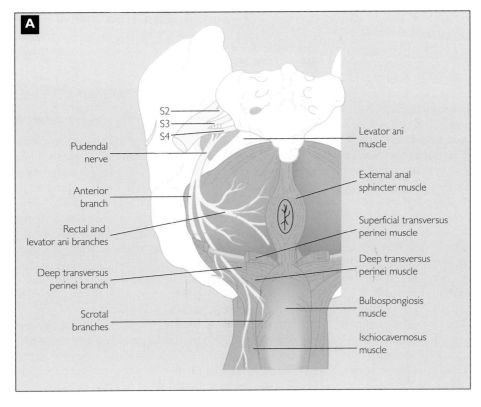

Figure 1.7 (A) Dorsal view of the somatic nerve supply of the prostate

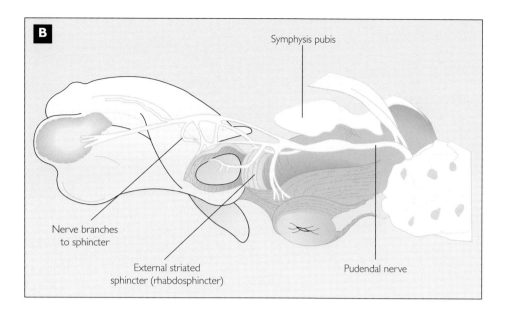

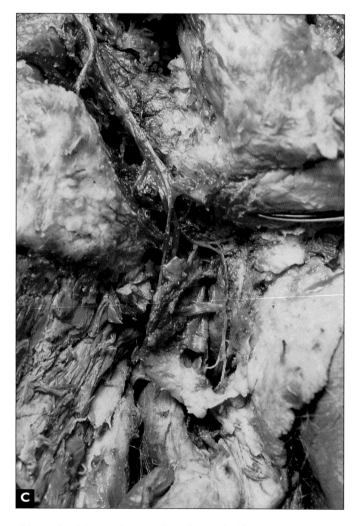

Figure 1.7 (B) Composite view of the pudendal nerve, its outer branches and sphincter nerve supply. (C) Anatomical dissection of the pudendal nerve with its branches to the external striated sphincter and other surrounding structures

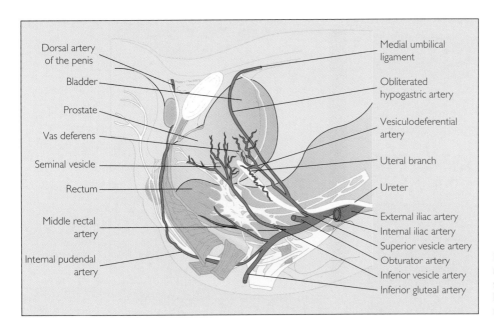

Figure 1.8 Lateral view of the nerve supply of the prostate, showing relationships of the hypogastric nerve plexus, somatic nerves, and pelvic plexus

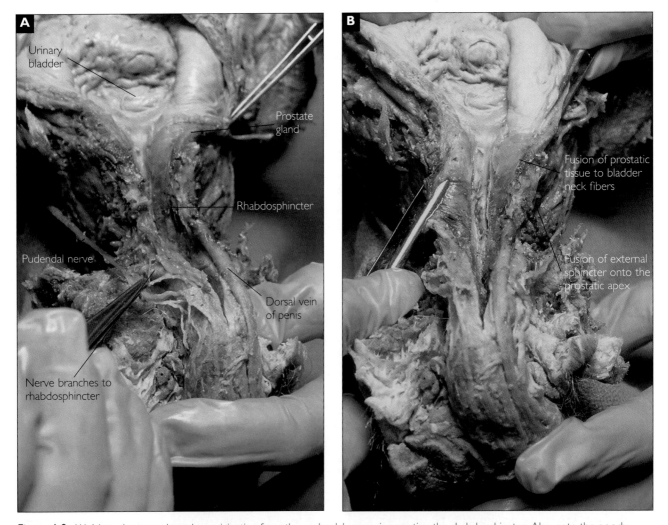

Figure 1.9 (A) Note the nerve branches originating from the pudendal nerve, innervating the rhabdosphincter. Also note the poorly defined and demarcated boundaries of the prostate gland and bladder and the prostate gland and rhabdosphincter. (B) Note the smooth continuation of the prostate with the external sphincter and bladder neck. Note the insertion of the rhabdosphincter into the perineal body

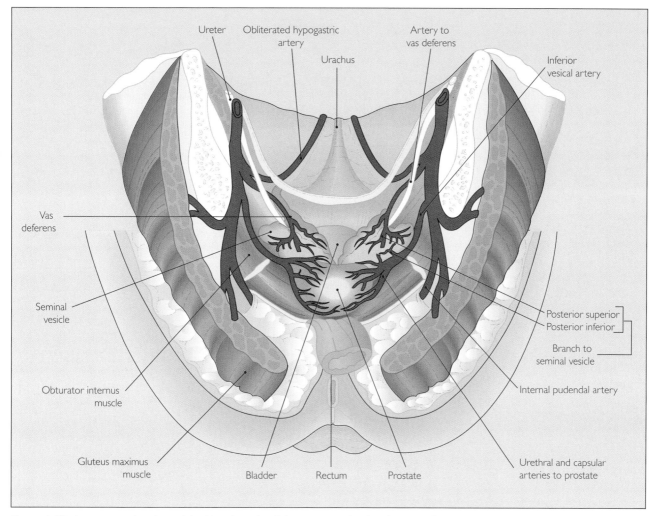

Figure 1.10 Anteroposterior view of the blood supply of the prostrate gland and surrounding structures

to the urethra. As it runs in the caudal direction, it gives off branches to supply the prostatic urethra, the periurethral glands, and the transition zone. In 1937, Flocks and associates noted that this artery is the major blood source for a developing adenoma (during BPH) in the transition zone. Of interest, during resection of the transition zone in patients with BPH, there is significant bleeding from the urethral artery, especially at the 4–8 o'clock positions where the vessels enter.

The second branch of the prostatic artery, the capsular artery (as its name says), supplies the prostatic capsule. This artery courses with the cavernous nerves (as the neurovascular bundle) to run in the posterolateral direction terminating at the pelvic diaphragm.

The venous outflow is extensive. The veins are wide, thin walled and course anterolaterally and posteriorly. The veins of the prostate coalesce to form the prostatic venous plexus (also known as periprostatic plexus), which has connections with the deep dorsal vein of the penis and the internal iliac (hypogastric) veins. This plexus surrounds the sides and base of the prostate, and is located between the true capsule of the prostate and its outer facial sheath. The prostatic venous plexus drains mainly into the internal iliac veins, but it does communicate with the vesical venous plexus and the deep dorsal vein (of the penis) to form the Santorini's venous plexus in the space posterior to the pubic bone, eventually emptying into the internal iliac veins (Figures 1.12 and 1.13) These plexuses are also connected to the presacral venous plexus, hemorrhoidal veins, and vertebral venous plexus. This latter plexus is of great clinical importance. Since prostate cancer spreads mainly via the hematogenous route, the communicating valveless vessels between the prostatic venous plexus in the pelvis and vertebral venous plexus in the vertebral column are the anatomical basis for metastasis of the cancer to the pelvis and spinal cord/brain. The main connections are via the pelvic and common iliac veins to the ascending lumbar veins. It is thought by some that straining to urinate may cause the blood draining the prostatic venous plexus to reverse its flow and pass via the lumbar plexus into the vertebral venous plexus to nest in the central nervous system (CNS).

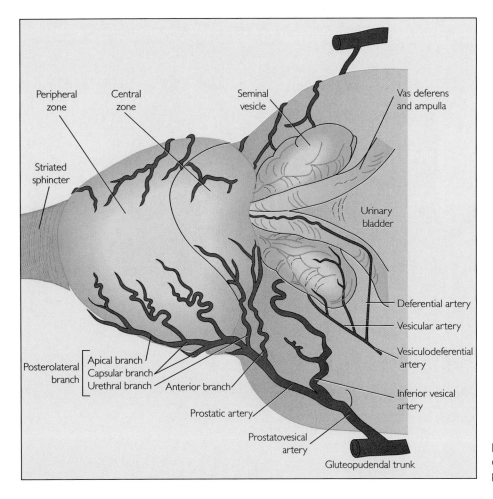

Figure 1.11 Anterolateral view of the blood supply to the prostate gland

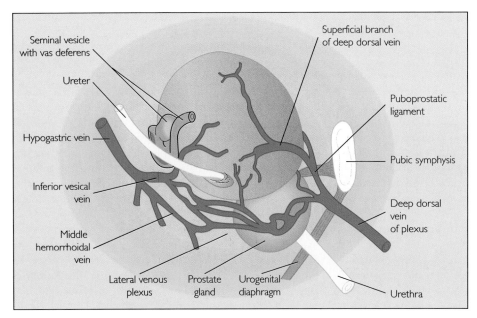

Figure 1.12 Lateral view of the venous drainage of the prostate gland. Note the relationship of the dorsal venous complex to the urethra and puboprostatic ligaments

Another route of metastases for prostate cancer is via the lymphatic system. The lymphatic vessels draining the prostate terminate chiefly in the obturator, internal iliac, and sacral lymph nodes (Figure 1.14). However, there are some lymphatic vessels draining the posterior aspect of the gland, that unite with the urinary bladder lymphatic vessels to drain into the external iliac lymph nodes. These lymph nodes from the internal iliac, vesical, external iliac, and

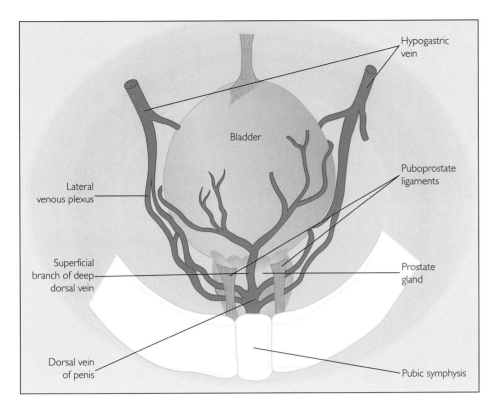

Figure 1.13 Anterior view of the venous drainage of the prostate gland

sacral regions subsequently drain into the inferior vena cava. This lymphatic route is also utilized by metastatic cells to the lungs and then to other parts of the body, such as the bone.

NERVE INNERVATION OF THE PROSTATE

The efferent nerve supply of the prostate arises from the prostatic nerve plexus, which lies at the base of the prostate on its posterior side; it lies there with the vascular supply, forming the neurovascular bundle. The prostatic plexus innervates the gland via the cavernous nerves. These nerves, following the capsular artery, branch into the glandular and stromal compartments of the gland. The prostatic nerve plexus receives innervation both from the thoracolumbar sympathetic (noradrenergic) nerves and sacral parasympathetic (cholinergic) nerves (Figures 1.8, 1.10, and 1.15).

The parasympathetic fibers feed into the prostate plexus via the pelvic splanchnic nerves (S2–S4), whereas the sympathetic fibers supply the prostatic nerve plexus via fibers that are derived from the inferior hypogastric plexus. Thus, within the prostate are contained both cholinergic and noradrenergic nerve cell bodies. It has been found that parasympathetic nerves, which terminate in the acini, promote secretion, whereas the sympathetic nerves cause contraction of the smooth muscles of the capsule and stroma. It is these latter nerves that are antagonized when treating BPH patients with α-blocker therapy; α-blockade diminishes the smooth muscle tone of the preprostatic sphincter, the capsule, and stroma, causing urethral lumen dilation and increased urinary flow rates.[21,26] This has formed the basis of

the therapeutic use of α-blockers in the medical management of BPH.

The autonomic nerves that supply the prostate enter the prostatic base from the posterior aspect. As the neurovascular bundle approaches the capsule, the majority of the nerves leave the bundle and penetrate the prostate to run in the medial direction. These nerves fan-out to form synapses with autonomic ganglions embedded in the layer of fatty tissue just beneath the capsule. These nerve fibers continue medially to supply not only the prostate base but also the central zone. Once within the prostatic parenchyma, the nerve fibers end in the walls of the ducts and acini, and the smooth muscle bundles of the stroma.

In 1983, Gosling reported that both sympathetic and parasympathetic nerves innervate the smooth muscles of the prostatic stroma, whereas the smooth muscle of the capsule is solely innervated by parasympathetic nerves.[27] Furthermore, from the studies by Smith and Lebeaux[28] and Brushini *et al.*[29] in the 1970s, it has been shown that parasympathetic stimulation increases the rate of secretion while sympathetic stimulation is responsible for the expulsion of prostatic fluid into the urethra (as seen in ejaculation).

EMBRYOLOGY

During the 8th week of gestation, the developing testis in the male fetus begins to produce androgens, mainly testosterone. Leydig cells secrete testosterone, which stimulates the wolffian (mesonephric) duct system to proliferate and differentiate. At the same time, the Sertoli cells secrete

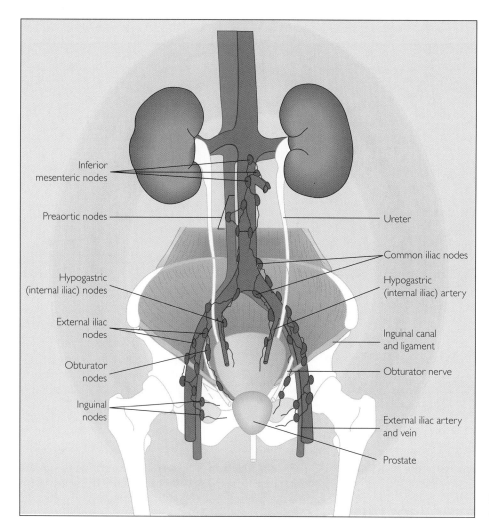

Figure 1.14 The lymphatic drainage of the prostate gland

müllerian-inhibiting substance which acts to suppress the development of the müllerian (paramesonephric) ducts.[30]

Approximately at a gestation age of 28 days, the cloaca, located at the caudal end of the hindgut (see Figure 1.16A), undergoes division by a coronal sheet of mesenchyme (the urorectal system), which develops in the angle between the allantois and the hindgut (Figures 1.16A and B). As this septum grows toward the cloacal membrane, the infolding of the lateral walls of the cloaca grow toward each other and fuse, dividing the cloaca into two parts: (1) the rectum and upper anal canal dorsally; and (2) the urogenital (UG) sinus ventrally.

By the end of the 6th week of gestation, the urorectal septum has fused with the cloacal membrane, dividing it into a dorsal anal membrane (which ruptures at the end of the 7th week to form the anal canal) and a larger ventral UG membrane. This primitive UG sinus proximal to the mesonephric duct becomes the vesicourethral canal (eventually forming the urinary bladder), whereas the region distal to the mesonephric ducts develops into the definitive UG sinus (which gives rise to the prostate gland and other male genital glands). The pelvic part of the UG sinus (Figures 1.16A and B), adjacent and inferior to the

bladder, develops into the lower portion of the prostatic and membranous urethra. Embryologically, the cranial half of the pelvic urethra is derived from the endodermal UG sinus, whereas the caudal half originates entirely from the UG sinus. Posteriorly, a component of the mesonephric mesoderm originating from the bladder becomes incorporated into the pelvic urethra, forming the superficial layer of the trigone. Later in development, this mesenchyme become smooth muscle that is continuous with the bladder trigone.[31,32] During the 10th week, the mesenchymal tissue associated with the urogenital sinus (UGS) responds to the 5α-reduced form of testosterone, 5α-dihydrotestosterone (DHT), which induces outgrowths of the nearby urothelium of the UGS.[33-35] During the 10th week of gestation, the endodermal UG sinus (caudal to the bladder, and above and below the origin of the mesonephric duct) begins to form multiple, solid endodermal outgrowths of the urethral epithelium (prostatic buds). The glandular epithelium of the prostate differentiates from the invaginated endodermal cells; the mesenchyme differentiates into stroma and smooth muscle fibers. According to several anatomical studies on the prostate, it is concluded that the formation of the fetal prostatic ducts occurs from a ventral, lateral, and

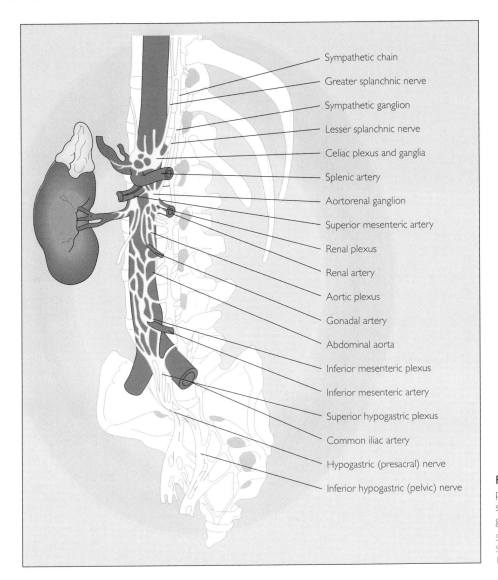

Sympathetic chain
Greater splanchnic nerve
Sympathetic ganglion
Lesser splanchnic nerve
Celiac plexus and ganglia
Splenic artery
Aortorenal ganglion
Superior mesenteric artery
Renal plexus
Renal artery
Aortic plexus
Gonadal artery
Abdominal aorta
Inferior mesenteric plexus
Inferior mesenteric artery
Superior hypogastric plexus
Common iliac artery
Hypogastric (presacral) nerve
Inferior hypogastric (pelvic) nerve

Figure 1.15 The prostatic nerve plexus with nerves from the sympathetic and parasympathetic ganglions

Source: From Hinman F, *Atlas of Urologic Surgery*, 2nd edn. Philadelphia: WB Saunders; 1998, with permission

dorsal aspect of the UGS.[36-38] These prostatic buds penetrate into the surrounding müllerian mesoderm to form the utricle and the mesonephric mesoderm, which, in turn, gives rise to the ejaculatory ducts.[39-43] These tubular outgrowths begin to lengthen rapidly, arborize, and canalize, forming five distinct groups by the end of the 11th week of gestation, and by the 13th week, 70 primary ducts are present. These outgrowths begin as solid epithelial buds, which branch extensively during late fetal growth to form a complex tubuloalveolar gland structure. This tubular outgrowth is completed by the end of the 16th week of gestation. The initial five distinct outgrowths are termed[43] the posterior, lateral (two), middle and anterior lobes. The majority of prostate ducts grow in a posterolateral direction. The buds of the middle (lobe) tubules originate from the posterior urethra between the bladder neck and the ejaculatory duct openings.[43] The predominant number of prostatic outgrowths occur in the lateral region (approximately 18 pairs), while the middle and posterior lobes average nine tubules opening into the prostatic urethra. The final size of the

prostate depends upon the degree of mesenchymal cell differentiation under the influence of the potent DHT.

Even though five lobes are widely separated to form distinct entities during fetal development, the distinct boundaries of these five lobes are abolished with no definite septa dividing them, as early as 2–5 months postnatally.[39,44] These five buds do not intermingle with each other, but simply lie side by side.

The glandular epithelium of the prostate differentiates from the endodermal cells of the prostatic buds, and the associated mesenchyme differentiates into the stroma and smooth muscle fibers on the prostate.[45] By the 22nd week, the muscular stroma is considered developed, and it continues to increase progressively until birth. Prior to term, the fetal prostate is composed of a few tubules that are widely separated by stroma. By term, the glandular epithelium proliferates and the stromal elements decline in amount.[46]

Some investigators[47] have examined the zonal histogenesis of the fetal prostate and concluded that the prostate undergoes three stages of histogenesis. During the bud state

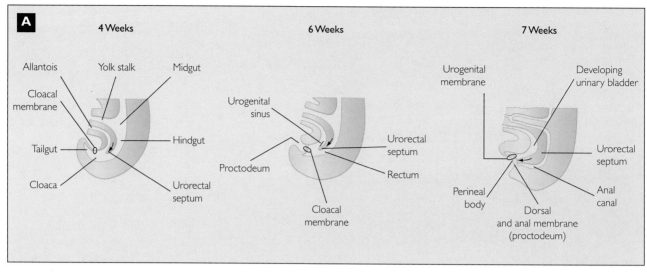

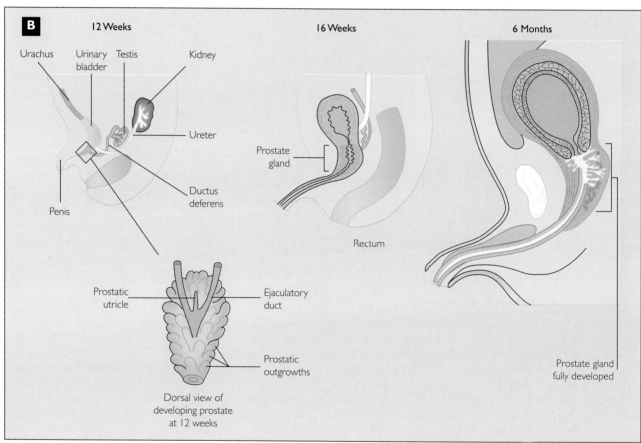

Figure 1.16 (A) Embryologic development of the prostate gland, beginning at week 4 of the gestational period. After the development of the urogenital membrane and sinus at week 7, the prostate and urinary bladder begin to develop. (B) Development of the prostate gland from week 12 to week 24 of gestation

(20–30 weeks of gestational age), the buds at the end of the ducts were simple, solid, and cellular with no lumen present; columnar cells were present basally and spindle-shaped cells were found near the bud centers. In the next stage, the bud-tubule state (31–36 weeks), there are small collections of cellular buds and acini. Further differentiation of the fetal prostate gland involves the development of

distinct acinotubular glands arising from the tubules with distinct lumina; this occurs during the 34–42 week gestational period, named the acinotubular state.

The most significant postnatal growth of the prostate gland occurs during puberty. During this maturation period, the ducts begin to branch extensively and form patent lumens within the terminal acini. Furthermore, the epithelial lining of the ducts and acini become highly differentiated with ciliated-columnar cells.

Although the entire prostate is thought to be derived from epithelium and mesenchyme of the embryonic UG sinus (mainly from the mesoderm), the ejaculatory ducts, a part of the verumontanum, the intraprostatic part of the vas deferens, and part of the acinar glands (the central zone) may be of wolffian duct origin. However, it has been suggested that the central zone (which is morphologically distinct from the adjacent peripheral zone) might also develop from the wolffian (mesonephric) duct.[48–50] Two pieces of evidence are present to support this claim. First, histologically, the central zone is similar to that of the seminal vesicle, suggesting a common origin. Secondly, the gastric proenzyme pepsinogen II is present within cells of both the central zone and the seminal vesicle, but not elsewhere within the prostate.[51] By contrast, plasminogen activator is not found within the cells of the peripheral zone.[52] These data suggest that tissues within and adjacent to the prostate are of different embryological origin. These differences could explain the susceptibility of certain parts of the prostate to specific disorders within different areas – namely BPH within the transition and periurethral zones and prostatic adenocarcinoma within the peripheral zone.

ZONAL ANATOMY OF THE PROSTATE

In 1912, Lowsley first presented a detailed description of the prostate, based on embryonic and fetal studies; he proposed that the prostate was an outgrowth of five lobes, namely two lateral, medial, anterior, and posterior.[43] In 1954, Franks[44] challenged this theory and revised the zonal anatomy of the prostate. This map of the prostate was modified many times by numerous others.[37,53–55] In 1972, McNeal proposed a concept of zonal anatomy based on histology and anatomy that is currently used as the basis for describing the location and perhaps the origin of neoplastic processes within the prostate.[31,37,53] McNeal defined four distinct regions of the prostate, each of which develops from a different segment of the prostatic urethra. According to this concept, there is a fibromuscular, non-glandular region (comprising 1/3 of the total gland) and the glandular portion of the prostate (comprising 2/3 of the gland); the latter region is composed of a large peripheral zone (70–80% of the total glandular area) and a small central zone, which together constitute about 95% of the glandular part of the gland. The other 5–10% of the glandular region is formed by the transition zone, located adjacent to the urethra at the verumontanum, and is composed of the periurethral glands. In 1975 Tissell was the first to describe the complex arrangement of prostatic ducts in an "onion pattern" with a central lobe in the centre and more lateral and posterior lobes in the periphery. The fourth region, described by McNeal as the largest, is the anterior fibromuscular (non-glandular) cap, which consists of stromal and muscular tissue, partially covering the urethra and bladder neck anteriorly; this region has no glandular epithelial cells (Figures 1.17A and B). This cap extends from the external longitudinal fibers of the bladder neck and is in contact with the distal prostatic urethra. The central and peripheral zones are not demarcated easily as separate regions, whereas the transition zone is well demarcated from the other two zones.

The stroma (collagen) and the smooth muscle of the anterior cap is continuous with the capsule. It encircles the entire gland, and the smooth muscle of the capsule contracts during ejaculation to expel the prostatic secretions into the urethra.

The peripheral zone of the glandular prostate forms the lateral and posterior part of the organ. It constitutes the

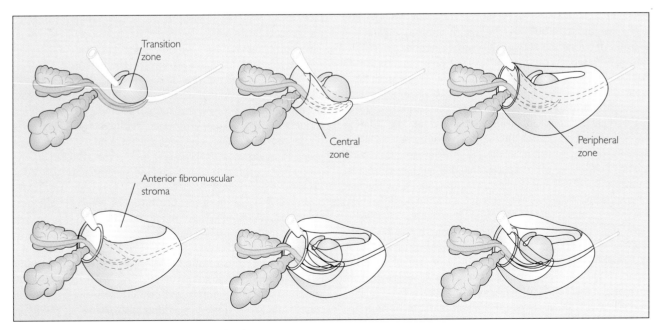

Figure 1.17 Zonal anatomy of the prostate gland

Source: Images were modified from Walsh *et al.* *Campbell's Textbook of Urology*, 7th edition. Philadelphia: WB Saunders 1998: 112

apex of the prostate and widens cranially to form a funnel-shaped structure; this open-end of the funnel fuses with the distal part of the wedge-shaped central zone. The ducts of this peripheral zone perforate into the distal prostatic urethra.

The cone-shaped central zone of the glandular prostate surrounds the ejaculatory ducts in the verumontanum with its apex and the bladder neck with its base. The seminal vesicles and ampulla of the vas deferens are embedded adjacently in the central zone to join together to form the ejaculatory ducts. Villers *et al.* have noted during several dissections that four separate ducts, two from the seminal vesicles and two from the vas deferens, penetrate the center zone for more than 3 mm before merging together to form two ejaculatory ducts.[56] The central zone surrounds the ejaculatory ducts as they course from the seminal vesicles to the verumontanum. Furthermore, just lateral to both of the ejaculatory ducts in the verumontanum, the ducts of the central zone glands open into the urethra. Owing to the closeness of the central zone ducts and ejaculatory ducts, it is believed that both have arisen from the same wolffian origin. The peripheral and central zones are incomplete structures anteriorly, where they are held in place and together by fibromuscular stroma; they are continuous structures posteriorly.

The transition zone is normally the smallest glandular part in young males; it consists of two independent lobes whose ducts drain into the posterolateral recess of the urethral wall at the point of urethral angulation and the inferior border of the preprostatic sphincter.

It has been shown through numerous studies by McNeal[53], Franks[44], and Tissell and Salander[54] that the transition zone is involved with BPH, whereas 70–80% of prostatic cancer occurs in the peripheral zone, 10–15% in the transition zone, and 5–10% in the central zone. In men without BPH, the border between the central gland and the peripheral gland is indistinct. As the transition zone (which can grow up to >90% of the gland volume) enlarges, a distinct demarcation between these two regions can readily be appreciated. With further enlargement, the transition zone can compress the central zone as well as the peripheral zone. The margin separating the transition zone hyperplasia from the peripheral zone is deemed the surgical capsule. Small calcifications are frequently seen at the surgical capsule. Further growth in the transition zone can allow visualization of multiple adenomas (often associated with cystic changes), or even capsular bulging, but never capsular infiltration.[57–59] Several studies have indicated that the size of the peripheral zone, central zone, and the non-glandular (anterior) zones of the prostate remain relatively constant in patients with BPH; it is the transition zone that varies in size and therefore determines the volume of the entire prostate. Although the zonal theory supports a concept of different zones with different diseases these distinctions are not inviolate. Ten to 20% of cancers occur in the transition zone and BPH has been noted in 15% of patients within the peripheral zone. Although some studies suggest that transition zone cancers may be dissimilar to peripheral zone cancers in biologic behaviour this is not yet proven.

ANATOMY OF THE PROSTATIC AND MEMBRANOUS URETHRA

The prostatic urethra is the widest and most dilated part of the entire male urethra; it is approximately 2.5–3.0 cm in length. As it passes through the prostate from the base to the apex, the urethra is divided into proximal (preprostatic) and distal (prostatic) segments of equal length (approximately 15 mm in each segment) by the 35° angulation of the posterior wall at the mid-point between the prostate apex and bladder wall. This angulation tends to be greater than 35° in men with nodular hyperplasia.[31] This angulation occurs just proximal to the verumontanum; the verumontanum belongs to the distal urethra. The urethra, as it extends through the prostate, lies nearer the anterior surface of the gland than the posterior surface. The proximal prostatic urethral wall is lined by transitional epithelium, and encircled by an internal (inner) longitudinal and a middle circular layer of smooth muscle of the vesical wall; these two muscle layers extend down the prostatic urethra to the verumontanum. The circular smooth muscle thickens to form the involuntary internal urethral (preprostatic) sphincter, whereas the longitudinal smooth muscle embeds the periurethral glands (which is also enclosed by the preprostatic sphincter). At the base of the prostate, the external (outer) longitudinal smooth muscle of the bladder blends with the fibromuscular stroma of the capsule to form the true involuntary sphincter of the posterior urethra in males (see Figures 1.3A and B).

The urethral segment, proximal to the anterior angulation of the posterior wall, is surrounded by an incomplete, concentrically arranged group of smooth muscles that form the preprostatic sphincter. This sphincter covers the entire posterior aspect of the proximal urethra from the bladder neck to the verumontanum; but anteriorly, its fibers do not form complete rings. From the posterior surface, the sphincter fibers migrate in a circular fashion to merge anteriorly with the anterior fibromuscular stroma. This sphincter serves two functions: (1) due to its high resting tone, it maintains closure of the proximal urethral segment to aid in the prevention of urinary incontinence; and (2) during ejaculation, it prevents the retrograde flow of seminal fluid from the distal parts of the urethra. Even though there are sparse number of ducts and acinar systems lying along the length of the proximal urethral segment, they are heavily concentrated in the confines of the preprostatic sphincter, forming what is called the periurethral gland region.

In a cross-section of the prostate, the lumen of the urethra has a characteristic crescentic shape with the convex side facing anteriorly (Figure 1.18); this unique shape is formed by an elevation of the mucous membrane, called the urethral crest. This crest forms a narrow median-longitudinal ridge at the midline of the posterior wall to course the length of the entire prostatic urethra. Furthermore, on each side of the crest, there lies a depressed groove on the floor, called the prostatic sinus, which is perforated by the openings of the glandular prostatic ducts. After the urethral angulation, the urethral crest widens and protrudes from

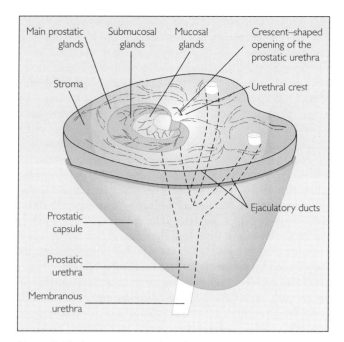

Figure 1.18 A transverse section of the prostate gland to show the crescent-shaped prostatic urethra and the surrounding related structures

the posterior wall to form the verumontanum; at the apex of the verumontanum, there lies a small orifice, called the prostatic utricle. The two ejaculatory duct openings lie on either side of the prostatic utricle, which is situated in the middle of the verumontanum in the middle lobe; this utricle a is blind-ended diverticulum of approximately 6 mm in length. It is a remnant of the (müllerian) para-mesonephric ducts that would develop into the female reproductive tract in the absence of androgens.

Smooth muscle cells (originating from the superficial trigone along the posterior wall of the preprostatic urethra) extend continuously into the proximal part of the urethral crest, and it continues anteroinferiorly as far as the prostatic utricle to unite with the smooth muscle of the ejaculatory ducts. Beyond the ejaculatory ducts, the smooth muscle of the distal prostatic urethra consists of two distinct orientated fibers – circular and longitudinal layers; these two muscle layers run distally to become continuous with the smooth muscle strands that permeate the prostate gland. Furthermore, distal to the apex of the prostate, the membranous urethra is also surrounded by a sphincter of striated muscle fibers (also known as the rhabdosphincter), which represent a proximal extension of the external sphincter located distal to the prostate apex.[60] Once again, similar to the proximal urethral sphincter, this sphincter (in the distal prostatic urethra) is incomplete posterolaterally, where the semicircular fibers anchor into the prostatic stroma.[60]

Distal to the apex of the prostate gland, the membranous urethra is suspended anteriorly to the pubis via the suspensory ligament of the penis, and posteriorly to the puboprostatic ligaments. The urethra leaves the prostate at the prostatic apex, where it passes through the muscle of the urogenital diaphragm as the bulbous urethra.

HISTOLOGY OF THE PROSTATE GLAND

PROSTATIC CAPSULE

The prostate is enveloped in a thin, dense fibromuscular stroma (called the true capsule), which is enclosed within a loose sheath derived from the pelvic fascia – called the prostatic sheath (also known as the false capsule). The prostatic venous plexus lies between this fibrous capsule and prostatic sheath. The capsule is composed of collagen, elastin, and smooth muscle. Anteriorly, the true capsule thickens abruptly via blending with the viscera of the endopelvic fascia to become the anterior fibromuscular stroma. The capsule does not exist at the 1 mm junction of the apex of the prostate and the membranous urethra, and in the midline anterior to this junction;[61] thus, the prostate gland extends into the striated sphincter (rhabdosphincter) at the membranous urethra without an intervening capsule. This capsule covers the base of the prostate at the posterior and lateral aspects; however, at the midline, the capsule invaginates to surround the ejaculatory ducts to form a longitudinal sheath, which contains bundles of smooth muscle. Microscopic bands of smooth muscle from the capsule extend from the posterior surface of the capsule to fuse with the muscular fibers of the periprostatic (Denonvillier's) fascia. Like the apex, no true capsule separates the prostate from the bladder (see Figures 1.9A and B).

Surrounding the prostate gland (exterior to the capsule) and its associating neighbors, there is a fatty fascia containing fibromuscular bundles and neurovascular structures; this fascia has been termed the hypogastric sheath.[62] It surrounds the terminal neurovascular branches emerging from the periaortic and pelvic autonomic neural plexus and hypogastric (iliac) vessels. This hypogastric sheath at the prostate base, adjacent to the distal portion of the seminal vesicle and bladder neck, is composed of thick adipose tissue and contains the superior pedicle of the prostate.[56] After the neurovascular structures enter the prostate gland from the posterolateral aspect, they extend towards the prostate apex to supply the membranous urethra and corpora cavernosa, which results in a posterolateral thickening of the hypogastric sheath; in this region, the sheath is renamed the lateral pelvic fascia. At the rectal surface of the prostate, the sheath is thin and contains numerous fibromuscular bundles that are more concentrated at the base and apex of the gland. This part of the hypogastric sheath is called the prostatoperitoneal fascia of Denonvilliers. Like the contents of the sheath at the rectal surface, the hypogastric sheath at the anterolateral surface is fused to the prostatic capsule. At the anterior aspect of the prostate, the hypogastric sheath contains the veins of the Santorini plexus; this fascia is now called the preprostatic fascia or Zuckerkandl's fascia.

HISTOLOGY OF THE ZONES

The glandular zones of the prostate contain duct-acini systems lined by columnar secretory cells. The ducts originate near the urethra and terminate near the capsule in acini that are saccular structures with undulating borders. The ducts of the prostate arise every 2 mm from the distal prostatic urethra. The ducts branch giving rise to acini. Acini appear uniformly along the ducts except close to the urethra. Each of the zones in the prostate gland shows a different histologic and biologic behavior. The central zone of the prostate constitutes 20% of the functioning glandular tissue and consists of large glands with papillary epithelium surrounded by a dense stroma (see Figures 1.17A and B). The ducts of these glands are wide and undergo extensive branching before terminating into the large, irregularly contoured acini. The stroma is long and compact, closely associated with these acini; it also has more smooth muscle than that of the peripheral zone. The epithelial cells in the central zone have granular darker cytoplasm and enlarged nuclei located at various levels from the basement membrane. Interestingly enough, this epithelium is similar to that of the seminal vesicle, suggesting that the central zone could be of wolffian duct origin. This possible theory does correlate with the uncommon occurrence of carcinoma in both the seminal vesicle and the central zone of the prostate gland.

The peripheral zone surrounds the central zone posteriorly, laterally, and inferiorly; it constitutes 70% of the total glandular mass (see Figure 1.6). Its glands are small and spherical, with a smooth epithelium and loose stroma. The ducts of these glands are narrow and straight, and branch into small, round, regular acini; these ducts, eventually, drain into the distal urethra on either side of the verumontanum and the crista urethralis. Unlike the central zone, where the stroma is compact, the stroma in the peripheral zone is loose and randomly associated. The epithelial cells have clear cytoplasm and small, dark nuclei located uniformly along the basal aspect of the basement membrane. This zone, the site of the majority of adenocarcinomas, is believed to be derived from the UG sinus. The peripheral zone can be easily visualized via computed tomography (CT) scan owing to the relatively higher water content than that of the central or transition zones; this leads to an exquisite display of prostatic zonal anatomy on magnetic resonance imaging (MRI), which is inherently sensitive to variations in tissue water content.[63]

The transition zone consists of two small periurethral lobes at the mid-level of the prostate. The glandular tissue in this zone constitutes only 5–10% of the total glandular mass. Their glandular system burrows along the axis, parallel to the proximal urethra, to open at the verumontanum just above the ejaculatory duct openings. The ducts from these glands are highly branched. The transition zone glands are identical to peripheral zone glands, but they are less numerous and are surrounded by a more dense and compact stroma.

Histologically similar to the transition and peripheral zones, the periurethral glands contain tiny ducts arising from the proximal urethral segment. These glands comprise less than 1% of the total glandular volume; although insignificant in size and function, the periurethral glands are a potential site of BPH development. As they are similar, the transition zone and the periurethral glands have a common embryonic UG sinus origin.

HISTOPATHOLOGY OF BENIGN PROSTATIC HYPERPLASIA

The earliest changes in BPH occur in the periurethral glands that open on to the verumontanum. The hyperplasia may be

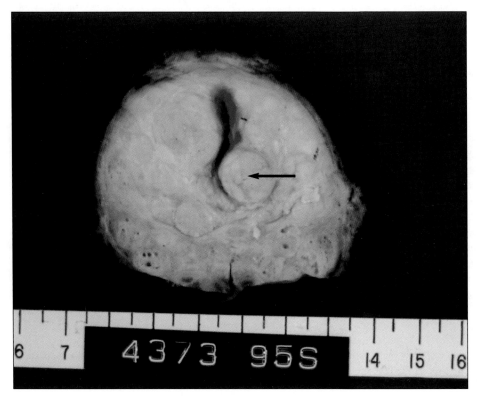

Figure 1.19 Note the numerous nodules (arrow) in this cross-section of a hyperplastic prostate gland and how they distort the shape of the prostatic urethra and compress it

manifested as stromal or glandular hyperplasia (fibro-muscular nodules, acinar nodules, or mixed nodules). The nodules can also have cystic areas within them. The stromal nodules (Figure 1.19) are composed of varying amounts of fibers and smooth muscle cells and may be infiltrated by lymphocytes. Stromal nodules in BPH originate predominantly from the transition zone. Most of the nodules arise from the central periurethral region but can be seen in the subcapsular areas in the transition zone. When the nodules protrude into the bladder lumen the lesion is referred to as median lobe hyperplasia. The hyperplastic nodules can also arise outside in the peripheral zone.

The role of inflammation in BPH is not known. However stromal nodules frequently have lymphoid cells that are variable in density and sometimes forming follicles within them they are initially mixed T & B cells but in later stages are helper T lymphocytes. It has been theorised that T cells may influence proliferation of stromal nodules. Mast cells have also been noted to be increased in BPH. The inflammation in BPH is limited to stromal nodules; when it involves glands the term prostatitis is more appropriate. The glandular hyperplasia may occur predominantly as acinar nodules or may be mixed with stromal hyperplasia nodules.

The glands are often large in epithelial hyperplasia within the infoldings of acini composed of tall columnar cells (Figures 1.20A–D). The nuclei of the glands, however, show no changes in malignancy. Epithelial variations seen in acinar hyperplasia include cystic changes secondary to obstruction, small acini lined by cuboidal cells, transitional epithelial variance, and cribriform patterns. The cribriform patterns of BPH may comprise somewhere between 10 and 60% of the gland in one-third of BPH specimens. This pattern may sometimes be confused with prostatic cancer, although the nuclei are benign and do not show large-sized chromatin and other features typical of malignancy. The frequent occurrence of atypical hyperplasia in malignancy, which may be as high as 80%, has led some to suggest that atypical hyperplasia may be a premalignant process; however, there are no conclusive data to confirm this.

Other variants of nodular hyperplasia include sclerosing adenosis and basal cell hyperplasia. Both sclerosing adenosis and atypical hyperplasia can be distinguished as being benign by the presence of basal cells. Other regressive changes seen in nodular hyperplasia include areas of infarction and congestion. Infarcts occur due to vascular compression. Congestion is a result of obstruction and

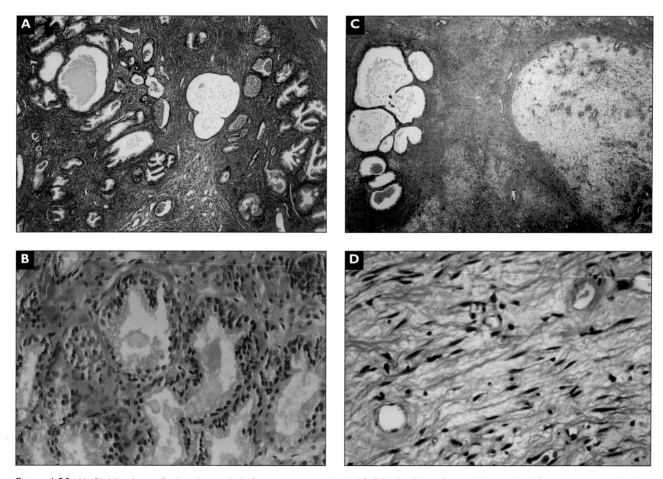

Figure 1.20 (A, B) Histology of acinar hyperplasia from a prostate gland. (C, D) Histology of stromal hyperplasia from a prostate gland. Magnifications: (A, C) ×10; (B, D) ×100

Source: Courtesy of Dr William Murphy, Department of Pathology at the University of Florida College of Medicine, Gainesville, FL

stasis. The stasis of secretions can also cause formation of luminal structures called corpora amylacecea.

The secretory cells are separated from the basement membrane and the stroma by a layer of basal cells. Basal cells are elongated with the long axis running parallel to the basement membrane. Basal cells also contain subsets of stem cells capable of differentiation into other cells.

Normal basal cells selectively stain positive for keratin 34beta-E12. Cancer cells stain negative for this antibody. This test is sometimes used to differentiate cancer from benign tissue. The epithelial cells of BPH are actively secreting cells and contain a variety of enzymes including prostate specific antigen, citrate, acid phosphatase, as well as other enzymes. The glandular nodules are believed to be derived from newly formed duct branches that bud-out from existing ducts leading to a totally new duct system within the nodule. Additionally, there appears to be true hypertrophy of individual cells in addition to the presence of new cells. McNeal has observed that during the initial two decades of BPH development, there is an increase predominantly in nodules whereas, during the subsequent decades, there is an increase in the already formed nodules but fewer new nodules occur. While there is considerable variation in the ratio of epithelium to stroma, in general, patients with BPH have a two to five times increase in stromal tissue compared with epithelial tissue. The prostatic smooth muscles represent a significant volume of stromal tissue in the gland. It is presumed that the contractile properties of these muscles are similar to those of other smooth muscles. It is believed, although not proven, that both passive and active forces in prostatic tissue play a role in the urethral spasm that causes symptoms of BPH. Apart from the epithelial and stromal tissue, there is also a significant volume of other tissue, which includes nerve tissue, extracellular matrix, and fibrous connective tissue. Recent data also suggest that the 5α-reductase enzyme is present in higher concentrations in stromal tissue and basal epithelial cells but not in acinar epithelial cells.

PROSTATIC NEUROENDOCRINE CELLS

Endocrine-paracrine or neuroendocrine (NE) cells are intraepithelial regulatory cells dispersed in the urethroprostatic region. They have both neuroendocrine and epithelial characteristics. Many of these cells will contain one or more biologically active amines, usually serotonin or chromogranin A, putting them in the category of amine precursor uptake and decarboxylation (APUD) cells.[64] These cells are known to regulate many cellular functions, including growth, differentiation, and exocrine secretory processes. Current evidence shows that NE cells lack androgen receptors but, since puberty stimulates proliferation, they may be indirectly affected by androgens. These cells are pleomorphic, including both open, flask-shaped cells with apical extensions into the ductal lumens, and closed cells with long processes that extend around and between epithelial cells, allowing NE cells to contact each other. The long extensions of the open cells may sample luminal contents as they regulate the epithelial secretory function of the adult prostate. They may accomplish this via various neuropeptides, including calcitonin, somatostatin, and bombesin-like peptides. NE cells are often closely associated with prostatic nerves, suggesting that they may be able to communicate with the CNS, indirectly affecting secretion.[64]

Mature nodules characteristic of BPH have substantially less NE cells and secretory products than normal prostate, although at what are apparently growth foci of proliferating nodules, the presence of NE cells is positively correlated with expression of Ki-67 and proliferating cell nuclear antigen.[64-67] In the periurethral zone of the prostate, which has fewer epithelial cells, a decrease in NE cells may alter the local hormonal equilibrium and may induce development of stromal BPH.[68]

Although the mechanism of regulation of NE cells is not understood, a recent study showed evidence of epidermal growth factor (EGF) expression in scattered cells from normal prostate tissue.[69] The positive cells also stained for chromogranin A, a polypeptide associated with most NE cells. This is the first report of a possible ligand-specific regulatory pathway for NE cells.

The effects of NE cell differentiation and regulation of production, secretion, and receptor status of NE products have not been well studied in relation to prostate cancer. However, it has been shown that NE cell differentiation is associated with a poor prognosis and that this population increases with malignancy and androgen withdrawal therapy.[70] Immunostaining has shown that normal and malignant human prostate tissue contains both androgen receptor positive (AR-positive) and AR-negative cells, which may have implications in androgen-independent tumor progression. New technologies currently under development that will allow simultaneous detection of several immunostains with high-resolution imaging may enable profiles of different tumor grades to be identified. Regulating the autocrine–paracrine functions of NE cells to prevent uncontrolled growth of either BPH or prostate cancer tumors is an area that demands further investigation.[64]

An additional type of cell seen in prostatic tissue in the paraganglial cells located near the neurovascular bundles. Paraganglia consist of clusters of cells that are variable in size with prominent nucleoli. They stain positive for norepinephrine markers and are negative for PSA.

Seminal vesicular tissue sometimes can be confused for malignant cells because they have large hyperchromatic cells with prominent nucleolii.

SEMINAL PLASMA COMPONENTS

Secretions of the sex accessory glands comprise about 99% of the ejaculate, with 1% of the total being spermatozoa. The majority of the ejaculatory fluid is contributed by the seminal vesicles, the prostate, and Cowper's glands, in order of decreasing volume. The contents of these glands are released sequentially during ejaculation. Prostatic secretions and sperm are released in the early fraction, while seminal vesicle secretions, which consist mostly of fructose, form the later fraction.[71-73]

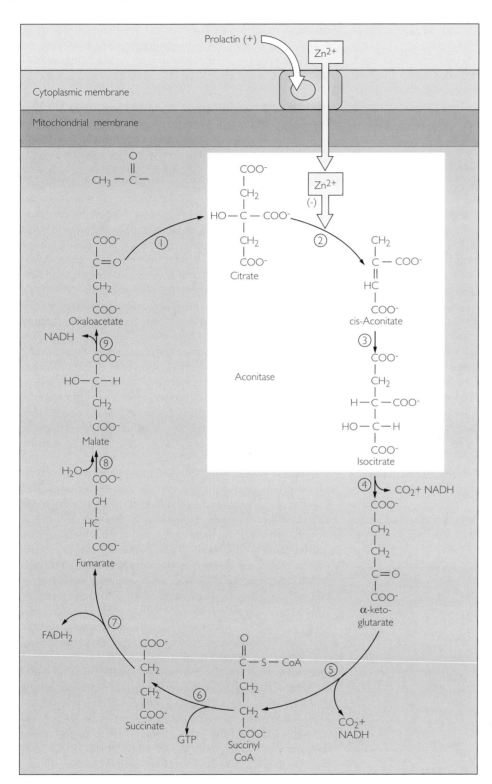

Figure 1.21 Effects of zinc and prolactin on citrate metabolism in the prostatic epithelium. The Kreb's cycle is depicted with the reactions catalyzed by the mitochondrial aconitase enzyme (inside box). In normal prostate cells, zinc is high, inhibiting enzyme activity at the first aconitase step. Citrate cannot be metabolized readily and accumulates to high concentrations. High levels of citrate are secreted into the seminal plasma. As a result of malignant transformation, zinc levels are reduced in the mitochondria, allowing the Kreb's cycle to proceed. Citrate is no longer present in large amounts. These metabolic changes seem to occur before cells show morphological evidence of carcinoma

Human seminal fluid is rich in zinc, potassium, citrate, fructose, polyamines, and free amino acids. Their functions are described in this section, although the roles of some components remain unknown.

CITRATE

Citrate is one of the major anions in human seminal fluid (~60 mEq L^{-1}). For comparison, the chloride ion concentration is 40 mEq L^{-1}. The major source of this citrate is the prostate, which contains the highest amount of any of the tissues of the body. Prostatic fluid levels can reach 40,000 to 150,000 nmoles g^{-1}.[74] Although citrate is present in such high quantities, its role in reproduction is not known. Some researchers have proposed that it acts as a buffering agent.

This unique citrate-accumulating aspect of the prostate has been the focus of many studies designed to understand

(and eventually inhibit) malignancy and BPH. Excellent reviews by Costello and Franklin[75,76] detail the specialized metabolism of prostatic secretory epithelium. Their work reveals that normal feedback mechanisms (such as regulation of phosophofructokinase and high ATP/ADP ratios), which are designed to decrease glycolysis (and citrate production) under conditions of high citrate levels, are not functional in these cells. As a result, the human peripheral zone epithelium is able to establish a citrate concentration of about 130,000 nmoles g^{-1}, compared with non-prostatic tissues containing 150–450 nmoles g^{-1}.[77]

Most cells use citrate as a major oxidizable energy source. An intermediate in the Kreb's cycle, it is converted to isocitrate by the mitochondrial enzyme aconitase, in a non-rate-limiting reaction (Figure 1.21). In typical mammalian cells, aconitase catalyzes the equilibrium reaction:

$$\text{citrate} \leftrightarrow \textit{cis}\text{-aconitate} \leftrightarrow \text{isocitrate}$$

which results in a steady-state citrate:isocitrate ratio of approximately 10:1. However, in the citrate-producing cells of the prostate, this ratio is closer to 30–40:1. Most cells are dependent upon "normal" aconitase activity for citrate oxidation, as evidenced by the cytotoxic effects of fluorocitrate, a specific enzyme inhibitor. However, the prostatic epithelium of humans and several other mammalian species are unique in that low aconitase activity allows them to produce, accumulate, and secrete very high quantities of citrate.[78]

In prostate cells, citrate becomes essentially an endproduct of intermediary metabolism, instead of an intermediate. By secreting, instead of oxidizing citrate, these cells sacrifice about 60% of the energy potentially available from glucose.[79] An additional energy cost is the metabolism of

aspartate to replenish Kreb's cycle intermediates such as oxaloacetate. Costello and coworkers have identified an energy-dependent aspartate transporter, which imports this amino acid from circulating plasma. Despite this inefficiency, ATP levels in citrate-producing cells of the rat prostate are typical of other types of cells, although ADP levels were lower.

Biochemical and molecular assays suggest that accumulation of citrate in the normal prostate occurs because aconitase *activity* is inhibited, effectively limiting oxidation, even though the *amount* of this enzyme is typical of citrate-oxidizing cells.[74,80–83] This led investigators to search for an inhibitor which would be unique to the prostate. Zinc was an obvious candidate, as it is present in high amounts in prostate cells and binds strongly to citrate, and it is now believed to play a role in aconitase inhibition (see Figure 1.21). During malignant transformation, intracellular zinc concentration in the prostate is decreased, permitting citrate oxidation to proceed at a rate similar to that of non-prostatic cells, presumably to meet the higher energy demands of the cancer. Several studies have confirmed that, without exception, prostate cancer cells have dramatically lower levels of citrate than normal or BPH cells.[84–86] Studies are under way in our laboratory to determine the mechanism of zinc inhibition of aconitase activity. For example, NMR experiments with prostate cancer cell lines reveal that increased zinc in the culture medium decreases ATP levels, indicating a drop in metabolic activity and cell viability (Figure 1.22).

There is recent evidence that mitochondrial zinc levels are positively regulated by prolactin and testosterone.[79,87,88] This exciting discovery has led us to initiate investigations into the effects of prolactin and zinc on the metabolism and growth rate of human prostate cancer in our laboratories, in collaboration with Costello and Franklin. Preliminary data suggest that these substances not only decrease citrate oxidation and slow cell division, but may also initiate programmed cell death (apoptosis).

Nuclear magnetic resonance imaging (MRI) and spectroscopy (MRS) techniques have been designed to take advantage of differences in citrate metabolism between normal, BPH, and malignant prostatic cells.[89–94]

Our research has resulted in the development of endorectal probes to acquire more precise information on the characteristics and location of suspected tumors (Figure 1.23).[89,90] We are currently developing innovative hardware and software to enable us to use the 3-tesla magnet at the University of Florida, one of only a few in the USA. Compared with the 1.5-tesla magnet in common use, we should be able to at least double the resolution. Data from our MRS studies *in vitro* will be used to identify how changes in citrate concentration changes with tumor stage, and after various treatments. We will then use this information to help distinguish prostate cancer from BPH, follow tumor progression, and search for recurrent tumors and metastatic lesions in human patients. Understanding the metabolic characteristics of progressive prostate cancer cells may lead to improved diagnostic tests and targeted treatment regimens.

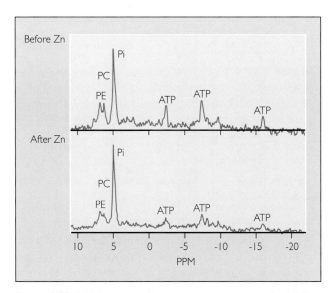

Figure 1.22 NMR spectra of human prostate cancer cells, PC-3, before and after administration of zinc. As expected, zinc inhibited energy metabolism in the cells, reducing ATP peaks. Cell viability was also lower. PC = phosphocholine, PE = phosphoethanolamine, Pi = inorganic phosphate, ATP = adenosine triphosphate

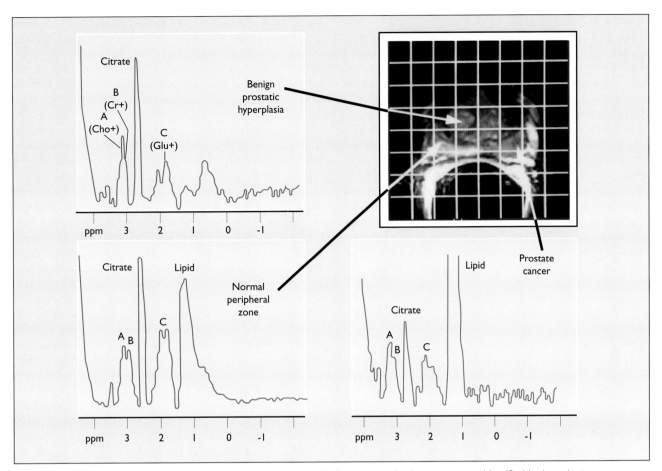

Figure 1.23 ¹H MRS and MRI alterations and prostatic pathology. Malignant areas in the prostate are identified by low citrate concentration. Note high concentrations of citrate in BPH tissues and normal peripheral zone tissue. There are also other metabolites detected by MRS that can be used in diagnosis and staging of prostate cancer. MRS and MRI are valuable tools in understanding the metabolic processes that occur within cells and in patients. The use of endorectal coils and newer, higher power magnets will improve resolution and decrease magnet time for patients

ZINC

Zinc levels in seminal fluid are quite high (140 μg mL⁻¹) and originate primarily from the prostate, which contains the highest amount of this divalent ion of any tissue.[95] BPH cells have stable or increased concentrations of zinc, while malignant cells have substantially lower amounts, as described in the preceding section.[96]

As well as binding to many metalloenzymes, zinc binds strongly to citrate and appears to act as an inhibitor of mitochondrial aconitase. Citrate oxidation, which provides energy for malignant cell growth, depends on adequate aconitase activity. In normal prostate cells, however, high zinc levels minimize aconitase activity, allowing citrate to accumulate for subsequent secretion into seminal fluid.

Recent studies[95,97] have begun to establish the roles of prolactin and testosterone in regulation of intracellular zinc concentrations in the prostate (Costello and Franklin, personal communication, 1998). In the rat, it is evident that effects are cell-type specific. Both hormones decrease zinc in the ventral lobes, increase zinc in the lateral lobes, and have no effect on the dorsal lobes. Therefore, zinc levels in specific cells can be regulated by the body. The human prostate, like the rat lateral lobes, increases intracellular zinc in response to prolactin and testosterone. This effect is also seen in malignant prostatic cell lines and may provide a clue to depriving cancer cells of needed energy by inhibiting citrate oxidation.[95]

The role of zinc in seminal fluid is not known, but it may play a direct role in preventing bacterial infections of the prostate.[98] Mann and Mann[71] found that prostatic fluid from patients with chronic bacterial prostatitis had a greater than 80% reduction in zinc.

FRUCTOSE

The seminal vesicles, under androgen regulation, produce and excrete fructose into the semen. Fructose is known to be an energy substrate for spermatozoa, although sperm are also capable of using glucose present in cervical mucus.[71] Fructose may also play a role in sperm motility and seminal viscosity.

Fructose levels in seminal fluid correlated with total antioxidant status, suggesting that seminal vesicle secretions contribute low molecular weight components with antioxidant capacity.[94] In addition, prostatic secretions also provide superoxide anion scavengers. Fructose levels in semen samples are known to be affected by storage, frequency of ejaculation, blood glucose levels, and nutritional status.[71]

POLYAMINES

These small, positively charged molecules (spermine, spermidine, and putrescine) are ubiquitous in nature and may be involved in many aspects of cell growth, proliferation, and differentiation. Prostatic fluid is the richest source of spermine in the body, resulting in seminal fluid concentrations of 50–350 mg (100 mL)$^{-1}$.[99]

Based on studies on tumors in rats, the administration of substances known to reduce polyamines, such as 3-hydroxy-4-methoxycinnamic acid or 3,4-dimethoxycinnamic acid, inhibit cancer growth in some tissues, including prostate, thymus, and stomach.[100] Treated rats were found to have lower spermidine-to-spermine ratios when compared with non-treated rats in various tissues, including seminal vesicles.

Changes in polyamine concentrations with malignant transformation have been identified. Cipolla et al.[101] propose that elevations in circulating polyamine levels be used as a diagnostic tool for prostate cancer. Their study suggests that erythrocyte spermine assays can predict tumor progression (lower levels indicate a better prognosis) and discriminate between hormone-sensitive and refractory metastatic prostatic carcinoma.

MRS can be used to identify these changes and provide insight into how various treatment regimens affect cellular metabolism and proliferation.[102]

LIPIDS

Phospholipids are a major component (67%) of the total lipids in homogenates of BPH cells, followed by cholesterol (29%) and glyceride glycerols (4%).[86] In this study, the lipid concentration of the epithelium was found to be two to threefold higher than the stroma, although on a per-cell basis, it was lower. The stroma had higher phospholipid and sphingomyelin but lower cholesterol and phosphatidylserine concentrations than the epithelium.

Changes in cellular membrane lipid characteristics as a result of BPH may affect activity of 5α-reductase, the enzyme that converts testosterone into its more potent metabolite DHT. Changes in lipid composition affect membrane fluidity, lipid-to-protein ratio, and, conceivably, post-translational activitation of transmembrane enzymes.[103] It is known that 5α-reductase must be embedded within the membrane to retain activity in both stroma and epithelial cells.[104]

In rat livers, levels of sphingomyelin are negatively correlated with mitotic activity.[105] Similarly, in human BPH tissue, stroma has higher sphingomyelin content and less mitotic activity than epithelial cells.[106] Further investigation needs to be done to determine whether this can be used as a mitotic index.

Phospholipids are a major component (67%) of the total lipids in homogenates of BPH cells, followed by cholesterol (29%) and glyceride glycerols (4%).[86] In this study, the lipid concentration of the epithelium was found to be two-to threefold higher than the stroma, although on a per-cell basis, it was lower. The stroma had higher phospholipid and sphingomyelin and lower cholesterol and phosphatidylserine concentrations than the epithelium. Weisser and Krieg

suggest that changes in membrane lipid composition may effect DHT production, resulting in alterations in the DHT-to-estrogen ratio. This ratio is known to be important in age-related changes in the prostate. The authors point out a need for further investigations on the impact of lipids on membrane-bound 5α-reductase and the effects of steroids on membrane lipid composition.

Recent evidence confirms that androgens coordinately enhance the expression of lipogenic enzymes that stimulate fatty acid and cholesterol synthesis.[107] Swinnen et al.[107] were able to show that androgens increase the expression and activation of transcription factors that affect the newly characterized sterol regulatory element binding proteins (SREBPs). The hormone-sensitive prostate cancer cell line, LNCaP, responds to androgen treatment by increased expression and activity of fatty acid synthetase (FAS) resulting in intracellular lipid.[108] Cancer cells that lack androgen receptors (PC-3 and DU-145) do not show this response. Androgen effects on LNCaP cells are inhibited by anti-androgens, such as Casodex (bicalutamide).

In prostate cancer, arachidonic acid protects cells from apoptosis induction by exogenous C2-ceramide, indicating a dual role of lipids in cell survival and death. However, when arachidonic is limiting, bcl-2 can provide the same protection.[109]

SEMINAL PLASMA SPERM MOTILITY INHIBITOR PRECURSOR

Recently, a 52-kDa protein was identified in seminal vesicle secretions.[93] Prostate-specific antigen (PSA) was able to digest the inhibitor precursor, resulting in a peptide whose sequence corresponds to that of semenogelin, a major structural component of semen coagulum. Intact semenogelin can immobilize spermatozoa. It is believed that it undergoes PSA digestion after ejaculation.

ANTIOXIDANTS

Various components of seminal plasma are proposed to have antioxidant (oxygen-scavaging) functions, including superoxide dismutase (SOD)-like activity. SOD-like activity was shown to be positively correlated with citrate, zinc, and acid phosphatase but not with fructose levels.[94] In fertilization studies on men, it was found that spermatozoa were able to generate the superoxide anion (O_2^-), which stimulated their capacitation. The free-radical scavenger SOD was able to inhibit the process of capacitation and may be a regulator of fertilization.[110]

HORMONAL CONTROL OF PROSTATE GROWTH AND FUNCTION

It has long been known that androgens are required for the development, maintenance, growth, and secretory functions of the prostate and other male sex accessory glands.[111] However, it has become clear that the interactions of androgens with prostate epithelium, stroma, neuroendocrine cells, and other hormones and growth factors (GF) form a complex system designed to regulate not only prostate growth, but also the relative numbers of epithelial and non-epithelial

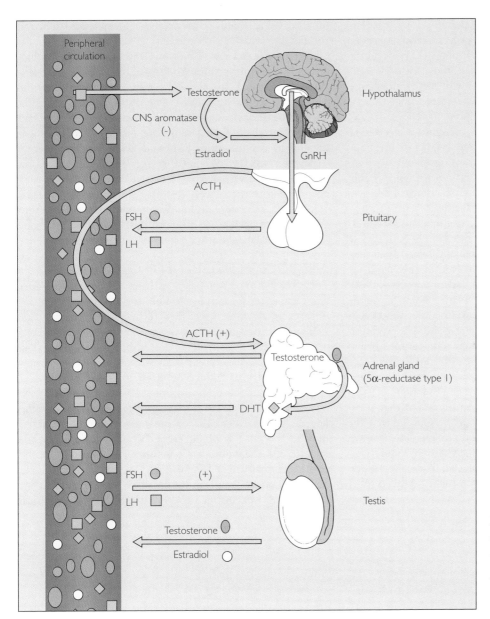

Figure 1.24 Hypothalamic–pituitary–gonadal axis. Hormone secretion by the testes is regulated in a feedback loop to the hypothalamus. Circulating androgens, estrogens from the testes, prostate and adrenals, and therapeutic agents such as LH, agonists, and antagonists produce a negative effect on GnRH release by the hypothalamus, limiting the release of androgen-stimulating hormones LH and FSH

cells.[112] This is accomplished by a precise balance of inhibition and stimulation of various GF. In addition, androgens modulate the availability of receptors, and the production of other cellular substrates. As more evidence is accumulated regarding these interactions at the subcellular level, new theories about the etiology and development of abnormal prostate growth, such as BPH and adenocarcinoma, are being put forth and tested. Many of these data have come from studies on rats and dogs, so we must remember that species differences can be quite extensive, especially when concerning a gland such as the prostate, where the various cell types arise from different embryological origins.[113] It is not yet clear, for example, which lobes of the rat prostate (which differ dramatically in metabolic patterns) correlate to areas of the human prostate. Nevertheless, some important conclusions have been drawn from animal models that have proven useful in understanding human prostate disorders.

HYPOTHALAMIC–PITUITARY–GONADAL AXIS

Studies from the early 1970s have shown that the hypothalamus, anterior pituitary, and the gonads (testes or ovaries) comprise an endocrine "loop" (Figure 1.24), which is responsible for maintaining the appropriate levels of steroid hormones in the serum and target tissues. In the female, the anterior preoptic nuclei of the hypothalamus is responsible for secreting gonadotropin-releasing hormone (GnRH) in a pulsatile, cyclic manner required for normal estrous cycles. It has been shown that neonatal male rats produce androgens that affect this nucleus, so that cyclic GnRH release will be inhibited later in life, while permitting tonic GnRH release from the ventromedial hypothalamic area.[114] There are some data to suggest that local aromatization of testosterone to estradiol is responsible for this action, as the non-aromatizable metabolite DHT is ineffective. However, it is thought that primates and other animals with longer gestational periods may respond differently. For example, male monkeys are known to retain the ability to release luteinizing hormone (LH) cyclically into adulthood.

That the feedback loop originates with the hypothalamus has been demonstrated with flutamide (anti-androgen) treatment in animals.[114] Flutamide-induced increases in LH secretion can be reversed by systemic administration of DHT (which also causes reduced testicular weight) or estradiol, while pituitary implants of DHT were ineffective in producing the same results. However, in humans, there is conflicting evidence as to the role of CNS aromatizable and non-aromatizable androgens on feedback mechanisms. Apparently, both estradiol and DHT can mediate a negative regulation of hypothalamus-induced testosterone production.

Other hormones, which may have autocrine, paracrine, or intracrine functions, are also involved in this feedback loop, although their exact roles may not yet be clear. Recently, it was shown that follicle-stimulating hormone (FSH) mRNA was present in the prostate, indicating that at least some of the FSH detected in this gland was produced locally. In addition, the dual-specificity receptor for LH and chorionic gonadotropin (LH/CG-R) and the FSH receptor (FSH-R) and their mRNA transcripts were both identified in prostate epithelial cells.[115,116] The function of this LH/CG-R in humans is unknown, but in rats, it may regulate secretory activity. Dirnhofer et al.[115] proposed that the prostate is an endocrine organ that can regulate its own endocrine activity. Their studies suggest that locally produced FSH can act on the producing cell, its neighbors, and also possibly influence the release of pituitary-derived FSH. The activated FSH-R initiates a cascade of events that result in increased aromatase activity, inducing increased estrogen production, which also feeds back to the hypothalamus.

In response to tonic release of GnRH from the hypothalamus, the anterior pituitary releases LH and FSH. As mentioned, receptors for these hormones are found in the prostate as well as the testes. The testes, in response, produce testosterone and estrogens that act on the prostate and feed back to the hypothalamus. There is known to be an age-dependent rise in serum FSH and LH in healthy, elderly males. As will be discussed in this section, there is an increase in the testosterone:estrogen ratio with increasing age, as testosterone levels decrease slowly, while estrogen levels remain the same. It has been proposed, although there is no conclusive data to support this, that if testosterone levels do not fall, abnormal prostate cell growth may result.

ANDROGEN EFFECTS ON PROSTATE CELLS

Testosterone, the principal circulating androgen, is released from the testes in response to FSH and LH stimulation and diffuses freely into cells. Two forms of the enzyme 5α-DHT reductase, present on the nuclear membrane of cells of many tissues, convert testosterone to 5α-DHT. The Type 1 isozyme is present in liver, skin, and other tissues and contributes to circulating levels of DHT. The Type 2 isozyme predominates in urogenital tissue. Individuals with inherited deficiencies in the Type 2 isozyme do not develop normal external genitalia or prostates.[117] In the prostate, most of the DHT is produced in the epithelium, while the majority of the androgen receptors (ARs) reside in the stromal compartment (Figure 1.25).

Immunohistochemical studies have shown staining for the Type 2 isozyme in prostate stromal tissue and basal

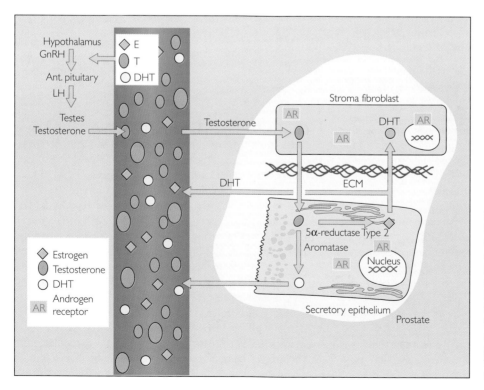

Figure 1.25 Prostate–hormonal interactions. Testosterone freely enters prostate cells, where it is converted to the more potent form, DHT. The action of DHT on epithelial cell proliferation in BPH is likely an indirect result of growth factor stimulation by DHT on the mesenchyme. DHT effects stromal and epithelial production of growth factors and their receptors to modulate the growth of all cell types

cells, with undetectable staining in the secretory epithelium.[118] BPH stroma and nodules and stroma around prostatic intraepithelial neoplasia (PIN) stain intensely, while no signal was evident in lymph node metastases. Normal, BPH, and malignant prostate extracts were found to contain nearly identical amounts of Type 2 reductase per microgram of protein, although the number of positively staining cells was greatest for BPH.[118] Several studies have confirmed higher levels of reductase staining in BPH nodules than in surrounding normal tissue.[119–121] Even with the drastic morphologic changes that occur with prostate cancer, the expression of the Type 2 reductase remains high in stroma, while androgen receptors predominate in the epithelium.[117] As the tumor progresses and the amount of stroma in relation to the epithelial component decreases, enzyme inhibitors are likely to have less of a role in regulating tumor growth.[122] These data bring to light the role of stroma in influencing epithelial cell growth and function. Data obtained by Chung and Cunha, who studied the regulation of prostate growth by cells of the mesenchymal compartment in rodents, support the hypothesis put forth by McNeal that pathological prostate growth (BPH) may be under stromal control.[32,37,123]

In rats, finasteride administration (which blocks Type 2 activity) results in a decrease in reductase mRNA in the ventral prostate, indicating that DHT stimulates enzyme synthesis via a feed forward mechanism. However, this may be different in humans, as biopsy samples from men on long-term finasteride treatment show only a slight decrease in enzyme activity after 3 years. Treatment with leuprolide, diethylstilbestrol, or flutamide abolished Type 2 expression in the epididymus, but not in the prostates of elderly men. It is important to remember that even under conditions of androgen blockade therapy, circulating DHT produced peripherally by the Type 1 isozyme can contribute to androgen-dependent prostate growth.[117,118]

The relative potencies of testosterone and DHT, when bound to the AR, vary with target tissue. In the prostate, DHT binds to the cytoplasmic AR more tightly than testosterone and has been shown to be about five times more potent.[111,113] BPH treatments are designed to prevent or reduce activation of the androgen receptor either by competing for ligand binding (flutamide), reducing testosterone production (LHRH-agonists or antagonists), or by limiting the synthesis of DHT (finasteride). Interestingly, recent studies do not show any increase in DHT levels in patients who develop BPH vs. elderly males that do not.[124] Type 2 long-term finasteride treatment results in a decrease in DHT, but an increase in testosterone, though the overall androgenic activity is thought to be lowered.

The AR, once thought to be predominately in the cytosol, has also been localized within the nucleus of the prostatic secretory epithelium.[121] However, it is not known whether these are functionally distinct receptors. Basal epithelial cells, in contrast, variably express the AR, are found to be predominantly androgen-independent (with a subset of potentially androgen-sensitive cells), and proliferate under estrogen exposure.[125] This may indicate that BPH may progress as the secretory cells are replaced from a pool of androgen-sensitive regenerative cells

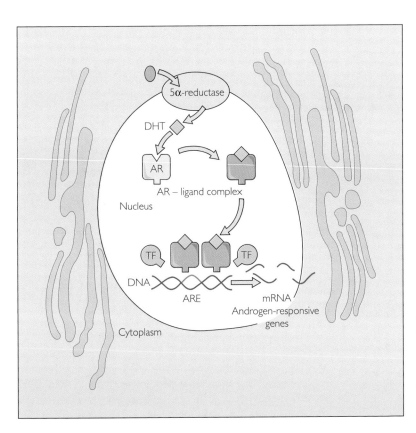

Figure 1.26 Transcription regulation by androgens. Once androgen binds to its receptor, located either in the cytosol or on the nuclear membrane, the activated complex enters the nucleus and binds to specific DNA sequences that make up the androgen response element in the upstream region of androgen-induced genes. Cell-specific transcription factors (TFs) are also present to finely tune gene expression further. ARE, androgen response element; AR, androgen receptor; TF, cell-specific transcription factor

from the basal cell population, as a result of stimulation by various growth factors.[126]

The results of seven studies were reviewed by Barrack and Tindall,[121] revealing that the presence of ARs is not a good measure of treatment response, as, of the treatment non-responders, 52% were AR-negative tumors while 48% were AR-positive. When only cytosolic ARs were analyzed, it was found that 87% of malignant AR-positive tumors responded to androgen blockade therapy. However, the response of AR-negative tumors was quite variable, with 63% responding to therapy.

The AR–ligand complex acts as a transcription regulator within the cell nucleus (Figure 1.26). The sequence recognizable by the AR closely resembles that of glucocorticoid and progesterone response elements.[127] The consensus sequence was found to be GGA/TACAnnnTGTTCT.[128] Work done by various groups to analyze the promoter region of the PSA gene has resulted in the identification of a putative androgen response element (ARE). There is supporting evidence that PSA expression is androgen-regulated in the human prostate cancer cell line LNCaP.[129]

There is no doubt that only a small portion of genes coding for the ARE have currently been identified. However, it is known that androgens have both direct and indirect effects on the cell cycle by regulating gene expression. A very early response of castrated rats to exogenous androgens is an increase in c-fos, c-Ha-ras, and c-Ki-ras synthesis.[112]

Ki-ras has been known to be activated in malignant prostate tissue and has shown some correlation with predicted metastatic potential. A later response includes increased expression of c-myc, c-myb, and actin, coinciding with DNA replication.[112] c-fos and c-myc are important cell cycle regulators and are increased during castration-induced apoptosis, an effect that also can be produced with exogenous estrogens. An increase in c-fos has been linked with androgen stimulation of prostate cancer cells in vitro. It is important to remember that the Fos protein has both transcription activation and inhibition domains.

After castration, the level of the AR falls, but the mRNA transcripts remain in the cytoplasm for a considerable time, so a single injection of androgens quickly restores the AR to normal levels.[113] Estrogens are also known to increase AR availability in humans and dogs.

Androgen response elements are similar to glucocorticoid (GC) response elements. The GC receptors, just recently identified in prostate cells, may only exert effects under conditions when AR levels are low, such as when androgen stimulation is lacking.[112,115]

Testosterone has been shown to affect the growth and metabolism of prostate cells in many ways (Figure 1.27), including regulating hormone synthesis (FSH), availability of GF receptors, DNA, RNA, and protein synthesis, and mRNA transcript stability.[113] Androgens are known to stimulate the production of GF such as prolactin, growth hormone, LHRH, bone morphogenetic proteins, nerve growth factor (receptors in epithelium, but has paracrine effects on stroma), insulin, insulin-like growth factor (mitogen), platelet-derived growth factor, epidermal growth factor (EGF) (increase growth of epithelial cells, receptor under control of androgens), fibroblast growth factor (FGF) (mitogenic, angiogenic), and transforming growth factor-β (decrease epithelium, increase stroma), that affect certain cells.[112] It is proposed that within the heterogeneous population of prostate cells, certain subpopulations will be inherently more sensitive to GF and hormones than others, possibly explaining why androgen-insensitive tumors arise even after androgen ablation therapy. GF receptor availability and intracellular metabolite concentrations are frequently under androgen control. Ligand binding to cell surface receptors triggers a second messenger cascade that could include protein kinases, membrane phospholipids, and G-protein pathways.[113] Although studies of the expression of many GF during embryological and neonatal development is ongoing, the role of these genes in the adult prostate is unclear. In studies of mature rodents, GF appear to play a homeostatic function on the cell cycle and on maintaining the extracellular matrix.[130] This calls into question conclusions about GF taken from experiments on prostates from elderly men or animals, where the growth of the prostate, even in BPH nodules is very slow.

Testosterone or androstenedione can maintain the prostatic epithelium, microvilli, golgi, and endoplasmic reticulum, while suppressing stromal growth and increasing secretory activity.[113] Although testosterone is sufficient to prevent involution and apoptosis, DHT is required for

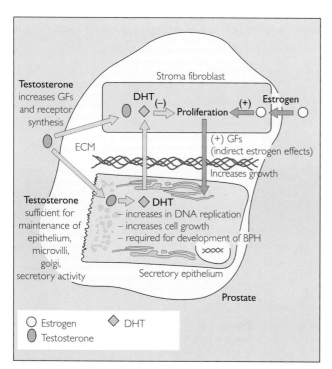

Figure 1.27 Growth factors – hormonal interactions in prostate cells. Testosterone and estrogen can have antagonistic effects on prostate cell growth. Although the stromal compartment is more sensitive to estrogen, it indirectly affects epithelial growth via stimulation of stroma-derived growth factors. The extracellular matrix (ECM) components also influence the action of growth factors on the various cell types

growth and for the development of BPH.[118,131] In humans, 10% of circulating androgens originate from the adrenal glands. Adrenal-derived steroids alone are able to maintain the prostate, as peripheral 5α-reductase (Type 1) produces sufficient DHT. This should be considered when Type 2 reductase inhibitors are considered for BPH treatment. The presence of functional testes during embryogenesis, puberty and, at least partly, during adulthood is required for the development of BPH or prostatic adenocarcinoma.

When men who were candidates for gender change surgery were given androgen blockade therapy prior to surgery, they had a decrease in serum testosterone and increased LH levels after 8 weeks.[132] Unlike rats and dogs, the prostates of these men were not reduced in size, although there was a decline in the secretory epithelium and acini concomitant with an increase in stromal tissue.

ESTROGEN EFFECTS ON PROSTATE CELLS

Estrogens, along with androgens, are involved in regulation of sexual behavior, gonadotropin secretion, and the growth of male accessory glands. In the CNS, estrogens are involved in differentiation of the hypothalamic cells responsible for cyclic, pulsatile release of GnRH. Exposure to androgens during development is essential for the embryo to masculinize. Even brief exposure of newborn rats to estrogen results in permanent suppression of prostate growth and a reduced response to testosterone in adulthood. The regressive effects of estrogen on the male sex accessory glands during development have stimulated interest in their possible therapeutic effects on abnormal prostate growth. Estrogens can act directly on the prostate, with similar effects as seen with castration, or can act indirectly via the hypothalamus or pituitary.[113] Estrogens can stimulate increased expression of the androgen receptor.

Testosterone is converted to estrogens in the CNS and target organs such as the prostate by aromatase enzymes.[114] Plasma levels of estrogens (derived from peripheral metabolism of testosterone and androstenedione) are low (estradiol, 1.6–4.5 ng mL^{-1}) compared with circulating testosterone (500 ng mL^{-1}). Plasma estradiol levels are known to be highly regulated by the hypothalamus, pituitary, and testes. As mentioned earlier, both estradiol and DHT may mediate negative hypothalamic feedback responses to high testosterone. Estrogen regulates testosterone secretion by reducing LH release at the level of the hypothalamus and anterior pituitary.

The effects of estrogen and testosterone on the sex accessory glands are antagonistic or can have no effect at all.[114] But, low doses of estrogens are known to potentiate secretory activity in dog prostate and bull seminal vesicles. In the mouse prostate, organ weight, acid and alkaline phosphatase, and citrate become elevated. In most animals, including primates, estrogen increases the fibromuscular tissues in the stroma of the seminal vesicles and prostate (see Figure 1.27). It is not known whether the epithelial cells are reduced in number. Human sex accessory glands, the anterior prostate of the rat, and the canine prostate contain high concentrations of estrogen receptors. This has led to investigations into the effects of this hormone under normal and androgen-deprivation conditions, when BPH is present. Estrogen has been shown to increase (but not initiate) BPH in dogs when given with testosterone. Additional estrogen is then produced by local aromatase activity.[124]

Several groups have shown that, in humans, in the seventh and eight decade of life, there is an increase in the estrogen:androgen ratio as testosterone levels decline slightly, while estrogen levels remain the same. In contrast, and perhaps due to small group numbers and wide age ranges, Krieg *et al.*[133] found that the increased estrogen:androgen ratio is due to an increase in estrogen with age and a decrease in DHT. They reported that estradiol and estrone increased with age in BPH stromal tissue to a greater extent that in BPH epithelium and in both cell types from normal prostates. In any event, the increased estrogen:androgen ratio with age may contribute to increased stromal growth, although estrogen alone cannot induce BPH.[114] The stroma is very estrogen-sensitive, as it is derived at least partially from the müllerian ducts.[111] The stroma is thought to contribute to the function of the epithelium and so may strongly influence the development of abnormal growth. For this reason, it has been thought that anti-estrogens may have a role in the treatment of BPH.

Administration of estrogen to normal males results in a decrease in size and function of the sex accessory glands' epithelial cells, probably by a reduction in testosterone synthesis via a negative feedback to reduce LH release. Estrogen can also directly block the action of testosterone on certain target tissues. A strong correlation was found between estradiol:testosterone ratio and prostate size, suggesting that an estrogen-dominant environment plays an important role in the development of BPH.[134]

PROLACTIN EFFECTS ON PROSTATE CELLS

Prolactin receptors have been detected in prostatic epithelial cells. In primary tissue cultures, proliferation of 5 of 19 BPH specimens was stimulated by prolactin.[135] However, when EGF was also added to the medium, either before or after prolactin treatment, growth was inhibited. When given alone, EGF stimulated cell division at least as well as DHT.

In the rat, prolactin has a synergistic action on androgen-induced weight gain and citrate secretion by the lateral prostate. It also stimulates accumulation of testosterone and DHT by the epithelial cells. In castrates, replacement androgens increase DNA, RNA, and protein synthesis. Prolactin can synergize these effects, although there is a significant response to it alone.[113] Transgenic mice overexpressing the prolactin gene were found to have dramatic enlargements of the prostates, increased DNA content, and increased secretory fluid.[136] The levels of testosterone and insulin-like growth factor I were also increased in these mice. This suggests that prolactin may play a role in prostatic hyperplasia through direct actions on the prostate or via stimulating increased circulating testosterone.

Recent biochemical assays of prostates cells in culture have revealed that prolactin plays a role in regulation of citrate metabolism (see section on "Citrate"). This is important in the energetics of cells that may be growing abnormally. Normal prostate epithelial cells produce and secrete citrate into the seminal plasma at a great energy cost.[79] During malignant transformation and even before morphological changes can be identified, these cells increase utilization of citrate, presumably to meet the new energy demands of stimulated cell growth.[74,80,81,83,137] In the prostate cell mitochondria, zinc helps modulate the activity of the enzyme aconitase, required for citrate metabolism. High zinc levels, as found in normal prostate tissue, inhibit aconitase activity. Zinc levels are dramatically reduced in malignant cells regardless of stage. There is new evidence, from our laboratory, in collaboration with Costello and Franklin, that prolactin regulates intracellular zinc levels. Experiments *in vitro* have shown that when supplemental zinc is added to the culture medium, citrate synthesis and cell proliferation are decreased (unpublished data). When prolactin is also added to the medium, this effect is greatly potentiated, providing exciting clues to regulation of abnormal prostatic cell growth.

OTHER HORMONES

In diabetic animals, insulin deficiency results in a decreased height of prostate epithelium and a decrease in secretory vesicles. Insulin supplementation is required for a response to testosterone.[113] Prostaglandin (PRG) receptors are located in the prostate and the action of PRG seems to be to maintain or stimulate weight, cellular structure, and secretory function.

EFFECTS OF AGE ON HORMONE LEVELS AND PROSTATE CELLS

The positive correlation between BPH volume and age has been well documented. It is attractive to theorize that changes in androgen levels with age influence the development of abnormal prostate growth such as BPH. However, several studies have shown no change over time in serum of tissue DHT levels in patients with BPH vs. healthy males,

although testosterone levels decline somewhat.[111,138] The decline in DHT and 5α-reductase with age appears to occur only in the epithelial compartment, while stromal levels remain the same over time.[86] Figure 1.28 shows the changes in hormone levels that occur over time. If these changes do not occur, the imbalance of hormones and GF may contribute to the development of BPH.

A long-term study of men with stage B prostate cancer and BPH, who eventually underwent radical prostatectomy, showed that, with age, there was a decrease in serum testosterone, androstenedione, and dihydroxyandrostenedione, with a concomitant increase in steroid hormone binding globulin (SHBG), FSH, LH, and estradiol.[138] In contrast to many published studies by various groups, Krieg *et al.*[133] compared the epithelial and stromal compartments of prostates from men with normal and BPH prostates and determined that DHT concentration in normal epithelium was higher than in normal stroma and higher than in epithelium and stroma from BPH. In addition, DHT in the epithelium, but not stroma, of both normal and BPH prostates decreased with age. They also found that estradiol increased in stroma, but not epithelium, with age. It is possible that their small population numbers (six normal and 19 BPH patients) and their wide range of ages (26–87 years) produced results different from other studies with more closely matched age groups and larger group sizes. This group also reported on the accumulation of DHT in the stroma of prostates from elderly men that may have been due to a decline in DHT-metabolizing enzymes.[106,139]

In a study designed to evaluate the risks of BPH surgery, gland size and symptoms had a poor correlation. There was also no clear relationship between severity of BPH symptoms and levels of either testosterone or DHT or the testosterone:DHT ratio.[111] Serum levels of estradiol were positively correlated and estrone slightly negatively correlated, when the data were adjusted for non-hormonal factors. Three risk factors became apparent when the data were age-adjusted. Diastolic blood pressure and moderate exercise were positively correlated, while alcohol consumption was negatively correlated. This study also confirmed that the estrogen:androgen ratio increases with age as testosterone levels decline, while estrogen remains the same. These findings led the authors to suggest that even though testosterone levels fall with age, androgens may be merely "permissive" for cell growth, and beyond a baseline amount, they have no further influence on BPH. It is possible that estrogens play more of a role at this time, too, as DHT in the epithelium declines while the stroma is accumulating more estrogens.[86]

In the rat, prostatic growth ceases after sexual maturity, and the level of androgen receptor has been shown to decrease by 30% in mature vs. 3-month-old rats.[140] However, in dogs, which may develop a form of stromal BPH as they age, there is no decrease in AR availability. Most of the AR immunoreactivity was found to be in the stromal compartment, rather than the epithelium. This supports the hypothesis that BPH may occur if the normal age-related decrease in testosterone does *not* occur.[124]

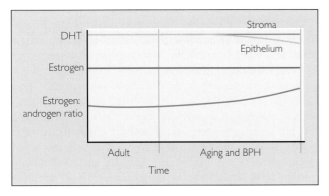

Figure 1.28 Changes in hormone concentrations in the prostate with age. During the normal aging process, DHT levels begin to decline, particularly in the epithelial cells, while estrogen levels remain constant. If the estrogen:androgen ratio does not increase, it may tilt the balance towards abnormal proliferation, which resembles a reawakening of embryonic cell growth

GROWTH FACTOR EFFECTS ON PROSTATE CELLS

Fibroblasts in the mesenchyme are known to be important regulators of development, differentiation, and proliferation of epithelium of many organs systems.[130] The mesenchyme also plays a role in the expression of tissue-specific secretory proteins. In the male sex accessory glands, the mesenchymal–epithelial interactions continue postnatally and are regulated by androgens. Since the 1900s it has been assumed that these two compartments communicated with each other via short-range signals.[123]

Recent improvements in cell culture techniques and development of relevant cell lines and strains have allowed researchers to investigate these interactions.[141] For example, by separating culturing stroma and epithelial cells from human BPH specimens, it was found that DNA synthesis in the epithelium was dependent on the presence of adjacent stromal and myoepithelial cells. That these two cell types must be in direct contact was discovered when attempts to place membrane filters between them abolished growth and morphogenesis in prostatic cultures. Studies by Thompson and Chung suggest that the microenvironment, including the vascular and neuroendocrine networks, may be crucial for proper secretory function in this gland.[142]

It appears that the reciprocal relationship between prostatic epithelium, where testosterone metabolism occurs, and the mesenchyme, with its neuroendocrine network, allows for a tight metabolic cooperation between the two tissue types.[141] The effects of on the secretory epithelium due to testosterone, then, likely occur as a result of stroma response to AR activation. The small peptide molecules collectively known as GF are thought to be the "currency" for this bidirectional communication. A series of elegant experiments by Chung *et al.*[141] using tumorigenic fibroblasts or marginally tumorigenic epithelial (LNCaP) cells implanted into normal rat prostates showed that the former could not induce normal epithelial cells to participate in tumorigenesis, while normal rat fibroblasts could induce tumor formation in LNCaPs. However, fibroblasts were found to be distinctly different, as co-implanted prostate or bone fibroblasts, but not human lung or mouse embryonic fibroblasts, were effective tumor-promoters in the study. The specificity of the fibroblasts may explain the propensity of prostatic tumors to metastasize to bone.

The mechanism of actions of epithelial and stromal cells on each other has been an area of intense research, as it may lead to an understanding of tumorigenesis, carcinogenesis, tumor progression, and metastasis.[143-147] It is now well accepted that, in the prostate, these actions are the result of the synthesis of polypeptide GF and their receptors, under the control and regulation of various hormones.[148] There are two broad categories of GF, autocrine and paracrine; however, they are not mutually exclusive (Figure 1.29). Paracrine factors originate in one cell type and affect another cell type, while autocrine factors originate and affect cells of the same type. GF are categorized into families based on structural homologies, despite names that

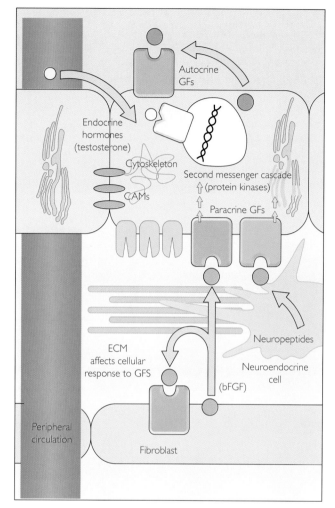

Figure 1.29 Stromal–epithelial interactions in the prostate. Hormonal control of the prostate is accomplished via a complex system of endocrine, autocrine, and paracrine growth factors that balance cell proliferation and programmed cell death (apoptosis). Any imbalance can tip the processes in an abnormal direction of uncontrolled growth

reflect a cell of origin or biological property.[149] They act predominantly on cell surface transmembrane receptors that are comprised of an aminoterminal extracellular domain for ligand binding, a hydrophobic transmembrane domain, and an intracellular carboxyterminal catalytic domain.[150] Of the six major GF families expressed in the prostate, the catalytic domains of three of them (insulin, EGF, and platelet-derived growth factor) are characteristic of tyrosine kinases. Protein kinases regulate many aspects of cell growth and differentiation, and biosynthetic and degradative pathways. Oncogenes that encode for these kinases have been implicated in malignancy and metastasis, although not much is yet known about these enzymes in prostate cancer. In addition, some oncogene products are similar to GF or their receptors. For example, the *erb*-B-2 (*neu*) oncogene is related to the truncated EGF receptor, *erb*-B. In addition, EGF recepter and *c-myc* expression, both induced by some GF, are elevated in malignant compared with BPH human

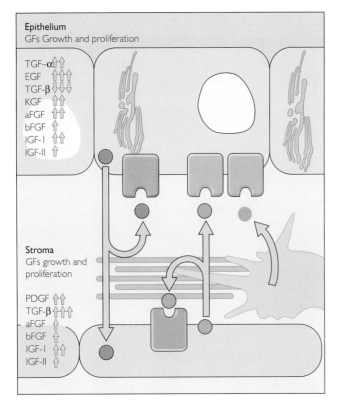

Figure 1.30 Growth factors (GF) in the prostate. GF are small peptides that have strong influences on the growth and secretory activities of specific cell types. The extracellular matrix (ECM) components such as cell–cell and cell–ECM adhesion factors influence cellular response to growth factors. A GF can have a stimulatory or inhibitory effect, depending on cell type and other hormonal influences. Under conditions of androgen deprivation, some GF are increased and some decreased. Since some receptors bind more than one GF, the lack of one GF can be compensated for by another that might be upregulated when androgens are low

prostatic tissue, possibly providing an autocrine pathway for androgen-independent tumor growth.

Although the major families of soluble prostatic GF will be described here, it is important to remember that direct contact of the cells with the extracellular matrix (ECM) is an integral part of tissue-specific growth and differentiation. ECM proteins such as fibronectin, laminin, collagen IV, vitronectin, tenascin, proteoglycans, and other cell adhesion molecules, such as the cadherins, can affect cell morphology and their response to GF.[151,152] The role of GF in the adult rodent, when prostatic growth ceases, may be on the ECM.[148]

OVERVIEW

The interactions of hormones, paracrine, autocrine, and extracellular matrix components act in a complex manner to support the normal prostate gland composition. Abnormal expression of any one of these factors may be enough to tip the balance towards aberrant growth or malignant transformation (Figure 1.30).[153] While there is much to be learned about all the players, it is known that in the normal prostate,

growth is regulated by peptide GF directly, and by androgens, indirectly via their effect on the stromal compartment. EGF and basic FGF (bFGF) provide most of the stimulation for prostate growth. TGF-β induces fibroblast proliferation, while inhibiting that of epithelium, and it can specifically abolish EGF activity. However, bFGF can prevent the inhibitory effects of TGF-β. Castration results in a decrease in EGF and FGF expression, while the EGF receptor is upregulated in an attempt to maintain growth. At the same time, TGF-β1 and its receptor levels are increased, thereby preventing epithelial cell proliferation and possibly initiating apoptosis, the net effect of androgen deprivation. In BPH, bFGF and TGF-β2 expression is elevated, while EGF, the EGF receptor, and TGF-β1 remain constant. bFGF is thought to be the major factor in BPH development, causing both the epithelium and mesenchyme to proliferate. Since TGF-β2 can stimulate the mesenchyme, induction of both these GF may result in a glandular nodule.

EPIDERMAL GROWTH FACTOR AND TRANSFORMING GROWTH FACTOR-α

A family of EGF growth factors, which includes TGF-α, has been identified and characterized. TGF-α and EGF have a 35% sequence homology, function via the same receptor, and have the same ability to bind and down-regulate the EGF receptor.[153, 154] Prostatic fluids contain high levels of EGF, suggesting that it is meant to be secreted.[155] Immunohistochemical studies have produced conflicting results regarding the relative amounts of EGF in BPH and malignant prostatic tissue,[156] although BPH tissue exhibits higher EGF binding than well-differentiated tumors. Not surprisingly, there was no correlation between EGF, Gleason score, or patient survival.

Both TGF-α and EGF have been found to promote proliferation and development of prostate epithelium. Androgens stimulate the production of EGF, which act in an autocrine manner to stimulate proliferation.[153] In malignant cells, EGF regulation may be lost, causing the induction of androgen-induced TGF-α mRNA, which binds to the EGF receptor to enhance growth further. It appears that EGF, not androgens, is required for growth of prostatic epithelial cells in vitro.[149]

The level of EGF receptors has been inversely correlated with the level of androgen receptors in human BPH tissue.[157] There are two families of EGF receptors which are tyrosine kinases. Products of the EGFr gene (c-erb-B-2 and HER-1) also appear to bind TGF-α with equal affinity, although the neu gene receptors (ERB-b2, HER-2, and NGL) do not.[149] The c-erb-B-2 receptor, actually a truncated form of the EGF receptor that is always active, even without the presence of a ligand, is thought to contribute to the malignant transformation of normal cells.[153] Castration in rats results in increased EGF binding to surface receptors, while human BPH specimens exhibited lower binding than normal or malignant tissues. There is some evidence that the phosphorylated EGF receptor is a substrate for prostatic acid phosphatase. This may be an important control pathway for the tyrosine kinase signaling cascade.[158]

Culture studies *in vitro* have shown that while prostatic stroma requires serum (or at least androgens) to grow, epithelial cells can be propagated in serum-free media containing selenium, glucocorticoid, cholera toxin, insulin, transferrin, EGF, and bovine pituitary extract (BPE). There are conflicting reports as to whether FGF could replace BPE and sustain growth.

PLATELET-DERIVED GROWTH FACTOR

Studies have shown that growth of isolated mesenchymal cells of the prostate and other tissues is stimulated by PDGF. Since receptors have not been identified in secretory cells, it is thought that PDGF may act as a paracrine factor, helping to organize the extracellular matrix in malignant tissues. It can induce expression of *c-fos* and *c-myc*; the latter may be required for an enhanced mitogenic response to PDGF.[159-163]

TRANSFORMING GROWTH FACTOR β

Three of the five isoforms of TGF-β are found in mammals. They share an 80% sequence homology, have similar biologic functions, and are found in a wide variety of tissues, including prostate.[164] The function varies from mitogen, to morphogen to inhibitor depending on the cell type and stage of differentiation.[165] Another member of this family, although more distantly related, comprise the bone morphogentic proteins, shown to stimulate prostate growth and thought to be a factor in successful metastasis.[166] TGF-β1 is fairly ubiquitous, while TGF-β2 and TGF-β3 have more restricted expression, and all may be controlled by steroid hormones.[167] The most-studied aspect of TGF-β action is on regulation of cell growth, but it is also an important modulator of the synthesis of ECM components such as collagen, fibronectin, and proteoglycans.[168] In addition, it can induce the production of inhibitors of plasminogen-activating factor, increase protease inhibitors, and decrease proteases.

TGF-β family of GF is known to be an inhibitory influence on non-neoplastic epithelial cells while promoting fibroblast development in many tissues, including prostate.[130,153,169] It strongly inhibits the expression of the AR in the androgen-responsive human cell line LNCaP.[170] At the same time, androgens regulate the expression of TGF-β1 and its receptor.[153] Proposed mechanisms of action include a cascade of factors, including retinoblastoma and *c-myc* genes. For an excellent review see Moses *et al.*[169]

TGF-β Types 1 and 2 show different binding affinities for the three types of receptors characterized to date, with the Type III receptor binding the most tightly to all TGF-β types. Receptor levels are known to increase after castration in the rat, but could be restored to normal levels with androgen therapy.[144] Androgen deprivation induces TGF-β expression in the prostate, which stimulates programmed cell death (apoptosis) in the epithelium.[153] In addition, it stimulates bFGF production in the stromal compartment, while inhibiting fibroblast proliferation. Readministration of androgens further increases bFGF while decreasing TGF-β, overcoming the growth inhibition of both cell types.[171] It is proposed, but not proven yet, that prostate cancer acquires autonomous growth by overcoming TGF-β inhibition.

In the normal rat prostate, TGF-β1 inhibits epithelial growth, which requires both EGF and FGF for growth. Even though EGF and TGF-α can stimulate the growth of slow-growing tumors, this effect is abolished by TGF-β.[172] Normal prostate growth does not appear to be affected by exogenous TGF-β administration, perhaps due to the overriding stimulatory effects of EGF. TGF-β1 is thought to inhibit only EGF-stimulated epithelial proliferation, which supports the concept that, at castration, when androgen-induced EGF expression is low, TGF-β1 inhibition is negligible.[153]

Expression of TGF-β2 and bFGF mRNA is elevated in human BPH. TGF-β1 expression also was elevated, particularly in the stromal compartment. It is thought that BPH may be a "reawakening" of embryonic growth, mediated by TGF-β stimulation of fibroblasts, which in turn stimulate epithelial hyperplasia, and by bFGF, which may stimulate both cell types.[153] The overall ratio of TGF-β2 and bFGF may determine whether the BPH is predominatly glandular or stromal.

FIBROBLAST GROWTH FACTOR (HEPARIN BINDING GROWTH FACTOR)

The FGFs are a large family of GF derived from cells of embryonic mesoderm or neurorectoderm origin. The two most predominant members of this family implicated in prostatic growth are acidic FGF (aFGF) and basic FGF (bFGF).[173,174] They share a 55% sequence homology, although bFGF is required for culture *in vitro* of prostatic epithelial cells.[172] Compared with normal prostate epithelial cells, those from slow-growing tumors require far less aFGF to elicit a maximal proliferative response. Interestingly, fast-growing tumors were found to be completely independent of exogenous FGF. Inhibitory effects of TGF-β on normal rat prostate growth in culture could be completely abolished in the presence of exogenous aFGF. It has not been shown conclusively that aFGF is present in human prostatic tissue.[166]

Although aFGF appears to predominate during the development of the young rat, bFGF plays a primary role in the adult human and rat.[153] The mitogenic effects of androgens are likely to be due to the indirect effect of stimulating bFGF production. The levels of bFGF mRNA have been found to be significantly higher in human BPH tissue compared with normal or malignant prostates.[175] In the prostate, bFGF is produced and secreted mainly by the fibroblasts and is thought to act in an autocrine fashion, in addition to its paracrine effects on the epithelium to stimulate growth.[153] It is also synthesized to a lesser degree by the secretory epithelial cells.

Culture studies *in vitro* have shown that, while prostatic stroma requires serum (or at least androgens) to grow, epithelial cells can be propagated in serum-free media containing selenium, glucocorticoid, cholera toxin, insulin, transferrin, EGF, and BPE. There are conflicting reports as to whether FGF could replace BPE and sustain growth.

Another FGF family member, keratinocyte growth factor (KGF), unlike other FGFs, codes for a secretory signal sequence and is found in the medium of cultured prostatic fibroblasts. Peehl and coworkers[176] found that KGF and aFGF could replace EGF and support almost maximal growth, while bFGF was less effective. These studies provide more evidence of the regulation of epithelial growth by paracrine factors produced by the stromal cells.

When epithelial cells from human BPH nodules were grown in primary culture with either exogenous EGF or aFGF, in the presence of 1 ng mL^{-1} TGF-β, growth was reduced to 90% of pretreatment rates, which remained unchanged with increasing EGF.[177] However, cells grown in aFGF and 1 ng mL^{-1} TGF-β showed increasing attentuation with additional aFGF treatment, down to less than 10% of initial rates. This effect was not seen in culture of normal prostate epithelium, which does not express aFGF, but may respond to paracrine secretion from fibroblasts. Detection of aFGF expression in transformed prostate epithelium led these workers to suggest that it may be involved in malignant tumor growth.

There is an increasing amount of evidence that both aFGF and bFGF bind to two recently identified high-affinity receptors that are found in rat prostatic epithelial as well as mesenchymal cells.[173] However, they may also be able to bind to the KGF receptor, with aFGF and KGF being bound more tightly than bFGF. It has yet to be determined whether receptor availability or binding affinity is altered in BPH or malignancy.

Although a putative role for FGFs is in angiogenesis, which has been demonstrated *in vitro*, most tissues expressing these GF do not show much endothelial proliferation. It is thought that perhaps they are complexed within the ECM, which is known to store GF as a mechanism of regulating growth. Heparinases, secreted by many tissues, including tumors, may degrade the ECM-releasing GF such as FGF.[178,179] Once released, they are free to bind to cell surface receptors. There is some evidence that proliferative response to bFGF could be an early feature of BPH initiation.[166]

INSULIN-LIKE GROWTH FACTOR

This family consists of at least three members: insulin, IGF-I, and IGF-II. There are specific receptors for each type, although all bind with low affinity to the insulin and IGF-I receptors, whereas insulin and IGF-I do not bind significantly to the IGF-II receptor.[180] Studies have shown that IGF-I can promote proliferation of both normal and tumor-derived epithelial and mesenchymal cells, while insulin and IGF-II are much less effective. Increased expression of IGF-I is detected during prostate regeneration after androgen treatment of castrated rats.

OTHER SECRETORY PROTEINS

Prostatic Acid Phosphatase

Many tissues contain several forms of acid phosphatase that can be separated by subfractionation of the tissue and may be associated primarily with either the lysosomal secretions or particular membrane fractions. Human PAP is a glycoprotein dimer of 102,000 MW and contains about 7% by weight of carbohydrate, which is composed of 15 residues per mole of neutral sugars (fucose, galactose, and mannose); 6 residues per mole of sialic acid; and 13 residues of N-acetylglucosamine.[181] The protein can be dissociated into two subunits of 50,000 MW.

In summary, many secretory proteins and enzymes are glycosylated after they have been synthesized, and it appears that this accounts for some of the isoenzyme patterns of PAP. The secretory enzyme is probably the major form in the prostate, and the lysosomal acid phosphatase form may be similar in properties to the acid phosphatase found in other tissue lysosomes. The genes for these two acid phosphatases are located on different chromosomes.

The high enzymatic activity of PAP is preferential to humans and is not found in accessory tissues of other species.

Prostate-Specific Membrane Antigen

Although it is not a secretory protein, prostate-specific membrane antigen (PSMA) is a very important membrane-bound protein of the prostatic epithelial cell. This transmembrane glycoprotein is found on the surface of prostatic epithelial cells and has a molecular weight of 100,000.[184] The cDNA for PSMA has been cloned and the amino acid sequence determined.[185] Based on the amino acid sequence, there are many glycosylation sites available, which suggests that the extracellular domain of this transmembrane peptide is heavily glycosylated.[184] A monoclonal murine IgG1 antibody (7E11-C5) was prepared against purified PSMA,[186] which recognizes the antigen on prostatic epithelial cells. 7E11-C5 immunoreacts weakly with normal and BPH prostatic epithelium and strongly with malignant epithelium from the prostate: 7E11-C5 does not react with most other tumors and other normal tissue.[186] PSMA expression in prostate tumors appears to correlate with the degree of differentiation of the tumor and not with tumor stage.[184] The monoclonal antibody to PSMA, 7E11-C5, has been covalently linked to indium (in-CYT-356) and is under investigation as an imaging tool to localize prostate cancer metastases and disease recurrence following radical surgery. Evidence has demonstrated that the cDNA sequence for PSMA and the cDNA sequence for N-acetylated α-linked acidic dipeptidase (NAALADase), an enzyme localized to the brain[187] that catalyzes the cleavage of glutamate from N-acetyl-L-aspartyl-L-glutamate (NAAG), are similar.[188] The clinical usefulness of PSMA for diagnosis, monitoring, and imaging of men with prostatic disease is under investigation.

Leucine Aminopeptidase

Leucine aminopeptidase is another product of prostatic epithelial cells. Its exact function is unclear. It is secreted into the lumen of acini. It has been noted that this enzyme has decreased activity in prostatic cancer tissues compared to BPH tissues and therefore may have a role as a marker for cancer.

Lactic Dehydrogenase

Lactic dehydrogenase is another enzyme that is being explored as a marker for prostatic cancer. Five isoenzymes of LDH are found in tissues. Their relative proportions vary depending on the type of tissue. Investigations have noted that increased levels of isoenzyme 4 and 5 are present in prostatic cancer.

Immunoglobulins and C3 Complement

There is considerable evidence that immunoglobulins are present in prostatic fluid. They may have a role in preventing infections and may function in other ways as immunologic barriers. Their concentrations in the seminal plasma is lower than that of the serum. It has been noted that in patients with chronic prostatitis IGA is increased along with a low molecular weight substance termed "prostatic antibacterial factor"[202]. C3 complement is another component present in seminal plasma. Its level increases in response to infection and prostatitis as well as in patients with prostate cancer.

APOPTOSIS[209]

Cell growth in the normal prostate is regulated by a delicate balance between cell death and cell proliferation (i.e. apoptotic vs. proliferative activity). Disruption of the molecular mechanisms that regulate these two processes may underline the abnormal growth of the gland leading to BPH. In this study, the incidence of programmed cell death (apoptosis) and cell proliferation was comparatively analyzed among the various cell subpopulations in the normal and benign hyperplastic human prostate. The authors also examined the relative expression of two proteins involved in the regulation of prostate apoptosis: (1) TGF-β1, a negative growth factor able to induce prostate apoptosis under physiological conditions; and (2) bcl-2, a potent apoptosis suppressor. Analysis of the

incidence of "spontaneous" apoptosis *in situ*, using the end-labeling terminal transferase staining technique for the detection of nucleosomal DNA fragmentation, revealed infrequent apoptotic staining in isolated basal and secretory prostate epithelial cells. The basal level of cell proliferation was determined on the basis of the Ki-67 nuclear antigen staining, a nuclear protein that appears primarily during the proliferative phases of the cell cycle. The Ki-67-positive nuclei were equally distributed among the basal and secretory epithelial cells of the hyperplastic prostatic acini. The apoptotic index of the secretory and basal cells of the prostate epithelium was higher in the normal prostate compared with BPH tissue, whereas there was a significant increase in the proliferative index of the respective cell populations in the hyperplastic prostate. Balancing the apoptotic vs. the proliferative activities revealed a substantial net decrease (fourfold) in the total number of cells dying via apoptosis in both the glandular and basal epithelial cell compartments of the hypertrophic prostate (BPH) when compared with the normal gland. TGF-β staining was exclusively identified in the secretory epithelial cells lining the prostatic lumen with minimal involvement of the basal cells and total lack of immunoreactivity among the stroma elements. Statistical analysis revealed a significant elevation in TGF-β expression in the epithelial cells of BPH tissue compared with the normal prostate ($P < 0.001$). Expression of bcl-2 was topographically restricted to the glandular epithelium of the prostate. In the normal prostate, bcl-2 immunoreactivity was predominantly identified in the basal cell layer. An increase in both the intensity of immunoreactivity for bcl-2 and the number of positive epithelial cells (basal and secretory) was detected in BPH specimens relative to the normal prostate ($P < 0.02$). These results suggest a potential involvement of enhanced expression of this anti-apoptosis protein in deregulation of the normal apoptotic cell death mechanisms in the human prostate, thus resulting in a growth imbalance in favor of cell proliferation that might ultimately promote prostatic hyperplasia.

REFERENCES

1 Althof V, Hoekstra CJ, Loo H. Variation in prostate position relative to adjacent bony anatomy. *Int J Radiat Oncol Biol Phys* 1996; **34**(3): 709–15.

2 Van Herk M, Bruce A, Kroes G *et al*. Quantification of organ motion during conformal radiotherapy of the prostate by three dimensional (3D) image registration. *Int J Radiat Oncol Biol Phys* 1995; **33**(5): 1311–20.

3 Beard CJ, Bussiere MR, Plunkett ME *et al*. Analysis of prostate and seminal vesicle motion. *Int J Radiat Oncol Biol Phys* 1993; **27** (Suppl 1): 451–8.

4 Melian E, Kutcher G, Leibel S *et al*. Variation in prostate position: quantitation and implications for three-dimensional conformal radiation therapy. *Int J Radiat Oncol Biol Phys* 1993; **27** (Suppl 1): 73–81.

5 Schild SE, Casale HE, Bellefontaine LP. Movements of the

prostate due to rectal and bladder distension. Implications for radiotherapy. *Med Dosim* 1993; **18** (Suppl 1): 13–15.

6 Ten Haken RK, Forman JD, Heidburger DK. Treatment planning issues related to prostate movement in response to differential filling of the rectum and bladder. *Int J Radiat Oncol Biol Phys* 1991; **20** (Suppl 6): 1317–24.

7 Hayek H. Das Faserkaliber in den Mm. Transversus perinei und Sphincter urethra. *Z Anat Entwick* 1960; **121**: 455–8.

8 Hayek H. Zur Anatomie des Sphincter urethrae. *Z Anat Entwickl* 1962; **123**: 121–5.

9 Henle J. *Handbuch der systematischen Anatomie des Menschen*, Bd. 2, *Eingeweidelehre*. Braunschweig: Friedrich 1873.

10 Williams PL, Warwick R, Dyson M, Bannister LH. *Gray's Anatomy*, 37th edn. Edinburgh: Churchill Livingstone 1989; 607–8.

11 Oelirich TM. The urethral sphincter muscle in the male. *Am J Anat* 1980; **158**: 229–46.

12 Walsh PC, Quinlan DM, Morton RA, Steiner MS. Radical retropubic prostatectomy. Improved anastomosis and urinary continence. *Urol Clin North Am* 1990; **17**: 679–84.

13 Myers PR, Goellner JR, Cahill DR. Prostate shape, external striated urethral sphincter and radical prostatectomy: the apical dissection. *J Urol* 1987; **138**: 543–50.

14 Walsh PC. Radical retropubic prostatectomy. Improved anastomosis and urinary continence. In: Walsh PC, Retik AB, Stamey TA, Vaughan ED, Jr (eds) *Campbell's Urology*, 6th edn, Vol. 3. Philadelphia: WB Saunders 1992; 2865–86.

15 Dorschner W. Der Streit um den Musculus sphincter urethrae. Histomorphologische Utersuchungen. *Akt Urol* 1992; **23**: 163–8.

16 Myers RP. Male urethral sphincteric anatomy and radical prostatectomy. *Urol Clin North Am* 1991; **18**: 211–27.

17 Tanagho EA. Anatomy of the lower urinary tract. In: Walsh PC, Retik AB, Stamey TA, Vaughan ED Jr (eds) *Campbell's Urology*, 6th edn, Vol 1. Philadelphia: WB Saunders 1992; 40–74.

18 Narayan P, Konety B, Aslam K *et al*. Neuroanatomy of the external urethral sphincter: implications for urinary continence preservation during radical prostate surgery. *J Urol* 1995; **153**: 337–41.

19 Zvara P, Carrier S, Kour NW, Tanagho EA. The detailed neuroanatomy of the human striated urethral sphincter. *Br J Urol* 1994; **74**: 182.

20 Lawson J. Pelvic anatomy I: pelvic floor muscles. *Ann R Coll Surg Engl* 1974; **54**: 244.

21 Donker PJ, Ivanovici F, Noach EL. Analyses of the urethral pressure profile by means of electromyography and the administration of drugs. *Br J Urol* 1972; **44**: 180.

22 Krahn HP, Morales PA. The effect of pudendal nerve anaesthesia on urinary continence after prostatectomy. *J Urol* 1965; **94**: 282–5.

23 O'Donnell P, Finan BF. Continence following nerve-sparing radical prostatectomy. *J Urol* 1989; **142**: 1227–9.

24 Helweg G, Strasser H, Knapp R *et al*. Transurethral sonomorphologic evaluation of the male external sphincter of the urethra. *Eur Radiol* 1994; **4**: 525–8.

25 Kokoua A, Homsy Y, Lavigne JF *et al*. Maturation of the external urinary sphincter: a comparative histophotographic study in humans. *J Urol* 1993; **150**: 617–22.

26 Furuya S, Kumamoto Y, Yokoyama E *et al*. Alpha-adrenergic activity and urethral pressure profilometry in prostatic zone in benign prostatic hypertrophy. *J Urol* 1982; **128**: 836.

27 Gosling JA. Autonomic innervation of the prostae. In: Hinman F (edn) *Benign Prostatic Hypertrophy*. New York: Springer 1983; 349–60.

28 Smith ER, Lebeaux MT. The mediation of the canine prostatic secretion provoked by hypogastric nerve stimulation. *Invest Urol* 1970; **7**: 313–18.

29 Brushini H, Schmidt RA, Tanagho EA. Neurologic control of prostatic secretion in the dog. *Invest Urol* 1978; **15**: 288–91.

30 Vom Saal FS, Montano MM, Wang MH. Sexual differentiation in mammals: chemically induced alterations in sexual and functional development. In: Colborn T, Clement C (eds) *The Wildlife–Human Connection*. Princeton, NJ: Princeton Scientific, 1992; 32.

31 McNeal JE. The prostate and prostatic urethra: a morphologic synthesis. *J Urol* 1972; **107**: 1008–16.

32 McNeal JE. Developmental and comparative anatomy of the prostate. In: Grayhack JT, Wilson JD, Scherbenske MJ (eds) *Benign Prostatic Hyperplasia. NIAMDD Workshop Proceedings* DHEW. Publ NIH 76–1113. Washington: US Government Printing Office 1976; 1–9.

33 Shannon JM, Cunha GR, Vanderslice KD. Autoradiographic localization of androgen receptors in the developing mouse prostate. *Anat Rec* 1981; **199**: 232.

34 Takeda H, Mizuno T, Lasnitzki I. Autoradiographic studies of androgen-binding sites in the rat urogenital sinus and postnatal prostate. *J Endocrinol* 1985; **104**: 87.

35 Takeda H, Chang C. Immunohistochemical and in-situ hybridization of androgen receptor expression during the development of the mouse prostate gland. *J Endocrinol* 1991; **129**(1): 83–9.

36 McNeal JE. Regional morphology and pathology of the prostate. *Am J Clin Pathol* 1968; **49**: 347–57.

37 McNeal JE. Origin and evolution of benign prostatic enlargement. *Invest Urol* 1978; **15**: 340–5.

38 Lee F, Torp-Pedersen ST, Siders DB *et al*. Transurethral ultrasound in the diagnosis and staging of prostatic carcinoma. *Radiology* 1989; **170**: 609.

39 Johnson FP. The later development of the urethra in the male. *J Urol* 1920; **4**: 447.

40 Kellokumpu-Lehtinen P. The histochemical localization of acid phosphatase in human fetal urethral and prostatic epithelium. *Invest Urol* 1980; **17**: 435–40.

41 Kellokumpu-Lehtinen P. Development of sexual dimorphism in human urogenital sinus complex. *Biol Neonate* 1985; **48**: 157.

42 Kellokumpu-Lehtinen P, Santti R, Pelliniemi LJ. Correlation of early cytodifferentiation of the human fetal prostate and Leydig cells. *Anat Rec* 1980; **196**: 263–73.

43 Lowsley OS. The development of the human prostate gland with reference to the development of other structures at the neck of the urinary bladder. *Am J Anat* 1912; **13**: 299–346.

44 Franks LM. Benign nodular hyperplasia of the prostate: a review. *Ann R Coll Surg Engl* 1954; **14**: 92–106.

45 Moore KL, Persaud TUN. The urogenital system. In: Moore KL, Persaud TUN (eds) *The Developing Human: Clinical Oriented Embryology*, 5th edn. Philadelphia: WB Saunders 1993: 288.

46 Zondek T, Zondek LH. The fetal and neonatal prostate. In: Goland M (ed) *Normal and Abnormal Growth of the Prostate*. Springfield: CC Thomas 1975: 5–28.

47 Xia BT, Blackburn XT, Gardner WA. Fetal prostate growth and development. *Pediatr Pathol* 1990; **10**: 527–37.

48 McNeal JE. The prostate gland: morphology and pathology. *Monogr Urol* 1983; **4**: 3.

49 McNeal JE. The prostate gland: morphology and pathobiology. *Monogr Urol* 1988; **9**: 3.

50 McNeal JE. Normal histology of the prostate. *Am J Surg Pathol* 1988; **12**: 619.

51 Reese FN, McNeal JE *et al*. Differential distribution of pepsinogen II between the zones of the human prostate and the seminal vesicle. *J Urol* 1986; **136**(5): 1148–52.

52 Reese JH, McNeal JE, Redwine EA *et al*. Tissue type plasminogen activator as a marker for functional zones, within the human prostate gland. *Prostate* 1988; **12**(1): 47–53.

53 McNeal JE. Anatomy of the prostate: an historical survey of divergent views. *Prostate* 1980; **1**: 3–13.

54 Tissell LE, Salander H. The lobes of the human prostate. *Scand J Nephrol* 1975; **9**: 185–91.

55 Tissell LE, Salander H. Anatomy of the human prostate and its three paired lobes. In: Kimball FA, Buhl AE, Carter DB (eds) *New Approaches to the Study of Benign Prostatic Hyperplasia*. New York: Alan R Liss 1984; 55–65.

56 Villers A, McNeal JE, Redwine EA *et al*. The role of perineural space invasion in the local spread of prostatic adenocarcinoma. *J Urol* 1989; **142**: 763.

57 Rifkin MD, Resnick M. Ultrasonography of the prostate. In: Resnick MI, Rifkin MD (eds) *Ultrasonography of the Prostrate*, 3rd edn. Baltimore: Williams & Wilkins 1991; 297.

58 Rifkin MD, Dahnert W, Kurtz AB. State of the art endorectal sonograph of the prostate gland. *Am J Roentgenol* 1990; **154**: 691.

59 Stamey TA, Hodge KK. Ultrasound visualization of the prostate anatomy and pathology. *Monogr Urol* 1988; **9**: 55.

60 Strasser H, Klima G, Poisel S *et al*. Anatomy and innervation of the rhabdosphincter of the male urethra. *Prostate* 1996; **28**(1): 24–31.

61 Villers A, Terris MK, McNeal JE *et al*. Ultrasound anatomy of the prostate: the normal gland and anatomical variations. *J Urol* 1989; **143**: 732–8.

62 Testut L, Latarjet A. Aponevroses du perinee chez l'homme. In: Testut L, Latarjet A (eds) *Traite d'Anatomie Humaine*, 9th edn, 5:XIII:6. Paris: G Doin 1949; 383–424.

63 Genenois PA, Salmon I, Stallenberg B *et al*. Magnetic resonance imaging of the normal prostate at 1.5 T. *Br J Radiol* 1990; **63**: 101–7.

64 Di Sant'Agnese PA. Neuroendocrine differentiation in human prostate carcinoma. *Hum Pathol* 1992; **23**: 287–96.

65 Cockett AT, diSant'Agnese PA, Gopinath P, Schoen SR, Abrahamsson PA. Relationship of neuroendocrine cells of prostate and serotonin to benign prostatic hyperplasia. *Urology* 1993; **42**(5): 512–9.

66 Bonkhoff H, Stein U, Remberger K. Androgen receptor status in endocrine-paracrine cell types of the normal, hyperplastic, and neoplastic human prostate. *Virchows Arch [A]* 1993; **423**: 291–4.

67 Di Sant'Agnese PA. Neuroendocrine differentiation in carcinoma of the prostate. Diagnostic prognostic, and therapeutic implications. *Cancer* 1992; **70**: 254–68.

68 Algaba F. Pathophysiology of benign prostatic hyperplasia: *Eur Urol* 1994; **25**(Suppl 1): 3–5.

69 Iwamura M, diSant'Agnese PA, Wu G *et al*. Overexpression of human epidermal growth factor receptor and c-*erb*B-2 by neuroendocrine cells in normal prostatic tissue. *Urology* 1994; **43**(6): 838–43.

70 Nakada SY, di Sant'Agnese PA, Moynes RA *et al*. The androgen receptor status of neuroendocrine cells in human benign and malignant prostatic tissue. *Cancer* 1993; **53**(9): 1967–70.

71 Mann T, Mann CL. *Male Reproductive Function and Semen*. New York: Springer 1981.

72 Amelar RD, Hotchkiss RS. The split ejaculate: Its uses in the management of male infertility. *Fertil Steril* 1965; **16**: 46–9.

73 Tauber PF, Zaneveld LJD, Propping D, Schumacher GFB. Components of human split ejaculate. *J Reprod Fertil* 1975; **23**: 249–67.

74 Costello LC, Fadika G, Franklin RB. Aconitase activity, citrate oxidation, and zinc inhibition in rat ventral prostate. *Enzyme* 1981; **26**: 281.

75 Costello LC, Franklin RB. Concepts of citrate production and secretion by prostate. 2. Hormonal relationships in normal and neoplastic prostate. *Prostate* 1991; **19**(3): 181–205.

76 Costello LC, Franklin RB. Concepts of citrate production and secretion by prostate. 1. Metabolic relationships. *Prostate* 1991; **18**(1): 25–46.

77 Costello LC, Franklin RB. The bioenergetic theory of prostate malignancy. *Prostate* 1994; **25**: 162.

78 Huggins C. The prostatic secretion: *Harvey Lect* 1947; **42**: 148.

79 Franklin RB, Costello LC. Intermediary energy metabolism of normal and malignant prostate epithelial cells. In: Naz RK (ed) *Prostate: Basic and Clinical Aspects*, Chap. 5. New York: CRC Press 1997; 115–150.

80 Costello LC, Franklin RB, Stacey R. Mitochondrial isocitrate dehydrogenase and isocitrate oxidation of rat ventral prostate. *Enzyme* 1976; **21**: 495.

81 Franklin RB, Costello LC. Isocitrate uptake and citrate production by rat ventral prostate fragments. *Invest Urol* 1976; **16**: 44.

82 Costello LC, Franklin RB. Novel role of zinc in the regulation of prostate citrate metabolism and its implications in prostate cancer. *Prostate* 1998; **35**(4): 285–96.

83 Kavanagh JP. Isocitric and citric acid in human prostatic and seminal fluid. *Prostate* 1994; **24**: 138.

84 Wenner CE. Regulation of energy metabolism in normal and tumor tissue. In: Becher FF (ed) *Cancer: Biology of Tumors*. New York: Plenum Press, 1975; 389–403.

85 Cooper JE, Farid I. The role of citric acid in the physiology of the prostate. A chromatographic study of citric acid cycle intermediates in benign and malignant prostatic tissue. *J Surg Res* 1963; **3**: 112.

86 Weisser H, Krieg M. Benign prostatic hyperplasia – the outcome of age-induced alteration of androgen–estrogen balance? *Urologe* 1997; **36**(1): 3–9.

87 Costello L. Intermediary metabolism of normal and malignant prostate: a neglected area of prostate research. *Prostate* 1998; **34**(4): 303–4.

88 Costello LC, Liu Y, Franklin RB. Testosterone stimulates the biosynthesis of m-aconitase and citrate oxidation in prostate epithelial cells. *Mol Cell Endocrinol* 1995; **112**(1): 45–51.

89 Hricak H, White S, Vigneron D *et al*. Carcinoma of the prostate gland: MR Imaging with pelvic phased-array coils versus integrated endorectal pelvic phased array coils. *Radiology* 1994; **193**: 703–9.

90 Narayan P, Presti J, Hricak H *et al*. Local staging of prostatic carcinoma: comparison of transrectal sonography and endorectal MR imaging. *Am J Roentgenol* 1966; **166**(1): 103–8.

91 Kurhanewicz J, Dahiya R, Macdonald JM *et al*. Citrate alterations in primary and metastatic human prostatic adenocarcinomas. 1H magnetic resonance spectroscopy and biochemical study. *Mag Reson Med* 1993; **29**: 149.

92 Schiebler ML, Miyamoto KK, White M *et al*. In vitro high resolution 1H-spectroscopy of the human prostate: benign prostatic hyperplasia, normal peripheral zone and adenocarcinoma. *Magn Reson Med* 1993; **29**: 285.

93 Robert M, Gagnon G. Purification and characterization of the active precursor of a human sperm motility inhibitor secreted by the seminal vesicles: identity with semenogelin. *Biol Reprod* 1996; **55**(4): 813–17.

94 Gavella M, Lipovac V, Vucic M, Rocic B. Superoxide anion scavenging capacity of human seminal plasma. *Int J Androl* 1996; **19**(2): 82–90.

95 Liu Y, Costello LC, Franklin RB. Prolactin and testosterone regulation of mitochondrial zinc in prostate epithelial cells. *Prostate* 1996; **30**(1): 26–32.

96 Brys M, Nawrocka AD, Miekos E *et al*. Zinc and cadmium analysis in human prostate neoplasms. *Biol Trace Elem Res* 1997; **59**(1–3): 145–52.

97 Harkonen PL, Isoltalo A, Santti R. Studies on the mechanism of testosterone action on glucose metabolism in the rat ventral prostate. *J Steroid Biochem Mol Biol* 1975; **6**: 1405.

98 Fair WR, Wehner N. The prostatic antibacterial factor: identity and significance: In: Marberger H *et al*. (eds) *Prostatic Disease*, Vol 6. New York: Alan R Liss 1976; 383–340.

99 Calandra RS, Rulli SB, Frungieri MB *et al*. Polyamines in the male reproductive system. *Acta Physiol Pharmacol Ther Latinoam* 1996; **46**(4): 209–22.

100 Watanabe S, Sato S, Nagase S, Shimosato K, Saito T. Polyamine levels in various tissues of rats treated with 3-hydroxy-4-methoxycinnamic acid and 3,4-dimethoxycinnamic acid. *Anticancer Drugs* 1996; **7**(8): 866–77.

101 Cipolla BG, Ziade J, Bansard JY *et al*. Pretherapeutic erythrocyte polyamine spermine levels discriminate high risk relapsing patients with m1 prostate carcinoma. *Cancer* 1996; **78**(5): 1055–65.

102 Czuba M, Smith IC. Biological and NMR markers for cancer. *Pharmacol Ther* 1991; **50**(2): 147–90.

103 Le Gimellec C, Friedlander G, El Yandouzi EH, Zlatkine P, Giocondi MC. Membrane fluidity in epithelial cells. *Kidney Int* 1992; **48**: 825–36.

104 Sargent NSE, Habib FK. Partial purification of human prostatic 5α-reductase (3-oxo-5α- steroid:NADP+ 4-ene-oxido-reductase; EC 1.2.1.22) in a stable and active form. *J Steroid Biochem Mol Biol* 1991; **38**: 73–7.

105 Camacho J, Rubalcava B. Lipid composition of liver plasma membranes from rats intoxicated with carbon tetrachloride. *Biochim Biophys Acta* 1984; **776**: 97–104.

106 Tunn S, Nass R, Ekkernkamp A *et al*. Evaluation of average life span of epithelial and stromal cells of human prostate by superoxide dismutase activity. *Prostate* 1989; **15**: 263–71.

107 Swinnen JV, Ultrix W, Heynes W, Verhoeven G. Coordinate regulation of lipogenic gene expression by androgens: evidence for a cascade mechanism involving sterol regulatory element binding proteins. *Proc Natl Acad Sci USA* 1997; **94**(24): 12975–80.

108 Swinnen JV, Esquenent M, Goossens K *et al*. Androgens stimulate fatty acid synthase in the human prostate cancer cell line LNCaP. *Cancer Res* 1997; **57**(6): 1086–9.

109 Herrmann JL, Menter DG, Beham A *et al*. Regulation of lipid signaling pathways for cell survival and apoptosis by bcl-2 in prostate carcinoma cells. *Exp Cell Res* 1997; **234**(2) 442–51.

110 Zhang H, Zheng RL. Promotion of human sperm capacitation by superoxide anion. *Free Radic Res* 1996; **24**(4): 261–8.

111 Gann PH, Hennekens CH, Longcope C, Verhoek-Oftedahl W, Grodstein F, Stampfer MJ. A prospective study of plasma hormone levels, nonhormonal factors, development of benign prostatic hyperplasia. *Prostate* 1995; **26**(1): 40–9.

112 Davies P, Eaton CL. Regulation of prostate growth. *J Endocrinol* 1991; **131**(1): 5–17.

113 Kumar VL, Majumder PK. Prostate gland: structure, functions and regulation. *Int Urol Nephrol* 1995; **27**(3): 231–43.

114 Mawhinney MG, Neubauer BL. Actions of estrogen in the male. *Invest Urol* 1979; **16**(6): 409–20.

115 Dirnhofer S, Berger C, Hermann M *et al*. Coexpression of gonadotropic hormones and their corresponding FSH and LH/CG receptors in the human prostate. *Prostate* 1998; **35**(3): 212–20.

116 Tao YX, Bao S, Ackermann DM *et al*. Expression of luteinizing hormone/human chorionic gonadotropin receptor gene in benign prostatic hyperplasia and in prostate carcinoma in humans. *Biol Reprod* 1997; **56**(1): 67–72.

117 Silver RI, Wiley EL, Davis DL *et al*. Expression and regulation of steroid 5α-reductase 2 in prostate disease. *J Urol* 1994; **152**: 433–7.

118 Thigpen AE, Silver RI, Guileyardo JM *et al*. Tissue distribution and ontogeny of steroid 5α-reductase isozyme expression. *J Clin Invest* 1993; **92**: 903.

119 Bruchovsky N, Rennie PS, Batzoid FH *et al*. Kinetic parameters of 5α-reductase activity in stroma and epithelium of normal, hyperplastic, and carcinomatous human prostates. *J Clin Endocrinol Metab* 1988; **67**: 806.

120 Hudson RW, Wherrett D. Comparison of the nuclear 5α-reduction of testosterone and androstenedione in human prostatic carcinoma and benign prostatic hyperplasia. *J Steroid Biochem* 1990; **35**: 231.

121 Barrack ER, Tindall DJ. A critical evaluation of the use of androgen receptor assays to predict the androgen responsiveness of prostatic cancer. *Current Concepts and Approaches to the Study of Prostate Cancer* 1987; 155–87.

122 Stamey TA, McNeal JE. Adenocarcinoma of the prostate. In: Walsh PC, Retik AB, Stamey TA, Vaughan ED Jr (eds) *Campbell's Urology*, 6th edn, Vol 1. Philadelphia: WB Saunders 1992; 1159–220.

123 Chung LW, Cunha GR. Stromal–epithelial interactions: II. Regulation of prostatic growth by embryonic urogenital sinus mesenchyme. *Prostate* 1983; **4**: 503–11.

124 Montie JE, Pienta KJ. Review of the role of androgenic hormones in the epidemiology of benign prostatic hyperplasia and prostate cancer. *Urology* 1994; **43**(6): 892–9.

125 Bonkhoff H, Remberger K. Differentiation pathways and histogenetic aspects of normal and abnormal prostatic growth: a stem cell model. *Prostate* 1996; **28**: 98–106.

126 Bonkhoff H, Remberger K. Widespread distribution of nuclear androgen receptors in the basal cell layer of the normal and hyperplastic human prostate: *Virchows Arch [A]* 1993; **422**: 35–8.

127 Luke MC, Coffey DS. Human androgen receptor binding to the androgen response element of prostate specific antigen. *J Androl* 1994; **15**(1): 41–51.

128 Roche PJ, Hoare SA, Parker MG. A consensus DNA-binding site for the androgen receptor. *Mol Endocrinol* 1992; **6**: 2229–35.

129 Montgomery BT, Young CY, Bilhartz DL *et al*. Hormonal regulation of prostate-specific antigen (PSA) glycoprotein in the human prostatic adenocarcinoma cell line LNCaP. *Prostate* 1992; **21**: 63–73.

130 Cunha GR, Hayashi N, Wong YC. Regulation of differentiation and growth of normal adult and neoplastic epithelia by inductive mesenchyme. *Cancer Surv Prostate Cancer* 1991; **11**: 73–90.

131 Walsh PC. Benign prostatic hyperplasia. In: Walsh PC, Retik AB, Stamey TA, Vaughan ED Jr (eds) *Campbell's Urology*, 6th edn, Vol. 1. Philadelphia: WB Sauders 1992; 1009–27.

132 De Voogt HJ, Rao BR, Geldof AA, Gooren LJG, Bouman FG. Androgen action blockade does not result in reduction in size but changes histology of the normal human prostate. *Prostate* 1987; **11**: 305–11.

133 Krieg M, Nass R, Tunn S. Effect of aging on endogenous level of 5 alpha-dihydrotestosterone, testosterone, estradiol, and estrone in epithelium and stroma of normal and hyperplastic human prostate. *J Clin Endocrinol Metab* 1993; **77**(2): 375–81.

134 Suzuki K, Ito K, Ichinose Y *et al*. Endocrine environment of benign prostatic hyperplasia: prostate size and volume are correlated with serum estrogen concentration. *Scand J Urol Nephrol* 1995; **29**(1): 65–8.

135 Janssen T, Petein M, van Velthoven R *et al*. Coregulatory effects of epidermal growth factor, dihydrotestosterone, and prolactin on benign human prostatic hyperplasia tissue culture proliferation. *Prostate* 1997; **30**(1): 47–52.

136 Wennbo H, Kindblom J, Isaksson OG, Tornell JP. Transgenic mice overexpressing the prolactin gene develop dramatic enlargement of the prostate gland. *Endocrinology* 1997; **138**(10): 4410–15.

137 Costello LC, Fadika G, Franklin RB. Citrate and isocitrate utilization by rat ventral prostate mitochondria. *Enzyme* 1978; **23**: 176.

138 Partin AW, Oesterling JE, Epstein JI *et al*. Influence of age and endocrine factors on the volume of benign prostatic hyperplasia. *J Urol* 1991; **145**(2): 405–9.

139 Tunn S, Haumann R, Hey J *et al*. Effect of aging on kinetic parameters of 3 alpha (beta)-hydroxysteroid oxidoreductases in epithelium and stroma of human normal and hyperplastic prostate. *J Clin Endocrinol* 1990; **71**(3): 732–9.

140 Prins GS, Jung MN, Vellanoweth RL *et al*. Age-dependent expression of the androgen receptor gene in the prostate and its implication in glandular differentiation and hyperplasia. *Dev Genet* 1996; **18**(2): 99–106.

141 Chung LW, Gleave ME, Hsieh JT *et al*. Reciprocal mesenchymal-epithelial interaction affecting prostate tumour growth and hormonal responsiveness. *Cancer Surv* 1991; **11**: 91–121.

142 Thompson TC, Chung LWK. Regulation of overgrowth and expression of prostatic binding protein in rat chimeric prostate gland. *Endocrinology* 1986; **118**: 2437–44.

143 Story MT, Livingston B, Baeten L *et al*. Cultured human prostate-derived fibroblasts produce a factor that stimulates their growth with properties indistinguishable from basic fibroblast growth factor. *Prostate* 1989; **15**: 355–65.

144 Kyprianou N, Isaacs JT. Identification of a cellular receptor for transforming growth factor-β in rat ventral prostate and its negative regulation by androgens. *Cancer Res* 1988; **123**: 2124–31.

145 Mydlo JH, Michaeli J, Heston WDW, Fair WR. Expression of basic fibroblast growth factor mRNA in benign prostatic hyperplasia and prostatic carcinoma. *Prostate* 1988; **13**: 241–7.

146 Thompson TC. Growth factors and oncogenes in prostate cancer. *Cancer Cells* 1990; **2**: 345–54.

147 Zhau HE, Wan D, Chung LWK *et al*. Expression of the HER-2/neu protooncogene in human prostate cancer. *J Urol* 1991; **145**: 348A (Abstract).

148 Cunha GR, Alarid ET, Turner T *et al*. Normal and abnormal development of the male urogenital tract: role of androgens, mesenchymal-epithelial interactions, and growth factors. *J Androl* 1992; **13**(6): 465–75.

149 McKeehan WL, Adams PS, Rosser MP. Direct mitogenic effects of insulin, epidermal growth factor, glucocorticoid, cholera toxin, unknown pituitary factors and possibly prolactin, but not androgen, on normal rat prostate tumor epithelial cells in serum-free primary cell culture. *Cancer Res* 1984; **44**: 1998–2010.

150 Ullrich A, Schlessinger J. Signal transduction by receptors with tyrosine kinase activity. *Cell* 1990; **61**: 203–12.

151 Fujita M, Spray DC, Choi H *et al*. Extracellular matrix regulation of cell-cell-communication and tissue-specific gene expression in primary liver culture. *Progr Clini Biol Res* 1991; **226**: 333–60.

152 Emerman JT, Enami J, Pitelka DR, Nandi S. Hormonal effects on intracellular and secreted casin in cultures of mouse mammary epithelial cells on floating collagen membranes. *Proc Natal Acad Sci USA* 1977; **74**: 4466–70.

153 Steiner MS. Role of peptide growth factors in the prostate: A review. *Urology* 1993; **42**(1): 99–110.

154 Massague J. Transforming growth factor-α. *J Biol Chem* 1990; **265**: 21393–6.

155 Gregory H, Wilshire IR, Kavanagh JP *et al*. Urogastrone – epidermal growth factor concentrations in prostatic fluid of normal individuals and patients with benign prostatic hypertrophy. *Clin Sci* 1986; **70**: 359–63.

156 Fowler JE Jr, Lau JLT, Ghosh L, Mills SE, Mounzer A. Epidermal growth factor and prostatic carcinoma: an immunohistochemical study. *J Urol* 1988; **139**: 857–61.

157 Lubrano C, Petrangeli E, Catizone A *et al*. Epidermal growth factor binding and steroid receptor content in human benign prostatic hyperplasia. *J Steroid Biochem* 1989; **34**: 499–504.

158 Hunter T. Protein-tyrosine phosphatases: the other side of the coin. *Cell* 1989; **58**: 1013–16.

159 Greenberg ME, Ziff EB. Stimulation of 3T3 cells induces transcription of the c-fos proto-oncogene. *Nature* 1984; **311**: 433.

160 Kelly K, Cochran BH, Stiles CD. Cell specific regulation of c-myc gene by lymphocyte mitogens and platelet-derived growth factor. *Cell* 1983; **35**: 603–10.

161 Fleming WH, Hamel A, MacDonald R *et al*. Expression of c-myc protooncogene in human prostatic carcinoma and benign prostatic hyperplasia. *Cancer Res* 1986; **46**: 1535–8.

162 Buttyan R, Sawczuk IS, Benson MC *et al*. Enhanced expression of c-myc protooncogene in high-grade human prostate cancers. *Prostate* 1987; **11**: 327–37.

163 Nag A, Smith RG. Amplification, rearrangement and elevated expression of c-myc in the human prostatic carcinoma cell line LNCaP. *Prostate* 1989; **15**: 115–22.

164 Miller DA, Pelton RW, Derynck R, Moses HL. Transforming growth factor beta. *Ann N Y Acad Sci* 1990; **593**: 208–17.

165 Nilsen-Hamilton M. Transforming growth factor-β and its actions on cellular growth and differentiation. *Curr Top Dev Biol* 1990; **24**: 95–136.

166 Story MT. Polypeptide modulators of prostatic growth and development. *Cancer Surv Prostate Cancer* 1991; **11**: 123–40.

167 Derynck R, Linquist PB, Lee A *et al*. A new type of transforming growth facto-beta, TGF-beta 3. *EMBO J* 1988; **7**(12): 3737–43.

168 Roberts AB, Sporn MB. Transforming growth factor beta. *Adv Cancer Res* 1988; **51**: 107–45.

169 Moses HL, Yang EY, Pietenpol JA. TGF-β stimulation and inhibition of cell proliferation: new mechanistic insights. *Cell* 1990; **63**: 245–7.

170 Gleave ME, Hsieh JT, Gao *et al*. Acceleration of human prostate cancer growth *in vivo* by factors produced by prostate and bone fibroblasts. *Cancer Res* 1991; **51**: 3753–61.

171 Katz AE, Benson MC, Wise GW *et al*. Gene activity during the early phase of androgen-stimulated rat prostate regrowth. *Cancer Res* 1989; **49**: 5889–94.

172 McKeehan WL, Adams PS. Heparin-binding growth factor/prostatropin attenuates inhibition of rat prostate tumor epithelial cell growth by transforming growth factor type beta. *In Vitro Cell Dev Biol Anim* 1988; **24**: 243–6.

173 Mansson PE, Adams P, McKeehan WL. Heparin-binding growth factor gene expression and receptor characteristics in normal rat prostate and two transplantable rat prostate tumors. *Cancer Res* 1989; **49**: 2485–94.

174 Gelmann EP. Oncogenes and growth factors in prostate cancer. *J NIH Res* 1991; **3**: 62–4.

175 Mori H, Maki M, Oishi K *et al*. Increased expression of genes for basic fibroblast growth factor and transforming growth factor type β-2 in human benign prostatic hyperplasia. *Prostate* 1990; **16**: 71–80.

176 Peehl DM, Stamey TA. Serum-free growth of adult human prostatic epithelial cells. *In Vitro Cell Dev Biol Anim* 1986; **22**: 82–90.

177 Matuo Y, McKeehan WL, Yan GC *et al*. Potential role of HBGF (FGF) and TGF-beta on prostate growth. In: Karr JP, Yamanaka H (eds) *Prostate Cancer and Bone Metastasis*. New York: Plenum Press: 1992; 107–114.

178 Baird A, Ling N. Fibroblast growth factors are present in the extracellular matrix produced by endothelial cells *in vitro*: implications for a role of heparinase-like enzymes in the neovascular response. *Biochem Biophys Res Commun* 1987; **142**: 429–35.

179 Baird A, Walicke PA. Fibroblast growth factors. *Br Med Bull* 1989; **45**(2): 438–52.

180 Czech M. Signal transmission by the insulin-like growth factors. *Cell* 1989; **59**: 235–8.

181 Chu *et al*. Enzyme markers in human prostatic carcinoma. *Cancer Treat Rep* 1977; **61**(2): 193–200.

182 Romas NA, Kwan DJ. Prostatic acid phosphatase; biomolecular features and assays for serum determination. *Urol Clin North Am* 1993; **20**(4): 581–8.

183 Lowe FC, Trauzzi SJ. Prostatic acid phosphatase in 1993; Its limited clinical utility. *Urol Clin North Am* 1993; **20**(4): 589–95.

184 Troyer JK, Beckett ML, Wright GL Jr. Detection and characterization of the prostate-specific membrane antigen (PSMA) in tissue extracts and body fluids. *Int J Cancer* 1995; **62**(5): 552–8.

185 Israeli RS, Powell CT, Fair WR, Heston WD. Molecular cloning of a complementary DNA encoding a prostate-specific membrane antigen. *Cancer Res* 1993; **53**(2): 227–30.

186 Horoszewicz JS, Kawinski E, Murphy GP. Monoclonal antibodies to a new antigenic marker in epithelial prostatic cells and serum of prostatic cancer patients. *Anticancer Res* 7(5B): 927–35.

187 Tsai GC, Stauch-Slusher B, Sim L *et al*. Reductions in acidic amino acids and N-acetylaspartylglutamate in amyotrophic lateral sclerosis CNS. *Brain Res*: 1991; **556**(1): 151–6.

188 Carter RE, Feldman AR, Coyle JT. Prostate-specific membrane antigen is a hydrolase with substrate and pharmacologic characteristics of a neuropeptidase. *Proc Natl Acad Sci USA* 1996; **93**(2): 749–53.

189 Mbikay M, Nolet S, Fournier S *et al*. Molecular cloning and sequence of the cDNA for a 94-amino-acid seminal plasma protein secreted by the human prostate. *DNA* 1987; **6**(1): 23–9.

190 Ulvsback M, Lindstrom C, Weiber H *et al*. Molecular cloning of a small prostate protein, known as beta-microsemenoprotein, PSP94 or beta-inhibin, and demonstration of transcripts in non-genital tissues. *Biochem Biophys Res Commun* 1989; **164**(3): 1310–5.

191 Lin MF, Clinton GM. Human prostatic acid phosphatase has phosphotyrosyl protein phosphatase activity. *Biochem J* 1986; **235**(2): 351–7.

192 Vafa AZ, Grover PK, Pretlow TG, Resnick MI. Study of activities of arginase, hexosaminidase, and leucine aminopeptidase in prostate fluid. *Urology* 1993; **42**(2): 138–43.

193 Mattila S. Further studies on the prostatic tissue antigens. Separation of two molecular forms of aminopeptidase. *Invest Urol* 1969; **7**(1): 1–9.

194 Niemi M, Harkonen M, Larmi TKL. Enzymic histochemistry of human prostate. *Arch Pathol* 1963; **75**: 528–37.

195 Kirchheim D, Gyorkey F, Brandes D, Scott WW. Histochemistry of the normal hyperplastic and neoplastic human prostate gland. *Invest Urol* 1964; **1**: 403–21.

196 Rackley RR, Yang B, Pretlow TG *et al*. Differences in the leucine aminopeptidase activity in extracts from human prostatic carcinoma and benign prostatic hyperplasia. *Cancer* 1991; **68**(3): 587–93.

197 Oliver JA, el-Hilali MM, Belitsky P, MacKinnon KJ. LDH isoenzymes in benign and malignant prostate tissue; the LDH V–I ratio as an index of malignancy. *Cancer* 1970; **25**(4): 863–6.

198 Grayhack JT, Wendel EF, Lee C *et al*. Lactate dehydrogenase isoenzymes in human prostatic fluid: an aid in recognition of malignancy? *J Urol* 1977; **118**(1 Pt 2): 204–8.

199 Denis L, Prout GR. Alterations in the isozymes of lactate dehydrogenase in canine prostate after androgenic stimulation. *Surgical Forum* 1962; **13**: 515–16.

200 Eihilali MM, Oliver JA, Sherwin AL, Mackinnon KJ. Lactate dehydrogenase isoenzymes in hyperplasia and carcinoma of the prostate: a clinical study. *J Urol* 1967; **98**(6): 686–92.

201 Flocks RH, Schmidt JD. Lactate dehydrogenase isoenzyme patterns of prostatic cancer and hyperplasia. *J Surg Oncol* 1972; **4**(2): 161–7.

202 Fair WR, Couch J, Wehner N. Prostatic antibacterial factor. Identity and significance. *Urol* 1976; **7**: 169–77.

203 Gahankari DR, Golhar KB. An evaluation of serum and tissue bound immunoglobulins in prostatic diseases. *J Postgrad Med* 1993; **39**(2): 63–7.

204 Friberg J, Tilly-Friberg I. Spontaneous spermagglutination in ejaculates from men with head-to-head or tail-to-tail spermagglutinating antibodies in serum. *Fertil Steril* 1977; **28**(6): 658–62.

205 Grayhack JT, Wendel EF, Oliver L, Lee C. Analysis of specific proteins in prostatic fluid for detecting prostatic malignancy. *J Urol* 1979; **121**(3): 295–9.

206 Fowler JE Jr, Mariano M. Immunologic response of the prostate to bacteriuria and bacterial prostatitis. II; Antigen specific immunoglobulin in prostatic fluid. *J Urol* 1982; **128**(1): 165–70.

207 Blenk H, Hofstetter A. Complement C3, coeruloplasmin and PMN-elastase in the ejaculate in chronic prostato-adnexitis and their diagnostic value. *Infection* 1991; **19**(Suppl 3): S138–40.

208 Grayhack JT, Lee C. Evaluation of prostatic fluid in prostatic pathology. *Prog Clin Biol Res* 1981; **75A**: 231–46.

209 Kyprianou N, Tu H, Jacobs SC. Apoptotic versus proliferative activities in human benign prostatic hyperplasia. *J Urol* 1994; **152**(6 Pt 1): 2120–4. *Hum Pathol* 1996; **27**(7): 668–675.

Epidemiology, Natural History, and Pathogenesis of Benign Prostatic Hyperplasia 2

P. Narayan, A. Tewari, and R. Makkenchery

INTRODUCTION

Benign prostatic hyperplasia (BPH) is one of the commonest neoplasms affecting men over 50 years of age. If untreated, it can result in acute urinary retention, infection, stones, and upper tract deterioration. Even though several associations and trends have been observed, the etiology, natural history, and pathophysiology of this disease are far from clear.

Natural history is variable and can range from a plateau and, at times, improvement in symptoms to ongoing progression and requirement of treatment. The lack of correlation between histologic BPH, clinical symptoms, and physical obstruction has been a major cause of ambiguity in the understanding of this disease. The understanding of natural history helps in management decisions and evaluation of response to various treatment modalities.

FACTORS AFFECTING INCIDENCE OF BENIGN PROSTATIC HYPERPLASIA

AGE

BPH is a disease of aging and Glynn et al.[1] have determined that the relative risk for developing clinical BPH or requiring surgical intervention for BPH almost doubles for each decade of life between the ages of 40 and 90 years. Sidney et al.[2] reported a similar relative risk for surgery. In men 30–50 years old, estimated doubling time is 4–5 years, while between 50 and 70 years of age it is 10 years. The mean prostatic size between age 40 and 79 years is 26.6 cm[3] with a 75th percentile of 35 cm.[3] Data suggest that there is a considerable proportion of undetected BPH in the general population.[3] Autopsy data in general yield higher age-specific prevalence figures than clinical series. Age per se has never been shown to be a direct causal agent of BPH.[4] However, the growth of BPH with age is attributed to synergistic interplay between androgenic and estrogenic stimulation, which creates permissive conditions for development of BPH. Recently, it has been suggested that with age there is a removal of a "brake", resulting in embryonic reawakening or a primary alteration in the regulation of stem cells in the prostate.[5]

FAMILY HISTORY

There is some suggestion that familial and genetic factors may play a role in the genesis of BPH.[6] Roberts et al.[7] studied a group of 2119 randomly selected men aged 40–79 years from Olmsted County, MN. In their study, the objective was to estimate the association between family history of BPH and prevalent signs and symptoms suggestive of BPH by using urinary symptom scores and peak urinary flow rates. These patients were administered a questionnaire that included questions with wording close to that of the American Urological Association Symptom Index (AUASI). Through a personal interview, a detailed family history of an enlarged prostate gland was obtained, and through a physical exam and uroflow assessment, peak urinary flow rates were measured for each participant. Twenty-one percent (440/2119) of the men reported a family history of an enlarged prostate gland. The age-adjusted odds of having moderate or severe urinary symptoms were elevated among those with a family history relative to those without (odds ratio=1.3). This suggests that the risk of having moderate-to-severe urinary symptoms (or impaired urinary peak flow rates) relative to mild-to-none was about 1.3 times in men with a family history compared with men without a family history. Furthermore, this association was stronger in men whose affected relative was younger than age 60 years at diagnosis, and strongest in men who had an affected brother as opposed to men with only an affected father. These findings suggest that, among men with a family history of an enlarged prostate gland, there may be an increased risk for development of symptoms and signs suggestive of BPH. In addition, this risk appears to be greater in men with relatives diagnosed at a younger age. Recognition of this association may help to target early interventions and may lead to further clues about the causes of BPH.

In order to clarify the role of genetic factors in BPH, Sanda and associates[8] performed a case-control study of men with early onset of symptomatic BPH. Men aged 64 years with large prostates (greater than 37 g resected tissue) who underwent surgery for BPH were identified as case probands from 909 consecutive prostatectomies for BPH. Control probands were selected because of the ability to distinguish treatment for benign prostate disease from treatment for malignant prostate disease and were women whose spouses underwent radical prostatectomy during the same interval.[8] Kaplan–Meier estimates of cumulative risk for BPH requiring surgery demonstrated that first-degree male relatives with early onset of BPH had a higher likelihood of undergoing prostatectomy for BPH than did control relatives. The cumulative lifetime risk for controls was 17%, while the lifetime risk of prostatectomy for BPH was 66% for first degree male relatives of case probands ($P=0.001$). Odds-ratio analysis showed that those first-degree male relatives of case probands had a fourfold greater risk of prostatectomy for BPH compared with first-degree male relatives of controls. Furthermore, the increase in age-adjusted relative risk was also noted when brothers and fathers were analyzed separately; brothers of patients with BPH had a sixfold increased risk of BPH requiring surgery ($P=0.0089$), while fathers showed a fourfold increased risk ($P=0.0003$). In the second part of this study, to determine the likelihood that genetic factors account for this familial aggregation of BPH, segregation analysis was done. Direct comparison of mendelian and non-genetic models showed that mendelian autosomal dominant transmission provided the best overall explanation of the observed familial aggregation. The autosomal dominant model suggested that a gene found in 7% of men in the study population carried 89% lifetime penetrance, and cumulative distribution analysis suggested that 9% of men undergoing surgery for BPH had an hereditary form of the disease.[8] Autosomal dominant inheritance raises provoking issues regarding the genes involved in the pathogenesis of BPH. This warrants the need for further investigation through DNA studies with or without linkage analysis.

Partin and associates[9] studied concordance rates of BPH. Concordance rates for benign prostatic disease among twins suggested hereditary influence among monozygotic (MZ) and dizygotic (DZ) twins who served in the US military in World War II and were followed by the Medical Follow-up Agency (of the Institute of Medicine of the National Academy of Science Research Council Twins Registry).[9] In 1985, questionnaires regarding BPH were sent to 15,948 twin pairs who had both served in the military, and 10,000 twins completed the questionnaire and subsequently were reviewed for evidence of prostatic disease. Five hundred and thirty-three (5.3%) of the questionnaires were identified as having had some form of prostatic disease. The average age of this group was 64 years (in 1985). After eliminating 39 men with known prostate cancer, there were 256 twin pairs that were informative for benign prostatic disease: both twins were concordant in 25 instances and discordant in 231, with only one twin mentioning benign prostatic disease. The pairwise concordance for MZ twins was 14.7% (19/129), and for DZ twins it was 4.5% (5/112). The relative risk for BPH for MZ twins was 3.3 ($P=0.008$). The proband-wise concordance rates, expressing the probability of BPH in a co-twin of an affected twin, were 25.7% for MZ twins and only 8.5% for DZ twins. Furthermore, a covariance analysis determined that approximately 49% of the observed variance between twins could be attributed to genetic factors, while 51% could be attributed to environmental influences. In summary, the results from this study show that the concordance rate for BPH is greater among MZ twins (who are genetically identical) when compared with DZ twins (who are (genetically) no more similar than other brothers and sisters), thus providing further evidence for the heritability of BPH.

Recently, Sanda and associates,[10] in an attempt to determine the clinical and biological characteristics of familial BPH, analyzed the relationship of family history of BPH to prostate size, urinary peak flow rates, symptom scores, circulating androgen levels, and PSA levels. Furthermore, the response of these variables to finasteride (in patients participating in a nationwide Merck Phase III finasteride clinical trial) were also analyzed. Sixty-nine men who were characterized as having familial BPH (as defined by having three or more family members with BPH, including the proband) were compared with those men (345) with no family history of BPH. Logistic regression analysis and multivariate regression were performed to evaluate the relationship of familial BPH and baseline parameters as well as response of these aforementioned parameters to the administration of 12 months of finasteride or placebo. Analysis of baseline parameters showed that familial BPH is associated with large prostate size. On the average, patients with familial BPH had prostate glands that were 50% larger than those with no family history of BPH. Mean prostate volume in men with familial and sporadic BPH was 82.7 and 55.5 mL, respectively ($P<0.001$). Stratification of patients according to prostate size demonstrated a progressive increase in the prevalence of familial BPH with prostate size greater than 50 ml. Familial BPH prevalence was greatest in men with prostate size greater than 106 mL (46%) compared with only 13% of the men with prostates smaller than 28 mL. Multivariate analysis was then done to confirm the association of prostate size and familial BPH. The analysis showed that PSA correlated with prostate size, and further suggested that familial BPH was more indicative of prostate size than PSA levels. No significant difference in responses to 5α-reductase blockade was noted in patients with sporadic or familial BPH, suggesting that familial BPH is not associated with abnormalities of dihydrotestosterone (DHT) metabolism. To conclude, this study demonstrated that familial BPH is characterized by large prostate size; almost 50% of the men with prostate size in the largest 10% of prostate size (>106 mL) had familial BPH with three or more family members affected. These findings suggest that hereditary factors responsible for familial BPH control prostatic growth, possibly through a genetic factor influencing androgen-independent control of prostatic growth.

This same group of investigators have also studied and characterized the histopathologic features of BPH in familial or genetically predisposed patients.[11] The prostate glands from 12 men previously determined to have hereditary BPH were obtained, and compared with 35 age-matched control prostate glands and 36 weight-matched control prostate glands. Via the use of a color video image analysis system, the researchers determined the stromal/epithelial ratios in several histologic sections taken of 12 prostates from men with hereditary BPH to 35 age-matched prostate glands, and 36 weight-matched prostate glands. The stromal/epithelial ratio was 2.6 in the men with hereditary BPH, 2.7 in age-matched control subjects, and 1.7 in weight-matched control subjects. Through the use of regression analysis (which took into account the differences in prostate weight or patient age between men with hereditary BPH and age-matched and weight-matched control subjects, respectively) significant differences between men with hereditary BPH and the weight-matched control subjects ($P=0.015$) were revealed. However, there was no difference between the hereditary BPH and the age-matched control subjects ($P=0.36$). From these findings, it is suggested that hereditary BPH may be more of a stromal disease than sporadic BPH; this finding gives rise to speculation that hereditary BPH is associated with an increase in stromal elements.

GEOGRAPHIC FACTORS

Over the past decade, evidence has begun to accumulate suggesting that racial and geographical variations in the incidence, prevalence, and mortality from BPH may not be marked as was thought historically. Much of the early evidence comes from anecdotal studies.[12-14] These studies suggested that BPH was most common in blacks, followed by whites, and is least common in orientals. However, methodological problems in the studies, such as lack of standardized diagnostic criteria, differences in case-ascertainment, and differences in the access, use, and quality of medical care confound these early impressions.[15] Race has not been found to be predictive for undergoing prostatic surgery for BPH in a large cohort of members of a prepaid health care plan in which there was equal access to medical care.[16] Several other analytical studies have confirmed that there is no statistically significant difference in the age-adjusted proportions of blacks and whites undergoing prostatectomies for BPH.[17,18] The preliminary results, however, from a study being conducted in Japan suggest that the prevalence of BPH may be lower in Japanese than in whites when the same definition of BPH is used.[19] A recent large cohort study by Chyou et al. among the Japanese-Americans in Hawaii suggests a 20% increase in risk for undergoing prostatectomy for BPH among men born in rural compared with urban areas.[20] The elevated risk just attained statistical significance. Armenian et al.[21] also reported a higher proportion of men with BPH living in smaller towns than the control group, but this difference was not statistically significant. The currently available age-specific mortality data for BPH from individual countries is of limited use for comparative purposes. This is because differences in recording and reporting practices may have a greater influence on the documented mortality rates than the actual occurrence of BPH.[22] At present, countries such as Singapore, Japan, and the USA have the lowest rates, while Norway and some Eastern European countries rank among the highest. The lack of quality in the mortality data is also highlighted by the fact that the age-specific autopsy prevalence is similar in many developing and developed countries.[23]

Tsukamoto and associates[24] studied the prevalence of prostatism in Japan. A total of 289 men (ranging in age from 40 to 79 years) completed a questionnaire similar to that of the international prostate symptom score and of the Olmsted County study questionnaire. (The protocol of this study was similar to the one used in the Olmsted County study to allow for comparability of the results between Japanese and American men.) A relatively high percentage of Japanese men in each age decade (40–49, 50–59, 60–69, and 70–79) reported frequency of symptoms; there was an increase with age for weak stream, nocturia, and urgency, but not for the other symptoms (such as dribbling, pain/burning, stopping and starting, straining, fullness feeling, frequency). The mean International Prostate Symptom Score (IPSS) increased with increasing age for Japanese men and similarly increased with age for American men, although the mean scores were nearly 3 points higher for the Japanese (8.0) than for the American men (5.0) in the Olmsted study. The incidence of men with moderate-to-severe symptoms was only 36.6% for Japanese men and 25.5% for American men after adjustment for non-response, but it still showed an increased trend with increasing age decade in Japanese men (41% in 40–49 years, 29% in 50–59 years, 31% in 60–69 years, and 56% in 70–79 years of age). This study revealed that lower urinary tract symptoms were common in Japanese men, with age-related increases similar to those of US men.

In a study from the UK, Jolleys and associates[25] reported the incidence of urinary symptoms associated with BPH (as defined by a Maine score of ≥ 11, a peak urinary flow rate of <15 mL s^{-1}, and failure to void ≥ 150 mL on three separate occasions) among men older than 40 years of age. According to these criteria, the prevalence of symptomatic BPH was 284/1000 for men greater than 40 years of age. When stratifying the data into age decade groups, the prevalence increased from 179/1000 in men of 40–49 years of age to 500/1000 in men of age 70 years or greater. Of the symptoms reported, terminal dribble, hesitancy, intermittency, and urgency were the most common. The symptoms that caused men the greatest degree of bother were frequency, nocturia, and those causing incontinence or social embarrassment.

In a Canadian study reported by Norman and associates,[26] a total of 508 men were enrolled to determine the prevalence of BPH. According to the age-group stratified data, 44% of the men were of age 50–59 years, 33% were 60–69 years, and 27% were 70 years or greater. After the data were adjusted for age differences, the most prevalent symptoms were nocturia (63%), weak stream (61%), and urinary frequency (46%). Urgency was reported by 18%, a sense of incomplete bladder emptying by 23%, intermittency by 18%, and hesitancy by 13%. The prevalence of men with a reduction in urine flow increased with age ($P<0.01$). In addition, the percentage of men who experienced nocturia, urgency, incomplete emptying, hesitancy, and intermittency increased with age, but not to a statistically significant degree. The severity of urinary frequency, incomplete emptying, and reduction in urinary flow rate increased with increasing age in a statistically significant manner ($P<0.05$, $P<0.05$, and $P<0.01$, respectively). Using predefined cut-off scores, 23% of the respondents experienced moderate-to-severe BPH symptoms, and this prevalence increased with age. Fifteen percent of men aged 50–59 years, 27% of men aged 60–69 years, and 31% of men 70 years and older had symptoms of BPH; the difference in prevalence between the age groups was statistically significant (50–59 ages vs. 60–69 ages, $P<0.05$). The clusters were grouped on the basis of the symptoms driving them, with one cluster designated as "moderates", two clusters designated as "irritatives" and two designated as "obstructives". The moderates cluster was driven by respondents who had lower symptom scores evenly distributed across all symptoms. The irritative and obstructive clusters were driven by respondents with higher scores for symptoms considered by convention to be irritative or obstructive in nature and, thus, were designated accordingly. Not all symptoms were discriminatory for irritative and obstructive symptom domains.[26]

In a recent study from Finland, 3143 men were enrolled to determine the prevalence of lower urinary tract symptoms due to BPH.[27] Among all responders, 89% reported at least one symptom, with postvoid dribbling and nocturia being the most prevalent symptoms. Furthermore, the proportion of men reporting symptoms increased with age: 84% among 50-year-old, 91% among 60-year-old and 94% among 70-year-old men. The prevalence of bothersome symptoms also increased with age.

The histological differences in the prostate glands from Chinese men in comparison with American men have been reported by Lepor and associates.[28] Surgical specimens of the prostate were obtained from 9 Chinese and 8 Caucasian-American men undergoing cystoprostatectomy for invasive transitional cell carcinoma. The mean ages of the Caucasian-American and Chinese men were 66.4 years and 66.8 years, respectively ($P=0.94$). The mean prostate weight of the Caucasian-American and Chinese men was 32.1 g and 53.4 g, respectively ($P=0.001$). Via the use of double-immunoenzymatic staining and computer-assisted color image analysis, the percent area density of smooth muscle (SM), connective tissue (CT), epithelium (E), and epithelial lumen (L) were determined from the transition zone of the prostate glands. The mean stromal:epithelial ratios of the prostates from Chinese and Caucasian-American men were 3.8 and 6.3, respectively. The mean percent area density of SM, CT, E, and L in the prostate of Chinese men was 32%, 9.1%, 10.8%, and 48.5%, respectively. The mean percent area density of SM, CT, E, and L in the prostate of Caucasian-American men was 52.5%, 27.9%, 12.8%, and 7%, respectively. The prostates of Caucasian-American men contained a significantly greater area density of smooth muscle and connective tissue, whereas that of Chinese men contained a significantly greater volume of epithelial lumen. This study demonstrated that the cellular composition of BPH in the prostates of Caucasian-American and Chinese men was different; and possibly, these cellular differences may account for the observed lower incidence of clinical BPH in Chinese men in comparison with American men.

INCOME

Two analytical studies suggest that men of higher socioeconomic status are significantly less likely to undergo prostatic surgery for BPH.[1,18] Chyou et al.[20] observed a small and non-significant association in the same direction. Educational level was used as a proxy for social status in the studies by Morrison[18] and Chyou et al.[20] Earlier studies report trends in the opposite direction for both surgical management and mortality from BPH.[21,29] Glynn et al.[1] reported no significant association between social class and the development of clinical BPH.

TESTICULAR FUNCTION

Androgens are essential to the pathogenesis of BPH, and it is the testis, under the influence of the pituitary gland, which is responsible for production of most of the testosterone. Castration or hypopituitarism prior to puberty appears to prevent the development of microscopic BPH, and before the age of 40 years prevents the development of clinical BPH.[5,30,31] Furthermore, enlarged prostates can regress following orchidectomy or anti-androgen therapy.[32,33] Additionally, patients with larger prostatic volumes have been found to have higher free testosterone and estrogen levels.[34] These findings suggest that BPH is under endocrine control. Changes in the hormonal milieu at the prostatic level are probably more important in the initiation and maintenance of BPH than the serum concentrations of the sex hormones in the peripheral circulation.[35] Whether the hormonal effect is active or merely permissive is undetermined.[5] It is interesting to note that symptomatic enlargement of the prostate occurs when testicular function is declining, resulting in a decrease in testosterone production, and when estrogen production is increasing. A synergistic relationship has been demonstrated in beagles, but the evidence in humans is less clear.[5,36]

Gann and associates[37] reported on a prospective study of participants in the Physicians' Health Study to determine the role that plasma hormones and other non-hormonal factors play in the development of BPH and with subsequent occurrence of surgical treatment for BPH. The Physicians' Health Study enrolled a total of 22,071 male physicians in 1982. After strict exclusion criteria, frozen plasma samples, collected at the onset of the study, were available for 320 men who developed BPH 9 years (or more) later, and to establish a control group, 320 age-matched blood samples were also taken. The blood samples were used to measure the plasma testosterone (T), dihydrotestosterone (DHT), androstenedione, estradiol (E2), and estrone (E1) levels. The age-matched odds ratio for BPH by quintile of individual plasma hormones and hormone ratio did not reveal any clear relationships between hormone levels and BPH. The DHT/testosterone ratio, which is considered an index of the efficiency of testosterone conversion to DHT, was also not materially related to BPH. Furthermore, odds ratios for non-hormonal factors such as blood pressure, body mass, smoking, exercise, and alcohol intake did show some strong age-adjusted correlations. Diastolic blood pressure, exercise, and alcohol intake showed a strong age-adjusted association with BPH. Systolic and diastolic blood pressure were positively associated with BPH, and diastolic pressure was more strongly related in the risk factor adjusted analysis. Body mass was not significantly related to BPH.

Smoking status and a history of diabetes were also not associated with BPH. Men who exercised most frequently were at higher risk compared with those who were sedentary, but there was an inconsistent pattern. When using multivariate analysis using a model simultaneously adjusted for exercise, alcohol intake, diastolic blood pressure, and estradiol, estrone, and DHT/testosterone ratio, the results for hormones were very different following adjustment for the non-hormonal factors. The estradiol level had a strong positive association with BPH ($P = 0.009$) in men with lower levels of plasma testosterone. The estradiol association emerged incrementally with adjustment for each extraneous factor and therefore was not due predominantly to adjustment for any single factor. Similar results were obtained for estradiol when androstenedione, testosterone, or DHT were included in the model individually. Estrone level displayed a weak, inverse relationship with BPH. The findings of this study indicate the circulating androgen levels are not associated with risk of BPH, but estradiol is related only in men with low circulating androgen levels.

OBESITY

Glynn et al.[1] reported an 18% reduction in risk for clinically developing BPH for each 5 kg m^{-2} increase in body mass index. This may in part be due to a detection bias, as it may be an easier diagnosis to make in less obese men. A graded decreasing relative risk, however, has also been observed with increasing obesity by Sidney et al.[2] for surgical intervention for BPH. Individuals in the highest quartile for body mass index had a 29% lower chance of surgery than individuals in the lowest quartile. Daniell,[38] on the other hand, reported that the more obese men in his case-control study had significantly larger prostatic volumes than leaner men, but were no more likely to undergo prostatectomy. It is biologically plausible that body mass index is related to the development of BPH, as adipose tissue is one of the main sites in which androgens are converted into estrogens. Furthermore, it has been shown that lean men have higher total plasma testosterone levels.[39]

Kupeli and associates[40] studied 68 men with BPH, to evaluate the association between obesity and prostatic enlargement, as well as changes in serum levels of estradiol, testosterone, dihydroepiandrosterone, and dihydroepiandrosterone sulfate. In spite of larger prostatic glands, no increase in the symptom score for BPH was observed with increasing obesity. However, the average weight of the prostate gland increased with increasing body weight, and increasing age from 46 to 80 g. They also found that the serum estradiol level was significantly elevated in obese men (51.3 pg mL^{-1}) who were 140% or over their recommended weight in comparison with underweight men (26.8 pg mL^{-1}); this was a statistically significant difference ($P<0.01$). This pattern was present in all age groups. From these findings, it was concluded that obesity is a risk factor for prostatic enlargement, but not for obstruction. In addition, the degree of obesity appeared to have a direct effect on estradiol levels, possibly from the effect of adipose tissue on the transformation of androgens to estrogens.

HYPERTENSION

Two recent cohort studies have found no significant relationship between hypertension and the development of BPH.[1,2] Two earlier case-control studies similarly found no association.[41] A relationship was first suggested by Bourke and Griffin[42] because they noted that men being admitted for elective prostatectomies had higher blood pressures than a control group of men who were being admitted for elective non-genitourinary surgery. However, it is now appreciated that BPH can cause high pressure chronic retention of urine, which may in turn cause hypertension.[43]

DIABETES MELLITUS

An association between diabetes and BPH was first postulated by Bourke and Griffin[42] in 1966. Glynn et al.[1] failed to substantiate this when they looked at fasting and 2-h blood glucose levels and the subsequent development of BPH in their cohort study. Interestingly, Sidney et al.[2] found a negative association between the highest quartile of blood glucose 1 h after the administration of an oral glucose load in their cohort study. Guess[15] attributed the higher prevalence of diabetes mellitus in the surgical series of Bourke and Griffin to detection bias.

LIVER CIRRHOSIS

Case-control studies using autopsy series have been used to investigate the relationship between liver cirrhosis and BPH. Only two of the studies have shown a small reduction in risk with cirrhosis.[44] Care with interpretation is required because of possible confounding factors.[4] An association between liver cirrhosis and BPH is biologically plausible because men with cirrhosis produce less testosterone and have lower testosterone and DHT levels.[45] Frea and associates[44] conducted a post-mortem study evaluating the prostates of 51 men who died with liver cirrhosis compared with a similar group without any hepatic disease. The data collected were categorized into three different age groups, namely 40–59, 60–69, and 70–80 years old. From histological examination, it was determined that the occurrence of BPH in cirrhotic subjects was diminished and delayed compared with the total population. The incidence of BPH is more frequent in the control group (patients without any liver disease) than in the group with liver cirrhosis; this difference in BPH incidence was especially evident in the age group 60–69, where 76.4% from the control group and 41.2% from the cirrhotic group had BPH. Upon microscopic examination, it was found that, in cirrhotic men, the appearance of BPH was delayed in comparison with the general population. Furthermore, in cirrhotic males, the hyperplastic prostate showed more stromal proliferation when compared with the histological sections of hyperplastic prostates from non-cirrhotic males.

VASECTOMY

Two studies reported the relationship between vasectomy status and the development of BPH.[1,46] Neither study found a significant relationship, but Jakobsen et al.[46] did find a higher prevalence of adenomatous prostates among their vasectomized men. Animal experiments have suggested that vasectomy causes a direct change in hormonal status, possibly mediated via the vas deferens, but human evidence is still lacking.[47,48] Jakobsen and associates conducted a study to determine the long-term influence of vasectomy on prostatic volume and morphology by comparing 56 men with vasectomies (done 8 years previously) to 56 age-matched control patients.[46] In the vasectomy group, 19.6% had ultrasonic signs of developing adenomas, while 30.3% of the control group showed developing adenomas. This difference was not statistically significant. Through the use of transurethral ultrasonography (TRUS), only one significant finding was observed. In vasectomized men with normal prostatic echopattern, the relative volume of the periurethral glands was found to be significantly larger than the corresponding value in the controls. The total prostatic volume, the volume of the periurethral gland, and the volume of the peripheral zone were not influenced by the vasectomy; nor was the growth rate of these zones affected.

SEXUAL ACTIVITY

In 1923, Gover first reported sexual activity as a possible etiological factor for the development of BPH, using marital status as a surrogate measure. Lytton et al.[17] and Glynn et al.,[1] however, found no association. More recently, Morrison reported a significant 49% reduction in the risk of surgery for BPH in widowed men compared with single men. Lower risks were also reported for married men and divorced and separated men, but they were not significant. Ekman postulates that the increase in the fibromuscular component of BPH may be the result of sexual activity.[18,49] However, as sexual activity declines with advancing age, a direct association between sexual activity and BPH is not immediately obvious. Further work is clearly required to increase the understanding in this area.

SMOKING

In the majority of studies there did not appear to be any evidence between intensity of smoking and the risk of BPH.[18] A cohort study by Seitter and Barrett-Connor[50] failed, however, to find a relationship between smoking status, the number of cigarettes smoked, and the number of years of smoking, with the risk for undergoing prostatectomy for BPH. It should be noted that any possible confounding effect of surgery not being performed because of the presence of a smoking-related disease is likely to be small, as medical ineligibility is not common.[18] Glynn et al.[1] found no association between smoking and the development of clinical BPH.

The case-control studies by Armenian et al.[21] and Araki et al.[29] similarly failed to demonstrate an association. Eldrup et al.[39] has shown no effect on testosterone levels by smoking status whilst Briggs[51] and Shaarawy and Mahmoud[52] reported higher levels of testosterone in non-smokers. Smoking also has an effect on estrogen production and metabolism, but as for the androgens, the findings are quite variable, and a firm conclusion cannot be drawn.[53] Additionally, the validity of

some of the studies is questionable because confounding variables were not always taken into account. At present, no conclusions can be drawn about the effect of smoking on the development of BPH.

ALCOHOL

Chyou et al.[20] reported a significant 36% reduction in the risk of prostatectomy for BPH in men who drink 25 oz or more of alcohol per month compared with non-drinkers. Morrison[18] noted a protective effect of one to three units of alcohol per day in his case-control study. Araki et al.[29] and Glynn et al.[1] failed to show any association. Anecdotal evidence exists; however, those men with symptomatic BPH may reduce their alcohol intake. Alcohol has been shown to reduce serum testosterone levels in men by reducing testosterone production rates and increasing its metabolic clearance, thereby giving biological plausibility to its possible protective effect.[54,55]

DIET

High-fat diets cause an increase in prolactin secretion, and prolactin has been shown directly to influence prostatic epithelial cell proliferation and may influence testosterone uptake.[56,57] A high soy and fiber content to the diet increases weak serum estrogenic compounds. Chyou et al.[20] looked at 33 dietary items in relation to undergoing prostatectomy for BPH. Only one dietary item, beef intake, attained significance, and this was just under the 5% level. Araki et al.[29] studied Japanese men, but used a clinical definition of BPH. This study reported an elevated risk for men who consume milk regularly, do not eat pickles at every meal, and who eat green and yellow vegetables irregularly. Several studies have reported no significant association between caffeine consumption and BPH.[1,18,29] There is no need for further investigation of dietary factors in the etiology of BPH.

OTHERS

There have been several other etiologic associations between BPH and wide variety of causative factors, including infection and immunological mechanisms. Zisman and associates[58] examined the possibility that BPH is an autoimmune disease by measuring titers of IgG antibodies toward PSA epitope (IgG anti-PSA antibodies). A total of 85 patients with BPH, 17 patients with chronic prostatitis, and 20 age-matched men with normal prostate glands (the control group) were enrolled in this study. Through the use of enzyme-linked immunosorbent assay, the mean titers of IgG anti-PSA antibodies in the BPH patients, chronic prostatitis patients, and the control group were 0.56, 0.23, and 0.17, respectively (for the BPH group vs. chronic prostatitis group, and the BPH group vs. the control group, $P<0.0005$). Furthermore, patients were categorized as responders to PSA when the antibody titers were equal to or greater than the mean ± 2 SD of the values of the control group. According to this definition, 59% of the patients with BPH responded to PSA by production of IgG antibodies compared with none in the control group ($P<0.0005$). This observation suggests that an autoimmune process might play a role in the pathogenesis of BPH. However, this hypothesis needs further validation in larger studies.

NATURAL HISTORY

Most of the relatively sparse evidence on the natural history of BPH comes from cohort studies of men presenting to urologists or primary care physicians. Studies of BPH defined at presentation to a physician probably miss a preclinical in the natural history of the condition but can provide valuable information. Symptoms of BPH are the most common reason for morbidity and the need for treatment. Approximately 30% of prostatectomies are performed solely for the relief of symptoms, and symptom relief is at least one of the indications for surgery in over 90% of operations. Patients considering treatment may want to know whether their symptoms will become worse, stay the same, or improve over time.

Girman and associates[59] studied the relationships among symptoms, prostate volume, and peak urinary flow rates in an age-stratified, community-based random sample of men with BPH. There were a total of 2115 men enrolled in this study who underwent TRUS for prostatic volume assessment and uroflow for peak urinary flow rates. Overall, the mean AUA symptom score was 6.0 with the mean prostatic volume of 26.4 mL, and a peak flow rate of 17.4 mL s^{-1}. Through the use of scatter graphs demonstrating the pairwise relationships, the correlation between prostate volume and AUA symptom score was similar in magnitude to the inverse relationship between prostate volume and peak urinary flow rates. All the pairwise correlations were statistically significant ($P<0.001$). The odds of moderate-to-severe symptoms increased with age from 1.9, 2.9, and 3.4 for men in the age groups 50–59, 60–69, and 70–79 years, respectively. Adjusting for age, the odds of moderate-to-severe symptoms were 3.5 times greater for men with prostatic enlargement (>50 mL) than for men with smaller prostates, while the odds were similarly increased (2.4-fold) for men not achieving a peak urinary flow rate of 10 mL s^{-1}. These results, based on randomly selected white men, suggest that a strong relationship exists among symptoms, prostate size, and urinary flow rate. The strength of these relationships is comparable with that found with other diseases.

Girman and associates[60] also conducted a study to assess the impact of urinary symptoms on health-related quality of life, which includes degree of bother, worry, interference with daily activities, psychological well-being, sexual function, and general health. This study enrolled 2115 men with BPH, and requested them to complete a questionnaire and to have an assessment of their prostatic volume and peak urinary flow rates. On the average, urinary symptoms and associated bother increased with age. Interference of urinary symptoms with daily activities and degree of worry and concern also increased with age. Sexual satisfaction, worry about sexual function, and general self-reported health ratings worsened with age. Only 8% of the men reported having none of the seven symptoms that make up the AUA

symptom score index, while 58% reported mild symptoms (AUASI=1–7) and 33% reported moderate-to-severe symptoms (AUASI=8–35). Men with moderate-to-severe voiding symptoms reported four to six times the degree of bother and interference with daily activities and twice the level of worry of men experiencing mild symptoms. Nearly five times the degree of bother and interference was reported in men with mild symptoms compared to those with no symptoms. A higher percentage of men with moderate to severe symptoms (26–33%) than mild symptoms (<8%) reported limiting fluids before going to bed, traveling for prolonged hours, or driving for 2 h. Receiver operating characteristic curves support the recommended symptom index cutpoint for moderate symptoms (=8) by differentiating men with and without bother, interference with daily living, or dissatisfaction with urinary condition. This study reveals that moderate-to-severe urinary symptoms have had a significant impact on men's lives in terms of their degree of bother, worry, interference with daily living, and psychological well-being.

Jakobsen and associates[46] reported the results of three contacts during the 42-month, Olmsted County Study of Urinary Symptoms and Health Status among Men. This study was designed as a longitudinal cohort study of men 40–79 years old, initiated in 1990 to describe changes in lower urinary tract symptom severity. Of the 2115 men enrolled in this study, there was an average increase in the AUA symptom score of approximately 0.18 points per year of follow-up. The average annual symptom score slope and variability in the slope increased with patient age, starting at a baseline of 0.05 per year in men aged 40–49 to 0.44 per year for men aged 60–69, and this rise decreased to 0.14 per year for men aged greater than 70 years. These results demonstrated a slow but measurable progression in the severity of urinary symptoms among men during a 42-month follow-up period.

Clarke[61] retrospectively examined the outcomes of 36 men who were felt to have definite BPH but did not have absolute indications for surgery at baseline. The diagnosis was based on symptoms, rectal examination, and cystoscopic findings. These men had a mean age of 64 years, and had duration of symptoms for an average of 3 years. These patients were followed for about 3.5 years. Over this period, 25 of the men had symptomatic improvement lasting about 2 years, and 31 men had either symptomatic improvement or stable symptoms over almost 3 years. Twelve men (33%) required prostatectomy.

In a Scottish study, Bosch and associates[62] conducted a study involving 502 men (55–74 years of age) with BPH to determine the relative impact on the prevalence rates of the inclusion of different parameters (and of different cut-off values for these parameters) on the case definition of BPH. There was an agreement that age was the dominant determinant of BPH. However, of 28 different case definitions that were formulated, only eight gave a statistically significant increase in the prevalence of BPH with age. The highest overall prevalence of 19% occurred using the definition of prostatic volume >30 cm^3 and an IPSS >7. The lowest prevalence rate of 4.3% occurred using the definition that combined a prostatic volume >30 cm³, an IPSS >7, a maximum flow rate <10 mL s⁻¹, and the presence of a postvoid residual urine volume >50 mL. From these findings, it is thought that prevalence rates depend on the defined parameters used in a case definition.

Birkoff and colleagues[63] reported outcomes for a small cohort of 26 men with prostatism but without absolute indications for surgery. These highly selected men had declined treatment with experimental drugs for BPH but were followed up none the less at 3–6-month intervals for 3 years. At the end of 3 years, 7 men (27%) had improvement in symptoms, 4 (15%) were unchanged, and 15 (58%) were worse.

Diokno and colleagues[64] studied the prevalence and progression of bladder-emptying symptoms by interviewing a random sample of 802 men aged 60 years and older living in Washtenaw County, MIC. Of men with no bladder-emptying symptoms at baseline, 12% had developed mild symptoms, 3% moderate symptoms, and 1% of patients with severe symptoms at baseline, 23% had no symptoms, 17% had mild symptoms, and 11% had moderate symptoms 1 year later.

In a UK study, Simpson and associates[65] examined the relationships between prostatic enlargement, urinary flow rates, and symptoms in 597 men with BPH. Of the 597 men in the study, 310 (52%) of them successfully underwent TRUS, 326 (55%) attended the clinic, and 367 (61%) completed the urinary symptom questionnaire form. The response rate for the 310 men who underwent the TRUS procedure were lower in the age group of 40–49 (45%) and of 70–79 years (42%) compared with the men aged 50–59 (55%) and aged 60–69 (62%). Age-specific prevalence rates for BPH (a prostate size of >20 g) per 1000 men were: 40–49 years, 615; 50–59 years, 776; 60–69 years, 892; and 70–79 years, 889, giving an overall rate for all ages of 765. According to the medical records, there was no statistically significant relationship between the size of the prostate and the symptoms present. Furthermore, no relationship was established between the prostate size and the peak urinary flow rates. However, men with a urinary flow rate >20 mL s⁻¹ were very unlikely to have prostate glands greater than 40 g in size. Age, weight, and PSA levels were the only independent variables associated with prostate gland size. From this study, it was shown that BPH was substantially more prevalent than assumed previously in the early 1990s. Furthermore, this study reinforces the need for the subtle and detailed evaluation of patients who have BPH in assigning them to intervention, medical or surgical, or non-intervention, or watchful waiting.

Placebo arms of randomized trials of pharmacological agents for the treatment of BPH have also provided information on the natural history of symptoms. In trials, 10–70% of men had symptomatic improvement over 1 month to 1 year of follow-up. Their results underscore the importance of including placebo-control-treatment arms in any evaluation of new treatment modalities for BPH.

Since many have reported that the AUASI is non-specific for BPH, Roberts and associates[66] examined the association between the AUASI and urinary incontinence in men and women. The study enrolled 1540 men and women aged 50 years and older from Olmsted County in Minnesota. They were asked to complete the AUASI questionnaire followed by a 12-month follow-up period to assess the prevalence of urinary incontinence. The mean AUASI scores increased with age, and were higher in those participants with urinary incontinence and men. All seven of the urologic items in the AUASI were more prevalent in those who had urinary incontinence and in men. Furthermore, nocturia was highly prevalent among the subjects with or without urinary incontinence, but urgency, frequency, and weak urinary stream were more prevalent in subjects with incontinence than subjects without incontinence. Upon multiple logistic regression analysis, it was determined that when urinary incontinence, gender, and age were considered simultaneously, the participants with urinary incontinence, men, and subjects older than 65 years of age were more likely to have moderate-to-severe urinary symptoms (the odds ratio is 4.4, 1.9, 1.5, respectively). Authors concluded that men and women with urinary incontinence and older men and women are significantly more likely to have moderate-to-severe urinary symptoms. These findings suggested that urinary incontinence might contribute to a high AUASI score in both sexes. Thus, these data indicate that the similarity in the distribution of the AUASI in men and women is, in part, an artifact introduced by the confounding effects of continence status.[66]

RISK FOR PROSTATECTOMY IN MEN WITH BENIGN PROSTATIC HYPERPLASIA

The cumulative incidence of prostatectomy over time was calculated by Craigen[67] using a life-table analysis to account for different durations of observation due to death or loss to follow-up. For men presenting with acute retention, the cumulative incidence of prostatectomy was projected to be 60% at 1 year and 80% at 7 years; for men presenting without retention, the cumulative incidence of prostatectomy was projected to be 35% at 1 year and 45% at 7 years. The indications for prostatectomy in these men were not specified, and no combinations of symptoms or rectal examination findings at baseline were significantly associated with prostatectomy.

In the Diokno series, the risk of prostatectomy for all men in the cohort was about 3% per year.[68] About two-thirds of men who underwent prostatectomy over 2 years of follow-up had BPH symptoms at baseline. The symptoms of urinating more than once, interrupted stream, hesitancy, and straining were all associated with subsequent prostatectomy during 2 years of follow-up. Although these associations were adjusted for age and overall health status, it is not clear to what extent individual symptoms are independent predictors of incident prostatectomy.

In the Baltimore Longitudinal Study on Aging (BLSA) symptom questionnaires and physical examinations were administered to 1057 men without a baseline history of prostatectomy or prostate cancer over up to 30 years of follow-up.[68] Multivariate proportional hazards regression analysis was used to predict prostatectomy, controlling for both variable length of follow-up and all factors that may be associated with prostatectomy. In this study, increasing age was the predominant risk factor for undergoing prostatectomy. Of specific symptoms sought by the BLSA questionnaire, change in the size and force of the urinary stream and a sensation of incomplete emptying were both, independently, positively associated with prostatectomy. Prostatic enlargement on rectal examination was also independently associated with prostatectomy. Of 464 men with none of these risk factors, only 3% eventually required surgery. For 303 men with one risk factor, the cumulative incidence of surgery was 9%; for 178 men with two risk factors it was about 16%; and for 112 men with all three, about 37%.

Overall, these studies concluded that an increasing burden of urinary symptoms as men age is an important source of morbidity in BPH as well as an important determinant of risk of prostatectomy.

REFERENCES

1 Glynn RJ, Campion EW, Bouchard GR et al. The development of benign prostatic hyperplasia among volunteers in Normative Aging Study. Am J Epidemiol 1985; 121: 78–90.
2 Sidney S, Quesenberry C, Sadler MC et al. Risk factors for surgically treated benign prostatic hyperplasia in a prepaid health care plan. Urology 1991; 38(Suppl 1): 13–19.
3 Garraway WM, Collins GN, Lee RJ. High prevalence of benign prostatic hypertrophy in the community. Lancet 1991; 338: 469–471.
4 Boyle P, McGinn R, Maisonneuve P et al. Epidemiology of benign prostatic hyperplasia. Urol Clin North Am 1990; 17: 495–507.
5 Walsh, PC. Why make an early diagnosis of prostate cancer. J Urol 1992; PC-147, 3(2): 853–4.
6 Roberts RO, Rhodes T, Panser LA et al. Association between family history of benign prostatic hyperplasia and urinary symptoms: results of a population based study. Am J Epidemiol 1995; 142(9): 965–73.
7 Roberts RO, Rhodes T, Paneser LA et al. Association between family history of benign prostatic hyperplasia and urinary symptoms: results of a population based study. Am J Epidemiol 1995; 142(9): 965–73.
8 Sanda MG, Beaty TH, Stutzman RE et al. Genetic susceptibility of benign prostatic hyperplasia. J Urol 1994; 152(1): 115–19.
9 Partin AW, Page WF, Lee BR et al. Concordance rates for benign prostatic disease among twins suggest hereditary influence. Urology 1994; 44(5): 646–50.
10 Sanda MG, Doehring CB, Binkowitz B et al. Clinical and biological characteristics of familial benign prostatic hyperplasia. J Urol Mar 1997; 157(3): 876–9.
11 Doehring CB, Sanda MG, Partin AW et al. Histopathologic characterization of hereditary benign prostatic hyperplasia. Urology 1996; 48(4): 650–3.
12 Movsas S. Prostatic obstruction in the African and Asiatic. Br J Surg 1996; 53(6): 538–43.
13 Lissoos I. Carcinoma of the prostate in the Bantu. S Afr J Surg 1973; 11(2): 89–90.
14 Kambal A. Prostatic obstruction in Sudan. Br J Urol 1977; 49(2): 139–41.
15 Guess HA. Benign prostatic hyperplasia antecedents and natural history. Epidemiol Rev 1992; 14: 131.
16 Sidney S. Vasectomy and the risk of prostatic cancer and benign prostatic hypertrophy. J Urol 1987; 138: 795.
17 Lytton B, Emery JM, Harvard BW. The incidence of benign prostatic obstruction. J Urol 1968; 99: 639–45.
18 Morrison AS. Risk factors for surgery for prostatic hypertrophy. Am J Epidemiol 1992; 135: 974.
19 Guess HA. Epidemiology and natural history of benign prostatic hyperplasia. Urol Clin North Am 1995; 22: 247–61.
20 Chyou PH, Nomura AM, Stemmermann GN, Hankin JH. A prospective study of alcohol, diet, and other lifestyle factors in relation to obstructive uropathy. Prostate 1993; 22(3): 253–64.
21 Armenian HK, Lilienfeld AM, Diamond EL, Bross ID. Epidemiologic characteristics of patients with prostatic neoplasms. Am J Epidemiol 1975; 102(1): 47–54.
22 Barry MJ. Epidemiology and natural history of benign prostatic hyperplasia. Urol Clin North Am 1990; 17: 495–507.
23 Bostwick DG, Cooner WH, Denis L et al. The association of benign prostatic hyperplasia and cancer of the prostate. Cancer 1992; 70(Suppl 1): 291–301.
24 Tsukamoto T, Kumamoto Y, Masumori N et al. Prevalence of prostatism in Japanese men in a community based study with comparison to a similar American study. J Urol 1995; 154(2 Pt 1): 391–5.
25 Jolleys JV, Donovan JL, Nanchahal K et al. Urinary symptoms in the community: how bothersome are they? Br J Urol 1994; 74: 551–5.
26 Norman RW, Nickel JC, Fish D, Pickett SN. "Prostate-related symptoms" in Canadian men 50 years of age or older: prevalence and relationships among symptoms. Br J Urol 1994; 74(5): 542–50.
27 Koskimaki J, Hakama M, Huhtala H, Tammela TL. Prevalence of lower urinary tract symptoms in Finnish men: a population-based study. Br J Urol 1998; 81(3): 364–9.
28 Lepor H, Shapiro E, Wang B, Liang YC. Comparison of the cellular composition of benign prostatic hyperplasia in Chinese and Caucasian-American men. Urology 1996; 47(1): 38–42.
29 Araki H, Watanabe H, Mishina T, Nakao M. High-risk group for benign prostatic hypertrophy. Prostate 1983; 4(3): 253–64.
30 Wilson JD. The pathogenesis of benign prostatic hyperplasia. Am J Med 1980; 68(5): 745–56.
31 Isaacs JT, Coffey DS. Etiology and disease processes of benign prostatic hyperplasia. Prostate 1989; 2(Suppl 2): 33–40.
32 McNeal JE. Origin and evolution of benign prostatic enlargement. Invest Urol 1978; 15: 340.
33 Peters CA, Walsh PC. The effect of nafarelin acetate, a luteinizing-hormone-releasing hormone agonist, on benign prostatic hyperplasia. N Engl J Med 1987; 317: 599–604.
34 Partin AW, Oesterling JE, Epstein JI et al. Influence of age and endocrine factors on the volume of benign prostatic hyperplasia. J Urol 1991; 145: 405–9.
35 Matzkin H, Soloway MS. Cigarette smoking: a review of possible associations with benign prostatic hyperplasia. Prostate 1993; 22(4): 277–90.
36 Walsh PC, Wilson JD. The induction of prostatic hypertrophy in the dog with androstanediol. J Clin Invest 1976; 57(4): 1093–7.
37 Gann PH, Hennekens CH, Longcope C et al. A prostatic study of plasma hormone levels, nonhormonal factors, and development of benign prostatic hyperplasia. Prostate 1995; 26(1): 40–9.

38 Daniell HW. Larger prostatic adenomas in obese men with no associated increase in obstructive uropathy. *J Urol* 1993; **149**: 315–7.

39 Eldrup E, Lindholm J, Winkel P. Plasma sex hormones and ischemic heart disease. *Clin Biochem* 1987; **20**(2): 105–12.

40 Soygur T, Kupeli B, Aydos K *et al*. Effect of obesity on prostatic hyperplasia: its relation to sex steroid levels. *Int Urol Nephrol* 1996; **28**(1): 55–9.

41 Greenwald P, Kirmss V, Polan AK, Dick VS. Cancer of the prostate among men with benign prostatic hyperplasia. *J Natl Cancer Inst* 1974; **53**(2): 335–40.

42 Bourke JB, Griffin JP. Hypertension, diabetes mellitus, and blood groups in benign prostatic hypertrophy. *Br J Urol* 1966; **38**(1): 18–23.

43 Ghose RR, Harindra V. Unrecognized high pressure chronic retention of urine presenting with systemic arterial hypertension. *BMJ* 1989; **298**(6688): 1626–8.

44 Frea B, Annoscia S, Stanta G *et al*. Correlation between liver cirrhosis and benign prostatic hyperplasia: a morphrlogical study. *Urol Res* **15**(5): 311–14.

45 Chopra IJ, Tulchinsky D, Greeway FL. Estrogen–androgen imbalance in hepatic cirrhosis. Studies in 13 male patients. *Ann Intern Med* 1973; **79**(2): 198–203.

46 Jakobsen H, Trop-Pedersen S, Juul N, Hald T. The long-term influence of vasectomy on prostatic volume and morphology in man. *Prostate* 1988; **13**(1): 57–67.

47 Pierrepoint CG, Davies P, Lewis MH, Moffat DB. Examination of the hypothesis that a direct control system exists for the prostate and seminal vesicles. *J Reprod Fertil* 1975; **44**(2): 395–409.

48 De la Torre B, Hedman M, Jensen F *et al*. Lack of effect of vasectomy on peripheral gonadotrophin and steroid levels. *Int J Androl* 1983; **6**(2): 125–34.

49 Ekman P. BPH epidemiology and risk factors. *Prostate* 1989; **2**(Suppl 2): 23–8.

50 Seitter WR, Barrett-Connor E. Cigarette smoking, obesity and benign prostatic hypertrophy: A prospective population-based study. *Am J Epidemiol* 1992; 135: 500.

51 Briggs MH. Cigarette smoking and infertility in men. *Med J Aust* 1973; **1**(12): 616–17

52 Shaarawy M, Mahmoud KZ. Endocrine profile and semen characteristics in male smokers. *Fertil Steril* 1982; **38**(2): 255–7.

53 Barrett-Connor E, Friedlander NJ, Khaw KT. Dehydroepiadrosterone sulfate and breast cancer risk. *Cancer Res* 1990; **50**(20): 6571–4.

54 Gordon GG, Altman K, Southren AL *et al*. Effect of alcohol (ethanol) administration on sex-hormone metabolism in normal men. *N Engl J Med* 1976; **295**(15): 793–7.

55 Nomura AM, Kolonel LN. Prostate cancer: a current perspective. *Epidemiol* 1991; **13**: 200–27.

56 Farnsworth WE, Slaunwhite WR Jr, Sharma M *et al*. Interaction of prolactin and testosterone in the human prostate. *Urol Res* 1981; **9**(2): 79–88.

57 Syms AJ, Harper ME, Griffiths K. The effect of prolactin on human BPH epithelial cell proliferation. *Prostate* 1985; **6**(2): 145–53.

58 Zisman A, Zisman E, Lindner A *et al*. Autoantibodies to prostate specific antigen in patients with benign prostatic hyperplasia. *J Urol* 1995; **154**(3): 1052–5.

59 Girman CJ, Jacobsen SJ, Guess HA *et al*. Natural history of prostatism: relationship among symptoms, prostate volume and peak urinary flow rate. *J Urol* 1995; **153**: 1510–15.

60 Girman CJ, Epstein RS, Jacobsen SJ *et al*. Natural history of prostatism: Impact of urinary symptoms on quality of life in 2115 randomly selected community men. *Urology* 1994; **44**(6): 825–31.

61 Clarke R. The prostate and the endocrines: a control series. *Br J Urol* 1937; **9**: 254–71.

62 Bosch JL, Hop WC, Kirkels WJ, Schroder FH. Natural history of benign prostatic hyperplasia: appropriate case definition and estimation of its prevalence in the community. *Urology* 1995; **46**(3 Suppl A): 34–40.

63 Birkoff J, Wiederhorn A, Hamilton M, Xinsser H. Natural history of benign prostatic hypertrophy and acute urinary retention. *Urology* 1976; **7**: 48–52.

64 Diokno A, Brown M, Goldstein N, Herzog A. Epidemiology of bladder emptying symptoms in elderly men. *J Urol* 1992; **148**: 1817–1821.

65 Simpson RJ, Fisher W, Lee AJ, Russell EB, Garraway M. Benign prostatic hyperplasia in an unselected community-based population: a survey of urinary symptoms, bothersomeness and prostatic enlargement. *Br J Urol* 1996; **77**(2): 186–191.

66 Roberts RO, Jacobsen SJ, Jacobson DJ *et al*. Natural history of prostatism: High American Urological Association Symptom scores among community dwelling men and women with urinary incontinence. *Urology* 1998; **51**(2): 213–219.

67 Craigen A, Hickling J, Saunders C, Carpenter R. Natural history of prostatic obstruction. A prospective survey. *J R Coll Gen Pract* 1969; **18**: 226–32.

68 Guess, HA, Arrighi HM, Metter EJ, Fozard JL. Cumulative prevalence of prostatism matches the autopsy prevalence of benign prostatic hyperplasia. *Prostate* 1990; **17**(3): 241–6.

Socioeconomics and Trends in the Management of Benign Prostatic Hyperplasia: United States Perspective

3

H.L. Holtgrewe

In addition to the patient and his physician, a third interested party is increasingly becoming a part of decision making in the management of benign prostatic hyperplasia (BPH). That third party is the payer of the costs of health care. Throughout the nations of the developed world, the overwhelming majority of patients have been relieved of the financial responsibility of their health care. Governments and private commercial health insurance or some related form of managed care organization (MCO) have assumed this responsibility. Table 3.1 depicts the ratios of public vs. private commercial health care funding in six nations of the developed world.[1] Understandably, these organizations are motivated to insure that the therapies they buy are effective and, more importantly, that these therapies are cost effective. This is particularly true of high cost and very common diseases and especially true of high cost and very common non-lethal diseases, where therapy is directed at improvement in the quality of life, not directed at the preservation of life. BPH is such a disease.

Economic issues surrounding the diagnosis and treatment of BPH are becoming a major area of concern for payers, in view of the prevalence of the disease, an aging population, and the attended increasing numbers of men in the BPH age range. The issue is further complicated by the recent explosion in the numbers of new emerging strategies of BPH management.

insular. Each must compete within the new world economy. Countries with disproportionately high health care costs are placed at a significant disadvantage when trading worldwide, compared with countries whose health care costs are less. Health care costs are a vital constituent of labor costs and have become a significant component in the price of those goods and services that are marketed into the global economy.

Judged by any standard, the USA spends more on health care than any other nation of the world. Table 3.2 depicts the per capita spending and health care spending as a percentage of gross domestic product among selected nations of the world.[1] The disadvantage suffered by nations with high health care costs, such as the USA, is exemplified by the following: the total aggregate health care costs contained in a mid-sized General Motors automobile manufactured in the USA in 1992 was $1100. Health care costs contained in a comparable Japanese import was $600.[2] In the competitive worldwide automotive industry, this constituted a severe disadvantage for American auto makers.

Motivated by thousands of similar situations and having experienced decades of uncontrolled escalating health care costs for their employees and retirees (costs over which they appeared to have no control), American businessmen

	% Public funds	% Private funds
USA	42	58
Japan	72	28
Canada	73	27
Germany	73	27
France	74	26
UK	84	16

Table 3.1 Health care spending: public vs. private funding selected nations, 1992

Source: Organization for Economic Cooperation and Development. OECD Health Data File. © OECD 1992

	Per capita (US$)[a]	% Gross domestic product	% Mean annual growth rate health spending 1980–92
Belgium	1485	8.2	8.3
Canada	1949	10.3	8.6
Denmark	1163	6.5	5.9
France	1745	9.4	7.9
Germany	1775	8.7	6.7
Italy	1497	8.5	8.4
Japan	1376	6.9	8.5
The Netherlands	1449	8.6	6.3
Spain	895	7.0	8.8
Sweden	1317	7.9	3.7
UK	1151	7.1	8.0
USA	3094	13.6	9.3

[a] On the basis of GDP purchasing power parities

Table 3.2 Health care spending, 1992

Source: Organization for Economic Cooperation and Development. OECD Health Data File. © OECD 1992

BACKGROUND

The world has become a giant trading community. No nation, irrespective of its economic strength or wealth, is

were driven to address the situation themselves, applying what they knew best – business. The result has been the commercialization of the world's largest single industry. Health care in the USA is a trillion dollar annual enterprise. Vanishing is the decades-old system where physicians made independent decisions for their patients and a third party paid the bills. That third party is demanding to participate. In the USA, this intrusion into patient care is by commercial MCOs and regulatory governmental agencies. In all nations of the world, some regulatory body or economically motivated agency is being increasingly involved in decisions regarding the diagnosis and management of this costly common disease of the aging male.

CURRENT COSTS OF BENIGN PROSTATIC HYPERPLASIA MANAGEMENT

There exist today no accurate data on the total costs of BPH evaluation and management in any nation. Focused record keeping and cost accounting is inadequate worldwide. This is particularly true for evaluation and treatment services rendered out of the hospital and in the physician's office setting, where retrieval of data is poorest and where the management of BPH becomes mingled with the concurrent management of other medical disorders.

The costs of BPH management must be divided into three components. Direct costs are actually those charges involved in perioperative and hospital events, including physician reimbursement, hospital charges, laboratory and imaging charges, as well as the charges for nursing services and medications. These charges are the most visible, are best chronicled, and receive the greatest attention. In fact, they are often used to serve incorrectly as surrogates for total BPH costs. They are not. There are also indirect costs that are much more difficult to assess but are of great importance. These are due to the lost incomes of patients and families, travel costs, and the numerous, miscellaneous expenses incurred during the patient's diagnosis and treatment. The third component of BPH costs are the intangible costs of pain, mental anguish, and suffering. In one of the few studies dealing with these latter costs, Standaert and Tarfs[3] measured the impact of BPH and its symptoms. They reported substantial adverse impact on patient quality of life and, thus, significant intangible costs.

The best existing economic data on BPH is for its surgical treatment. Transurethral resection of the prostate (TURP) is the most widely utilized form of surgery for BPH (constituting over 95% of all prostatectomies in the USA in 1994).[4] Charges (direct costs) for TURP in selected nations are depicted in Table 3.3 along with mean durations of hospitalization.[5] While hospital stay in the USA was shortest, charges were the highest. The enormous worldwide magnitude of costs of the surgical management of BPH is depicted in Table 3.4. Six nations of the developed world spent over US$3 billion for the surgical treatment of BPH in 1990.[6]

In a study from Sweden, Carlsson[7] reported that of total prostatectomy costs, 80% were direct and 20%

	US$	Duration of hospital stay mean or range (days)
USA	6889	2.7
Japan	5000	10
Denmark	3218	5
Sweden	3045	5–7
UK	2217	7
Belgium	1842	4–7

Table 3.3 Total charges for TURP, 1995

Source: Holtgrewe L, Writing Committee. The economics of BPH. In: Cockett, ATK, Khoury S. Aso Y et al. (eds) *The 3rd International Consultation on Benign Prostatic Hyperplasia (BPH), Monaco, 1995 June 26–28.* Jersey: Scientific Communications International 1996: 53–70

	US$	Population
USA	2,304,485,000	259,571,000
Japan	459,600,000	123,540,000
UK[a]	96,430,000	42,370,000
Belgium	55,670,000	9,993,000
France	37,800,000	56,735,000
Sweden	24,906,000	8,566,000
[a]England only		

Table 3.4 Estimates of direct costs of surgical treatment of BPH 1990

Source: Holtgrewe L, Writing Committee. The economics of BPH. In: Cockett ATK, Aso Y, Chatelain C et al. (eds) *The 2nd International Consultation on Benign Prostatic Hyperplasia (BPH), Paris, France, 1993 June 27–30.* Jersey: Scientific Communications International 1993: 35–44

indirect. A further assessment of direct costs by Ahlstrand et al.[8] found that 15% of direct costs were incurred prior to the surgical event, 70% were perioperative, and the remaining 15% were incurred in the 5 years following surgery and were required for the management of complications and surgical failures.

Further confounding the economics of BPH and its surgical management is the ratio of urologists to population or, more specifically, urologists to men in the BPH age range. Does the mere availability of increased numbers of urologists lead to increased numbers of prostatectomies? There exist no data conclusively to confirm such a fact, but it is of interest to note that between 1976 and 1988 the number of urologists in Belgium increased 37% (153 to 270). During this same interval the number of TURPS for BPH increased 75%, while the male population over 65 years of age grew by a minimal 1.3%.[9]

For nearly a century following the first successful surgical removal of the adenoma of BPH,[10] surgery was the only effective treatment. Medical therapy was first suggested by Caine et al.[11] with their description of the symptom improvement achieved with the use of the α-blocker, phenoxybenzamine. The advent of the selective long-acting α-1 blockers, terazosin, doxazosin, and tamsulosin have witnessed alpha blockade's rapid adoption in BPH therapy.

A 1994 survey of the practice patterns of American urologists commissioned by the American Urological Association (AUA) and conducted by the Gallup Organization of Princeton, NJ, asked these urologists questions concerning their methods of diagnosis and management of BPH.[12] Excluding those patients who presented with the recognized mandatory indications for surgery – refractory retention, recurrent infections, recurrent bleeding, bladder calculi, or bladder or renal complications due to BPH (patients who would normally be candidates for surgery), the respondees were asked their first recommendation of management based upon the patient's AUA Symptom Index score[13] (with a possible sum ranging from 0 to 35). Based upon severity of symptoms, patients were divided into three groups: mild (0–7), moderate (8–19), and severe (20–35). The results of the survey are depicted in Table 3.5 and reveal that 77% of American urologists do not treat men with mild symptoms. Most significant is that 71% employed medical management as their first recommendation for men with moderate symptoms, and 34% continued to recommend medical therapy as their first recommendation even for men with severe symptoms.

A repeat similar poll was conducted in 1997 by the AUA and the Gallup Organization.[14] It revealed that in the 3-year interval the percentage of American urologists recommending medical management as their first choice for the man with moderate symptoms had risen from 77% to 85% and medical management for men with severe symptoms had risen from 34% to 55%.

This trend toward medical management is documented by the rapid rise in the number of prescriptions written for BPH between 1992 and 1994 in the USA (Table 3.6).[15] Table 3.7 reveals the dollar value of BPH prescriptions and their relative positions among the top 20 medications prescribed by American urologists in 1994.[16]

	Number of prescriptions per year for BPH in USA (thousands)		
	1992	1993	1994
Finasteride	317,000	1,345,000	2,040,000
Alpha-blockers	1,075,000	1,512,000	2,940,000

Table 3.6 Medical therapy for BPH

Source: Abbott Methodology Applied to NPA Plus™ and NDTT™ Data. IMS America 1995; methodology on file at Abbott

Product	Ranking within top 20 prescriptions written by US urologists	Total sales (US$)
Cipro (ciprofloxacin)	1	28,789,000
Proscar (finasteride)	2	27,917,000[a]
Hytrin (terazosin)	4	22,034,000[a]
Cardura (doxazosin)	17	2,508,000[a]

[a]Total of $52,459,000 for three BPH pharmacologicals

Table 3.7 Prescriptions written by urologists, USA 1994

Source: Medical Economics Research Group. Urologists facts about their practices. Walsh America/PMSI Alpha Data, Jan–Oct 1994. Five Paragon Dr., Montvale, NJ 1995

Clearly, medical management has made an enormous penetration into the treatment of BPH, and the trend is increasing. The question remaining regarding medical treatment is its durability. Will failures eventually develop that require surgical or other treatment in large numbers of patients previously treated by medical means? Lepor[17] reports durability of beneficial outcomes of terazosin treatment over an observed interval of 4 years. Yet the number of men upon whom we have 4-year data remain very small. Reporting on the longer-term outcomes of finasteride treatment, Stoner[18] has reported that in a sub-group contained within a large trial, dihydrotestosterone levels remain persistently suppressed, that observed prostate volume reductions were maintained, and that observed symptom improvements were maintained at 36 months. One could speculate whether, over time, the initial beneficial effect of alpha-blockers upon the dynamic component of the patient's obstruction will eventually be overcome by continuing prostatic growth, producing an ever-increasing static component of his obstruction. Further long-term trials are required to resolve this question and to establish the durability and the definitive cost effectiveness of all varieties of medical therapy.

AUA score 0–7 (mild)	%
Watchful waiting	77
Alpha-blockers	17
Other	4
Finasteride	1
No response	1
AUA score 8–19 (moderate)	
Alpha-blockers	65
Other	15
Watchful waiting	6
Finasteride	6
Transurethral resection	4
Laser	2
No response	2
AUA score 20–35 (severe)	
Transurethral resection	41
Alpha-blockers	31
Other	16
Laser	6
Finasteride	3
No response	3

Table 3.5 First treatment recommendations for BPH patients not in retention (with no major complications)

Source: Gee W, Holtgrewe L, Albertsen P et al. Practice trends in the diagnosis and management of benign prostatic hyperplasia in the United States. J Urol 1995; 154: 205–6

The recently published Proscar Long-term Efficacy and Safety Study (PLESS) of McConnell and co-workers[19] revealed BPH to be a progressive disease, with men in the study's placebo group experiencing a mean 14% increase in their prostate volumes over the 4 years of the study, while men on finasteride experienced about an 18% decrease in prostate volumes, which was sustained over 4 years. These data suggest that finasteride may possess the ability to arrest BPH growth.

There currently do not exist, however, any data to confirm that the prophylactic use of this agent would be cost effective over the long term, despite the fact that over the 4 years of the PLESS study men on finasteride experienced a 57% reduction in the risk rate of acute urinary retention and a 54% reduction in the risk rate of prostatic surgery for their BPH.

The recent explosion in device treatment includes transurethral electrovaporization of the prostate (TUEP), visual laser ablation of the prostate (VLAP), high-frequency intensity focused ultrasound (HIFU), transurethral needle ablation of the prostate (TUNA), transurethral microwave thermal therapies, and the placement of permanent alloy stents within the prostatic urethra.

Most reports dealing with these device treatments are of 12 months or less follow-up. Most report outcomes approaching, but not equaling, TURP, and most report lower mortality, lower complications, fewer blood transfusions, and substantially shorter durations of hospitalizations than TURP. All of these have the potential for enormous costs savings. In the only reported double-blinded randomized trial of device therapy (VLAP) vs. TURP, Dixon *et al.*[20] found marked symptom improvement at 6 months in 76% of the TURP patients vs. only 35% in the VLAP patients. These authors concluded that TURP was more effective but VLAP was safer.

The largest study and the one with the longest duration of follow-up dealing with device therapies is that of Kabalin.[21] He reported data on 227 VLAP patients, which included 24-month data on 45 patients and 36-month data on 10 patients. His study confirmed outcomes similar to those achieved with TURP. It also confirmed durability of outcomes within the very small numbers of patients followed to 2 and 3 years.

The unknown factor in 1998 is the long-term durability of these newer therapies. History reminds us that, only a few years ago, balloon dilation emerged and was heralded as a safe and effective strategy of BPH management. Time revealed it to not be durable, a reminder that we must not rush to judgment regarding new therapy until longer-term data become available.

CHANGING TREATMENT PATTERNS AND THEIR IMPACT ON UROLOGISTS

Prostatectomy and BPH have been central to the profession of urology for decades. Indeed, it was surgery of the prostate gland that set urologists apart from general surgeons in the early years of the twentieth century. Prostatectomy for BPH

accounted for over 50% of American urologists' major surgery in 1962.[22] In 1986, while other major surgery was becoming increasingly important, TURP still represented 38% of their major procedures.[22] The number of TURPs reached an annual peak of 253,000 in the USA under its Medicare program (men aged 65 years and over) in 1987.[4] Since that year, the numbers have progressively fallen 43% to 145,000 in 1994, the most recent year for which data are available (Figure 3.1).[4] Similar reductions are occurring worldwide (Table 3.8).[5]

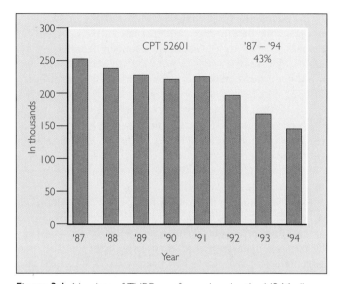

Figure 3.1 Number of TURPs performed under the US Medicare program (men aged 65 years and older) over the 8 years 1987–94. These represent actual numbers of operations performed not taking into account the increased number of men enrolled into the Medicare program during these years

Source: United States Government Health Care Financing Administration (HCFA). *B.E.S.S. Data.* Washington, DC 1994

	Prostatectomies per 1000 men age 55 years and over	
	1990	1993
USA	13	10.3
Sweden	11	7.8
Japan	9	8.7
UK[a]	5.9	6

[a]Men aged 45 years and older

Table 3.8 Incidence of prostatectomy for BPH, selected nations 1990 and 1993

Source: Holtgrewe L, Writing Committee. The economics of BPH. In: Cockett ATK, Khoury S, Aso Y et al. (eds) *The 3rd International Consultation on Benign Prostatic Hyperplasia (BPH), Monaco, 1995 June 26–28.* Jersey: Scientific Communications International 1996: 53–70

Medical management, device therapies and, perhaps, a renewed awareness of the strategy of watchful waiting are dramatically altering the need for surgery. Not only is BPH being increasingly treated medically, but 1994 data reveal that 59% of terazosin prescriptions and 55% of finasteride prescriptions for BPH were written by primary physicians.[15] Once within the exclusive domain of the urologist, BPH patients are now being managed by their primary physicians. These shifts in BPH management patterns combined with the major dependence of urology upon this one disease are creating inevitable economic vulnerability for urologists – especially those reimbursed on a system of fee for service.

FUTURE COSTS OF BENIGN PROSTATIC HYPERPLASIA

In the properly selected patient, no treatment of BPH provides the probability of symptom relief as does surgery.[23,24] Prostatectomy incurs much greater initial cost than most device therapies and certainly all medical therapy. Those monies saved by the avoidance of surgery can be retained within the nation's health care delivery system and can be invested at interest or directed into other areas of need. But, these initial savings do not constitute the entire scenario.

During the era when surgery was the only therapy for the obstructive uropathy induced by BPH, many men avoided or postponed medical evaluation, realizing that a surgical operation would be the ultimate outcome. Fear of surgery, its pain, and potential complications induced many men to reject prostatectomy even after an initial evaluation resulted in the recommendation for prostatectomy. The dread of an operation outweighed their desire for symptom relief.

The advent of effective medical therapy and the lesser invasive device therapies provides the former "silent sufferer" with new options. Not only will men previously averse to surgical treatment accept daily oral medication, they will actively seek such treatment, even if that medical therapy provides a lesser degree of symptom relief than would surgery. They willingly accept a lesser outcome in exchange for a lesser risk.

Coupled with this increased demand for medical therapy will be increased public awareness of the disease, its symptoms, and its treatment options. The pharmaceutical industry and the medical device industry seeking return on their investments in research and development will insure that men of BPH age and their families are made aware of their products through promotions and lay advertising. The improved management of cardiovascular and other diseases has been attended with greater longevity. Men are living longer, and more are living to the BPH age range. The multiple forces of an aging male population, enhanced public awareness, and increasing patient demand for the new medical and less invasive treatments will combine to create a huge increase in the total number of men undergoing evaluation for and receiving treatment of BPH. The total aggregate cost of the foregoing will overwhelm and greatly exceed any savings derived from the reduced volumes of surgery currently being experienced worldwide. The final result will be a dramatic increase in total BPH expenditure

that will have to be borne by the health delivery systems of the nations of the world owing to the vast increase in the total numbers of men under treatment. The opposing forces of BPH management costs are depicted in Figure 3.2.

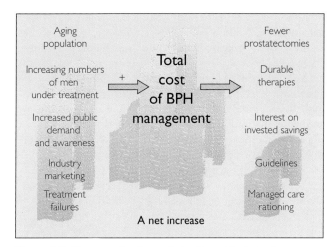

Figure 3.2 The opposing forces that will contribute to the increasing total future costs of the management of BPH in developed nations

MEANS OF COST CONTAINMENT

Confronted with the inevitable foregoing economic forces and the resultant dramatic rising costs of BPH treatment, it is equally inevitable that cost-containment measures will be imposed by the payers of health care – that third party at the decision-making table. Outright rationing through availability of access to the urologist or denial of medications for BPH patients are obvious options.

As there exists economic competition between nations of the world, so too there exists competition within the health delivery systems of a single nation – competition between diseases, and competition between the various specialties of medicine. Each vies for its proper allocation of those finite resources at the disposal of the nation's health care delivery system. In light of this reality, it must be asked: what obligation does the public purse have through its tax revenues or its collective insurance premiums to improve the symptoms of an older man suffering from a disease which, if properly evaluated and managed, is nonlethal? What obligation does the public purse have to reduce an older man's urinary frequency, nocturia, and urgency, thus improving, to whatever extent, his quality of life? Could the same resources be better transferred to prenatal care, infant immunization programs, cancer screening for younger adults, or for any one of an array of other worthy health needs.

Arbitrary rationing is often implicit and indiscriminate. No distinction as to value, true cost efficacy, and cost savings is made, thus creating distortions within the quality of care. Far better is the determination of the quality, durability, and cost efficacy of BPH treatments through the use of clinical guidelines, and based upon these data, making available only those therapies of established value. Such an effort was undertaken by the US government's Agency for Health Care Policy and Research (AHCPR) when, in 1994, they released guidelines for the diagnosis and management of BPH.[23] The AHCPR guidelines were produced by a multidisciplinary panel with representation from urology, internal medicine, family medicine, radiology, and nursing. Central to the guidelines is the seven-question, self-administered AUA Symptom Index.[13] Recommendations for the evaluation of the BPH patient contained within the AHCPR guidelines have the potential for achieving great cost savings. Based upon the world's peer-reviewed literature, the guidelines recommend that imaging of the upper urinary tracts by radiographic or sonographic means not be routinely performed and that these studies should be reserved for complicating factors such as hematuria, uremia, a history of stone disease, flank pain, previous renal trauma, previous renal surgery, or other coexisting disease, all of which in their own right constituted an indication for the study. Likewise, a purely diagnostic routine cystoscopy is not recommended, since there is no literature-based evidence that the procedure provides any useful information in treatment decision making. Once the decision for surgical treatment has been made, cystoscopy is often useful in planning the type of surgery to be undertaken.

Despite their lack of utility, urologists of the world continue to employ routine diagnostic upper tract imaging and cystoscopy, thus wasting enormous health care resources, as depicted in Tables 3.9 and 3.10.[5,24] These vast amounts of health care resources could be saved by adherence to AHCPR guideline principles.

The use of urodynamics to predict the probability of favorable outcomes with various BPH management strategies remains controversial. Abrams et al.[25] feel pressure-flow studies should be performed routinely prior to prostatectomy. They correctly state that symptom indices and uroflow rates cannot discriminate the obstructed from the unobstructed patient. McConnell,[26] citing the modest additional value of routine, invasive, and costly urodynamics as a predictor of outcomes, reserves urodynamics for those patients who are symptomatic but whose peak flow rates are greater than $15 \ cm^3 \ s^{-1}$ or where there is suspicion of a

	% of urologists performing routine diagnostic cystoscopy in the evaluation of the BPH patient
Sweden	55
Belgium	52
Denmark	45
USA	41
Japan	10

Table 3.10 BPH evaluation practices, selected nations

Source: Holtgrewe L, Writing Committee. The economics of BPH. In: Cockett ATK, Khoury S, Aso Y et al. (eds) The 3rd International Consultation on Benign Prostatic Hyperplasia (BPH), Monaco, 1995 June 26–28. Jersey: Scientific Communications International 1996: 53–70

coexisting urological disorder or some other comorbidity. The ACHPR guidelines regard pressure-flow studies and urodynamics as optional. The discriminate rather than the routine use of urodynamics is another potential source for enormous cost savings in the evaluation of the BPH patient.

The most effective cost-containment effort will be to confine public payment to those therapies that have a defined and proven durability and low failure rate, thus avoiding the compounding of costs intrinsic to a "cascade" of treatments. Failure rates reported in the AHCPR guidelines are depicted in Table 3.11. Failure rates of device therapies are not included since, at the time of the AHCPR guidelines development, there was insufficient peer-reviewed literature of adequate duration of follow-up to make any judgment upon these. The AUA is planning an independent revision and modernization of these BPH guidelines in the very near future (HI Kona, personal communication, 1996).

What use health care planners, governmental bureaucrats, and health ministers of other nations may, or may not, make of the US AHCPR guidelines is impossible to determine. Given their potential for substantial and consistent cost savings achieved in a scientific and logical

	% of urologists routinely obtaining IV urogram or renal sonogram in the evaluation of the BPH patient
Japan	60
UK	29
Belgium	25
USA	18
Sweden	5
Denmark	0

Table 3.9 BPH evaluation practices, selected nations

Source: Holtgrewe L, Writing Committee. The economics of BPH. In: Cockett ATK, Khoury S, Aso Y et al. (eds) The 3rd International Consultation on Benign Prostatic Hyperplasia (BPH), Monaco, 1995 June 26–28. Jersey: Scientific Communications International 1996: 53–70

Treatment modalities	High estimate	Low estimate
Watchful waiting		38% (90% CI 15–65%)[a]
Alpha-blocker	39% (90% CI 23–70%)[b]	13% (90% CI 4–31%)[a]
Finasteride	27% (90% CI 25–29%)[b]	10% (90% CI 9–12%)[a]
TUIP		9% (90% CI 1–28%)[a]
TURP		10% (90% CI 9–11%)[c]
Open surgery		2% (90% CI 1–4%)[c]

[a]Reported initial failure rate with subsequent period up to 5 years assumed to have 20% of the initial failure rate, modeled after the study by Craigen et al.[27]
[b]Reported initial failure rate assumed to be linear up to 5 years
[c]Single point estimates and confidence intervals (CI), devised from large clinical series out to and past 5 years

Table 3.11 Five-year projected treatment failure rates

Source: McConnell JD, Barry MJ, Bruskewiz RC et al. Benign Prostatic Hyperplasia: Diagnosis and Treatment. Clinical Practice Guidelines, No. 8. AHCPR Publication No 94–0582. Rockville, MD: Agency for Health Care Policy and Research, Public Health Service, US Department of Health and Human Services 1994

manner, it is difficult to believe they can totally ignore such an important resource.

CONCLUSIONS

Clearly, the most costly aspect of any strategy of BPH management is its failure rate and lack of durability. Ineffective treatments, even marginally effective treatments, although initially less costly than prostatectomy, become very expensive when the costs of definitive therapies such as surgery must be inevitably added to costs incurred during the course of the ineffective or unsuccessful treatment. Such a "cascade" of treatments inevitably increases the costs over those that would have been experienced had the initial therapy been definitive. Proven clinical effectiveness and cost effectiveness, documented in properly performed prospective randomized clinical trials, are essential. Only when such BPH therapies have been documented to have beneficial impact on the quality of life, over time, should the payment for these therapies come from the communal purse, either public or private. The costs of new therapies should be documented in their presentation in the world's peer-reviewed literature, and those costs should be compared with existing established treatments and with other competing, new, emerging strategies of management. Such cost data have often been lacking in previous world literature dealing with BPH treatment. The Committee on the Economics of BPH of the World Health Organization's Third Consultation on BPH, held in Monaco in June of 1995,[5] admonished the editors of the world's peer-reviewed medical and urological journals to reject those manuscripts dealing with new BPH treatments lacking such economic data, just as they would reject manuscripts lacking proper important clinical data.

	Population in millions	
	Aged 65 years and over	Aged 85 years and over
1990	3	0.13
1930	6	0.27
1960	18	0.9
1990	33	3
2000[a]	37	4
2020[a]	65	6
2050[a]	80	18
[a]Estimates		

Table 3.12 US population trends

Source: US Decennial Life Tables. State Life Tables, Vol. 1 ALMO 2 MT-WY. Life Expectancy; Mortality (U.S.), PHS 90–1151. Hyattsville, MD: US Department of Health and Human Services, Public Health Service, National Center for Health Statistics 1990

Given the enormous future increase in the numbers of men in the BPH age range (Table 3.12),[28] most of whom will be coming into treatment in this new era of alternative managements, it is essential that cost effectiveness be an integral part of payment considerations.

The urologist can help! He or she should reserve their diagnostic and management strategies to those shown to be cost effective, based on proper clinically constructed guidelines and upon proper economic documentation in the world's peer-reviewed literature. It is a sobering fact that BPH constitutes an enormous world health care expense. Its costs will grow dramatically in the years ahead. Physician- and urologist-induced cost containment is vital lest bureaucrats and businessmen impose upon our patients poorly conceived, non-scientific, and totally arbitrary economies.

REFERENCES

1 Organization for Economic Cooperation and Development (OECD). *OECD Health Data File*, OECD 1992.

2 McAlinden S. *Competitive Survival: Private Initiatives, Public Policy and the North American Automotive Industry*. Transportation Research Institute, Report 92–3. Ann Arbor, MI: University of Michigan 1992.

3 Standaert B, Tarfs K. Economics of BPH: measuring the intangible costs. In: Kurth K, Newling D (eds) *Benign Prostatic Hyperplasia, EORTC Genitourinary Monograph 12*. New York, Wiley–Liss 1994: 409–18.

4 United States Government Health Care Financing Administration (HCFA). *B.E.S.S. Data*. Washington, DC 1994.

5 Holtgrewe L. Writing Committee. The economics of BPH. In: Cockett ATK, Khonty S, Aso Y *et al.* (eds) *The 3rd International Consultation on Benign Prostatic Hyperplasia (BPH), Monaco, 1995 June 26–28*. Jersey: Scientific Communications International 1996; 53–70.

6 Holtgrewe L. Writing Committee. The economics of BPH. In: Cockett ATK, Aso Y, Chatelain C *et al.* (eds) *The 2nd International Consultation on Benign Prostatic Hyperplasia (BPH), Paris, France, 1993 June 27–30*. Jersey, Scientific Communications International 1993; 35–44.

7 Carlsson P. Diffusion and economic effects of medical technology in treatment of peptic ulcer, prostatic hyperplasia and gall bladder diseases. *Likoping Studies in Art and Science* 1987; No. 12 diss.

8 Ahlstrand C, Carlsson P, Jonsson B. An estimate of the life-time cost of surgical treatment of benign prostatic hyperplasia in Sweden. *Scand J Urol Nephrol* 1996; 30(1): 37–43.

9 Holtgrewe L. Writing committee. The economics of BPH. In: Cockett ATK, Aso Y, Chatelain C *et al.* (eds) *The International Consultation on Benign Prostatic Hyperplasia (BPH), Paris, France, 1991 June 26–27*. Jersey: Scientific Communications International 1991; 261–7.

10 Freyer P. A new method of performing prostatectomy. *Lancet* 1900; 1: 774–6.

11 Caine M, Pfau A, Perlberg S. The use of alpha adrenergic blockers in benign prostatic obstruction. *Br J Urol* 1976; 48: 255–63.

12 Gee W, Holtgrewe L, Albertsen P *et al.* Practice trends in the diagnosis and management of benign prostatic hyperplasia in the United States. *J Urol* 1995; 154: 205–6.

13 Barry MJ, Fowler FJ Jr, O'Leary MP *et al.* The American Urological Association Symptom Index for benign prostatic hyperplasia. *J Urol* 1992; 148: 1549–57.

14 American Urological Association. *Gallup Poll of American Urologists*. Baltimore, MD: American Urological Association 1997.

15 *Abbott Methodology Applied to NPA Plus™ and NDTT™ Data*. IMS America 1995; methodology on file at Abbott.

16 Medical Economics Research Group. Urologists facts about their practices. *Walsh America/PMSI Alpha Data, Jan–Oct 1994*. Five Paragon Dr., Montvale, NJ 1995.

17 Lepor H. Long term safety and effectiveness of terazosin in patients with BPH. *Urology* 1995; **45**: 406–13.

18 Stoner E. Three year safety and efficacy data on the use of finasteride in the treatment of benign prostate hyperplasia. *Urology* 1994; **43**: 284–92.

19 McConnell JD *et al*. The effect of finasteride on the risk of acute urinary retention and the need for surgical treatment among men with benign prostatic hyperplasia. *N Engl J Med* 1998; **338**: 557–63.

20 Dixon C, Machi G, Theune C *et al*. A prospective, double blind randomized study comparing the safety, efficacy and cost of laser ablation of the prostate and transurethral prostatectomy for treatment of BPH. *J Urol* 1994; **151**: 229A.

21 Kabalin J, Bite G, Doll S. Neodymium: YAG laser coagulation prostatectomy: 3 years of experience with 227 patients. *J Urol* 1996; **155**: 181–5.

22 Holtgrewe L, Mebust W, Dowd J *et al*. Transurethral prostatectomy: practice aspects of the dominant operation in American urology. *J Urol* 1989; **141**: 248–53.

23 McConnell JD, Barry MJ, Bruskewitz RC *et al*. *Benign Prostatic Hyperplasia: Diagnosis and Treatment. Clinical Practice Guidelines*, No 8. AHCPR Publication No. 94–0582. Rockville, MD: Agency for Health Care Policy and Research, Public Health Service, US Department of Health and Human Services 1994.

24 Holtgrewe HL. Transurethral prostatectomy. In: Lepor H (ed) *Urologic Clinics of North America*, Vol. 22, No. 2. Philadelphia: WB Saunders 1995; 357–68.

25 Abrams P, Blaivas J, Griffiths D *et al*. The objective evaluation of bladder outflow obstruction (urodynamics). In: Cockett A, Aso Y, Chatelain C *et al*. (eds) *The 2nd International Consultation on Benign Prostatic Hyperplasia (BPH), Paris, France, 1993 June 27–30*. Jersey: Scientific Communications International 1993; 151–209.

26 McConnell J. Why pressure flow studies should be optional and not mandatory for evaluating men with benign prostatic hyperplasia. *Urology* 1994; **44**: 156–8.

27 Craigen A, Hickling J, Saunders C *et al*. Natural history of prostatic obstruction. *J R Coll Gen Pract* 1969; **18**: 226–32.

28 *US Decennial Life Tables. State Life Tables*, Vol 1 ALMO 2 MT-WY. *Life Expectancy; Mortality (U.S.)*, PHS 90–1151. Hyattsville, MD: US Department of Health and Human Services, Public Health Service, National Center for Health Statistics 1990.

Socioeconomics and Trends in the Management of Benign Prostatic Hyperplasia: European Perspective

4

B. Standaert and L. Denis

INTRODUCTION

As defined in other chapters, benign prostatic hyperplasia (BPH) is a common, chronic disease mainly affecting the aging man in the western world.[1]

Benign prostatic hyperplasia may cause several complications including acute retention, bladder decompensation, hydronephrosis, and urinary tract infections. These, in turn, may lead to irreversible bladder and kidney damage.[2]

It is unclear, however, how these events are being avoided when treating BPH. A man suffering from obstruction is likely to be at risk of these complications if no therapy is given. Today, it is difficult to measure appropriately the individual risk at the moment the patient seeks medical advice for his lower urinary tract symptoms (LUTS). No clear working definition of BPH is yet available, although attempts have been made by different international working groups during the last decade.[3] These attempts have resulted in definition proposals that still lack the necessary sensitivity and specificity.[4]

The availability of a clear-cut definition for BPH is, however, a prerequisite for managing the disease efficiently. A good description would enable us to test values of variables that at certain levels would identify patients at risk of complications related to BPH. These complications could be avoided with preventive treatment. Today, mixed feelings remain on "over"-diagnosing and "over"-treatment. Often when the new treatment is applied, only part of the problem, such as symptom relief, is resolved, while the bladder outflow obstruction remains.[5]

The International Consultation Meetings organized by the International Consultation on Urological Diseases (ICUD) revealed that at least three properties summarize well the clinical definition of BPH: symptoms of "prostatism", enlargement of the prostate gland, and bladder outflow obstruction.[3] It reflects the entities of subjective, objective, and physiological effects of the disease. Moreover, these workshops have also highlighted that BPH and "prostatism" should not be used for the clarification of the symptoms that a patient has when his prostate gland is enlarged.[6] BPH is a pathological and not a clinical description of the disease entity, and "prostatism" is not specific for prostate-related complaints. New terms are now being used, such as LUTS, "voiding", and "storage" symptoms instead of "irritative" and "obstructive" symptoms. The former may outline better what is going on with the patient.

The symptoms, the prostate enlargement and the obstruction of the bladder outflow, may appear independently from each other or in combination. Very weak correlations have been found between the reported symptoms and prostate enlargement or between the symptoms and the bladder outlet obstruction.[7] Therefore, when conducting epidemiological surveys, one may investigate the symptoms and signs supposedly related to BPH, measure the enlargement of the prostate gland with digital rectal examination (DRE) or transrectal ultrasonography (TRUS), and observe the decrease in urine flow rate with electronic devices. This represents a huge effort, which does not always procure the epidemiological benefit that is sought.[8]

Additionally, when the treatment of BPH management is investigated, the variety of treatment options range from drug treatment to non-invasive devices. Some of these treatments focus on the effect of symptom relief, others on obstruction relief. As a result of the wide variation in treatment possibilities, a worldwide search to identify potential candidates for specific types of treatment has taken place.[9]

Cross-sectional and small cohort studies at the community level and in selected, clinic-based environments have been published during the past 10 years, mentioning that BPH is an importantly underreported disease.[10] A shift was also observed regarding the evaluation of the treatment effect. The main trend in clinical research is from risk reduction for acute complications toward an increase in the level of quality of life (QoL) of the BPH sufferers. New questionnaires have therefore been developed that investigate not only the symptoms and signs of BPH, but also the degree of bother caused by the symptoms reported.[11] The latter effect is then investigated and related to the QoL level of the patient. It is important to note that, so far, these instruments have not been validated regarding the value of their scores as clinical, objective parameters.[12]

The international community of experts is aware of these weaknesses, which make today's BPH disease management a difficult task. The physician is not always certain of treating patient in the most efficient way. The authorities, most of which in Europe subsidize the health care systems, do not know whether they reimburse treatment procedures that prevent important complications or only increase the QoL of some patients. Thus, the patient will have to pay "out of pocket" in some settings, depending on local health policy, in order obtain treatment for his LUTS.

We report here on the studies that have investigated the magnitude of the BPH problem in Europe. An overview will be given of what has been reported so far in the change of treatment patterns of BPH during the past decade in a number of European countries. We also discuss the limited possibility of comparing data between the different countries in Europe, where the organization of the health care systems may differ considerably.

THE MAGNITUDE OF THE PROBLEM

At least two levels concerning the magnitude of the BPH problem in Europe could be investigated.

The first is related to the collection of countrywide annual data of specific diagnostic tests and of treatment interventions related to BPH. These data procure an overall, rough estimate of the BPH problem in a country and, related to it, the money spent on resolving it. The data are, however, insufficiently representative to give a clear picture of the disease's prevalence in a country.

The second approach concerns the collection of more specific data regarding symptoms, prostate enlargement measurements, and/or urine flow measurements. This may occur in specific health care settings or at the community level. Most data regarding urine flow measurements are gathered during prostate cancer screening trials, as recently occurred in the Netherlands and in Belgium.[7,13] The collection of both sorts of data, at the community level and in hospital settings, is important, as it may be of interest to observe the discrepancy between what comes to light in clinics and what is obscurely present in the community. In other words, the degree of "under"- or "over"-reporting of BPH as a particular health care problem is of interest. Also, the collection of normative, reference values, if the community study is unbiased, to which the clinic-based values could be referred is warranted if no absolute reference value exists. This could, for instance, be the case for the symptom scores reported for BPH.

COUNTRYWIDE DATA

So far, national data in Europe regarding BPH specific medical intervention strategies have been reported in the *Proceedings of the International Consultation on BPH*.[3,14,15] Tables 4.1–4.3 summarize the kind of information collected during these sessions.

Table 4.1 presents the health care spending in different European countries for 1995. Table 4.2 reports the number of urologists available in those countries in 1993–95. Table 4.3 reports the trends in transurethral resection of the prostate (TURP) performed over periods of 3–4 years in some of the countries.

Health care spending varies considerably among the different countries in Europe, from 6.4% of the gross domestic product (GDP) in Denmark to 10.4% in Germany.[16] Moreover, it may also be surprising to consider the different number of urologists available in those countries and the different rates of TURPs performed per country per 1000 men aged 55 years and over.

Country	Total expenditure on health as % of GDP	Total expenditure on health per capita in US$ (PPP[a])
Austria	7.9	1634
Belgium	8	1665
Denmark	6.4	1370
France	9.9	1975
Germany	10.4	2136
Netherlands	8.8	1731
Spain	7.6	1088
Sweden	7.2	1353
UK	6.9	1237

[a]PPP purchasing power parity

Table 4.1 Health care spending for different countries in Europe (OECD 1995)
Source: © OECD 1995

Country	One urologist per number of men aged >55 years
Belgium	34,000
Denmark	37,500
France	65,000
Germany	31,000
Netherlands	36,000
UK	250,000

Table 4.2 Urological manpower in some countries in Europe, 1993–95

Country	1990	1993
Belgium	11	12
Netherlands	12.7	13.1
Sweden	11	7.8
UK	5.9	6

Table 4.3 Rates of TURPs performed for BPH in 1990 and 1993 per 1000 men aged 55 and over

The data perfectly illustrate the well-known phenomenon that the health care activities performed in a country reflect a situation that is more complex than just the simple medical answer to a health care problem. The real needs and the demands of the health care problem are not always adequately covered. The medical care delivered is the result of a complex and entangled interaction of different issues. These issues concern the availability and accessibility of medical resources or facilities in a country, linked to the perception of what the health care problems mean for the community and for the health care providers, clustered into the frame of the disease prevalence under study.[17]

The following example illustrates well the dynamic process of this phenomenon applied to BPH. It concerns a data review of the Belgian situation over a 10-year period,

1985–96.[18] The number of urologists available per 100,000 men aged 55 years and over is compared with the population at risk and the rate of TURPs performed among the population at risk.

Figure 4.1 depicts first a steep rise in the number of TURPs performed per year from 1985 until 1993. This rise does not follow the slower trend increase of the potential target population over a same period. After 1993, a spectacular fall in the number of TURPs can be observed, despite the continuous increase in both the number of urologists arriving on the market and the target population.

Several factors may explain these spectacular changes in trends within this decade. One factor is the availability of new treatment options for BPH on the Belgian market since the early 1990s. Another factor is the market compensation reaction after a period of "over"-consumption during previous years. What matters more is that the average number of TURPs performed per urologist is now decreasing. It leaves a group of surgeons with less experience in operational skills for patients who, when submitted to TURP, are more likely to be exposed to an increased risk of complications.

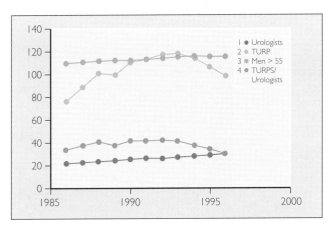

Figure 4.1 Trend lines of numbers of urologists available per 100,000 men aged >55 years (1); TURP performed per 10,000 men aged >55 years (2); the number of men aged >55 years (× 10,000); (3) average TURP performed per urologist per year in Belgium (1985–96) (4)

Source: RIZIV–INAMI, Ministry of Public Health, Belgium. *Annual Activity Reports*, 1985–1996. Belgium: Brussels

COUNTRY SPECIFIC

In a disease like BPH, where symptoms and "bothersomeness" scores may reflect the subjective importance of the health problem a man experiences, cultural differences may explain the differences observed in reporting BPH complaints among countries. One may need, therefore, to compare the results of the "in-depth" investigations of BPH symptom scores and of prostate gland measurements that have taken place recently in different community settings in Europe. Table 4.4 gives an overview of symptom scores regarding moderate and severe complaints reported from Scotland, France, Denmark, Belgium, and the Netherlands for the different age groups considered.[7,13,19–21] All the studies

Source	Age ≤ 59	Age 60–69	Age ≥ 70
Garaway *et al*. 1991, Scotland[19]	24	43	40
Sagnier *et al*. 1995, France[20]	8	14	27
Sommer *et al*. 1990, Denmark[21]	18	23	
Bosch *et al*. 1995, Netherlands[22]	25	29	35
Standaert *et al*. 1997, Belgium[13]	17	27	28

Table 4.4 Age-specific prevalence rates of symptom scores in men with moderate-to-severe complaints in different countries in Europe (%)

were performed at the community level on men who were not treated for prostate diseases. It is important to note that different questionnaires were used to measure the symptom scores. The results suggest that important differences exist between the countries investigated if no sample bias is present in the studies performed. Moreover, it may be concluded that age is a determinant factor for the increase in the reported BPH complaints, and that the percentage of complaints in the population is much higher than the percentage of medical interventions performed so far for BPH.

The next question, then, is what clinical value should be given to these symptom scores registered? Is a patient with a moderate-to-high score on a symptom questionnaire susceptible to being more at risk for acute diseases potentially caused by BPH, or should this selection be more focused?

In that respect Bosch and co-workers in Rotterdam did an interesting analysis.[22] They investigated a series of test combinations to identify clinical BPH in a community population free of prostate cancer and free of treatment for BPH. Their starting points were twofold.

The first was to use cut-off points of variables that could easily be investigated in clinical practice. The second was that the test combination should discriminate different rates of BPH among the different age groups considered. In other words, a combination of tests that could not identify an increased trend of BPH with increasing age was rejected.

The selected cut-off points of the variables used to suspect a man of BPH had the following values:

- on the International Prostate Symptom Score (IPSS) questionnaire that evaluated the symptom scores, a score >7 points on a scale of 0–35 points;
- the prostate volume measured with TRUS was a prostate gland >30 cm^3;
- the Q_{max} value for urine flow measurement evaluated with a portable electronic device was <15 mL s^{-1};
- the residual urine volume in the bladder measured by suprapubic echography was >50 mL.

Table 4.5 shows the results of some combinations of applied tests. There is a spectacular decrease in the percentage of patients that are susceptible to having BPH when more than two tests are combined: from 35% in the older age group, when only symptom scores were considered, to a rate as low as 8% if strict criteria were applied with at least four selection variables.

Test	N	Age (years)			
		55–59	60–64	65–69	70–74
A	494	9	20	19	27
B	494	6	16	14	17
C	326	5	2	9	13
D	326	1	2	3	8

A Volume >30 cm^3 + IPSS >7 + Q$_{max}$ <15 mL s^{-1}
B Volume >30 cm^3 + IPSS >7 + Q$_{max}$ <10 mL s^{-1}
C Volume >30 cm^3 + IPSS >7 + Q$_{max}$ <15 mL s^{-1} + PVR >50 mL
D Volume >30 cm^3 + IPSS >7 + Q$_{max}$ <10 mL s^{-1} + PVR >50 mL

Table 4.5 Percent of men with positive test results over different age groups with different test combinations

Source: Adapted from Bosch JLHR, Hop WCJ, Kirkel WJ, Schröder FH. *Natural history of benign prostatic hyperplasia: appropriate case definition and estimation of its prevalence in the community. Urology* 1995; 46: 34–46, with permission from Elsevier Science

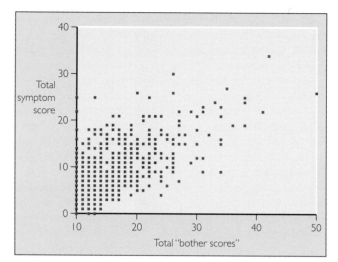

Figure 4.2 Plotted values of "bother scores" and symptom scores of 1419 men aged 55–74 years in Antwerp, using the modified IPSS questionnaire. Each of the 10 symptoms has a score range from 0 to 4; Each bothersome value on each symptom has a score range from 1 to 5

Source: Standaert B, Denis L. *Reports on the Prostate Disease Screening Studies in Antwerp.* Brussels, Belgium: Flemish Ministry of Public Health 1993–97

These figures, however, are more in line with what is clinically performed as frequent medical interventions for BPH. But as the authors correctly point out in their conclusion, these study results are "open-ended", because no follow-up information has been reported about who has requested a work-up and a treatment for BPH. Therefore, it is difficult to state correctly what the true rates of BPH are in a population, as long as no clear figures are obtained regarding the man who needs or will seek treatment, after establishing selection criteria of those suitable for it.

Are the symptom questionnaires useless then, or how should we appreciate them? It is interesting to note that the symptom scores correlate well with the "bothersomeness" scores the patients declared. In a study performed in Antwerp (Belgium) where 1419 men aged 55–74 were interviewed with a modified International Prostate Symptom Score (IPSS) questionnaire, the Pearson correlation coefficient between symptom scores and "bothersomeness" scores was 0.69 ($P<0.001$).[13] It indicates that if the patient reports a severe symptom, it bothers him equally badly and vice versa.

That conclusion is also well illustrated in Figure 4.2, where the values of the "bother scores" are plotted against the symptom scores. Moreover, the symptom weighted "bother scores" of the same group of men are also well linked to the only QoL question of the IPSS questionnaire (Spearman correlation coefficient=0.52 ($P<0.001$)) (see

Table 4.6). But again, the QoL figures measured cannot in a representative way be compared with the QoL situations of other health care problems. The QoL scores of IPSS have a stand-alone value that is only related to the situation of BPH. It is to be hoped that better-validated instruments will soon be available that measure the QoL and the symptom score of each relevant and specific clinical BPH situation. What has been produced so far, however, is the first step in elucidating a BPH puzzle that seems more complex than at first thought.

SUMMARY

One may conclude that the magnitude of the BPH problem investigated so far in Europe, based on the criteria most frequently employed in the literature, is equivalent to the numbers reported elsewhere in the western world.[1] We must also be aware of a cultural component regarding the symptom scores reported in different countries.

But it is hard to see the relevance of what has been measured.[10] Men became patients who, in the past, were unaware that they might be sick. They should now seek

IPSS	0	1	2	3	4	5	6
Low	296 (83%)	452 (77%)	156 (43%)	12 (13%)			
Moderate	58 (16%)	130 (22%)	171 (47%)	48 (51%)	9 (51%)		
Severe	2 (0.6%)	3 (0.5%)	34 (9%)	34 (36%)	8 (49%)	2 (100%)	2 (100%)
Total	356 (25%)	585 (41%)	361 (25%)	94 (6%)	17 (1%)	2 (0.1%)	2 (01.%)

Table 4.6 Distribution of 1419 men aged 55–74 years reporting their "bothersomeness" scores weighted with their symptom scores over the different QoL scales of the IPSS questionnaires (Fisher exact test P <0.001)

Source: Standaert B, Denis L. *Reports on the Prostate Disease Screening Studies in Antwerp.* Brussels, Belgium: Flemish Ministry of Public Health 1993–97

medical advice and treatment for their BPH-related complaints. The authorities see their health care budgets rising and spend large amounts of money on a disease that evades definition, classification and, hence, correct treatment. Finally, the health care provider's role has changed from a specialist confronted with urgent urological problems that, in the past, needed adequate and clear medical care. Now he has become a regulating force of delicate situations weighing prevention against cure and assessing risk of BPH based on insufficiently solid criteria, such as symptom scores and uroflow measurements.

Measurements carried out during the last decade have helped in discovering a hidden and neglected health care problem amongst elderly men. The approach has, however, insufficiently tackled the real focus of BPH: to obtain a clear definition of the disease, which under certain circumstances should be avoided with adequate treatment measures.

DISEASE MANAGEMENT

Only a few papers in the literature report global country-specific data covering the management and evolution of the BPH treatment in Europe. These data are from Sweden, UK, Austria, the Netherlands, and Belgium. Other information collected about the European situation is related to cost evaluations of clinical trials that compare new with only a few treatment options over a limited period of time. As the duration of these trials is too short for a correct evaluation of the treatment effect of BPH, the trial results are modeled into decision trees that procure insight into future prospects. We will not report on these studies, because the data are only partial. They do not reflect the "evidence based" medical practice of BPH management in the countries where the trials are conducted. However, study of this literature, which contains valuable information on unit cost and resource use in particular countries related to the management of BPH is recommended.[23,24]

SWEDEN

The data on Sweden are interesting for many reasons. The authors studied countrywide data over a period of at least 8 years (1987–94).[25] During that period, less-invasive treatment options than TURP were introduced on to the Swedish market, such as transurethral microwave therapy (TUMT) and medical treatment.

Until the introduction of 5α-reductase (SAR) agents and the α-blocker agent therapy in 1992, there was a slight annual increase in the treatment budget for BPH, while the target population remained constant. After that, a budget decrease was observed, which can be explained by the decrease in surgery that resulted in less in-hospital care and fewer procedures in ambulatory care (Figure 4.3). Drug costs increased rapidly, but in 1994 the direct costs for BPH accounted for only 0.3% of the total direct health care costs and for 8.6% of the direct costs for urogenital diseases in Sweden. Compared with TUMT, which disappeared as rapidly from the market as it appeared, the drug therapy is a success story. Facility of evaluation, not complex in

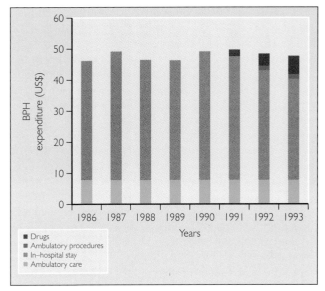

Figure 4.3 Total direct medical cost from 1987 to 1994 (million US$, 1994 prices) in Sweden

Source: Blomqvist P, Ekbom A, Carlsson P *et al.* Benign prostatic hyperplasia in Sweden 1987 to 1994: changing patterns of treatment, changing patterns of costs. *Urology* 1997; **50**(2): 214–20, with permission of Elsevier Science.

administration, reduced risk, compatible with the current set of treatment values, and lower initial costs are elements facilitating the introduction of "product"-based treatments on the market. This is in contrast to "procedure"-based treatment, such as TUMT or laser therapy.

Also reported by the authors is the suspicion that a wider range of men aged 55 years and over is now reached and offered treatment for BPH since the introduction of the drug therapy on the market. Additional to that is the shift of physicians treating patients with BPH complaints. With the drug therapy on the market, the general practitioner is now also likely to be consulted by the target population. What is missing in the Swedish report is the long-term evaluation of these market changes, and an evaluation of the indirect cost benefit after the introduction of the drugs on the market. Systematic follow-up is a prerequisite for correctly estimating the true benefit of the new treatments once they appear on the market.[26]

UNITED KINGDOM

Indirect cost estimates of BPH disease that reflect the cost of loss in production due to disease disability have been estimated by Drummond and co-workers for the UK for the year 1990.[27] These calculations were part of a study that estimated total cost related to BPH in the UK, including direct, indirect, and intangible costs. The latter are, however, very difficult to value in money and were not reported. But as the Swedish data mentioned, the data from the UK estimated that the direct medical cost for treating BPH in the UK, including primary care and hospital care, represents a maximum of 0.4% of the total health care budget of the

NHS spent in 1990. Compared with other common, chronic diseases, such as arthritis, Parkinson's disease, or depression, these cost estimates for BPH are on the low side of the NHS budget. Only the treatment of migraine in the UK has lower cost figures compared with BPH (£23 million vs. £67 million). The estimate of the indirect cost ranged from £3 million to £14 million. This wide cost range is explained by the method of indirect cost calculation. The lower range included only the public expenditure, while the upper value also estimated the loss in production time of the people being treated surgically for BPH. These cost figures represent 5–15% of the total measurable treatment cost of BPH in the UK in 1990.

Also interesting about the UK is the study of Vale and co-workers, who tried to compare the cost effectiveness of different treatment procedures available for BPH in their hospital (St Mary's Hospital, London).[28] As an effect measure of the treatment intervention, they evaluated two parameters. One is the cost per unit of milliliters per second increase in the Q_{max}, and the other is the cost per unit of percentage reduction in the symptom scores. Surprisingly, the two cost-effectiveness measures calculated for the different treatment options selected do not follow a parallel course (Figure 4.4). What is most cost effective in the symptom score is therefore not most cost effective when evaluating the urine flow of the patient. This presents the physician with a difficult dilemma: should he/she first treat the symptoms and then the obstruction or vice versa? In his discussion, Vale points out the difficulties in assembling correctly the unit costs for the different treatment procedures considered, as well as what effect measure should adequately represent the obstruction in the case of BPH. For instance, one may criticize the selection of his effect measures as short-term evaluations, not including the long-term failure

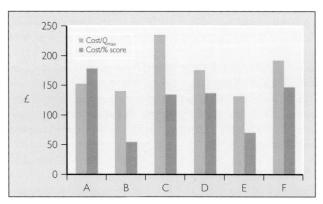

Figure 4.4 Comparison of two cost-effectiveness measures for different treatment options in BPH. A TURP; B transurethral microwave treatment (Leo); C transurethral microwave treatment (Prostatron); D visual laser ablation of the prostate; E terazosin (5 mg day⁻¹ for 1 year); F finasteride (for 1 year). The cost-effectiveness values of the symptom scores are multiplied by a constant factor 10 in order to facilitate comparison between all the measurements

Source: With permission from Yale JA, Bdesha AS, Witherow RON. An analysis of the costs of alternative treatments for benign prostatic hypertrophy. *J R Soc Med* 1995; **83**: 644–8

rates that could be present among the drug therapies and the newer, less-invasive device therapies.

AUSTRIA

The Austrian data review published in 1993 concerns the report of the direct medical cost for 1990 of hospital care expenses related to BPH. A total of 9742 new BPH sufferers were treated that year in hospital care.[29] That number represents 1.3% of the total morbidity of BPH estimated for Austria. The authors believe there is a huge underreporting of the burden of illness related to BPH in Austria due to a lack of adequate information. It is interesting to note that with these precise numbers of patients being treated for BPH in Austria in 1990, the country arrives at a 25% lower rate of surgical intervention for BPH compared with Belgium, which has the same number of population at risk.

THE NETHERLANDS

The study conducted in 1992–94 by the University of Rotterdam concerns the collection of data for 670 new patients aged 50 years and over with BPH complaints, in 12 different urologic centers in the Netherlands.[30]

The variation in diagnostic tests used and in the treatment offered to the patients was the object of the study. An explanation for the observed variation was related to the patient selection as well as to characteristics of the treating urologist, such as age, degree of experience, and the type of hospital where he was practicing. The most applied diagnostic tests with the least variation among the centers were DRE, blood, and urine tests.

In contrast, a huge variation was observed in all other tests used, such as uroflow measurement, echography of the bladder and the prostate, cystoscopy, intravenous urography (IVU), and urodynamic evaluation. The variation ranged from 35% for urodynamic evaluation up to 90% for echography of the prostate.

The best explanation for the variation in the used diagnostic tests was whether the patient was an emergency case, and the amount of experience the physician had. The more experienced he was, the less likely the specialist would use the echography of the prostate gland, but he would be more willing to use the echography of the kidney.

Regarding the selection of the treatment that was applied, here also a wide variation could be observed among the centers, although it was less pronounced compared with the variation in diagnostic tests used. The variation could usually be explained by the degree of observed bladder outflow obstruction. A higher degree resulted in a lower treatment variation. Moreover, in the case of less severe obstruction, the more experienced physician would prefer to follow a watchful waiting strategy instead of using drug therapy, except for the use of finasteride. The latter could be explained by the fact that the use of the drug has limited but clear indications.

From the study results, it is clear that not only is the variation in disease management of BPH patient specific, like the severity of the symptoms, but also the physician's characteristics as well as the hospital setting may play a role. The authors conclude that having management guidelines available for BPH in the Netherlands is no guarantee that the management variation of the disease will therefore be reduced. Many factors play a role, of which the most important one is the regular introduction of new tools for achieving diagnosis and treatment of the BPH patient. More diagnostic and treatment options will invariably cause greater management variation.

BELGIUM

An investigation of the diagnosis and treatment of BPH by the urologists in Belgium was performed in 1994 through a mailed questionnaire.[31] Urologists in Belgium represent 1.7% ($N=280$ for 1994) of all the practicing specialists. Some 130 urologists (47%) responded to the double mailing organized by the Provincial Institute of Hygiene in Antwerp.

Regarding the diagnostic tests normally used, the symptom questionnaires was limited to 35% of the physicians interviewed, as was the IPSS. About 60% responded that they never took it. These data are in contrast with other countries, such as the USA and/or Denmark, which report a lower application of the questionnaires. Positive correlations were observed between the use of the questionnaire, the age of the physician, and the size of his practice ($P<0.0001$). Compared with his colleague in the Netherlands, the Belgian urologist is more likely to use echography of the prostate and less cystoscopy (Table 4.7).

As in the Netherlands, a huge variation is observed in the type and numbers of tests used for defining the diagnosis of BPH. Of the Belgian urologists, 50% employ at least four to five diagnostic tests per case to define the disease and its status. However, regarding treatment of BPH, their handling seems to be more clearly defined, depending on the type of patient (Table 4.8). Despite the fact that reimbursement of drug therapy for BPH in Belgium is still

	A	B	C
Patient (<55 years) and IPSS >7 ≤17	66	33	1
Patient (≥55 years) and IPSS >7 ≤17	23	72	5
Patient (<55 years) and IPSS >17	2	53	45
Patient (≥55 years) and IPSS >17	–	5	95

A watchful waiting; B drug therapy; C TURP

Table 4.8 Response rates of the Belgian urologists regarding what treatment they may select when confronted with four types of patients (Fisher exact test: 431, P <0.001) (%)

Source: Standaert B, Van Loon J. *Evaluation of Health Care Practices of Urologists in Belgium 1994. Report*. Antwerp, Belgium: Provincial Institute of Hygiene 1995: 1–32

not accomplished, drugs such as α-blockers, which could also be prescribed for hypertension, gain market share. The use of other treatment devices, such as laser therapy, is limited. The urological world in Belgium is, in this respect, rather conservative. Belgium is, therefore, in comparison with other small countries in Europe, not different regarding its disease management of BPH. The market is, however, confronted with two problems. Drug therapy for BPH is not yet reimbursed, and an important reduction in surgical interventions has been observed during the last few years, which is not explained by a reduction in the numbers of urologists on the market or by a decrease in the target population. This raises the question of whether the "surplus" in urologists will make efficient management of the disease affordable in this particular market?

CONCLUSION

Disease management of patients presenting BPH-related symptoms varies in the different countries in Europe. However, the severity of BPH is, in general, measured through symptom scores and urine flow measurements. Although the former does not always happen systematically, the latter sometimes causes difficulties in interpreting the results correctly. Physicians will therefore do additional testing. They will not limit the evaluation to one problem, one test, one result, one diagnosis. Moreover, the treatment applied to a patient with the same sort of BPH problem may also vary among countries, and among hospital settings in the same country. One explanation for that difference is that the patient's requirement for medical intervention after the onset of his symptoms could be individually determined. The way he will respond to his treatment seems also individually dependent. Some patients will benefit more from relieving the obstruction, others from care of the symptoms.

If all these forms of variability are a fact, is it then still possible to identify parameters that predict patients at risk for the different outcomes considered including a substantial decrease in QoL and/or a reduction in the risk for acute complications, such as retention and hydronephrosis? In other words, can one reconsider the problem of BPH as a

Test	Netherlands	Belgium[a]
DRE	97.9	98
Blood test	92.3	95
Urine test	86.6	75
Uroflow	84.4	57.7
Echography bladder	72.1	
Echography prostate	48.6	74
Cystoscopy	51	33
Echography kidney	46.9	36
Rx abdomen	30.8	
IVP	23	23
Urodynamic evaluation	14	5

[a]In the Belgian survey, the application of Rx abdomen and echography of the bladder were not asked for

Table 4.7 Comparison of the routine use of diagnostic tests for BPH between the Netherlands and Belgium among urologists (%)

Source: Standaert B, Van Loon J. *Evaluation of Health Care Practices of Urologists in Belgium 1994. Report*. Antwerp, Belgium: Provincial Institute of Hygiene 1995: 1–32

disease to be classified in different entities with specific profiles on which a therapy could be tailored accordingly?

It is an option that one should really consider when there are so many different diagnostic tools and therapeutic options available. It could then encourage efficient disease management of BPH that will support the physician, the authorities, and the patient. The latter is usually insufficiently informed, and he is not aware of what is going on in himself, his prostate gland, and his health. "Over"-diagnosis and "over"-treatment should be avoided, certainly in an age group that is already targeted for the consumption of so many different therapies.

REFERENCES

1 Napalkov P, Maisonneuve P, Boyle P. Worldwide patterns of prevalence and mortality from benign prostatic hyperplasia. *Urology* 1995; **46**(Suppl 3A): 41–6.

2 Ekman P. Outcome studies in begnin prostatic hyperplasia. In: Chisholm G (ed) *Handbook on Benign Prostatic Hyperplasia*. New York: Raven Press 1994; 137–52.

3 Cockett ATK, Khoury S, Aso Y *et al*. (eds) *The 3rd International Consultation on Benign Prostatic Hyperplasia (BPH) Monaco, 1995, June 26–28*. Jersey: Scientific Communication International 1996.

4 Guess HA. Population studies in benign prostatic hyperplasia. *Prospectives* 1993; **2**(2): 1–4.

5 Kirk D. How should new treatments for benign prostatic hyperplasia be assessed?: symptomatic measurements are not enough. *BMJ* 1993; **306**: 1283–4.

6 Abrams P. New words for old: lower urinary tract symptoms for prostatism. *BMJ* 1994; **308**: 929–30.

7 Bosch JLHR, Hop WCJ, Kirkels WJ, Schröder FH. The IPSS in a community-based sample of men between 55 and 74 years of age. *Br J Urol* 1995; **75**(5): 622–30.

8 McKelvie GB, Collins GN, Hehir M, Rogers AC. A study of BPH: challenge to British urology. *Br J Urol* 1993; **71**(1): 38–42.

9 Peeling WB. Patient selection and evaluation. In: Chisholm G (ed) *Handbook on Benign Prostatic Hyperplasia*. New York: Raven Press 1994; 53–72.

10 Barry MJ, Boyle P, Fourcroy J *et al*. Epidemiology and natural history of BPH. In: Cockett ATK, Khoury S, Aso Y *et al*. (eds) *The 3rd International Consultation on Benign Prostatic Hyperplasia (BPH), Monaco, 1995, June 26–28*. Jersey: Scientific Communication International 1996; 21–36.

11 Mebust WK, Ackerman R, MJ Barry, *et al*. Symptom evaluation, QoL and sexuality. In: Cockett ATK, Khoury S, Aso Y *et al*. (eds) *The 3rd International Consultation on Benign Prostatic Hyperplasia (BPH), Monaco, 1995, June 26–28*. Jersey: Scientific Communication International 1996; 257–61.

12 Barry MJ. The BPH impact index. In: Cockett ATK, Khoury S, Aso Y *et al*. (eds) *The 3rd International Consultation on Benign Prostatic Hyperplasia (BPH), Monaco, 1995, June 26–28*. Jersey: Scientific Communication International 1996; 275–6.

13 Standaert B, Denis L. *Reports on the Prostate Disease Screening Studies in Antwerp*. Brussels, Belgium: Flemish Ministry of Public Health 1993–97.

14 Holtgrewe L, Ackerman R, Bay-Nielsen H *et al*. *The economics of BPH*. In: Cockett ATK, Aso Y, Chatelain C *et al*. (eds) *The International Consultation on BPH, Paris, 1991, June 26–27*. Jersey, Scientific Communication International 1991; 26–27.

15 Holtgrewe L, Ackerman R, Bay-Nielsen H *et al*. The economics of BPH. In: Cockett ATK, Khoury S, Aso Y *et al*. (eds) *The 2nd International Consultation on Bening Prostatic Hyperplasia (BPH), Paris, 1993; 27–30 June*. Jersey: Scientific Communication International 1994; 35–45.

16 OECD Health Data 96. *A Software for the Comparative Analysis of 27 Health Systems*. Paris, France 1996.

17 Wagstaff A, Van Doorslaer E. Equity in the delivery of health care: methods and findings. In: Van Doorslear E, Wagstaff A, Rutten F (eds) *Equity in the Finance and Delivery of Health Care*. New York: Oxford Medical Press 1993; 49–87.

18 RIZIV–INAMI, Ministry of Public Health, Belgium. *Annual Activity Reports, 1985–1996*. Belgium: Brussels.

19 Garraway WM, Collins GN, Lee RJ. High prevalence of benign prostatic hypertrophy in the community. *Lancet* 1991; **338**: 469–71.

20 Sagnier PP, MacFarlane G, Teillac P *et al*. Impact of symptoms of prostatism on the level of bother and QoL of men in the French Community. *J Urol* 1995; **153**: 669–73.

21 Sommer P, Nielsen KK, Bauer T *et al*. Voiding patterns in men evaluated by a questionnaire survey. *Br J Urol* 1990; **65**: 155–60.

22 Bosch JL, Hop WC, Kirkels WJ, Schroeder FH. Natural history of benign prostatic hyperplasia: appropriate case definition and estimation of its prevalence in the community? *Urology* 1995; **46**(3): 34–40.

23 Baladi JF, Menon D, Otten N. An economic evaluation of finasteride for treatment of benign prostatic hyperplasia. *Pharm Econ* 1996; **9**(5): 443–54.

24 Lowe F, McDaniel RL, Chmiel JJ, Hillman AL. Economic modeling to assess the costs of treatment with finasteride, terazosin, and TUP for men with moderate to severe symptoms of BPH. *Urology* 1995; **46**: 477–83.

25 Blomqvist P, Ekbom A, Carlsson P *et al*. Benign prostatic hyperplasia in Sweden 1987 to 1994: changing patterns of treatment, changing patterns of costs. *Urology* 1997; **50**(2): 214–20.

26 Kortt MA, Bootman JL. The economics of benign prostatic hyperplasia treatment: a literature review. *Clin Ther* 1996; **18**(6): 1227–41.

27 Drummond MF, McGuire AJ, Black NA *et al*. Economic burden of treated benign prostatic hyperplasia in the United Kingdom. *Br J Urol* 1993; **71**(3): 290–6.

28 Vale JA, Bdesha AS, Witherow RON. An analysis of the costs of alternative treatments for benign prostatic hypertrophy. *J R Soc Med* 1995; **83**: 644–8.

29 Schwarz B, Vutuc C, Kunze M. Gesundheitsoekonomische Aspecte der benignen prostatahyperplasie in Osterreich. *Wien Med Wochenschr* 1993; **143**(22): 571–3.

30 Stoevelaar HJ, Beek C Van De, Casparie AF *et al*. Variatie in diagnostiek van benigne prostaathyperplasie in de urologische praktijk. *Ned Tijdschr Geneeskd* 1996; **140**(15): 837–42.

31 Standaert B, Van Loon J. *Evaluation of Health Care Practices of Urologists in Belgium 1994. Report*. Antwerp, Belgium: Provincial Institute of Hygiene 1995: 1–32.

Health-related Quality of Life in Men with Benign Prostatic Hyperplasia

5

M.J. Barry and M.P. O'Leary

WHAT IS BENIGN PROSTATIC HYPERPLASIA?

Benign prostatic hyperplasia (BPH) is fundamentally a histologic condition commonly found among aging men worldwide. Based on data from autopsy studies, about 80% of men have some evidence of histologic BPH by the time they are in their 70s.[1] Remarkably, the histologic prevalence of BPH has been similar in autopsy studies of men from around the world, across many cultures and ethnicities.[2] In some men, through a poorly understood causal pathway, histologic BPH can lead to lower urinary tract symptoms (LUTS) and other BPH complications (such as acute urinary retention or obstructive uropathy) that can affect the health of the men who have it, giving this condition its morbidity, and a small but finite mortality. Without these manifestations, BPH would be more of a histologic curiosity than a disease.

Because material for histologic examination is not usually obtained in clinical and epidemiologic studies, because the mechanisms by which histologic BPH ultimately leads to LUTS have not been well delineated, and because other disease processes can cause or exacerbate LUTS (even in the presence of histologic BPH), there is no widely accepted working definition of "clinical BPH" for use in epidemiologic or clinical research.[3] Abrams has suggested reserving the term "benign prostatic hyperplasia" for the histologic condition, while using the terms "lower urinary tract symptoms", "benign prostatic enlargement", and "benign prostatic obstruction" to describe the clinical, anatomic, and physiologic manifestations of BPH, respectively (recognizing that other diseases besides BPH can produce LUTS).[4]

One problem with this terminology, which is certainly a step in the right direction, is that it tends to sacrifice sensitivity for specificity. Theoretically, the diagnosis of physiologic bladder outflow obstruction due to BPH can only be made using simultaneous recordings of intravesical pressure and uroflow. However, the cost and degree of invasiveness of these studies makes them impractical for epidemiologic research on large populations.[3] Indeed, most clinicians do not use these studies in day-to-day practice in the diagnosis of BPH for the same reasons. For example, in a survey of a nationwide random sample of urologists in the USA in 1995, 86% of respondents reported rarely or never using pressure-flow studies in the diagnosis of BPH.[5]

In fact, men aged 50 years and older with LUTS and a physician diagnosis of BPH, who undergo pressure-flow studies at referral centers are shown to be physiologically obstructed 60–80% of the time in recent studies,[6-11] with the higher proportions being reported in studies that exclude men with other conditions (especially neurologic diseases) that raise the probability of an alternative diagnosis, such as a primary hypocontractile bladder. The term "lower urinary tract symptoms" sounds too generic for men with such a relatively high likelihood of being physiologically obstructed, while, in truth, they have not yet been definitely proven to have bladder outlet obstruction. Many epidemiologic researchers and clinicians seem willing to sacrifice some specificity for sensitivity, preferring a term like "clinical BPH" for men with LUTS who would have a relatively high probability of bladder outlet obstruction if they underwent a pressure-flow study.

In addition, this discussion assumes that lower urinary symptoms are linked to the histologic process of BPH solely through the development of physiologic bladder outlet obstruction. The poor correlation of LUTS severity with the physiologic severity of bladder outlet obstruction, which will be reviewed subsequently, even among men that can be shown to be physiologically obstructed, makes this tight relationship unlikely. Moreover, while men who are physiologically obstructed have the best response of their LUTS to treatments aimed at reducing outflow obstruction, such as prostatectomy, similar men who do not appear to be physiologically obstructed often have been reported to have a satisfactory response to prostatectomy.[7,12-14] Although these responses may in part reflect a placebo effect, other explanations include false negative pressure-flow studies, reduction of symptoms by means other than reducing obstruction (such as heat injury to sensory afferent nerves in the prostate and bladder neck), or improvement in symptoms of a hypocontractile bladder through surgical "after-load reduction" even with normal outflow resistance preoperatively.

WHAT ARE THE GOALS OF TREATMENT FOR BENIGN PROSTATIC HYPERPLASIA

The uncertainty about the relationship between histologic BPH, benign prostatic enlargement, bladder outlet obstruction, and LUTS should not cause the reader to lose sight of the fact that it is the LUTS associated with BPH, along with the possibility of complications over time, that affect the health of men who have this condition. Men are treated to reduce their LUTS, or reduce the future risk of complications. Other outcomes, such as reduction in postvoid residual urine, or reduction in measurements of the severity of physiologic outflow obstruction, are not primary outcomes of treatment themselves, but potential intermediate steps toward what really matters to patients: reduction in symptoms and the risk of complications.

Since symptom severity can be measured directly, there is little reason to measure intermediate outcomes instead of symptom severity as an outcome of treatment. However, BPH complications such as acute urinary retention and obstructive uropathy are uncommon, and studies would have to be extraordinarily large to capture clinically important differences in these outcomes between arms. Measures of the physiologic severity of bladder outlet obstruction, such as peak urinary flow rates or pressure at peak flow, might be measured as a "proxy" for the probabilities of these complications; however, the relationship between physiologic severity and long-term complications has not been established in prospective studies.

WHAT IS HEALTH-RELATED QUALITY OF LIFE AND HOW IS IT MEASURED?

Some domains of quality of life that have been proposed include symptoms, functional status, role activities (work and household management), social functioning, emotional status, cognition, sleep and rest, energy and vitality, health perceptions, sexuality, and general life satisfaction. Health-related quality of life (HRQOL), or health status, encompasses not only disease state and the presence or absence of disabilities, but functional status (social and cognitive as well as physical performance), mental condition, and prognosis.[15]

With growing recognition that a disease and its treatments can affect not only the quantity but also the quality of life, measurements of HRQOL have been assuming increasing importance in clinical research and practice in recent years. Measurements of health status usually take the form of questionnaires that explore the different domains of health status of interest in that clinical situation. As the measurement of health status is a relatively new field, there is little consensus on exactly how best to measure it in a particular clinical situation or study.

In general, question sets exploring each topic are developed to generate scales that are intended to improve the psychometric properties of the measurement, its reliability, and validity.[16–18] Reliability simplistically means that the instrument being used is measuring something reproducible. Whether the instrument is actually measuring what it is intended to measure is the concept of validity. Multi-item scales are generally used because they can cover the different aspects of a particular domain of health status more thoroughly, and the effect of measurement error associated with each item is dampened when multiple items are considered together. The development of the optimal instrument for a particular purpose often involves making trade-offs between an instrument's length, which helps determine its comprehensiveness and reliability, and its burden for respondents, who may not tolerate completing a long questionnaire, particularly multiple times in follow-up.

The reliability of a multi-item scale is usually assessed in two ways: its internal consistency reliability and its test–retest reliability.[17,18] Internal consistency refers to the inter-correlation of the different items making up the scale. High levels of internal consistency reliability help ensure that irrelevant items not addressing that domain of health status are not included. Test–retest reliability helps ensure that reproducible results are obtained in stable patients over time. In general, longer questionnaires improve reliability measures, and when instruments are shortened to reduce respondent burden and eliminate redundancy, attention must be paid to any resulting deterioration in the scale's reliability.

Validity is more difficult to assess, as a "gold standard" assessment of what is intended to be measured is not often available.[17,18] Usually, investigators will want to be sure important concepts that are related to the health status domain of interest are covered ("construct" validity), through input from clinicians and, most importantly, patients. Then, one may examine correlations between an existing, "gold standard" instrument and a new, shorter, more practical instrument ("criterion" validity). More commonly, in the absence of a gold standard, the new measure will be correlated with other measures or categorizations, which would be hypothesized to relate in a certain way to the new measurement if it were indeed valid ("construct" validity). Of particular note, establishing the validity of an instrument in the absence of a gold standard is an ongoing process. Investigators or clinicians choosing an instrument should not simply ask themselves whether a particular scale has been validated, but how extensively it has been validated. "Validity" is really a continuous, rather than a dichotomous, variable.

Health status scales can be used for different purposes. Depending on the purpose, different aspects of reliability and validity assume greater or lesser importance. Kirshner and Guyatt have proposed that health status measures can be used for three purposes: discrimination, prediction, and evaluation.[19] Discriminative indices separate individuals on an underlying dimension when no gold standard exists (such as an "intelligence" test), and predictive instruments classify individuals into categories that can be confirmed with a gold standard test (such as the CAGE questionnaire for alcohol abuse). Evaluative instruments measure change over time in the health status domain of interest. In outcomes research focusing on disease prognosis and response to therapy, evaluative instruments are employed. Of note, specificity for the concept of interest is very important for discriminative and predictive instruments, but unimportant for evaluative instruments. On the other hand, responsiveness to change, while unimportant for discriminative and predictive instruments, is critical for evaluative instruments.[20]

DISEASE-SPECIFIC AND GENERIC MEASURES OF HEALTH STATUS

Disease-specific health status measurement scales are comprised of items that have relevance to patients with the disease or condition of interest. Questions usually explore disease symptoms, and the impact of those symptoms and the possibility of future disease progression on function, mental health, and perceptions of general health. Generic health status measurements, on the other hand, contain questions designed to be answered by anyone, regardless of their particular disease burden. These questions ask about function, mental health, general health perceptions, and other domains of health status directly. A number of these instruments are already in wide use, especially the Short Form Health Surveys arising from work related to the RAND Health Insurance Experiment and the subsequent Medical Outcomes Study.[21] Disease-specific instruments often allow a more intensive focus on how a particular disease affects health and may be more responsive than generic instruments when disease status changes; for example, in response to treatment. However, generic instruments allow comparisons of disease impact and the effect of treatment across conditions, and can allow the integration of the therapeutic and adverse affects of a treatment into a common currency. Because of the synergistic strengths of these two types of instruments, they are often combined in outcomes research studies.

BENIGN PROSTATIC HYPERPLASIA-SPECIFIC MEASURES OF HEALTH STATUS

Simplistically, one can outline a model relating different aspects of BPH to overall health status (Figure 5.1).[22] Through a poorly understood mechanism, the anatomic and physiologic changes in the lower urinary tract that can accompany the histologic process of prostatic hyperplasia, including increased outflow resistance and hypertrophy of

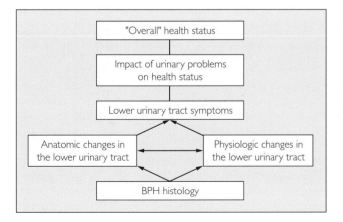

Figure 5.1 A conceptual model of the impact of BPH on health

Source: Adapted from Barry MJ, Fowler FJ. The methodology for evaluating the subjective outcomes of treatment for benign prostatic hyperplasia. *Adv Urol* 1993; **6**: 83–99, with permission

the detrusor muscle, can lead to the development of symptoms. These symptoms include a weak stream, hesitancy, intermittency, incomplete emptying, frequency, urgency, and nocturia. These LUTS can of course also be caused by other pathologic conditions of the lower urinary tract in the absence of BPH.

Although it makes pathophysiologic sense to categorize these symptoms as voiding and filling (or storage) symptoms, as suggested by Abrams,[4] our understanding of their genesis is poor enough that it may be best to avoid further splitting. The psychometric and urodynamic evidence for different categories of LUTS is relatively weak. In addition, these anatomic and physiologic changes in the lower urinary tract increase the risk of future BPH complications, again through uncertain mechanisms. The LUTS and the risk of future complications can, in turn, impact the health status of men with this condition. Treatments administered for BPH may also affect overall health status, either by modifying symptoms or the probability of complications, or by causing adverse effects, which impact on health status directly.

Disease-specific health status measures for men with BPH include instruments designed to measure the frequency and severity of LUTS, the degree of bother caused by these symptoms, or the impact of the condition (both symptoms and the potential for complications) on various domains of health status. The American Urological Association (AUA) Symptom Index,[23] known internationally as the International Prostate Symptom Score (IPSS),[24] is currently the most widely used instrument for measuring symptom burden among men with BPH in clinical practice and research. Sagnier and colleagues have described a process of linguistic validation for accurate translation of the IPSS into French.[25] Seven items, each with six ordered categorical responses, comprise the index (Figure 5.2). Total scores on the index range from 0 to 35. This instrument was developed for the predictive purpose of determining which patients were bothered to a greater or lesser degree by their urinary condition; and for the longitudinal evaluation of BPH patients over time, particularly to assess treatment outcomes, an evaluative purpose. For these purposes the instrument has been shown to be reliable and valid, and for the latter use, responsive to clinically important changes in patient status. Of note, the AUA index was not developed to discriminate men from women, men with greater from men with lesser degrees of physiologic bladder outlet obstruction, or men with LUTS due to BPH from men with symptoms due to other conditions, all uses for which the AUA index has been demonstrated to perform poorly.[9,26–29]

The conceptual parents of the AUA index include the Boyarsky and Madsen–Iversen symptom indices,[30,31] and the Maine Medical Assessment Program (MMAP) symptom index.[32] Another BPH symptom index was developed and validated by researchers at Merck Research Laboratories,[33] and has been subsequently used in clinical trials of medical therapy for BPH,[34,35] as well as a number of population-based studies of BPH epidemiology.[36]

Questions	Not at all	<1 time in 5	<1/2 the time	About 1/2 the time	>1/2 the time	almost always
1. Over the past month or so, how often have you had a sensation of not emptying your bladder completely after you finished urinating?	0	1	2	3	4	5
2. Over the past month or so, how often have you had to urinate again less than 2 hours after you finished urinating?	0	1	2	3	4	5
3. Over the past month or so, how often have you found you stopped and started again several times when you urinated?	0	1	2	3	4	5
4. Over the past month or so, how often have you found it difficult to postpone urination?	0	1	2	3	4	5
5. Over the past month or so, how often have you had a weak urinary stream?	0	1	2	3	4	5
6. Over the past month or so, how often have you had to push or strain to begin urination?	0	1	2	3	4	5
7. Over the past month or so, how many times did you most typically get up to urinate from the time you went to bed at night until the time you got up in the morning?	0	1	2	3	4	5
AUA symptom score = sum of questions 1–7 = _____ _____						

Figure 5.2 The American Urological Association Symptom Index

Source: From Barry MJ, Fowler F Jr, O'Leary MP et al. The American Urological Association Symptom Index for benign prostatic hyperplasia. *J Urol* 1992; **148**: 1549–57

(During the PAST MONTH, how often have your urinary problems interfered in the following activities?). If you do not have any urinary problems mark "none of the time"	None of the time	A little of the time	Some of the time	Most of the time	All of the time
1. Drinking fluids before you travel	0	1	2	3	4
2. Drinking fluids before you go to bed	0	1	2	3	4
3. Driving for 2 hours without stopping	0	1	2	3	4
4. Getting enough sleep at night	0	1	2	3	4
5. Going places that may not have a toilet	0	1	2	3	4
6. Playing sports outdoors such as golf	0	1	2	3	4
7. Going to movies, shows, church, etc	0	1	2	3	4

Figure 5.3 BPH-Specific Interference with Activities Index

Source: From Epstein RS, Deverka P, Chute CG et al. Validation of a new quality of life questionnaire for benign prostatic hyperplasia. *J Clin Epidemiol* 1992; **45**: 1431–45, with permission from Elsevier Science

Other BPH-specific measures of health status seek to quantify how much of a problem a set of symptoms is from the respondent's perspective. The Symptom Problem Index (SPI) was developed in parallel to the AUA Symptom Index for this purpose;[37] with this instrument the degree of problem associated with each of the seven symptoms represented in the AUA index is elicited, using a five-point ordered categorical response frame from "no problem" to "big problem". Another instrument, the Danish Prostate Symptom Score (DAN-PSS-1), assesses both the frequency and bother of 12 symptoms, and multiplies the frequency and bother ratings for each question to obtain an overall score.[38–40] Despite having a greater number of items than either the AUA index or SPI, the internal consistency reliability of the DAN-PSS-1 is lower, with an alpha statistic of 0.73 as opposed to about 0.85 for the other two instruments, indicating greater heterogeneity. A related instrument, the ICS male questionnaire, includes 20 questions about LUTS and 19 questions about the degree of problem due to individual symptoms. This instrument has also been demonstrated to have acceptable measures of psychometric reliability and validity.[41]

Questions	None	Only a little	Some	A lot	
1. Over the past month, how much physical discomfort did any urinary problems cause you?	0	1	2	3	
2. Over the past month, how much did you worry about your health because of any urinary problems?	0	1	2	3	
3. Overall, how bothersome has any trouble with urination been during the past month?	0	1	2	3	
4. Over the past month, how much of the time has any urinary problem kept you from doing the kinds of things you would usually do?	0 / None of the time	1 / A little of the time	2 / Some of the time	3 / Most of the time	4 / All of the time
BPH Impact Index = sum of questions 1–4 = _____ _____					

Figure 5.4 The BPH Impact Index

Source: From Barry MJ, Fowler FJ, O'Leary MP et al. Measuring disease-specific health status in men with benign prostatic hyperplasia. *Med Care* 1995; **33**: AS145–55, with permission

---

Physical/functional subscore

Question 2: When you are driving, you need to stop to urinate seldom (0 cm) or frequently (10 cm)
Question 3: At night, you sleep well (0 cm) or badly (10 cm)
Question 4: Currently your appetite is good (0 cm) or poor (10 cm)
Question 5: Your sexual drive is currently strong (0 cm) or poor (10 cm)
Question 9: When you feel the need to urinate and you cannot go to the toilet immediately, the time seems to pass quickly (0 cm) or slowly (10 cm)
Question 11: Currently, you can achieve an erection easily (0 cm) or with difficulty (10 cm)

Mental subscore

Question 6: You have losses of memory rarely (0 cm) or often (10 cm)
Question 7: You feel tired, weary, and lifeless rarely (0 cm) or often (10 cm)
Question 12: You have difficulties in paying attention or concentrating that are negligible (0 cm) or significant (10 cm)
Question 13: Your energy and vitality are high (0 cm) or low (10 cm)
Question 15: Currently, your mood changes are rare (0 cm) or frequent (10 cm)
Question 18: You are worried and anxious rarely (0 cm) or often (10 cm)

Social subscore

Question 1: Your social life is impaired very little (0 cm) or a lot (10 cm)
Question 8: You take part in activities with family and friends often (0 cm) or rarely (10 cm)
Question 10: Your recreational activities are affected not at all (0 cm) or a lot (10 cm)
Question 14: You adapt to new situations easily (0 cm) or with difficulty (10 cm)
Question 17: You are satisfied with your sexual life frequently (0 cm) or rarely (10 cm)
Question 20: In your relationships with other people, you feel comfortable (0 cm) or uneasy (10 cm)

Global assessment

Question 16: Currently, your love life is intense (0 cm) or weak (10 cm)
Question 19: Overall, considering your current life, you are satisfied (0 cm) or dissatisfied (10 cm)

Figure 5.5 BPH-Specific Health Related Quality of Life Questionnaire. Subjects respond by marking a 10-cm linear analog scale

Source: From Lukacs B, Leplege A, Thibault P, Jardin A. Development, validation and application of a BPH-specific health-related quality of life questionnaire: results of a BPH medical outcome study. In: Cockett ATK, Khoury S, Aso Y et al. (eds) *Proceedings of the 3rd International Consultation on Benign Prostatic Hyperplasia, Monaco, 1995, June 26–28.* Jersey: Scientific Communication International 1996; 277–80, with permission

Three additional BPH health status instruments include the BPH-Specific Interference with Activities Index (Figure 5.3),[42] the BPH Impact Index (Figure 5.4),[37] and the BPH-Specific HRQOL Questionnaire (Figure 5.5).[43] Another instrument was developed for a Veterans Administration trial of prostatectomy vs. watchful waiting.[44,45] These instruments were designed to measure how urinary symptoms and potential BPH complications affect various domains of patients' health status. The BPH-Specific HRQOL Questionnaire combines questions that are BPH specific with generic health status questions. All three instruments have undergone studies documenting their reliability and validity. However, the performance of these instruments has not been compared in the same patients.

HOW DOES BENIGN PROSTATIC HYPERPLASIA IMPACT HEALTH-RELATED QUALITY OF LIFE?

The interrelationships among the various levels of health in men thought to have BPH can be explored by correlating measurements of anatomic, physiologic, and health status measures among these men.

RELATIONSHIP BETWEEN ANATOMIC AND PHYSIOLOGIC MEASURES OF BENIGN PROSTATIC HYPERPLASIA SEVERITY WITH LOWER URINARY TRACT SYMPTOMS

Studies have consistently shown weak or absent correlations between prostate size, peak urinary flow rate, residual volume, and symptom severity among men with a clinical diagnosis of BPH.[6,46–49] Interestingly, Kaplan and colleagues have recently reported a relative high correlation ($r=0.75$) between symptom frequency as measured by AUA scores and the transition zone index, which represents the ratio of transition zone volume to total gland volume, as well as a similarly strong inverse relationship between peak flow rates and this index.[50] In community-based studies that correlate these measurements among all older men in a population, regardless of a clinical diagnosis of BPH, correlations are somewhat stronger, probably owing to the wider range of the key variables within these populations, though the relationships are still weak in an absolute sense.[51,52] Results from several representative studies are presented in Table 5.1. In the study by Barry and colleagues, conducted among men with a clinical diagnosis of BPH by a urologist, there was no statistically significant correlation between AUA symptom score and peak flow, postvoid residual, or prostate size.[47] In the community-based studies by Bosch and colleagues[51] and Girman and colleagues,[52] peak flow rate was modestly negatively correlated with AUA symptom score, while prostate size was modestly positively correlated with symptom level. Residual volume was also significantly but modestly correlated with symptom score in the former study.

Parameter	Clinical settings		Community settings	
	Barry[47] et al (N=196)	El Din[49] et al (N=803)	Bosch[51] et al (N=502)	Girman[52] et al (N=471)
Peak flow rate	−0.07	−0.20**	−0.18*	−0.35*
Prostate size	−0.09	+0.03	+0.19*	+0.18*
Postvoid residual	+0.01	+0.18**	+0.25*	–
Significant correlation: * $P<0.001$; ** $P<0.05$				

Table 5.1 Correlations of AUA/IPSS scores with other non-invasive measures of BPH severity

Many experts feel the best measures of the physiologic severity of bladder outflow obstruction are extracted from simultaneous pressure-flow studies.[4,53,54] Several studies, all performed among men given a clinical diagnosis of BPH by a urologist, also document no, or at best a weak, correlation between presence or degree of physiologic obstruction and LUTS severity.[8–11,55]

Interestingly, patients' perceptions of the frequency and severity of their LUTS as reflected in responses to symptom questionnaires show poor-to-modest agreement with the same symptoms as reflected in symptom diaries[41,56] or even 24-h home uroflowmetry recordings.[57] However, how much these discrepancies are due to a true disconnect between perceived and actual symptomatology as opposed to different recording periods (questionnaires often use a 1-month recall period, while diaries often cover a week and home uroflowmetry recordings a day) remains unclear.

RELATIONSHIP BETWEEN LOWER URINARY TRACT SYMPTOMS, BENIGN PROSTATIC HYPERPLASIC-SPECIFIC HEALTH STATUS, AND OVERALL HEALTH STATUS

In general, a higher burden of LUTS reflects poorer health status as measured by both disease-specific and overall measurements of health-related quality of life. These findings have been consistent both among men who carry a diagnosis of BPH in a clinical setting,[32,47] and among older men in the community.[58–62]

Among men with a diagnosis of BPH by a urologist participating in an outcomes study of prostatectomy, Fowler and colleagues described a significant relationship between subjects' MMAP symptom scores and two validated, generic health status measures: a General Health Index and a Mental Health Index ($r=0.22$ for both).[32,63] In the same study, scores on a three-question "global problem index" (a forerunner of the BPH Impact Index described previously) of the impact of the subjects' prostate condition on their overall health were even more highly correlated with the generic measures ($r=0.40$ and 0.36, respectively). In a follow-up study, the same investigators correlated disease-specific (AUA Symptom Index) and generic measures of health status, again among men diagnosed with BPH in a number of urologic practices, with the General Health and Mental Health indices from the previous study, as well as a generic Activity Index capturing functional status.[37] Table 5.2 displays these results, along with the results of the validation study of the Symptom Problem and BPH Impact Indices, which also correlated prostate-specific with overall measures of health status. A similar picture emerges, with AUA Symptom scores being significantly correlated with overall health status, but the measures of BPH impact on health status being even more strongly correlated with overall health-related quality of life. In this study, data on subjects' peak flow rates, residual volumes, and prostate sizes were also available; none of these measurements correlated with any of the domains of overall health status. Measures

	AUA Symptom score	Symptom Problem score	BPH Impact Index
AUA symptom score	1.00	–	–
Symptom Problem score	0.74*	1.00	–
BPH Impact score	0.76*	0.81*	1.00
General Health Index	–0.32*	–0.47*	–0.61*
Mental Health Index	–0.46*	–0.63*	–0.61*
Activity Index	–0.21	–0.38**	–0.49*

N = 57 BPH patients with complete answers to all questions in these indices
Significant correlation: * P<0.001; ** P<0.05

Table 5.2 Correlations of BPH-specific and generic health status scores among men with BPH

of the presence and severity of urodynamic obstruction do not appear to correlate with measures of health status either.[55] Clearly, it is the symptoms associated with BPH that directly affect health, rather than the anatomic or physiologic severity of disease.

A number of studies have documented that the severity of LUTS, and particularly ratings of symptom bother, are correlated with men seeking consultation with a physician for their condition.[64–66] However, Jolleys and colleagues have reported that many men with LUTS in the UK generally tolerated them quite well.[67] In one study, a single rating of symptom bother was the dominant predictor of whether men consulting a US urologist subsequently underwent a prostatectomy.[68]

CHANGES IN LOWER URINARY TRACT SYMPTOMS AND HEALTH STATUS WITH TREATMENT FOR BENIGN PROSTATIC HYPERPLASIA

Transurethral prostatectomy has an impressive effect, on average, in reducing urinary symptoms when they are measured objectively.[23,32,44,69–71] Fewer studies have measured the impact of prostatectomy on higher-order measures of BPH-specific or generic health status measures. Scores on the BPH Impact Index have been demonstrated to be about as responsive as symptom scores in measuring improvement in men following surgery.[37] Fowler has described statistically significant improvements in an Activity Index, a General Health Index, and a Mental Health Index, all generic health

status measures, following prostatectomy for men with moderate-to-severe symptoms, though not for men with mild symptoms.[63] In a similar outcomes study from the UK, patients had statistically significant improvements in a number of domains of the Nottingham Health Profile (NHP),[71,72] another generic health status measure, to complement substantial improvements in their LUTS. These domains included energy, pain, emotional reaction, sleep, and mobility.

Another prospective cohort study from the UK evaluated men undergoing transurethral resection of the prostate (TURP) with the Euro QoL (EQ) quality-of-life measure and the NHP.[73] These instruments were administered at 6 weeks, 6 months, and 12 months post-operatively. Younger, fitter, and more symptomatic men experienced the greatest benefit from surgery.

In two randomized trials, finasteride has been reported to result in a trend toward improvement in several BPH-specific health status measures, including measures of troublesomeness of symptoms, interference with activities, and worry about urinary problems.[74] However, consistent with its modest impact on symptoms, finasteride did not improve measures of generic health status in these studies. In a large placebo control trial of terazosin, BPH Impact Index scores improved by about 40% with active treatment, compared with about 20% improvement for the placebo; these proportional improvements were similar to the degrees of improvement seen in AUA symptom scores in trial subjects.[75]

CONCLUSION

Men with LUTS have decrements in both disease-specific and generic measures of health-related quality of life. LUTS levels correlate better with these higher-order health status measures than measures of the anatomic or physiologic severity of BPH. These findings document the morbidity of this common condition. Treatment can result in improvement in disease-specific measures of health status, and treatment with prostatectomy results in improvements in generic measures of health status as well.

ACKNOWLEDGMENT

The assessments underlying this chapter were funded by a Patient Outcome Research Team-II grant (No. HS 08387) from the Agency for Health Care Policy and Research.

REFERENCES

1 Berry SJ, Coffey DS, Walsh PC, Ewing LL. The development of human benign prostatic hyperplasia with age. *J Urol* 1984; **132**: 474–9.

2 Isaacs JT, Coffey DS. Etiology and disease process of benign prostatic hyperplasia. *Prostate* 1989; (Suppl 2): 33–50.

3 Barry MJ, Boyle P, Fourcroy J *et al*. Epidemiology and natural history of BPH. In: Cockett ATK, Khoury S, Aso Y *et al*. (eds) *The 3rd International Consultation on Benign Prostatic Hyperplasia*

(BPH), *Monaco, 1995, June 26–28*. Jersey: Scientific Communication International 1996; 17–34.

4 Abrams P. New words for old: lower urinary tract symptoms for "prostatism". *BMJ* 1994; **308**: 929–30.

5 Barry MJ, Fowler FJ, Bin L, Oesterling JE. A nationwide survey of practicing urologists: current management of benign prostatic hyperplasia and clinically localized prostate cancer. *J Urol* 1997; **158**: 488–92.

6 Schou J, Poulsen AL, Nordling J. The anatomy of a prostate waiting list: a prospective study of 132 consecutive patients. *Br J Urol* 1994; **74**: 57–60.

7 Kaplan SA, Bowers DL, Te AE, Olsson CA. Differential diagnosis of prostatism: a 12-year retrospective analysis of symptoms, urodynamics, and satisfaction with therapy. *J Urol* 1996; **155**: 1305–8.

8 Van Venrooij GEPM, Boon TA. The value of symptom score, quality of life score, maximal urinary flow rate, residual volume and prostate size for the diagnosis of obstructive benign prostatic hyperplasia: a urodynamic analysis. *J Urol* 1996; **155**: 2014–18.

9 Ezz El Din K, Kiermeney LALM, deWildt MJAM *et al*. The correlation between bladder outlet obstruction and lower urinary tract symptoms as measured by the international prostate symptom score. *J Urol* 1996; **156**: 1020–5.

10 Netto NR, D'Ancona CAL, deLima ML. Correlation between the international prostatic symptom score and a pressure-flow study in the evaluation of symptomatic benign prostatic hyperplasia. *J Urol* 1996; **155**: 200–2.

11 Yalla SV, Sullivan MP, Lecamwasam HS *et al*. Correlation of American Urological Association Symptom Index with obstructive and nonobstructive protatism. *J Urol* 1995; **153**: 674–80.

12 Bruskewitz R, Jensen KM, Iversen P, Madsen PO. The relevance of minimum urethral resistance in prostatism. *J Urol* 1983; **129**: 769–71.

13 McConnell JD, Barry MJ, Bruskewitz RC *et al*. *Benign Prostatic Hyperplasia: Diagnosis and Treatment. Clinical Practice Guideline.* No. 8. AHCPR Publication No. 94–0582. Rockville, MD: Agency for Health Care Policy and Research, Public Health Service, US Department of Health and Human Services 1994.

14 McConnell JD. Why pressure-flow studies should be optional and not mandatory studies for evaluating men with benign prostatic hyperplasia. *Urology* 1994; **44**: 156–8.

15 Bergner M. Quality of life, health status, and clinical research. *Med Care* 1989; **27**(Suppl 3): S148–56.

16 Guyatt GH, Veldhuyzen Van Zanten SJO, Feeny DH, Patrick DL. Measuring quality of life in clinical trials: a taxonomy and review. *Can Med Ass J* 1989; **140**: 1441–8.

17 McDowell I, Newell C. *Measuring Health: a Guide to Rating Scales and Questionnaires*. New York: Oxford University Press 1987.

18 Streiner DL, Norman GR. *Health Measurement Scales: a Practical Guide to their Development and Use*. New York: Oxford University Press 1989.

19 Kirshner B, Guyatt G. A methodological framework for assessing health indices. *J Chron Dis* 1985; **38**: 27–36.

20 Deyo RA, Diehr P, Patrick DL. Reproducibility and responsiveness of health status measures: statistics and strategies for evaluation. *Control Clin Trials* 1991; **12**: 142S–58S.

21 Ware JE, Snow KK, Kosinski M, Gandek B. *SF-36 Health survey: Manual and Interpretation Guide*. Boston: Nimrod Press 1993.

22 Barry MJ, Fowler FJ. The methodology for evaluating the subjective outcomes of treatment for benign prostatic hyperplasia. *Adv Urol* 1993; **6**: 83–99.

23 Barry MJ, Fowler FJ Jr, O'Leary MP *et al*. The American Urological Association Symptom Index for benign prostatic hyperplasia. *J Urol* 1992; **148**: 1549–57.

24 Cockett AT, Aso Y, Denis L *et al*. International prostate symptom score (IPSS) and quality of life assessment. In: Cockett ATK, Khoury S, Aso Y *et al*. (eds) *Proceedings of the 3rd International Consultation on Benign Prostatic Hyperplasia (BPH) Monaco, 1995, June 26–28*. Jersey: Scientific Communication International 1996; 626–39.

25 Sagnier PP, MacFarlane G, Botto RH, Teillac P, Boyle P. Results of an epidemiological survey using a modified American Urological Association symptom index for benign prostatic hyperplasia in France. *J Urol* 1994; **151**: 1266–70.

26 Lepor H, Machi G. Comparison of AUA Symptom Index in unselected males and females between fifty-five and seventy-nine years of age. *Urology* 1993; **42**: 36–41.

27 Chancellor MB, Rivas DA. American Urological Association Symptom Index for women with voiding symptoms: lack of index specificity for benign prostatic hyperplasia. *J Urol* 1993; **150**: 1706–9.

28 Chai TC, Belville WD, McGuire EJ, Nyquist L. Specificity of the American Urological Association Voiding Symptom Index: comparison of unselected and selected samples of both sexes. *J Urol* 1993; **150**: 1710–13.

29 Chancellor MB, Rivas DA, Keeley FX *et al*. Similarity of the American Urological Association Index among men with benign prostatic hyperplasia (BPH), urethral obstruction not due to BPH and detrusor hyper-reflexia without outlet obstruction. *Br J Urol* 1994; **74**: 200–3.

30 Boyarsky S, Jones G, Paulson DF, Prout GR. A new look at bladder neck obstruction by the Food and Drug Administration regulators: guidelines for investigation of benign prostatic hypertrophy. *Trans Am Assoc Genitourin Surg* 1977; **68**: 29–32.

31 Madsen PO, Iversen P. A point system for selecting operative candidates. In: Hiniman F (ed) *Benign Prostatic Hyperplasia*. New York: Springer 1983; 763–5.

32 Fowler FJ, Wennberg JE, Timothy RP *et al*. Symptom status and quality of life following prostatectomy. *JAMA* 1988; **259**: 3018–22.

33 Bolognese JA, Kozloff RC, Kunitz SC *et al*. Validation of a symptoms questionnaire for benign prostatic hyperplasia. *Prostate* 1992; **21**: 247–54.

34 Gromley GJ, Stoner E, Bruskewitz RC *et al*. The effect of finasteride in men with benign prostatic hyperplasia. *N Engl J Med* 1992; **327**: 1185–91.

35 Stoner E, Members of the Finasteride Study Group. Three-year safety and efficacy data on the use of finasteride in the treatment of benign prostatic hyperplasia. *Urology* 1994; **43**: 284–94.

36 Guess HA, Jacobsen SJ, Girman CJ *et al*. The role of community-based longitudinal studies in evaluating treatment effects. *Med Care* 1995; **33**(Suppl): AS26–35.

37 Barry MJ, Fowler FJ, O'Leary MP *et al*. Measuring disease-specific health status in men with benign prostatic hyperplasia. *Med Care* 1995; **33**: AS145–55.

38 Hald T, Nordling J, Andersen JT *et al*. A patient weighted symptom score system in the evaluation of uncomplicated benign prostatic hyperplasia. *Scand J Urol Nephrol* 1991; **138**(Suppl): 59–62.

39 Meyhoff HH, Hald T, Nordling J *et al*. A new patient weighted symptom score system (DAN-PSS-1). *Scand J Urol Nephrol* 1993; **27**: 493–9.

40 Hansen BJ, Flyger H, Brasso K *et al*. Validation of the self-administered Danish Prostatic Symptom Score (DAN-PSS-1) system for use in benign prostatic hyperplasia. *Br J Urol* 1995; **76**: 451–8.

41 Donavan JL, Abrams P, Peters TJ *et al*. The ICS-"BPH" Study: the psychometric validity and reliability of the ICS male questionnaire. *Br J Urol* 1996; **77**: 554–62.

42 Epstein RS, Deverka P, Chute CG *et al*. Validation of a new quality of life questionnaire for benign prostatic hyperplasia. *J Clin Epidemiol* 1992; **45**: 1431–45.

43 Lukacs B, Comet D, Grange JC, Thibault P. Construction and validation of a short-form benign prostatic hypertrophy health related quality of life questionnaire. *Br J Urol* 1997; **80**: 722–30.

44 Wasson JH, Reda DJ, Bruskewitz RC *et al*. A comparison of transurethral surgery with watchful waiting for moderate symptoms of benign prostatic hyperplasia. *N Engl J Med* 1995; **332**: 75–79.

45 Wasson JH, Bruskewitz RC, Elinson J *et al*. A comparison of quality of life with patient reported symptoms and objective findings in men with benign prostatic hyperplasia. *J Urol* 1993; **150**: 1696–1700.

46 Bosch R. Use of the International Prostate Symptom Score (IPSS) in epidemiological studies and clinical practice – a review. In: Cockett ATK, Khoury S, Aso Y *et al.* (eds) *Proceedings of the 3rd International Consultation on Benign Prostatic Hyperplasia (BPH), Monaco, 1995, June 26–28.* Jersey: Scientific Communication International 1996; 262–76.

47 Barry MJ, Cockett ATK, Holtgrewe HL *et al.* Relationship of symptoms of prostatism to commonly used physiological and anatomical measures of the severity of benign prostatic hyperplasia. *J Urol* 1993; **150**: 351–8.

48 Ko DSC, Fenster HN, Chambers K *et al.* The correlation of multi-channel urodynamic pressure-flow studies and American Urological Association Symptom-Index in the evaluation of benign prostatic hyperplasia. *J Urol* 1995; **154**: 396–8.

49 EI Din KE, Kiemeney LALM, de Wildt MJAM *et al.* Correlation between uroflowmetry, prostate volume, postvoid residue, and lower urinary tract symptoms as measured by the international prostate symptom score. *Urology* 1996; **48**: 393–7.

50 Kaplan SA, Te AE, Pressler LB, Olsson CA. Transition zone index as a method of assessing benign prostatic hyperplasia: correlation with symptoms, urine flow and detrusor pressure. *J Urol* 1995; **154**: 1764–1769.

51 Bosch JLHR, Hop WCJ, Kirkels WJ, Schroder FH. The international prostate symptom score in a community-based sample of men between fifty-five and seventy-four years of age. *Br J Urol* 1995; **75**: 622–30.

52 Girman CJ, Jacobsen SJ, Guess HA *et al.* Natural history of prostatism: relationship among symptoms, prostate volume and peak urinary flow rate. *J Urol* 1995; **153**: 1510–15.

53 Reynard J, Abrams P. Symptoms and symptom scores in BPH. *Scand J Urol* 1995; (Suppl): 137–57.

54 Abrams P. Objective evaluation of bladder outlet obstruction. *Br J Urol* 1995; **76**(Suppl 1): 11–15.

55 Van Venrooji GEPM, Boon TA, de Gier RPE. International prostate symptom score and quality of life assessment versus urodynamic parameters in men with benign prostatic hyperplasia symptoms. *J Urol* 1995; **153**: 1516–19.

56 Russell EBAW, Lee AJ, Garraway WM, Prescott RJ. Use of a 7-day diary for urinary symptom recording. *Eur Urol* 1994; **26**: 227–32.

57 Matzkin H, Greenstein A, Prager-Geller T *et al.* Do reported micturition symptoms on the American Urological Association Questionnaire correlate with 24-hour home uroflowmetry recordings? *J Urol* 1996; **155**: 197–9.

58 Tsang KK, Garraway WW. Impact of benign prostatic hyperplasia on general well-being of men. *Prostate* 1993; **23**: 1–7.

59 Garraway WM, Russell EBAW, Lee RJ *et al.* Impact of previously unrecognized benign prostatic hyperplasia on the daily activities of middle-aged and elderly men. *Br J Gen Pract* 1993; **43**: 318–321.

60 Girman CJ, Epstein RS, Jacobsen SJ *et al.* Natural history of prostatism: impact of urinary symptoms on quality of life in 2115 randomly selected community men. *Urology* 1994; **44**: 825–31.

61 Sagnier PP, MacFarlane G, Teillac P *et al.* Impact of symptoms of prostatism on level of bother and quality of life of men in the French community. *J Urol* 1995; **153**: 669–73.

62 Hunter DJW, McKee M, Black NA, Sanderson CFB. Health status and quality of life of British men with lower urinary tract symptoms: results form the SF-36. *Urology* 1995; **45**: 962–71.

63 Fowler FJ. Patient reports of symptoms and quality of life following prostate surgery. *Eur Urol* 1991; **20**(Suppl 2): 44–49.

64 Jacobsen SJ, Guess HA, Panser L *et al.* A population-based study of health care-seeking behavior for treatment of urinary symptoms. *Arch Fam Med* 1993; **2**: 729–35.

65 Roberts RO, Rhodes T, Panser LA *et al.* Natural history of prostatism: worry and embarrassment from urinary symptoms and health care-seeking behavior. *Urology* 1994; **43**: 621–28.

66 MacFarlane GJ, Sagnier PP, Richard F *et al.* Determinants of treatment-seeking behavior for urinary symptoms in older men. *Br J Urol* 1995; **76**: 714–18.

67 Jolleys JV, Donavan JL, Nanchahal K *et al.* Urinary symptoms in the community: how bothersome are they? *Br J Urol* 1994; **74**: 551–5.

68 Barry MJ, Fowler FJ, Mulley AG *et al.* Patient reactions to a program designed to facilitate patient participation in treatment decisions for benign prostatic hyperplasia. *Med Care* 1995; **33**: 771–82.

69 Lepor H, Rigaud G. The efficacy of transurethral resection of the prostate in men with moderate symptoms of prostatism. *J Urol* 1990; **143**: 533–7.

70 Flood AB, Black NA, McPherson K *et al.* Assessing symptom improvement after elective prostatectomy for benign prostatic hypertrophy. *Arch Intern Med* 1992; **152**: 1507–12.

71 Doll Ha, Black NA, Flood AB, McPherson K. Patient-perceived health status before and up to 12 months after transurethral resection of the prostate for benign prostatic hypertrophy. *Br J Urol* 1993; **71**: 297–305.

72 Thorpe AC, Cleary R, Coles J, Neal DE. Nottingham health profile measurement in the assessment of clinical outcome after prostatectomy. *Br J Urol* 1995; **76**: 446–50.

73 Mac Donagh RP, Cliff AM, Speakman MJ *et al.* The use of generic measures of health related quality of life in the assessment of outcome from transurethral resection of the prostate. *Br J Urol* 1997; **79**: 401–8.

74 Girman CJ, Kolman C, Liss CL *et al.* Effects of finasteride on health-related quality of life in men with symptomatic benign prostatic hyperplasia. *Prostate* 1996; **19**: 83–90.

75 Roehrborn CG, Oesterling JE, Auerbach S *et al.* The Hytrin Community Assessment Trial study: a one-year study of terazosin versus placebo in the treatment of men with symptomatic benign prostatic hyperplasia. *Urology* 1996; **47**: 159–68.

Section II

DIAGNOSIS AND EVALUATION

DIAGNOSIS AND EVALUATION

P. Narayan

The diagnosis and evaluation of BPH has undergone considerable changes secondary to several related developments in the field over the last 5 years. These include, first, the advent of clinical practice guidelines in many countries, designed to streamline the various tests in evaluation and management of BPH; secondly, the availability of medical agents that are safe, efficacious, and long-acting has allowed patients to seek relief of symptoms without fear of surgery; and thirdly, the recognition that quality-of-life issues are paramount in evaluation of therapies for BPH has led to a decrease in the use of TURP and an increase in the use of minimally invasive therapies. This has translated into more use of instruments such as symptom scores to assess patient complaints objectively and to reduce the number of cystoscopies; finally, as noted in the commentary to Chapter 10, there has been increasing recognition of the central role the detrusor plays in patients with prostatic obstruction. All of these developments have not necessarily been beneficial to the patient with BPH. Certainly the practice guidelines have allowed practicing urologists to avoid unnecessary tests while providing some reproducible assessment of symptom scores for evaluating therapy. However, as stated in the commentary sections of Chapters 6–9, most urologists are still not using symptom scores for management. This, unfortunately, is also true for European urologists, as noted by Denis and others. The changes that have occurred have been mostly related to decreases in the number of TURPs, and this has been driven mostly by patient recognition of the fact that BPH is not a life-threatening disease and that avoiding surgery does not necessarily mean that the patient has to live with symptoms. The AHCPR guidelines have certainly set a standard for urologists to measure their tests against, and most certainly it is hoped that, with the passage of time, the number of urologists who perform upper tract imaging and cystoscopy solely for diagnosis of BPH will diminish. In a recent review, Dr Holtgrewe noted that even the cost of performing uroflow using a stopwatch to the Medicare system was $542 million annually and one can easily surmise from this data that the cost of cross-sectional imaging and unnecessary cystoscopies would be higher.[1] We as urologists have seized the leadership in establishing guidelines for BPH evaluation and therapy and should remain in the forefront of cost-effective management of patients with BPH. However, we have to temper cost-effectiveness with science and improvements in understanding of disease. Therefore, the observations of Drs McGuire, Elbadawi and others on performing relevant urodynamic studies in order to provide better care to patients with the constellation of LUTS is a dilemma for which we have to continue to strive to find a proper answer.

1 Holtgrewe L. Editorial: benign prostatic hyperplasia. *J Urol* 1997; **157**: 184.

Symptom Evaluation, Clinical Presentation, and Differential Diagnosis

M.R. Feneley and R.S. Kirby

6

INTRODUCTION

Lower urinary tract symptoms (LUTS) are acquired by both men and women as they grow older. They may reflect age-dependent physiological changes but can declare the presence of lower urinary tract pathology. Benign prostatic hyperplasia (BPH) is one of the most prevalent conditions to affect the aging, human male, progressing with advancing years and dependent on circulating androgens. Therefore, LUTS and BPH commonly coexist in older men and must be carefully evaluated before appropriate therapy can be recommended.

Men with LUTS who seek urological advice usually do so because they have experienced some degree of functional disturbance that is either bothersome or affecting their quality of life. Many others do not do so, and there is tremendous variation between individuals in the tolerability of symptoms and associated inconvenience. Clinical presentation may be influenced by concerns about overall health and, in particular, the possibility of underlying prostatic malignancy. Cultural attitudes and experience of prostate disease within a family may also affect the decision to discuss urinary difficulties. The relationship between each of these issues is subtle and unique for each patient. With the increasing profile of male health issues in western society, men are often well informed about both benign and malignant prostatic diseases and their treatment before seeking expert opinion.

PROSTATIC ENLARGEMENT, SYMPTOMS, AND BLADDER OUTFLOW OBSTRUCTION

BPH is characterized by abnormal patterns of proliferation and atrophy within the epithelium and stroma of the prostate. It begins to develop in men in their third decade, manifest as ductal branching followed by proliferation of stromal and glandular elements, which is ultimately responsible for the benign prostatic enlargement (BPE) evident in many elderly men. It may give rise to LUTS but their severity does not correlate with the degree of prostatic enlargement.

Prostatic enlargement may cause increased resistance to bladder emptying, termed bladder outflow obstruction (BOO). Demonstrated by low flow rate in relation to normal or high voiding pressures, BOO has been shown to be a critical factor in distinguishing men whose symptoms are likely to respond well to operative treatment.[1,2] It has both static and dynamic components, corresponding respectively to the mechanical effect of prostatic enlargement and smooth muscle tone in the prostatic and bladder neck mechanisms. Though these elements cannot be separated diagnostically, their relative contribution may determine the response to alternative treatments, such as α-1 receptor blockade, 5 α-reductase inhibition, or surgery.[3-5] BOO is also responsible for many of the pathophysiological complications of untreated BPH.

BOO gives rise to a spectrum of urinary symptoms, of which reduced uroflow and hesitancy are the most reliable.[6] Sometimes it is associated with incomplete bladder emptying. This is traditionally attributed to failure of the detrusor to compensate with increased voiding pressure or its eventual "decompensation." Incomplete emptying may, however, reflect primary failure of the detrusor muscle in sustaining contraction. This may be a consequence of structural changes in the bladder wall or abnormality within the micturition reflex, as in neurological disease. An increase in the amount of connective tissue, atrophy of smooth muscle, and axonal degeneration has been observed,[7] and this may also account for both changes in bladder compliance and development of detrusor instability, which may occur either secondary to BOO or with aging.[8] This leads to trabeculation, sacculation, and eventually diverticula formation. Incomplete emptying may predispose some patients to recurrent urinary tract infections and produce an environment conducive to calculus formation. Impaired bladder emptying is ultimately responsible for urinary retention. Chronic retention with high intravesical pressures may lead to bilateral hydronephrosis, impaired renal function, and eventually irreversible renal damage.

LUTS correlate poorly with specific abnormalities of lower urinary tract function and are an unreliable indicator of BPH, BPE, and BOO.[9,10] Furthermore, retention is infrequently observed in men with symptomatic BPH.[11] Although BPH may be associated with LUTS or BOO, components of this triad can occur independently. Symptoms may be due to a variety of other causes, including detrusor instability, detrusor hypocontractility, poor voiding habits, advancing age, or other acquired lower urinary tract pathology, any of which may exist alongside BPH. The term "prostatism," which implies causality in this context, is therefore quite misleading and should be avoided.[12]

The clinical assessment of patients with symptomatic BPH has been extensively debated by expert panels. Guidelines have been developed by the US Agency for Health Care Policy[13] and by the International Consultations on Benign Prostatic Hyperplasia, sponsored by the World Health Organization. While certain investigations can be recommended, the value of others may be considered optional, to be undertaken according to the discretion of the urologist.

DIFFERENTIAL DIAGNOSIS

The differential diagnosis of BPH includes conditions that give rise to altered lower urinary tract physiology (e.g. abnormal bladder compliance, capacity, instability, obstruction, etc.), as well as benign and malignant pathological processes that can develop within the urinary tract.

BOO is frequently secondary to BPH, particularly in older men, but may be due to a variety of other causes, including urethral stricture or tumor, meatal stenosis, and phimosis. Bladder neck obstruction or dysynergia may be suspected in younger men without significant prostatic enlargement, and definite diagnosis requires demonstration of contrast entrapment between the bladder neck and external sphincter on video-urodynamic investigation. Detrusor–external sphincter dysynergia may be similarly demonstrated as failure of sphincteric relaxation while voiding and distinctive flow pattern.

Detrusor motor instability also commonly occurs secondary to BOO, but may be idiopathic and associated with the aging bladder. Sensory instability, characterized by heightened bladder sensation without pressure abnormalities, may be due to other pathologies, including carcinoma *in situ*, invasive malignancy, stones, etc., but it can be idiopathic. The possibility of urinary tract infection must always be evaluated, and though this may be secondary to BPH, other causes need to be excluded.

Neurological disease may present with changes in lower urinary tract function and should be recognized. Detrusor hypocontractility or instability, altered bladder capacity and compliance, sphincter dysynergia, and urinary incontinence may develop in men with neurological disease and can be characterized by urodynamic investigations.

Urethrocystoscopy may reveal causes of outflow obstruction other than BPH, including urethral stricture, tumor, calculus, and foreign bodies. These may sometimes be suspected because of dysuria, urethral pain, or previous urological history. Endoscopy is an invasive investigation, mandatory for patients with hematuria but also useful in patients with irritative bladder symptoms to exclude other lower urinary tract pathology. Prostatic obstruction, however, cannot be reliably assessed visually, and such investigation is therefore not usually informative in uncomplicated BPH.

CLINICAL PRESENTATION

The presentation of BPH is varied and has been strongly influenced in recent years by increasing awareness of the importance of prostatic disease among patients and their partners, and a growing armamentarium of medical and minimally invasive therapies. Many men seek medical advice after becoming conscious of minor urinary symptoms, and sometimes concern is precipitated because of subtle changes in sexual function. Some mindful of the risks and insidious presentation of prostate cancer hope for reassurance or benefit from serendipitous treatment. Others may tolerate symptoms of varying severity, sometimes for considerable periods of time, before recognizing the need for medical consultation.

The most dramatic presentation of BPH is acute urinary retention with a painful, tender, distended bladder, and a strong desire but inability to void. It is commonly preceded by relatively minor symptoms, but hesitancy with a full bladder is frequently reported. Sometimes there is an obvious precipitant, such as a surgical operation, painful perineal condition, constipation, imprudently deferred voiding (e.g. after drinking alcohol), or medications, particularly diuretics, anticholinergics, and opiate analgesics. Chronic retention is in contrast characteristically painless, associated with frequent voiding of small urinary volumes, or incontinence. Acquired nocturnal enuresis may indicate high pressure chronic retention.

Complications that present primarily may point to BPH as the underlying cause, though in these situations the possibility of other pathology needs to be investigated. These would include hematuria, urinary tract infection, and bladder calculus. Renal failure with bilateral hydronephrosis and hydro-ureter may be due to high pressure chronic retention. Bladder calculi may cause an intermittent ability to void, sometimes related to posture, recurrent urinary tract infections, and their presence (in industrialized countries) frequently indicates bladder outflow obstruction. Incomplete bladder emptying may promote urinary tract infection and encourage further calculus formation.

SYMPTOM EVALUATION

Lower urinary tract symptoms relate to bladder filling, storage, and voiding of urine. Their traditional classification as either "obstructive" or "irritative" correlates poorly with the urodynamic diagnoses and, therefore, may be both inaccurate and misleading. Symptoms should be assessed carefully to determine their cause, the diagnosis as BPH should be confirmed, and other pathology excluded as appropriate. Factors that determine the need for treatment and influence therapeutic outcome should also be evaluated to give the patient reliable advice on management.

The importance of a careful medical history cannot be overstated. Urinary symptoms, their frequency, severity, duration, and course require specific assessment, and should be recorded. Certain symptoms may alert the clinician's suspicions to other pathological conditions. However, the bladder is renowned as an unreliable witness. Coexisting disease, concurrent medication, and previous surgery, not uncommon in men with BPH, may have an important bearing on management recommendations.

LUTS should be considered in relation to underlying urodynamic abnormalities as well as functional aspects of urine storage and transport, not only for understanding symptomatology but these factors may also influence therapeutic outcome. Nocturia is one of the commonest presenting symptoms in men with BPH but the mechanisms responsible are often poorly understood. It may be due to nocturnal polyuria, associated with loss of diurnal control of urine production, and this is most readily revealed by the voiding diary.[14] In other cases, it may be attributed to irritation or sensory changes in the bladder. Hesitancy and weak urinary stream have a proven correlation with BOO.[6] However, these associations are not sufficiently reliable to allow a confident pathophysiological diagnosis in the individual patient, and a weak urinary stream is not infrequently associated with detrusor hypocontractility. Instability may be associated with daytime frequency and urgency, but is not specific for this urodynamic diagnosis, which may be more strongly suspected in men with urge incontinence.

Incontinence due to BPH may be classified as urge incontinence, overflow incontinence, and nocturnal incontinence. Urge incontinence is often associated with detrusor instability or hyperreflexia (due to neurological abnormality). Overflow incontinence occurs with chronic retention and sometimes frequent voiding of small urinary volumes. Nocturnal incontinence is commonly due to chronic retention, with high detrusor pressures that may also lead to progressive renal parenchymal damage. The presence and etiology of incontinence has important implications for treatment and its timing.

Voiding habit can be examined most objectively by asking the patient to complete a voiding diary. This may offer useful insight into an individual's urinary symptoms, their

variability, and particular circumstances that may provoke them. Urinary frequency, nocturia, and episodes of incontinence are timed and recorded, and voided volumes measured to give an estimate of functional bladder capacity. Symptoms sometimes vary according to the patient's environment and emotional state, and this may be difficult to recognize without objective evaluation.

Symptom scores provide a quantitative assessment of the overall severity. Several scoring systems have been developed, differing in method of administration, symptom evaluation and quantification, and validation. The most widely used are the Boyarsky,[15] the Madsen–Iversen,[16] and the AUA or International Prostate Symptom Score (IPSS).[17] Of these, the AUA symptom score is now the most widely used in both clinical practice and research. It is designed to be self-administered, consisting of seven standardized questions concerning specific urinary symptoms. Scores for each question are added, giving an overall range from 0 to 35, with total scores of 0–7 classified as mild, 8–19 as moderate, and 20–35 as severe. The questionnaire has been well validated and shown to be reproducible and responsive to symptom severity in men with BPH.

Symptom scores enable comparisons to be made between patients, and may be particularly useful for monitoring symptom severity in individual patients or evaluating therapeutic outcome. They are neither disease-specific for BPH nor sex-specific in discriminating symptoms of aging men from those of women, which is entirely compatible with their design and purpose. They do not, however, have prognostic value or aid decisions on appropriate therapy: though less-invasive therapies may be reserved for men with lower symptom scores, patients with severe symptoms may also benefit significantly.

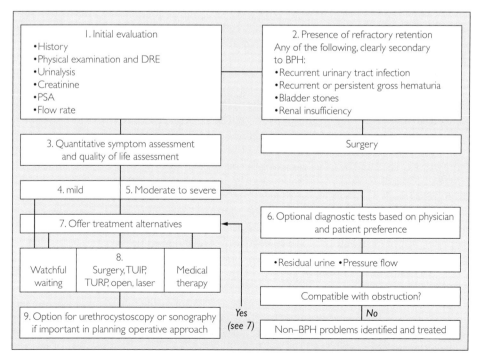

Figure 6.1 Decision diagram. Although PSA and flow rate studies are considered optional by the CPG guidelines, these tests are relatively simple, inexpensive, and helpful in clinical management of most patients

Source: Adapted and reproduced with permission from McConnell JD, Barren MJ, Bruskewitz RC et al. *Benign Prostatic Hyperplasia: Diagnosis and Treatment. Clinical Practice Guideline,* No. 8. AHCPR Publication No. 94-0582. Rockville, MD: Agency for Health Care Policy and Research, US Department of Health and Human Services, 1994

The use of symptom scores has been recommended in both the US Clinical Guidelines and the International Consultation on BPH. For the individual patient with BPH, the need for treatment is often driven by the "bothersomeness" of his symptoms, and similarly this may be the most important criteria for successful therapeutic outcome. This degree of bother can differ dramatically between patients with similar symptom severity and further impact on quality of life.[17]

CLINICAL EXAMINATION

Focused clinical examination is essential for evaluating urinary symptoms in the individual patient. Coexisting conditions may influence subsequent therapeutic decisions. Occasionally, retention may be diagnosed, and findings such as a palpable kidney would merit specific investigation. The possibility of underlying neurological disease must also be considered. Perianal sensation, anal sphincter contraction and tone can be examined alongside digital rectal examination for abnormalities affecting the S2–4 segments that also innervate the bladder. Neurogenic bladder dysfunction is, however, more commonly due to disease at a suprasacral level affecting higher centers responsible for control of micturition reflexes or connecting tracts.

Digital rectal examination of the prostate is mandatory in patients with LUTS. Induration or a nodule may alert the clinician to the possibility of prostatic malignancy and, less commonly, tenderness may indicate underlying prostatitis. Digital assessment of prostate volume is often misleading, because the length and anterior extent of the gland cannot be assessed.[18] Transrectal ultrasonography (TRUS), now generally available, provides a reasonably accurate measurement when required, but is not routine outside the context of research of clinical trials. Gland volume assessment may be relevant when selecting medical or surgical therapy most appropriate to the individual. Size alone, however, does not correlate with symptom severity or the degree of outflow obstruction, and should not influence a decision on need for treatment.

INVESTIGATIONS FOR THE EVALUATION OF BENIGN PROSTATIC HYPERPLASIA

URINE AND BLOOD TESTS

Urine testing is recommended in men with LUTS. Dipstix testing of a mid-stream urine sample offers cost advantages over conventional microscopy and culture, as well as providing an immediate result. It is sensitive for hematuria, though ideally this should be confirmed by microscopic examination of spun urine. Positive finding merits careful investigation of both the upper and lower urinary tract. Proteinuria may alert the clinician to the possibility of renal disease. Infection may require careful assessment and treatment according to the organism(s) responsible.

Serum creatinine is usually recommended in patients with urinary symptoms for baseline evaluation. Raised creatinine indicates significant impairment of overall renal function and may demand further investigation. It is also associated with increased morbidity of surgical treatment.[19] Impaired function with chronic retention and bilateral hydronephrosis is associated with an unpredictable reversible component that can only be determined by relieving the obstruction.

Serum prostate-specific antigen (PSA) testing is not required for the evaluation of BPH but is an important test for early detection of prostate cancer. The greater than normal amount of prostatic epithelium in BPH causes considerable overlap in the PSA levels between these patients and those with early prostate cancer. Discrimination may be improved by measuring the ratio of free to total PSA, as the proportion of PSA that is bound to α-1 antichymotrypsin and α-2 macroglobulin is significantly higher in men with cancer. PSA testing increases the diagnosis of prostate cancer in men with clinically benign prostate on digital rectal examination, particularly in the context of prostate cancer screening. Unfortunately, significant, transient increase in PSA levels may be observed with urinary retention, after instrumentation, and in other benign prostatic diseases, particularly prostatitis and infarction. Thus, PSA measurements are most likely to be representative in men without complications of BPH.

UROFLOW MEASUREMENT

The symptom of impaired urinary flow is associated with BOO, but it is also subjective. Uroflow traces provide an objective and non-invasive assessment of urinary flow and pattern. Reduced uroflow may also be due to detrusor hypocontractility, and therefore definitive assessment of the cause of poor urinary flow requires voiding cystometrography. An intermittent, poor flow without a sharp end-point may distinguish patients with BOO due to BPE from those with urethral stricture, characterized by a more prolonged uroflow, sharp cut-off, and sometimes abdominal straining.

Reduced maximum flow rate (Q_{max} < 15 mL s^{-1} can be a useful means of distinguishing bladder outflow obstruction among symptomatic men[20] and identifying those most likely to benefit from surgical treatment.[1,21] BOO is more common at lower maximum flow rates and as many as 90% of men with Q_{max} less than 5 mL s^{-1} may be obstructed.[22] Some symptomatic patients, however, have a high flow with increased voiding pressures with outflow obstruction. Surgery is less successful in those men with instability[1] or underactive detrusor,[2] but in 30% of men with BOO, the instability may be relieved. Patients with LUTS who do not have reduced uroflow are less likely to have BOO, more likely to have detrusor instability, and therefore merit further investigation.

We evaluated the variability of uroflow measurements in 147 men with clinical evidence of BPH prior to recruitment into a study of the efficacy and safety of the α-1 selective adrenoceptor blocker, doxazosin, in the treatment of BPH.[23] Uroflow was measured twice at the initial screening visit and again twice 2 weeks later. The differences in maximum and mean uroflow between these measurements were calculated at each visit, and the within-patient variability assessed using the intraclass correlation coefficient (ICC): the ICC is the ratio of the between-patient variation to the total variation, where the total variation is the sum of the between-patient variation and the within-patient variation. Thus, an ICC equal to 1 indicates that all the variability is accounted for by differences between patients rather than that within individuals. We observed intraclass correlation coefficients for the mean and maximum flow rate between 0.70 and 0.82, indicating that intra-individual variation accounted for a substantial component of the total variation in uroflow.

A single uroflow in an individual patient, therefore, may not be reliable, and should be interpreted with caution. Clinically important test–retest variation may be observed in some patients. In this study,[23] variation of at least 2.0 mL s^{-1} was observed in up to 40% of patients and as many as 32% of uroflows improved and 40% declined with respect to a cut-off of 12 mL s^{-1} at either of the two visits. The variability of uroflow, particularly in men with BPH, has been addressed in other studies.[24-26] Age and circadian changes may contribute, together with differences in voided volume (particularly in normal men with normal lower urinary tract function). Psychological and learning factors also may influence flow-rate measurements.

ULTRASOUND ASSESSMENT OF THE URINARY TRACT

Ultrasound is a readily available means of assessing structural aspects of both lower and upper urinary tracts. It provides an opportunity for objective measurement of bladder emptying, and this may be worthwhile, because incomplete emptying is a notoriously unreliable and subjective symptom, and furthermore chronic retention may exist without bothersome urinary symptoms.[27,28]

Ultrasound provides a reasonably accurate and non-invasive method of assessing bladder emptying,[29] as well as an estimate of functional capacity. Though catheterization with careful attention to technique offers a more accurate method, this is invasive and incurs risks of sepsis and trauma. Bladder wall thickness can be examined with ultrasound, though this has no particular clinical value in the evaluation of BOO. Incomplete bladder emptying may alert the clinician to the possibility of hydronephrosis, easily diagnosed at the same examination. Ultrasound may also detect concomitant pathology, including calculi, diverticula, and larger bladder tumors. Renal ultrasound may be indicated for loin pain or mass, urinary tract infection, hematuria or renal insufficiency, but though not necessary in uncomplicated BPH, it may be done as a complementary test to identify unsuspected, coexisting pathology.

The clinical significance of incomplete emptying depends on the quantity of residual urine itself and its relationship to the patient's symptoms and bladder function. It may reflect the degree of BOO, detrusor decompensation secondary to BOO, detrusor failure, or sensory abnormalities.[27,30-32] Incomplete emptying, however, does not correlate with symptoms[28] and does not necessarily indicate BOO.[31] A risk of retention or renal impairment in men with incomplete emptying is generally recognized, but difficult

to quantify or relate to a residual threshold. The events that determine how incomplete emptying leads to acute retention, low pressure chronic retention, or high pressure chronic retention with renal impairment are not understood. Residual volumes greater than 200–300 mL are taken somewhat arbitrarily to be significant, and lesser volumes may be relevant in men with neuropathic bladder or recurrent urinary tract infection.

Assessment of residual volume is unfortunately not a precise test, owing to significant test–retest variability, and several measurements may be required for a representative estimate. We examined post-micturition bladder urine volumes using transabdominal ultrasound among 40 men aged between 55 and 82 years awaiting TURP.[33] Measurements were taken on six occasions over a 3-month period, ensuring a full bladder before voiding, and a voided volume of at least 150 mL. In two-thirds of patients, these measurements varied by over 150 mL, and in one-third it was less than 120 mL. The variation was related to the mean residual, with reasonable test–retest reliability seen only in those men with a mean residual less than 100 mL. The unphysiological circumstances in which this investigation is often carried out, together with the patient's anxiety and unfamiliarity with procedure may account for some variation, but age and diurnal variation may also contribute.[28]

Unless chronic retention is diagnosed, postvoid residual does not offer any substantial insight into a patient's clinical condition or prognosis (either treated or untreated). Postvoid residual is not suitable for monitoring individual patients, and serial changes are unlikely to provide information that reflects the course of BOO.

URODYNAMIC STUDIES

Pressure-flow studies provide the most reliable means of assessing bladder outflow obstruction and relating lower urinary tract symptoms to functional abnormalities of the bladder. Pressure-flow studies are of particular value in the assessment of symptomatic patients who have already had treatment, and those in whom neurological disease is suspected or lower urinary symptoms persist after treatment. Ambulatory urodynamics may be worthwhile in men requiring more detailed assessment of symptomatology. These investigations are merited for research, but are invasive and not usually necessary for the routine assessment of BPH.[13]

CONCLUSION

Growing numbers of men are seeking advice and treatment for LUTS, BPE, and prostate cancer. Presentation varies considerably between individuals, and management decisions must be based on careful clinical evaluation. A diagnosis of BPH requires thorough symptomatic assessment, appropriate clinical examination, and exclusion of other significant prostatic or lower urinary tract pathology. A wide range of medical therapies are available that improve symptoms, quality of life, and urodynamic parameters, and surgery can generally be reserved for men with complications of BOO or persistent and bothersome symptoms.

REFERENCES

1 Jensen KME, Jorgensen JB, Mogensen P. Urodynamics in prostatism: I. Prognostic value of uroflowmetry. *Scand J Urol Nephrol* 1988; **22**: 109–17.

2 Neal DE, Ramsden PD, Sharples L *et al.* Outcome of elective prostatectomy. *BMJ* 1989; **299**: 762–7.

3 Shapiro E, Hartanto V, Lepor H. The response to alpha blockade in benign prostatic hyperplasia is related to the percent area density of prostate smooth muscle. *Prostate* 1992; **21**(4): 297–307.

4 Boyle P, Gould AL, Roehrborn CG. Prostate volume predicts outcome of treatment of benign prostatic hyperplasia with finasteride: meta-analysis of randomized clinical trials. *Urology* 1996; **48**: 398–405.

5 Dorflinger T, England DM, Madsen PO, Bruskewitz RC. Urodynamic and histological correlates of benign prostatic hyperplasia. *J Urol* 1988; **140**: 1487–90.

6 Reynard JM, Abrams P. Bladder-outlet obstruction – assessment of symptoms. *World J Urol* 1995; **13**: 3–8.

7 Elbadawi A. BPH-associated voiding dysfunction: detrusor is pivotal. *Contemp Urol* 1994; **6**: 21–38.

8 Holm NR, Horn T, Hald T. Detrusor in ageing and obstruction. *Scand J Urol Nephrol* 1995; **29**: 45–9.

9 Girman CJ, Jacobsen SJ, Guess HA *et al.* Natural history of prostatism: relationship among symptoms, prostate volume and peak urinary flow rate. *J Urol* 1995; **153**: 1510–5.

10 Rosier PFWM, de la Rosette JJMCH. Is there a correlation between prostatic size and bladder outlet obstruction? *World J Urol* 1995; **13**: 9–13.

11 Ball AJ, Feneley RCL, Abrams PH. The natural history of untreated "prostatism". *Br J Urol* 1981; **53**: 613–16.

12 Abrams P. New words for old: lower urinary tract symptoms for "prostatism". *BMJ* 1994; **308**: 929–30.

13 McConnell JD, Barry MJ, Bruskewitz RC *et al. Benign Prostatic Hyperplasia: Diagnosis and Treatment. Clinical Practice Guideline*, No. 8. AHCPR Publication No. 94–0582. Rockville, MD: Agency for Health Care Policy and Research, Public Health Services, US Department of Health and Human Services 1994.

14 Reynard JM, Cannon A, Yang Q, Abrams P. A novel therapy for nocturnal polyuria: a double-blind randomized trial of frusemide against placebo. *Br J Urol* 1998; **81**: 215–18.

15 Boyarsky S, Jones G, Paulson DF, Prout GR. A new look at bladder neck obstruction by the Food and Drug Administration regulators: guidelines for investigation of benign prostatic hypertrophy. *Trans Am Assoc Genitourin Surg* 1977; **68**: 29–32.

16 Madsen PO, Iverson P, Hinman F Jr (eds) A point system for selecting operative candidates. In: *Benign Prostatic Hypertrophy*. New York: Springer 1983: 763–5.

17 Barry MJ, Fowler FJ Jr, O'Leary MP *et al.* The American Urological Association symptom index for benign prostatic hyperplasia. *J Urol* 1992; **148**: 1549–57.

18 Roehrborn CG, Girman CJ, Rhodes T *et al.* Correlation between prostate size estimated by digital rectal examination and measured by transrectal ultrasound. *Urology* 1997; **49**: 548–57.

19 Mebust W, Holtgrewe H, Cocket APC, Peters PC. Transurethral prostatectomy: immediate and post operative complications. A comparative study of 13 participating institutions evaluating 3885 patients. *J Urol* 1989; **141**: 243–7.

20 Neal DE, Styles RA, Powell PH, Ramsden PD. Relationship between detrusor function and residual urine, in men undergoing prostatectomy. *Br J Urol* 1987; **60**: 560–6.

21 Abrams P. Prostatism and prostatectomy: the value of urine flow rate measurement in the preoperative assessment for operation. *J Urol* 1977; **117**: 71–4.

22 van Mastright R. Is it really necessary to do a pressure-flow study in each patient? *Neurourol Urodyn* 1993; **12**: 419–20.

23 Feneley MR, Dunsmuir WD, Bryan J, Kirby RS. Reproducibility of uroflow measurements: experience during a double blind placebo controlled study of doxazosin in benign prostatic hyperplasia. *Urology* 1996; **47**: 658–71.

24 Drach GW, Layton TN, Binard WJ. Male peak urinary flow rate: relationships to volume voided and age. *J Urol* 1979; **122**: 210–4.

25 Golomb J, Lindner A, Siegel Y, Korczak D. Variability and circadian changes in home uroflowmetry in patients with benign prostatic hyperplasia compared to normal controls. *J Urol* 1992; **147**: 1044–7.

26 Barry MJ, Girman CJ, O'Leary MP *et al.* BPH Treatment Outcomes Study Group. Using repeated measures of symptom score, uroflow, and prostate specific antigen in the clinical management of prostate disease. *J Urol* 1995; **153**: 99–103.

27 Andersen JT, Nordling J, Walter S. Prostatism. 1. The correlations between symptoms, cystometric and urodynamic findings. *Scand J Urol Nephrol* 1979; **13**: 229–36.

28 Bruskewitz RC, Iverson P, Madsen PO. Value of postvoid residual urine determination in evaluation of prostatism. *Urology* 1982; **20**: 602–4.

29 Birch NC, Hurst G, Doyle PT. Serial residual volumes in men with prostatic hypertrophy. *Br J Urol* 1988; **62**: 571–5.

30 Turner-Warwick R, Whiteside CG, Arnold EP *et al.* A urodynamic view of prostatic obstruction and the results of prostatectomy. *Br J Urol* 1973; **45**: 631–45.

31 Abrams PH, Griffiths DJ. The assessment of prostatic obstruction from urodynamic measurements and from residual urine. *Br J Urol* 1979; **51**: 129–33.

32 Parys BT, Machin DG, Woolfenden KA, Parsons KF. Chronic urinary retention – a sensory problem? *Br J Urol* 1988; **62**: 546–9.

33 Dunsmuir WD, Feneley MR, Corry DA *et al.* The day-to-day variation (test–retest reliability) of residual urine measurement. *Br J Urol* 1996; **77**: 192–3.

COMMENTARY

In this chapter, Drs Feneley and Kirby have described in detail the role of, and controversies surrounding, each of the symptom indices and tests commonly used to diagnose, evaluate, and treat patients with symptoms of BPH and LUTS. They have also discussed the differential diagnosis of BPH and LUTS and various conditions that may mimic BPH.

It has become obvious in recent years that men with LUTS or BPH seek therapy for the relief of symptoms. Objective tests to document obstruction, such as pressure-flow studies, do not correlate well with symptoms, and relief of obstruction does not always relieve symptoms. There is even less significant association between symptoms and tests such as uroflow and residual urine measurements. One area where pressure-flow studies in men with symptoms of prostatism may be useful is in the patient who has a peak uroflow over 15 mL s^{-1}. Such patients may have overcompensating detrusor muscles that force urine out despite obstruction. By documenting high pressure urine flow corrective measures can be employed. Otherwise detrusor failure and urinary retention may eventually occur. The key index, however, for assessment of BPH from a patient's point of view is the symptom score. The IPSS or AUA score, while not perfect, has been validated and found to be reproducible for determining progression and response to therapy. The drawback of the AUA symptom score is that it increases in all men with aging[1] and also in women, suggesting that the symptoms are not disease-specific for BPH. Nevertheless, the AHCPR has recommended an algorithm of diagnosis and treatment of BPH (see Figure 6.1 and Chapter 7 – "AHCPR (US) Guidelines in BPH") and symptom scores are a key part of it. This algorithm is useful as a guide for avoiding unnecessary tests and for determining in a sequential manner which patients need further evaluation.

Recently, the adherence to these guidelines in the US by urologists in four states was assessed.[2] It was found that, of 1828 cases evaluated, only 7.5% of cases had documentation of AUA symptom scores, and among recommended tests of UA, DRE, and preoperative serum creatinine only 26% had documentation that these tests were performed. Furthermore, only 36% of sonograms had indications documented, while 76% of IVPs had indications documented.

This survey suggests that more education of urologists is needed to implement AHCPR guidelines. It was also noted that there was a 32% decrease in the number of TURPs from 1992 to 1994, based more on the advent of medical therapy than on the AHCPR guidelines.

It is interesting also to note that, in a recent study by the International Continence Society of symptoms of LUTS reported in 12 countries, significant differences were found in the types of symptoms reported between European countries.[3] For example, while decreased stream and intermittency were very common in most European countries, terminal dribbling was the most common symptom reported in Israel. Symptoms common in European countries were not common at all in others. Moreover, the differences were not explainable, even controlling for confounding variables. Additionally, the symptom differences appeared more pronounced between far eastern countries and Europe and the US data. Similar findings were also noted in a study from Singapore.[4]

These findings suggest that country-specific symptoms may need to be developed and evaluated. However, a common theme in all these data was that efficacy of various therapies was most pronounced with "bothersomeness" of symptoms.[5] The bother score may, therefore, be the critical index that should be used to evaluate need for therapy as well as its efficacy. The AUA Bother Index is also further discussed in Chapter 5.

1 Kojima M, Naya Y, Inoue W. *et al*. The American Urological Association Symptom Index for benign prostatic hyperplasia as a function of age, volume, and ultrasonic appearance of the prostate. *J Urol* 1997; **157**: 2160–5.

2 Hood H, Burgess PA, Holtgrewe HL. *et al*. Adherence to Agency for Health Care Policy and Research Guidelines for benign prostatic hyperplasia. *J Urol* 1997; **158**: 1417–21.

3 Witjes WPJ, de la Rosette JJMCH, Donovan JL. *et al*. International Continence Society "Benign Prostatic Hyperplasia" Study Group. The International Continence Society "Benign Prostatic Hyperplasia" Study: international differences in lower

urinary tract symptoms and related bother. *J Urol* 1997; **157**: 1295–1300.

4 Tan HY, Choo WC, Archibald C, Esuvaranathan K. A community based study of prostatic symptoms in Singapore. *J Urol* 1996; **157**: 890–3.

5 Peters TJ, Donovan JL, Kay HE *et al*. International Continence Society "Benign Prostatic Hyperplasia" Study Group. The International Continence Society "Benign Prostatic Hyperplasia" Study: the bothersomeness of urinary symptoms. *J Urol* 1997; **157**: 885–9.

The Agency for Health Care Policy and Research Clinical Guidelines for the Diagnosis and Treatment of Benign Prostatic Hyperplasia

7

C. G. Roehrborn

RATIONALE FOR THE BENIGN PROSTATIC HYPERPLASIA GUIDELINES

The Agency for Health Care Policy and Research (AHCPR) in the US Department of Health and Human Services (HHS) was established in 1989 under the Omnibus Budget Reconciliation Act to enhance the quality, appropriateness, and effectiveness of health care services, and the access to these services. AHCPR attempted to carry out its mission by facilitating the development of clinical practice guidelines, and disseminating them to health care providers, policy makers, and the public.

The topics for guideline development were selected based on a variety of criteria: the condition had to be a significant public health problem, significant health care costs had to be associated with the problem, and a variance in current medical practice with regard to the treatment of the problem had to be present.

Among the first eight topics selected was the diagnosis and treatment of benign prostatic hyperplasia (BPH). BPH is a condition with a very high prevalence in elderly men, and its treatment is associated with significant health care expenses. Most importantly, however, at the time the guideline process was initiated, there was great uncertainty regarding the etiology and natural history of the disease process, the indications *for* and the timing and choice *of* treatment, as well as the outcomes expected *from* treatment. The Prostate Outcomes Research Team (PORT) observed significant variations in practice pattern in a small geographic area in New England with regard to treatment for BPH as well as other common diseases.[1,2] Concerning the treatment choices available, the "gold standard" of transurethral resection of the prostate (TURP) had come under increasing criticism. It was observed that up to 20% of patients were dissatisfied with the outcome of the intervention, that many patients with mild or moderate symptoms did not benefit at all from the intervention,[3] and, lastly, there were concerns about increased delayed mortality following TURP.[4,5]

Parallel to these developments, new medical and device-oriented therapies for BPH became available, most notably α-receptor blockade and 5 α-reductase inhibitor treatment, as well as balloon dilation of the prostatic urethra. Although time has proven balloon dilation not to have a lasting beneficial effect on the signs and symptoms of prostatism above and beyond simple cystoscopy,[6] other minimally invasive treatment modalities such as hyperthermia, thermotherapy, stents and spirals, laser ablation of the prostate and others, entered the research and testing stage, and occasionally the market place. While the first edition of the BPH guidelines addresses the data available on balloon dilation of the prostate at the time of its writing, a treatment now all but obsolete, other device-oriented treatment strategies can be analyzed and compared in a similar fashion in future editions of the BPH guideline documents.

BPH, its high prevalence, the uncertainties concerning its natural history, the high health care cost associated with its treatment, and the rapidly changing and sometimes confusing field of treatment alternatives, made it a perfect target for one of the early AHCPR-sponsored treatment guidelines.

THE GUIDELINES PANEL AND PROCESS

The AHCPR convened a multidisciplinary panel, which reviewed the entire available literature on BPH and then formulated guidelines for the diagnostic evaluation and treatment of the disease.[7] The entire process of the guideline development followed the so-called explicit approach, championed and described by David Eddy in a series of articles in the *Journal of the American Medical Association*.[8-22] This particular approach calls for a comprehensive review of all available literature and data on the intervention in question. The data are then taken at face value and analyzed with regard to the benefits and harms associated with the intervention. Costs are taken into consideration if there are limits on resources. Preferences of patients, based on their interpretation of the benefits and harms and, if present, the net benefit of the intervention, are taken into account, and the guidelines are formulated. Thus, the guideline process in its purest form is explicit in that all supporting data are clearly laid out, evidence and preference based. In areas of uncertainty or where no data are available, expert opinion of the panel might be utilized instead of data, as long as it is clearly labeled as such in an explicit manner.

There are three components to the BPH guidelines, which are available through the AHCPR Publications Clearinghouse at (800)358–9295 or by writing to PO Box 8547,

Silver Spring, MD 20907, USA. The three components are the *Clinical Practice Guideline* (AHCPR Publication No. 94–0582), the *Quick Reference Guide for Clinicians* (AHCPR Publication No. 94–0583), and the *Patient Guide* (AHCPR Publication No. 94–0584).[7,23,24]

TARGET POPULATION

The BPH guidelines are intended to apply only to men over the age of 50 with lower urinary tract symptoms (LUTS) suggestive of BPH, but no other severe or confounding comorbidities or other known causes of voiding dysfunction. Patients to whom the guidelines apply should be overall in good health and not at increased risk for a possible surgical procedure.

Patients with one or more of the following exclusion criteria would, in general, not follow the suggested diagnostic and treatment algorithms:

- patients who have been diagnosed to have cancer of the prostate;
- patients who either have already been treated for BPH, or who are currently being treated and have failed to improve;
- patients under the age of 50 years;
- patients with diabetes mellitus and diabetic neuropathy;
- patients whose history is suggestive of a neurological disorder;
- patients with a history of pelvic surgery or trauma;
- patients taking drugs that have the potential to affect the function of the detrusor muscle, the function of the bladder outlet and sphincter muscle, or to alter the patient's voiding habits.

The work-up of such patients is expected to be more in-depth and tailored to the individual patient's problem. It usually will involve more urodynamic and imaging studies than is recommended for the "standard" patient.

DIAGNOSTIC EVALUATION

INITIAL EVALUATION

As part of the initial evaluation of a patient presumed to have BPH, the following tests and procedures should be conducted (Figure 7.1):

(1) obtain a careful medical history;
(2) focused physical examination including a digital rectal examination (DRE) and a focused neurological examination;
(3) urinalysis by using a dipstick method or microscopic examination of the urinary sediment;
(4) measurement of serum creatinine as a measure of renal function;
(5) measurement of serum prostate-specific antigen (PSA) (optional test).

These tests serve to confirm the presumed diagnosis of BPH and to exclude other conditions that might mimic the non-specific LUTS.

(1) Medical History

A detailed medical history focusing on the urinary tract, previous surgical procedures, general health issues, and fitness for possible surgical procedures is recommended.

Specific areas to discuss when taking the history of a man with BPH symptoms include a history of hematuria, urinary tract infection, diabetes, nervous system disease (for example, Parkinson's disease or stroke), urethral stricture disease, urinary retention, and aggravation of symptoms by cold or sinus medication. Current prescriptions and over-the-counter medications should be examined to determine if the patient is taking drugs that impair bladder contractility (anticholinergics) or increase outflow resistance (sympathomimetics).

(2) Physical Examination

DRE and neurologic examination are done to detect prostate or rectal malignancy, to evaluate anal sphincter tone, and to rule out any neurologic problems that may cause the presenting symptoms. The presence of induration is as important a finding as the presence of a nodule.

The outcomes of these tests are not entirely known, and the specificity of the rectal examination for the detection of prostate cancer is limited. Only 26–34% of men with suspicious findings on DRE have positive biopsies for cancer.[25–27] The sensitivity is equally low and in one study was found to be only 33%.[28]

Nevertheless, given the minimal expense, discomfort, and time involved, most patients would opt to have the DRE done. Although the Preventive Services Task Force[29] could not recommend for or against inclusion of the DRE in periodic health examinations, that recommendation applies to screening of asymptomatic men and not specifically to aging men with LUTS.

Furthermore, the rectal examination establishes the approximate size of the prostate gland. In patients who choose or require invasive therapy such as surgery, estimation of prostate size is important for selecting the most appropriate technical approach. DRE provides a sufficiently accurate measurement in most of these cases.

However, the size of the prostate should not be considered in deciding whether active treatment is required. Prostate size does not correlate with symptom severity, degree of urodynamic obstruction, or treatment outcomes.[30,31] If a more precise measurement of prostate size than can be obtained from a DRE is needed, to determine whether to perform open prostatectomy rather than TURP, ultrasound (transabdominal or transrectal) is more accurate than intravenous urography or urethrocystoscopy.

(3) Urinalysis

There is insufficient evidence that urinalysis is an effective screening procedure for asymptomatic men.[29] Because serious urinary tract disorders are relatively uncommon, the positive predictive value of screening for

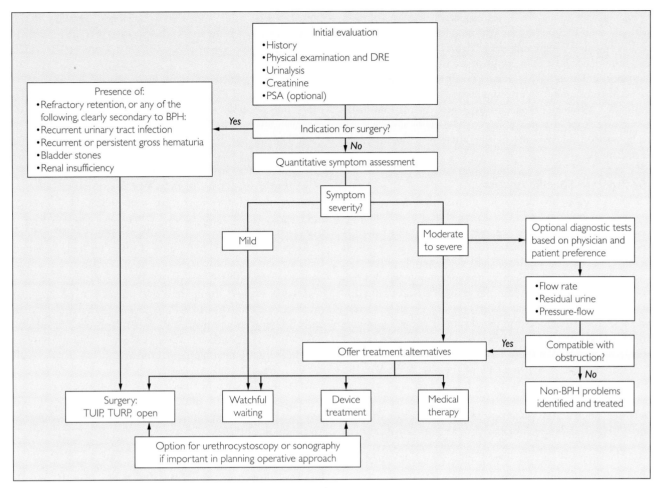

Figure 7.1 Decision diagram for the diagnosis and treatment of BPH

Source: Adapted from McConnell JD, Barry MJ, Bruskewiz RC *et al. Benign Prostatic Hyperplasia: Diagnosis and Treatment. Clinical Practice Guideline,* No. 8. AHCPR Publication No. 94–0582. Rockville, MD: Agency for Health Care Policy and Research, US Department of Health and Human Services 1994

them is low, and the effectiveness of early detection and intervention is unproven.

However, in older men with BPH and a higher prevalence of these disorders, the benefits of an innocuous test such as urinalysis clearly outweigh the harms involved. The test permits the selective use of renal imaging and endoscopy for patients with the greatest chance of benefiting from them. More important, urinalysis assists in distinguishing urinary tract infections and bladder cancer from BPH. These conditions may produce urinary tract symptoms (such as frequency and urgency) that mimic BPH.

The positive predictive value of urinalysis for cancer or other urologic diseases is 4–26, depending on the patients screened and the rigor of follow-up studies.[32–34] If a dipstick approach is used, a test that includes leukocyte esterase and nitrite tests for the detection of pyuria and bacteriuria should be utilized.[29]

(4) Creatinine Measurement (Assessment of Renal Function)

There are many reasons for recommending creatinine measurement. One is the percentage of BPH patients who may have renal insufficiency. An analysis of the basis of BPH treatments contained seven studies in which the percentage of patients with renal insufficiency is mentioned.[7] In these studies, the percentage of patients with renal insufficiency ranges from 0.3 to 30%. The mean is 13.6%. This may be an overestimation, because the reports contain information only on patients eventually receiving treatment. Still, the number of patients with renal insufficiency, in a population of patients seeing a physician for symptomatic prostatism, may be as high as 1 in 10.

It is well established that BPH patients with renal insufficiency have increased risk of postoperative complications. The risk is 25% for patients with renal insufficiency, compared with 17% for patients without the condition.[35] Moreover, the mortality increases up to sixfold for BPH patients treated surgically if they have renal insufficiency.[36,37] Of 6102 patients evaluated in 25 studies by intravenous urography prior to prostate surgery, 7.6% had evidence of hydronephrosis. Of these patients, 33.6% had associated renal insufficiency.

Elevated serum creatinine in a patient is a reason for recommending appropriate imaging studies to evaluate the upper urinary tract. In a retrospective analysis of 345 patients who had undergone prostatectomy, 1.7% ($n = 6$) had occult and progressive renal damage.[38] These patients had minimal or no urinary symptoms and presumably fit the category of patients with "silent prostatism." Measurement of serum creatinine is one modality for identifying such patients. Although renal insufficiency from minimally symptomatic BPH is probably rare, the probability has yet to be defined. Meanwhile, routine creatinine measurement is reasonable.

(5) Prostate-Specific Antigen

PSA was initially discovered in seminal plasma by Hara *et al.* in Japan in 1971.[39] In 1979, Wang *et al.* isolated an antigen from prostatic tissue, purified it, and demonstrated its specificity for prostatic tissue.[40] Although it was identified in all types of prostatic tissue (normal, benign hyperplastic, and malignant), it could not be found in any other human tissue. Concentrations of PSA per gram of tissue do not differ significantly among the three types of prostatic tissue, and PSA can be detected in the serum of young men with small, non-hyperplastic prostates, older men with BPH, and men with localized or metastatic prostate cancer.

With regard to the discussion of the role of PSA in the diagnostic work-up of patients with LUTS, it is of greatest importance to know how well PSA is able to separate between benign and malignant prostatic diseases. In four series reported in the literature,[41–44] 191 of 688 (28%) of men with histologically proven BPH had a PSA level of only >4.0 ng mL^{-1} (Tandem-R PSA), thus above the currently accepted upper limit of normal.

Since PSA is not specific for prostate cancer, but rather for all types of prostate tissue, it is certainly not the ideal tumor marker. If PSA is to be of value as a detector of early prostate cancer and to be used for this purpose in the evaluation of patients presenting with LUTS, it must be capable of identifying and distinguishing patients with curable disease from men with purely benign conditions of the prostate. In other words, PSA must have a high sensitivity and specificity, a low false negative and false positive rate, as well as a high negative and positive predictive value for detecting and distinguishing prostate cancer from BPH. These are clearly the ideal characteristics of any screening test for prostate cancer.

Since BPH tissue contributes to the serum PSA concentration and has a high prevalence in men more than 50 years old, a method of evaluating PSA as a reliable detector of early, curable prostate cancer is to compare the PSA values of patients with organ-confined prostate cancer (CaP) (patients who have the greatest likelihood of cure with definitive therapy) with those men who have BPH only. When combining data reported by three independent investigators,[43,45,46] 136 of 319 (43%) of patients with prostate cancer had a PSA value within the normal range (<4.0 ng mL^{-1}) and 148 of 597 (25%) of men with BPH had a PSA value above the reference range (0.0–4.0 ng mL^{-1}). When one evaluates these data statistically, PSA has a 64% diagnostic accuracy (efficiency) for CaP if the serum concentra-

tion is >4 ng mL^{-1}, and a 70% diagnostic accuracy if the serum value is >10 ng mL^{-1}. The positive predictive value is 49 and 75% for serum PSA values >4 and 10 ng mL^{-1}, respectively.

Recently, additional data were presented making a mandatory use of PSA in the evaluation of men with LUTS more questionable. Sershon *et al.*[47] compared retrospectively PSA values in 200 men with BPH vs. 199 men with CaP. The median PSA was 4.0 (0.2–76.0) ng mL^{-1} in the BPH group, vs. 5.9 (0.4–58.0) ng mL^{-1} ($P<0.01$) in the CaP group. At a cut-off point of 4.0, PSA had a sensitivity of 71, but a specificity of only 49% for distinguishing the two groups. Furthermore, the area under the receiver operating characteristic (ROC) curve for PSA, which estimates the probability that a randomly chosen CaP patient would have a higher PSA value than a randomly selected BPH patient, was only 0.64 (a non-informative test would have a value of 0.5).

Monda *et al.*[48] compared the prevalence of stage A prostate cancer in 499 TURP specimens from a pre-PSA era with 532 specimens from a PSA era. The prevalence was 8.6 vs. 9.3%, respectively. These data argue against a patient benefit from the mandatory routine use of PSA in men with LUTS, particularly when considering that a large number of patients (28%) with histological BPH only would undergo unnecessary further studies (transrectal ultrasound and prostate biopsy) with added costs and morbidity because of an elevation of PSA.

One important subgroup of patients are those patients, who are potential candidates for curative treatment for localized prostate cancer (life expectancy over 10 years), and who are interested in treatment with finasteride (Proscar). Finasteride is a 5α-reductase inhibitor, which was approved recently for the treatment of BPH in the USA by the FDA and in other European countries. It inhibits the conversion of testosterone to dihydrotestosterone (DHT). Over the course of 6–12 months treatment, the prostate shrinks in over 50% of patients by >20%. During the same time interval, the serum PSA level falls by about 50%, independent of the pretreatment level.[49,50] It is not known whether or not this fall in PSA levels is identical in men harboring prostate cancer at the time of initiating treatment, and neither is it known whether the lower level represents a new baseline for monitoring of the patient. A patient who has been on finasteride for 6 months and presents with a PSA level of 4.0 ng mL^{-1} might have had a level of 8.0 ng mL^{-1} – which is clearly abnormal – prior to the treatment. Thus, it is imperative to obtain a PSA baseline level in this particular subgroup of men. However, it is still unknown how to interpret the results of PSA measurements during treatment with finasteride if the level does not drop by 50% or more. No reliable information is available to give guidance to health care providers as to the critical level to which it must fall before more invasive testing needs to be instituted to rule out prostate cancer.

The single cut-off level for serum PSA measurement has come under scrutiny. Oesterling *et al.*[51] randomly selected a sample of 471 men between 40 and 79 years of age from the

Olmsted County population for a detailed preliminary examination, including serum PSA measurement, DRE, and transrectal ultrasonography (TRUS). Regression models were used to assess the association between PSA concentration and age, and the derived age-specific reference ranges. After analyzing these data, they recommended an upper limit of normal for serum PSA using the Tandem-R PSA assay for men age 40–49 years of 3.0 ng mL^{-1}; 50–59 years of age, 4.1 ng mL^{-1}; 60–69 years of age, 5.6 ng mL^{-1}; and 70–79 years of age, 7.6 ng mL^{-1}. By decreasing the reference range in younger men, the sensitivity for the detection of prostate cancer will be increased, while by increasing the cut-off level in elderly men, the specificity will be increased, thus reducing the number of unnecessary biopsies in elderly men. While the basic underlying concept of age-specific reference ranges has been corroborated by other investigators,[52,53] it should be noted that these reference ranges established in normal men may differ considerably between racial and ethnic groups.

PSA is capable of forming complexes with serine protease inhibitors found in serum, most readily with α1-antichymotrypsin (PSA-ACT) and α2-macroglobulin (PSA-MG). Of the three possible forms of PSA in serum, only the uncomplexed and PSA-ACT can be measured by immunoassays – the sum of these two thus representing the total (T-PSA) in serum.[54]

Although considerable overlap exists, several investigators have reported that the proportion of PSA-ACT is higher in men with prostate cancer than in men with BPH. Therefore, by calculating either the ratio of PSA-ACT/T-PSA[55] or the ratio of free PSA/total PSA (F-PSA/T-PSA),[56] the two disease processes might be better differentiated than by the T-PSA alone.

The two measurable forms of PSA vary in their concentration values depending on the assay used to measure them. For example, if two samples contains exactly the same amount of PSA, but in the first sample it is present in 100% F-PSA form, and in the second in 100% PSA-ACT form, an equimolar-response assay would result in an identical measurement. A skewed-response assay would, however, result in different concentrations for both samples, depending whether it "favors" the F-PSA or the PSA-ACT. Length of incubation time and the characteristic of the antibody reagent contribute to the skewed response. Specific assays for F-PSA and PSA-ACT should help in sorting out these differences, and thus improve the statistical performance of PSA testing in differentiating between prostate cancer and BPH.

Christensson et al.[56] measured F-PSA and PSA-ACT in the serum of 144 men with BPH and 121 with prostate cancer. The mean F/T (F-PSA/T-PSA) ratio was 0.18 in men with prostate cancer and 0.28 in men with BPH ($P<0.0001$), indicating a greater proportion of PSA-ACT in men with prostate cancer. Using a cut-off of 5 ng mL^{-1} for T-PSA, the specificity for T-PSA to differentiate prostate cancer and BPH at a sensitivity of 90% was 55%, while it was 73% for the F/T ratio. One caveat of this study is that some of the patients with prostate cancer were diagnosed

based only on fine needle aspiration, while others had undergone hormonal treatment already, the effect of which on the various forms of PSA is unknown.

Catalona et al.[57] studied 96 men with presumed BPH who had at least three negative TRUS biopsies, 84 men with cancer (20 small glands <40 mL and 64 large glands >40 mL), and 96 age-stratified controls with a PSA of <4.0 ng mL^{-1}. Men with BPH had lower percent F-PSA (8.6 and 13.4%, respectively, with small and large glands) vs. men with BPH (20.3%) and controls (23.0%). ROC curve analysis showed that, using a cut-off of <18% of F-PSA or a suspicious DRE, 93% of all cancers would have been detected while eliminating 39% of the negative biopsies.

Partin et al.[58] measured various ratios of F-PSA and T-PSA in the preoperative sera of 87 men, 41 of whom had BPH confirmed by TURP or prostatectomy, and 46 had prostate cancer by TRUS biopsy or radical prostatectomy. By ROC curve analysis, they found that the ratio of F/T PSA best detected cancer in men with a T-PSA between 4.0 and 10.0 ng mL^{-1} ($n=50$) with an area under the curve (AUC) of 0.77 vs. 0.59 for T-PSA. Sensitivity and specificity were 72% and 71%, respectively.

The problems with these two preliminary studies are that, in one, the absence of cancer was assumed based on negative biopsies without ultimate histological proof, while, in the other, a limited number of patients were available for ROC analysis.

Most recently, Oesterling et al.[59] examined stored sera from 422 healthy men 40–79 years of age in Olmsted County, MN, in whom the diagnosis of prostate cancer was excluded by DRE, T-PSA, and TRUS. Based on their findings, reference ranges were proposed for F-PSA, T-PSA, and PSA-ACT (c-PSA), as well as for the F/T, C/T, and F/C ratios.

Because of the limited diagnostic sensitivity and specificity of serum PSA in differentiating men with BPH from those with localized prostate cancer, the panel classified the measurement of serum PSA as an optional test. Whether or not this recommendation will change in future editions of the guidelines, based on additional data, remains to be seen.

INDICATION FOR SURGERY

An immediate indication for surgery is present in men with one or more of the following conditions attributable to BPH (see Figure 7.1):

- refractory retention;
- recurrent urinary tract infection;
- recurrent or persistent gross hematuria;
- bladder stones;
- renal insufficiency.

Patients falling in any one of these categories identified during the initial evaluation should be considered for any one of the available surgical treatment options, usually transurethral incision or resection of the prostate (TUIP or TURP) or open surgical enucleation of the prostate. The choice of the surgical treatment depends on the size and configuration of the prostate itself.

EVALUATION OF ABNORMAL FINDINGS DURING INITIAL EVALUATION

Abnormal findings detected during the initial evaluation should be pursued outside the scope of the BPH guidelines, e.g. microscopic hematuria should be evaluated by upper tract imaging, endoscopy, and cytology, an elevated serum PSA should trigger a transrectal ultrasonography-guided biopsy in patients in which the diagnosis of prostate cancer would be of clinical significance.

If after appropriate evaluation no other therapeutic action is required, these patients may re-enter the diagnostic decision algorithm.

QUANTITATIVE SYMPTOM ASSESSMENT

In the past most physicians have attempted to judge the severity of lower urinary tract symptoms by asking the patient a set of questions they were most familiar with in an unstructured interview style. Given the high prevalence of such symptoms in an unselected population of men over the age of 50 years,[60,61] such unstructured, randomly chosen, qualitative questions regarding symptoms do little in terms of identifying patients in need of treatment. Recently, Diokno et al.[62] provided estimates of LUTS in 802 non-institutionalized men aged 60 years and older in the USA. The prevalence of one or more symptoms was 35%, while the annual incidence rates during year 1 and 2 of follow-up was 16.4% and 16.1%, respectively (based on 68.2% and 63.4% who were reinterviewed).

Concerning the global assessment of symptoms by physicians and/or patients, one has to keep in mind that patients and physicians do not always agree in their assessment. In a structured interview of 385 patients and their treating physicians, disagreement in terms of irritative and obstructive symptoms was found in 41% and 25% of cases prior to surgery.[63] Following surgery, disagreement was found in terms of various irritative symptoms in between 33% and 47%, and in terms of obstructive symptoms in 21–42% of cases. In most of these cases, the disagreement arose because patients reported symptoms which were not reported by the physician. Of particular interest is the fact that 16% of patients reported sexual dysfunction following surgery, of which the surgeon was not aware.

To overcome these assessment problems, several attempts have been made to develop standardized symptom score instruments.[64,65] Both of these questionnaires are based on a set of nine questions regarding LUTS believed to be associated with BPH. The patient receives a certain number of points, based on his answers, which are then added to a total score, which ranges from 0 to 27 points. Neither of the questionnaires was ever formally operationalized (put into a question format for self-administration by the patient) or validated. Nevertheless, the use of these questionnaires made it possible to compare the results of different treatment trials for BPH. The American Urological Association (AUA) Measurement Committee has developed a Symptom Index (AUA-SI) which has been tested and validated (Figure 7.2).[66-68] The questionnaire was reduced from originally 73 to finally seven questions, and operationalized for self-administration by the patient. Each

Questions	Not at all	<1 time in 5	<1/2 the time	About 1/2 the time	>1/2 the time	almost always
1. Over the past month or so, how often have you had a sensation of not emptying your bladder completely after you finished urinating?	0	1	2	3	4	5
2. Over the past month or so, how often have you had to urinate again less than 2 hours after you finished urinating?	0	1	2	3	4	5
3. Over the past month or so, how often have you found you stopped and started again several times when you urinated?	0	1	2	3	4	5
4. Over the past month or so, how often have you found it difficult to postpone urination?	0	1	2	3	4	5
5. Over the past month or so, how often have you had a weak urinary stream?	0	1	2	3	4	5
6. Over the past month or so, how often have you had to push or strain to begin urination?	0	1	2	3	4	5
7. Over the past month or so, how many times did you most typically get up to urinate from the time you went to bed at night until the time you got up in the morning?	0	1	2	3	4	5
AUA symptom score = sum of questions 1–7 = _____ _____						

Figure 7.2 American Urological Association Symptom Index

Source: Barry MJ, Fowler FJ Jr, O'Leary MP et al. The American Urological Association Symptom Index for benign prostatic hyperplasia. J Urol 1992: **148**(5): 1549–57

question can be answered on a scale from 0 to 5 and the total score therefore ranges from 0 to 35 points. The 1991 and 1993 WHO-sponsored International Consultations on BPH adopted the AUA-SI and termed it International Prostate Symptom Score (IPSS).

Patients with AUA-SI scores from 0 to 7 points are considered mildly symptomatic, those with scores from 8 to 19 moderately, and those with scores from 20 to 35 points severely symptomatic.

Over the last few years the AUA-SI has been the most widely utilized assessment tool in BPH treatment trials, and validated translations in multiple languages have made it applicable virtually worldwide.

Moon et al.[69] have applied the IPSS to 2245 men participating in the cancer awareness week, and found that the index was not affected by educational and ethnic (72% white and 13% African-American participants) differences, while there were differences in the mean IPSS between different geographic locales (New Orleans 6.24, New York 7.18, and Madison 8.58). Similarly, in over 2000 men participating in the HYCAT (Hytrin Community Assessment Trial) trial, mean AUA-SI (IPSS) were not significantly different when the patients were stratified by educational or socioeconomic status (unpublished data).

A further useful contribution to the IPSS was made by its developers.[70] In a placebo-controlled BPH treatment trial, 1218 men were given the AUA-SI at baseline and at 13 weeks, and were asked to rate their improvement globally at the same time point. Mean changes in AUA-SI for each level of self-rated global improvement were calculated for those men with a AUA-SI from 8 to 19 points, and those with an AUA-SI from 20 to 35 points (Table 7.1).

While the presentations and publications that utilize the AUA-SI are numerous, several investigators have criticized it as being not specific for BPH.[71-73] These authors have administered the AUA-SI to men and age-matched women and showed a similar symptom level within each age stratum in both sexes. To be useful as a measure of symptom severity in a given patient, however, an instrument does not have to be disease specific, e.g. it is immediately evident, that patients with severe arthritis would score poorly on the

Karnofsky performance score, commonly used to assess the impact a cancer has on a patient's everyday activities. This does not mean, that these patients suffer from cancer, but rather that their illness impacts on their everyday activities in a way similar to an advanced cancer disease. Despite these observations, improvements of performance following effective cancer treatment can still be measured by using the Karnofsky performance index, and different treatment regimens can be compared by comparing the resulting changes in the Karnofsky score. This is precisely the appropriate indication for the AUA-SI, namely to measure the baseline severity or frequency of symptoms and allow monitoring of these symptoms during and/or after treatment in men who, on the basis of a comprehensive evaluation, have been diagnosed with BPH. The lack of disease specificity has led some authorities to suggest that the term LUTS should be used rather than BPH until the diagnosis of BPH has been confirmed or established as the causative pathogenic mechanism responsible for the symptoms.

Symptom severity and frequency alone do not sufficiently explain health care-seeking behavior of men. While some men are bothered enough by mild symptoms to consult a physician, others tolerate much more severe symptom frequency and severity before seeking help. In general, a high degree of correlation has been found between symptom severity or frequency and bother. Jacobsen et al.[74] found in a population-based study of men aged 40–79 in Olmsted County, MN, a tight correspondence between the two measures ($r^2 = 0.71$). The AUA Measurement Committee developed and validated an AUA symptom problem index (SPI) as a companion to the AUA-SI.[75] Instead of inquiring about the frequency or severity of symptoms, the seven questions are aimed at the degree to which the present symptoms are a problem for the patient. The answer scheme ranges from "no problem"=0 to "big problem"=4 points for a total score from 0 to 28 points. Baseline data from a medical treatment trial for BPH revealed a correlation of $r=0.74$ between the AUA-SI and the SPI in 1990 men with an AUA-SI of at least 13 points (unpublished data). A comparison of populations in North America and Scotland demonstrated that similar symptom severity levels have a similar impact on and degree of bother in both American and Scottish men.[76] The degree to which patients are bothered by symptoms is more important in the decision whether or not to seek help and undertake treatment, and in fact, men with a bother index greater than predicted from their symptom index were more likely to have sought health care.[74] These men were older, poorer, more anxious, and had a lower general well-being score than those with a bother index closer to that predicted from their symptom index. Moreover, worry and embarrassment about urinary symptoms have also been shown to be important in determining health care-seeking behavior beyond symptom frequency and severity alone.[77] In recognition of these facts, the AUA Measurement Committee has recently also developed and validated a BPH Impact Index (BII) which measures how much the urinary problems affect various domains of health.[75] Both have excellent test–retest

	Mean absolute changes ± SEM in AUA-SI	
	Lower baseline (8–19)	Higher baseline (20–35)
Marked	−7.4 ± 0.29	−15.3 ± 0.76
Moderate	−4.0 ± 0.29	−8.7 ± 0.62
Slight	−1.9 ± 0.29	−6.1 ± 0.54
None	−0.2 ± 0.35	−2.0 ± 0.62
Worse	+3.3 ± 1.09	+1.2 ± 1.79

Table 7.1 Mean absolute changes in AUA-SI for each level of self-rated global improvement in 1218 men enrolled in a medical treatment trial for BPH

Source: Barry MJ, Williford WO, Chang YC et al. BPH-specific health status measures in clinical research: how much change in AUA Symptom Index and the BPH Impact Index is perceptible to patients? J Urol 1995; **154**: 1770–4, with permission

($r=0.88$ for both) reliabilities, correlate with AUA-SI ($r=0.86$ and 0.77), and discriminate between men with BPH and controls (ROC areas under the curve of 0.87 and 0.85).[75] In the aforementioned 1990 men with BPH, a correlation of $r=0.519$ was found between the AUA-SI and the BII.

A single question concerning the disease-specific quality of life was recommended by the 1st and 2nd International Consultations ("If you were to spend the rest of your life with your urinary condition just the way it is now, how would you feel about that?"). The answers to this question range from "delighted" ($=0$ points) to "terrible" ($=6$ points). The combined patient assessment can be expressed as $IPSS_{0-35}$ and QoL_{0-6}.

Other tools have been developed parallel to those discussed above by different groups of investigators, which might serve the same purpose.[78–83]

Assessment of sexual function and dysfunction, an important part of general quality of life, has also become increasingly more important. Several groups are currently developing questionnaires for quantitative evaluation of several domains of sexual function.[84,85]

Linguistic and cultural validated translations of the AUA-SI are available,[86–88] allowing researchers all over the world to utilize this instrument, and permitting a direct comparison of population study data,[89] as well as treatment outcome data between different cultural and ethnic groups.

The guidelines suggest that, for men with mild symptoms (0–7 points), watchful waiting should be the preferred management option (see Figure 7.1). This recommendation is based on the fact that these men usually do not stand to experience any benefit from either medical or surgical treatment for BPH.[3,90] Yearly follow-up using the tests recommended during the initial evaluation is recommended for these patients.

Patients with moderate-to-severe symptoms (8–35 points) may be offered the available treatment alternatives without any further testing (see Figure 7.1). However, certain optional tests may be performed based on physicians' and patients' preferences.

OPTIONAL DIAGNOSTIC TESTS

Urodynamic Studies

Postvoid Residual Urine

Di Mare et al.[91] found that 78% of normal male volunteers have postvoid residual urine volumes of <5 mL, while all of them had residuals of <12 mL. Thus, the presence of significant amounts of residual urine indicates in a non-specific way either the inability of the detrusor muscle to empty the bladder or an increased outlet resistance. For the measurement of residual urine, the least invasive method with acceptable accuracy should be utilized, which is transabdominal ultrasonography.[92,93] The intra-individual day-to-day and circadian variation in the amount of residual urine have been shown to be sometimes greater than the error of transabdominal ultrasonography in measuring that

amount.[94,95] Jensen et al.[96] examined the prognostic value of postvoid residual (PVR) and 14 other variables in relation to postoperative outcome. They found that pressure-flow plots were the best predictor of outcome, and PVR was the second best predictor for differentiating between favorable and unfavorable outcome of surgery. Unfortunately, even a combination of these two best predictors did not allow the authors correctly to predict a single one of the 14 patients who in fact had an unsuccessful outcome in their population of 120, while all successfully treated patients were correctly predicted. Even a combination of all 15 examined parameters allowed only an overall 87.4% correct prediction, and a 33.3% correct prediction of patients destined to fail. A bladder capacity of <300 mL indicated a poorer outcome in this study. The patients with smaller bladder capacity also had a higher incidence of uninhibited detrusor contraction, which is known to be associated with a high rate of failure to improve symptoms.

Data from the BTOPS trial[30] indicate that there is no correlation between residual urine volume and symptom severity or "bothersomeness," prostate size, or PSA, while there is a weak inverse correlation to peak flow rate. Furthermore, there is no correlation between changes in residual urine and changes in either peak flow rate or AUA-SI in 82 men completing a 6-months follow-up visit in the BTOPS BPH Treatment Outcomes Pilot Study trial (Table 7.2).

Similarly, in 274 men in the HYCAT study with an AUA-SI of 13 or greater, no correlations were found between symptom severity, "bothersomeness," or quality of life, and residual urine or peak flow rate (Table 7.3). When the patients were stratified by a peak flow rate of over or under 10 mL s^{-1}, none of the symptom indices was significantly different between these two groups, again demonstrating an absence of correlation between residual urine, flow rates, and symptom severity, bother, and disease-specific quality of life.

Guess et al.[97] evaluated the correlation between peak urinary flow rate, residual urine volume, and degree of renal impairment (defined as a serum creatinine of >1.2 mg dL^{-1}). To address this question, 474 men aged 40–79 years underwent urological examination as part of the Olmstead County study of urinary symptoms. While initially it appeared that residual urine volumes of >100 mL were associated with renal impairment in men with peak flow rates of <10 mL s^{-1}, statistical significance was not reached during the second year of follow-up, and thus the conclusion was that, in this population-based study, no correlation between residual urine volume and renal function compromise could be found.

Rosier et al.[98] evaluated the urodynamic findings of 242 men with ultrasound-confirmed BPH. They found that residual urine volume was associated with bladder outlet obstruction to a much greater degree than with impaired detrusor contractility. Of men with a residual urine oleum of >50 mL 75% were obstructed.

Wasson et al.[99] reported on the failure rates of in-patients randomized to either watchful waiting or TURP. One of the criteria of failure was a PVR urine volume of >350 ml. The

Symptom measure	Mean ± SEM	Correlations (P values) between changes in measures		
		AUA-SI	Q_{max}	Residual urine
AUA-SI	−7.33 ± 0.80	1.00		
Q_{max}	+7.17 ± 1.23	−0.35 (0.001)	1.00	
Residual urine	−48 ± 11.5	0.17 (0.16)	−0.23 (0.05)	1.00

Table 7.2 Correlations between improvements in measurements of disease severity among 82 men enrolled in BTOPS at 6 months follow-up

Source: Adapted with permission from Barry MJ, Cockett AT, Holtgrewe HL et al. Relationship of symptoms of prostatism to commonly used physiological and anatomical measures of the severity of benign prostatic hyperplasia. J Urol 1993; **150**(2 Pt 1): 351–8

	Peak flow rate	Residual urine
AUA-SI (Symptom Index)	−0.16[a]	0.05
AUA-SPI (Symptom Problem Index)	−0.08	0.09
AUA-BII (BPH Impact Index)	−0.06	0.00
Quality of Life score	−0.08	−0.01
[a]$P < 0.05$		

Table 7.3 Correlations between symptom indices and peak flow rate and residual urine volume in 274 men with AUA-SI of 13 or greater in the HYCAT trial

Source: Roehrborn CG, Oesterling, JE, Auerbach S et al. for the HYCAT Investigator Group: The Hytrin Community Assessment Trial study: a one-year study of terazosin versus placebo in the treatment of men with symptomatic benign prostatic hyperplasia. Urology 1996; 47: 159–168, with permission of Elsevier Science

failure rate in the watchful waiting group was 6.1 per 100 person-years vs. 3.0 in the TURP group. One of the reasons for the higher failure rate in the watchful waiting group was a high volume of residual urine (5.8 vs. 1.1%). The most common indication for surgery in the watchful waiting arm was high residual urine volume.

Despite the questionable value of PVR as an important outcome prognosticator, it may play a role as a safety parameter. It is not known whether residual urine volumes above a certain threshold lead to progressive deterioration of the upper urinary tract[97]. Another concern has traditionally been that increased amounts of residual urine lead to bacteriuria and urinary tract infections. Riehmann et al. recently studied risk factors for bacteriuria in 99 institutionalized elderly men[100]. The presence of bacteriuria in 30/99 men was not associated with age, residual urine volume, previous diagnosis of BPH, or any LUTS.

Thus, at present there are no convincing data available that would suggest that the measurement of residual urine should be a mandatory test in the evaluation of patients with LUTS. The measurement of residual urine as a safety parameter is also still an unresolved issue. The least invasive method should be employed when it is measured, and two or more baseline measurements are recommended.

Flow-rate Measurement

Uroflowmetry is the recording of the urinary flow rate throughout the course of the micturition. It is one of the basic non-invasive urodynamic tests in the diagnostic evaluation of patients presenting with symptoms of, or suspected to have, bladder outlet obstruction. The flow-rate recording represents the interaction between the expelling force of the detrusor muscle and the resistance of the outflow channel (urethra). Thus, the results of uroflowmetry are nonspecific, i.e. an abnormally low flow rate may be the result of an obstruction (bladder neck, prostate, scar tissue, urethral stricture, meatal stenosis, etc.) or the result of weakness of the bladder muscle. All modern uroflowmeters measure the peak urinary flow rate (Q_{max}), the voided volume, and the micturition time reliably. However, due to unavoidable technical artifacts, machine-read flow-rate recordings tend to overestimate Q_{max} by 1.5 mL s^{-1} when compared with visual (physician or technician) interpretation of the recordings as shown in a database of over 23,000 repeated recordings from 1645 patients.[101] A difference of 2 mL s^{-1} or greater occurred in 20% of recordings, while in 9% the difference was >3 mL s^{-1}. This is due to the spike phenomenon occurring in some of the recordings.

Flow-rate recordings are also associated with significant intra-individual variability. A recent contribution to this issue was made by Golomb et al.[102] In 32 men with BPH, 476 home flow-rate recordings were obtained (mean of 14.9/patient), and a great variability was observed. This variability was >1 SD in 87% of patients, and >2 SD in 47% of patients. In 65.6%, the highest recorded flow rate was greater than the −2nd SD on the Siroky nomogram (see below), while the lowest was below the −2nd SD (by definition pathologic). None of the 100 recordings obtained by repeated voiding in 16 healthy volunteers was below the −2nd SD. Circadian changes in Q_{max} occurred in both the BPH patients and controls; however, they did not reach statistical significance.

	Void #1–void #2	Void #1–void #3	Void #1–void #4
Q_{max} (mL s^{-1}) criterion: >3 mL s^{-1}	27	52	69
Volume (mL) criterion: >50 mL	37	40	28
RU (mL) criterion: >50 mL	25	20	22

Table 7.4 Percentage of men with lower urinary tract symptoms who experience changes as specified in peak flow rate, voided volume, and residual urine in four consecutive voiding episodes

Source: Adapted with permission from Reynard J, Lim C-S, Abrams P. The value of multiple free-flow studies in men with lower urinary tract symptoms (LUTS). *J Urol* 1995: **153**: 397A

Other evidence in this regard was presented by Reynard *et al.*,[103] who studied the effect of repeated flow rates in 164 men with LUTS. The mean peak flow rate increased significantly from void #1 to void #4, and a substantial percentage of patients experienced an increase in peak flow rate from void #1 to void #2, void #3, and void #4 of over 3 mL s^{-1} (Table 7.4). The significance of this latter finding is that medical treatment trials for BPH often present the percentage of patients who achieved an improvement in peak flow rate of over 3 mL s^{-1}, and designate this outcome as "success".

Repeated measures flow rates ($n=231$) were also analyzed by Barry *et al.*[104] Rather than determining the likelihood for the peak flow rate to increase, they determined the variabiltiy of the measure from one to another assessment time point. The estimated critical differences bounding the middle 80% of an assumed normal distribution of changes were ±4.1 mL s^{-1} for the peak flow rate. Not unlike Reynard's findings, these authors also pointed out the significant variability of these measures from one assessment point to another, and the inherent danger when relying on one measurement alone in clinical decision making.

Urinary flow-rate recordings were obtained from 2113 participants in the Olmsted County study, and normal reference ranges stratified by age and voided volume have been established.[105,106] The median maximum flow rate decreased from 20.3 in men 40–44 years old to 11.5 mL s^{-1} in men 75–79 years old. The decrease in maximum flow rate was 2 mL s^{-1} per decade of life. Between 24% (40–44 years) and 69% (75–79 years) of men between these age strata had a maximum flow rate of less than 15 mL s^{-1}, while between 6 and 35% of men had a maximum flow rate of less than 10 mL s^{-1}. Keeping this age-dependent decline of the maximum flow rate in mind, it is understandable that this parameter by itself is not specific for the diagnosis of BPH.

There is substantial evidence that Q_{max} in normal men depends on the volume voided. The correlation between Q_{max} and volume has been described by various authors using various mathematical models. No agreement exists about the drop-off in Q_{max} observed by some investigators if volumes over 500 mL are voided. Disagreement also exists about the lowest admissible volume voided that may permit accurate interpretation of the flow-rate measurement. Most authors who addressed this issue found a decrease in Q_{max}

with increasing age even in patients who did not volunteer urological symptoms (which is not to say those patients had no bladder outlet obstruction!). Because of the complexity of this issue, a general recommendation about the use of a nomogram to correct Q_{max} for age and/or volume voided cannot be made. However, it is advisable to relate an individual flow-rate recording to some form of nomogram to determine whether the patient falls within two standard deviations of the normal population for the volume he voided. Age correction does not appear to be warranted, since most patients with symptoms suggestive of BPH will be in a higher age group. Some of the nomograms are based on volunteers over 60 years of age, who are in an age bracket similar to the patient population under consideration.

Recently, data derived from the Merck Phase III Finasteride Study Database were presented that would indicate that the volume dependency of the Q_{max} may be not as pronounced or even absent in men with BPH (P. Grino, MSD, personal communication). In this database, several consecutive voidings in over 1000 participating men with BPH, the correlation between voided volume and Q_{max} was almost a straight line.

The most significant drawback of flow-rate recording is that a given Q_{max} does not discriminate between men with impaired detrusor strength and those with outlet obstruction.[107] Thus, a decision for or against certain therapies for BPH cannot be entirely based on the Q_{max} alone.

A cut-off value for Q_{max} of less or greater than 15 mL s^{-1} has been found to be a useful predictor of treatment outcome. Subjective improvement is noted in 70.6% of patients with a Q_{max} of >15 mL s^{-1} vs. 91.5% of patients with a Q_{max} of <15 mL s^{-1}.[108]

To highlight the ongoing debate in this area, two recent contributions from recognized experts in the field of urodynamics may be juxtaposed. Krah *et al.*[109] reported on 139 patients with BPH who underwent flow-rate recordings and pressure-flow studies. Using the passive urethral resistance ratio (Schäfer) (PURR), no difference was found between three groups of patients stratified by peak flow rate (<10 mL s^{-1}; 10–15 mL s^{-1}; >15 mL s^{-1}), and patients in the stratum with the lowest peak flow rate were as obstructed as those in the stratum with the highest peak flow rate. Abrams[110] presents a somewhat different analysis of the situation (Table 7.5), suggesting that men with a peak flow

	Peak flow rate		
	<10 mL s⁻¹	10–14 mL s⁻¹	>14 mL s⁻¹
Obstructed	88	57	33
Not obstructed	12	43	67

Table 7.5 Correlation between peak flow rate and results of pressure-flow studies (%)

Source: Abrams P. Objective evaluation of bladder outlet obstruction. *Br J Urol* 1995; **76**: 11–15, with permission of Blackwell Science

rate of <10 mL s⁻¹ are obstructed by pressure-flow criteria in 88% of all cases.

At the time of the first edition of the guidelines, no convincing data were available to support the use of flow-rate measurements as a mandatory test in the evaluation of men with LUTS. When used, two separate baseline recordings with a voided volume of >125–150 mL each should be obtained for validity. No corrections for age and voided volume are presently recommended. The peak flow rate is the most useful parameter obtained.

Pressure-flow Studies

Pressure-flow studies measure intravesical pressure at the time of voiding, thus attempting to discern between those patients with a low Q_{max} primarily because of a detrusor muscle failure and those with an obstructed outlet. The data can be plotted into a nomogram of Q_{max} vs. detrusor pressure, allowing the physician to diagnose the patient as being obstructed or not obstructed.[111] By operating only on patients clearly identified as obstructed, the subjective failure rate was reduced from 28% to 12% following TURP.[112]

Schäfer *et al.*[113,114] have used sophisticated computerized analysis of pressure-flow data, and defined passive and dynamic urethral resistance measures (PURR and DURR). In all their reports, they document that in fact approximately 25% of the patients undergoing TURP are *not* obstructed based on their criteria, although they may have a low Q_{max}. The objective improvement rate (residual urine and Q_{max}) was 100% in those patients categorized as severely obstructed, while it was lower in the mildly obstructed and non-obstructed patients. However, direct health outcome data have not been reported by these investigators.

Schäfer's model has been utilized and expanded by other investigators,[115] but correlation of the results to direct health outcomes is lacking. The technical details of the analysis would be outside the purpose of this discussion.

Others have employed computer programs to analyze pressure-flow plots.[116–119] In a series of publications, Rollema has described a computer program (CLIM) and its usefulness in the evaluation and selection of patients with BPH for treatment. He repeatedly demonstrated that >25% of patients undergoing TURP are not obstructed prior to treatment based on the CLIM analysis. In the most comprehensive publication to date, he showed that the parameters U/I (maximum extrapolated rate of increase in isometric

pressure, W m⁻¹) and URA (intersection of quadratic urethral resistance relation with pressure axis of pressure flow plot, cmH₂O) were able clearly to separate obstructed from non-obstructed patients with symptoms of BPH. Also, those patients classified as obstructed had improvement in their symptoms in a higher percentage of cases than those classified as non-obstructed. These results need to be confirmed in (1) a larger number of patients, and (2) by different investigators, before they can be accepted and translated in recommendations for clinical practice.

One particular use of pressure–flow studies deserves special comment. Seaman *et al.*[120] studied 129 patients with post-TURP voiding symptoms (i.e. symptomatic failures), and found that 38% were still obstructed, 25% had impaired detrusor contractility, and 8% intrinsic sphincteric deficiency. They concluded that urodynamic evaluation was an important part of the work-up of patients who failed standard surgical treatment for BPH.

At the time of the first edition of the guidelines, there were no convincing data to support the mandatory use of pressure-flow studies in the evaluation of men with LUTS. If utilized, the detrusor pressure at peak flow rate is the most useful parameter. Pressure-flow studies are useful in men with complicating factors (e.g. neurologic disorders), and in those men who failed prior therapy

Other Tests

Other urodynamic tests, such as filling cystometry and urethral pressure profile measurement, currently have no role in the evaluation of men with LUTS

Urethrocystoscopy

Urethrocystoscopy is not recommended for determining the need for treatment in men presenting with LUTS. The test is recommended for men with LUTS who have a history of microscopic or gross hematuria, urethral stricture disease (or risk factors, such as history of urethritis or urethral injury), bladder cancer, or prior lower urinary tract surgery (especially prior TURP). To help the surgeon determine the most appropriate technical approach, urethrocystoscopy is an optional test in men with moderate-to-severe symptoms who have chosen (or require) surgical or other invasive therapy

Endoscopy of the lower urinary tract (urethrocystoscopy) provides visual documentation of the appearance of the prostatic urethra and bladder in men with BPH. Historically, many urologists believed that the visual appearance of the lower urinary tract defines the severity of disease or predicts the outcome of treatment. However, this common urologic procedure has been poorly studied. No data are available on the sensitivity, specificity, or predictive value of the test.

Urethrocystoscopy is associated with certain potential benefits and harms (although they are not quantified in the literature). Potential benefits include the ability to demonstrate prostatic enlargement and visual obstruction of the urethra and the bladder neck; identification of specific anatomic abnormalities that alter clinical decision making;

identification of bladder stones, trabeculation, cellules, and diverticula; measurement of PVR; and the ruling out of unrelated bladder and urethral pathology. Potential harms include patient discomfort, anesthetic or sedative risk, urinary tract infection, bleeding, and urinary retention.

The probability of any harm occurring is uncertain. Except for discomfort, its occurrence is likely to be infrequent. Nevertheless, potential harms must be balanced against potential benefits of this invasive procedure.

The endoscopic appearance of the bladder and prostate is often felt to be helpful in the decision to treat. Although the linkage between the endoscopic appearance of the lower urinary tract and treatment outcome is poorly documented in the literature, available information suggests that the relationship is minimal. Bladder trabeculation may predict a slightly higher failure rate in patients managed by watchful waiting, but does not predict the success or failure of surgery. Urethrocystoscopy may, nevertheless, be useful in determining the technical feasibility of specific invasive therapies. For example, if urethrocystoscopy reveals a large middle lobe, balloon dilation and TUIP are unlikely to be successful. The decision to perform an open prostatectomy may be appropriately influenced by the shape of the gland, as well as its size. In all of these cases, however, the patient and his physician have already selected invasive therapy. Urethrocystoscopy is therefore performed to select (or rule out) specific techniques, not to determine the need for treatment.

The remote probability of identifying, by urethrocystoscopy, lower urinary tract complications possibly due to BPH in men without hematuria, urinary tract infection, or a history of risk factors makes the routine use of this procedure for all men with prostatism questionable. Available data suggest there is a minimal relationship between the endoscopic appearance of the lower urinary tract and treatment outcome. However, urethrocystoscopy may be useful in determining the technical feasibility of specific invasive therapies.

Imaging Studies of the Upper Urinary Tract

Imaging of the urinary tract prior to prostate surgery has been an integral part of the urological work-up of patients with benign prostatic obstruction over the last decades. A very recent survey of 24 urological centers in the UK showed that 21/24 (79%) used either intravenous urography (IVU) or sonography in the routine preoperative evaluation of patients with BPH[121]. This is surprisingly similar to the number of urologists ordering an IVU prior to treatment for BPH in the USA.[122] However, the reasons why such a policy would benefit the patient are rarely discussed. A common belief appears to be that the imaging study is performed in order "not to miss an important lesion." It is obvious that such statements have their roots in "defensive medicine" – the practice of performing all tests necessary to make sure that nothing is wrong with the entire urinary tract.

More recently, the decision to image the urinary tract prior to prostatectomy has been questioned by several authors.[123–126] Each of these authors base their recommendation on

eliminating the routine imaging policy on an analysis of a series of patients with BPH. Other authors recommend an alternative imaging modality to IVU, namely sonographical evaluation of the urinary tract.[127–130] Their recommendation is based on the fact that sonography is superior in assessing renal lesions seen on IVU and is harmless and non-invasive. Nevertheless, other investigators maintain that routine imaging by IVU should remain part of the perioperative workup of patients with BPH, and present data on screened patient populations to support their views.[131–133] In the last few years, two additional studies argued against the routine use of imaging studies. Wilkinson and Wild[134] found in 175 patients with BPH, but not in retention, no abnormality on screening plain films of the abdomen and pelvis or ultrasonography of the urinary tract that would alter the management. Böss and Knönagel[135] examined the value of IVU and sonography in 79 patients with BPH and did not find any abnormality that altered the treatment plan.

A comprehensive analysis of the available literature pertinent to this subject demonstrated that, for the majority of men with LUTS, an imaging study of the upper urinary tract is not warranted based on the relatively low yield of significant findings.[136] Imaging should be reserved for men with a history of urinary tract infection, hematuria, urinary retention, history of previous urinary tract surgery, urolithiasis, or renal insufficiency, since in these men a better yield may be expected.

BENIGN PROSTATIC HYPERPLASIA TREATMENT GUIDELINES

At the time of the guideline development, there was adequate evidence in the literature to estimate outcomes for the following treatments:

- *Watchful waiting* – A strategy of management in which the patient is monitored by his physician, but receives no active intervention for BPH.
- *α-blocker therapy* – Treatment using any of the class of α_1-adrenergic receptor blockers (including doxazosin, prazosin, and terazosin) that inhibit α-adrenergic mediated contraction of prostatic smooth muscle.
- *Finasteride therapy* – Treatment using the drug finasteride, an inhibitor of the enzyme 5α-reductase, which lowers prostatic dihydrotestosterone levels and can result in some decrease in prostate size.
- *Balloon dilation* – A procedure for treating BPH in which a catheter with a balloon at the end is inserted through the urethra and into the prostatic urethra. The balloon is then inflated to stretch the urethra where narrowed by the prostate.
- *Transurethral incision of the prostate* (TUIP) – An endoscopic surgical procedure limited to patients with smaller prostates (30 g or less of resected weight) in which an instrument is passed through the urethra to make one or two cuts in the prostate and prostate capsule, reducing constriction of the urethra. This procedure can be done on an out-patient basis.

- *Transurethral resection of the prostate* (TURP) – Surgical removal of the prostate's inner portion by an endoscopic approach through the urethra, with no external skin incision. This is the most common active treatment for symptomatic BPH and usually requires a hospital stay.
- *Open prostatectomy* – Surgical removal (enucleation) of the inner portion of the prostate via a suprapubic or retropubic incision in the lower abdominal area. The procedure is rarely done through the perineum. Open prostatectomy requires a longer hospital stay than the other surgical procedures do.

Treatment modalities such as hyperthermia, thermal therapy, laser prostatectomy, prostatic stents, and hormonal manipulation are considered investigational in the first edition of the BPH guidelines. With the exception of laser prostatectomy, and most recently thermotherapy (Prostatron, Technomed), few of these treatments are available for routine clinical practice. As these modalities become widely available, appropriate outcome data will be analyzed and incorporated in updates of the guidelines. It is most likely that they will fall in a category of "device treatments" (see Figure 7.1) which in the original guideline text was labeled "balloon dilation".

Based upon the US AHCPR BPH Guideline Panel's review of treatment options available in clinical practice, as well as on the preferences of patients, the following practice recommendations were made.

Patients with mild symptoms of BPH (IPSS score ≤ 7) should be followed in a strategy of watchful waiting. The patient's symptoms and clinical course should be monitored, usually annually. He should be instructed on behavioral techniques to reduce symptoms, such as limiting fluid intake after dinner and avoiding decongestants. Probabilities of disease progression or the development of BPH complications are uncertain. Until research defines these probabilities, patients in a strategy of watchful waiting should be monitored periodically by reassessment of symptom level, physical findings, routine laboratory testing, and optional urologic diagnostic procedures. If the patient's symptoms progress to moderate or severe levels, as defined by the IPSS, it is appropriate to rediscuss the symptoms with the patient to determine whether the condition is bothersome or is interfering with his health and to offer him other treatment options if applicable.

Patients with moderate and severe symptoms (IPSS score ≥ 8) should be given information on the benefits and harms of watchful waiting, α-blocker therapy, finasteride therapy, balloon dilation, and surgery. This information should be presented to the patient in an unbiased format, which expresses not only the probabilities of benefits and harms, but the range of uncertainty associated with those probabilities. The physician's opinion about optimal treatment should not be the only information communicated to the patient. Actual outcome data should be presented, to allow the patient to determine the best treatment for himself. However, health care providers should be cautious of using educational materials developed by groups with a vested interest in a particular form of treatment.

If patients initially choose watchful waiting or treatments other than surgery and later experience symptom progression or deterioration, it is appropriate to rediscuss surgery as a treatment option. However, failure to respond to medical or balloon dilation therapy is not an absolute indication for surgery. Many patients who fail to benefit from medical therapy, for example, will elect to return to a strategy of watchful waiting rather than accept the risks of surgery.

On the other hand, surgery should not be "reserved" for those men who fail medical or device therapy. If the patient has been fully informed, it is appropriate for him to have the option of electing surgery as his initial treatment. Choice of type of surgery (TUIP, TURP, or open prostatectomy) is primarily a technical decision; this choice should be based on the surgeon's experience and judgment and should be discussed with the patient. The panel noted, however, that TUIP is an underutilized procedure that should be strongly considered for patients in whom the estimated resected tissue weight (if done by TURP) would be 30 g or less.

The following types of BPH patients should be treated surgically: (1) those with refractory urinary retention who have failed at least one attempt at catheter removal; (2) those who have recurrent urinary tract infections, recurrent gross hematuria, bladder stones, or renal insufficiency clearly due to BPH. There is little evidence to suggest that treatment options other than surgery benefit patients with any of these BPH complications. Nevertheless, if patients refuse surgery, or if they have sufficient medical comorbidity to present an unacceptable risk for surgery, alternative therapies may be considered.

The foregoing treatment recommendations should not diminish the pivotal role of a caring physician in reaching an optimal treatment decision. Rather, it should expand the physician's counseling role by providing the patient with sufficient information to permit his participation in the decision-making process to the extent he desires. In those cases where the patient wants the physician's opinion on the optional treatment strategy, or even "surrenders" the decision completely to the physician, it is appropriate for the physician to recommend the most optimal treatment and to act as the patient's proxy in the decision-making process if necessary. The physician should take this prerogative, however, only at the patient's request.

BALANCE SHEET OF BENEFITS AND HARMS

Depending on the criteria utilized, rather different estimates for the prevalence of BPH have been suggested. Autopsy studies have shown that about 50% of men in the sixth decade of life have histologic evidence of BPH, and that the prevalence increases to 70% by the seventh and to 90% by the ninth decade of life.[136] As histologic presence of BPH does not necessarily imply an enlarged prostate,

LUTS, a reduced flow rate, or the need for prostate surgery, the prevalence estimates are lower when any of these criteria are utilized. Aside from those patients with an immediate indication for surgical treatment for BPH, the vast majority of men are treated for this condition because of their symptoms.[122] Health care-seeking behavior is difficult to analyze, and factors such as worry and embarrassment have been shown to play an important role in an individual patient's decision to seek medical attention.[137] However, when patients were asked which of 15 outcomes (probability and magnitude of symptom improvement, incontinence, surgical complications, adverse events of medications, operative mortality, complications requiring surgery, impotence, requirement of blood transfusion, retrograde ejaculation as a result of the treatment, pain due to treatment, retreatment for recurrent disease, duration of recovery time, loss of work time, duration of hospital stay, and cost of treatment), the overwhelming majority of patients indicated that the probability and magnitude of the expected symptom improvement was the most important factor in choosing a particular treatment approach.[7]

Based on the ranking of these outcomes in order of importance by patients, the panel proceeded to develop the balance sheet of benefits and harms (Table 7.6). The concept of the balance sheet is one that we utilize whenever we make major decisions or purchases, e.g. which college to go to, which car, which major appliances to buy, etc.: we weigh the advantages and disadvantages of the products available, and make a decision based on this analysis. Our own preferences enter heavily into the decision-making process. While for some the most important issue in buying a car is its power and speed, for others it is the gas mileage, and for others yet the cargo space, etc. When faced with decisions concerning our health, it is reasonable to use a similar approach, namely to compare the benefits and harms of various alternative treatments available.[14]

Such a balance sheet was developed for the BPH guidelines, listing in tabular format the benefits and potential harm of those treatments available at the time when the guidelines were conceived: namely, watchful waiting, drug treatment with α-blockers and 5α-reductase inhibitors, balloon dilation, and surgical treatments, i.e. TUIP, TURP, and open enucleation of the adenoma (Table 7.6). A comprehensive literature review was conducted, focusing on outcome data for these treatment choices. Analysis of the outcomes was performed by the Confidence Profile Method (CPM), a form of meta-analysis developed by David Eddy for situations in which there is a paucity of randomized controlled studies that would lend themselves to a more classic type of meta-analysis.[138,139] The choice of the outcomes analyzed is based on a prioritization of a list of possible outcomes as described above. The probability of symptom improvement and the expected magnitude of improvement were clearly the most important outcomes on every patient's mind. Adverse outcomes as listed in Table 7.6 were also of great significance to the polled individuals. Some other outcomes such as hospitalization time, time off work, and especially the need for retreatment

because of a failure to relieve symptoms are of enormous economic consequences.

The following is a line-by-line explanation of the rows in Table 7.6.

Line 1:   Likelihood that a patient will experience some symptom improvement. This likelihood is greater if the pretreatment symptoms are more severe (higher symptom score).

Line 2:   Expected drop in symptom score in percent (e.g. a drop in mean symptom score from 18 to 12 represents a 30% improvement).

Line 3:   Morbidity and adverse events resulting from the treatment are necessarily vastly different in nature and scope for surgical treatments and drug treatments. This should be kept in mind when analyzing the presented likelihood data.

Line 4:   The chance of a man dying within 90 days following any treatment depends on the treatment and his age. As a baseline value, the probability of dying is listed for an average patient with BPH at age 67 years, based on the US Life Tables.

Line 5:   Total urinary incontinence is a feared complication of surgery. Despite improvements in techniques, there are still a finite number of patients experiencing this problem. It must be noted, however, that incontinence is also very prevalent in untreated aging men.

Line 6:   Bladder neck contracture and urethral stricture are also well-documented long-term complications of surgery. The risk of such complications requiring another surgical intervention is clearly higher than that of incontinence.

Line 7:   The older literature supports a rather high risk for developing impotence following prostate surgery. Newer studies deny, for the most part, any association.[99] Although this issue is unresolved at present, it probably is safe to inform the patient about this potential risk.

Line 8:   Retrograde ejaculation is very common after prostate surgery. This outcome was the least important one of 15 possible outcomes for the proxy patients. However, patients who have not been informed about this possibility prior to surgery, are usually quite concerned when they notice the absence of ejaculate during orgasm following surgery.

Line 9/10: These are estimates based on Medicare data, and projected number of out-patient office visits on a drug therapy regimen or conservatively followed patients.

One outcome which is both important to patients and of considerable economic consequence is the probability of treatment failure over time. Treatment failure in its strictest sense is the lack of improvement in symptoms or the recurrence of symptoms at some point in time after the

Direct treatment outcomes	Surgical options				Conservative options		
	Balloon dilation	TUIP	Open surgery	TURP	Watchful waiting	Alpha blockers	5α-reductase inhibitor
1. Chance for improvement of symptoms (90% confidence interval)	37–76	78–83	94–99.8	75–96	31–55	59–86	54–78
2. Degree of symptom improvement (% reduction in symptom score)	51	73	79	85	?	51	31
3. Morbidity/complications associated with surgical or medical treatment (90% confidence interval), about 20% of all complications assumed to be significant	1.78–9.86	2.2–33.3	6.98–42.7	5.2–30.7	1–5 Complications from progression of BPH	2.9–43.3	13.6–18.8%
4. Chance of dying within 30–90 days of treatment (90% confidence interval)	0.72–9.78 (Patients treated were high risk/elderly)	0.2–1.5	0.99–4.56	0.53–3.31	0.8 — Chance of death 90 days for 67-year-old man		
5. Risk of total urinary incontinence (90% confidence interval)	?	0.06–1.1	0.34–0.74	0.68–1.4	? Incontinence due to aging		
6. Need for operative treatment for surgical complications in the future (90% confidence interval)	?	1.34–2.65	0.6–14.1	0.65–10.1	0		
7. Risk of impotence (90% confidence interval)	(See watchful waiting, no long-term follow-up available)	3.9–24.5	4.7–39.2	3.3–34.8	About 2 (1/50) of men age 67 become impotent per year. Long-term data on α-blocker treatment are not available		2.5–5.3 (Also decreased volume of ejaculate)
8. Risk of retrograde ejaculation (% of patients)	?	6–55	36–95	25–99	0	4–11	0
9. Loss of work time (days)	4	7–21	21–28	7–21	1	3.5	1.5
10. Hospital stay (days)	1	1–3	5–10	3–5	0	0	0

Table 7.6 Balance sheet of benefits and harm

Source: McConnell JD, Barry MJ, Bruskewitz RC et al. Benign Prostatic Hyperplasia: Diagnosis and Treatment. Quick Reference Guide for Clinicians. AHCPR Publication No. 95–0583. Rockville, MD: Agency for Health Care Policy and Research, Public Health Service, US Department of Health and Human Services 1994

intervention. Treatment failure in itself is not of particular concern to those who pay for health care. However, an undetermined number of patients who experience treatment failure will seek help and undergo retreatment, which in turn will cost additional resources. Solid data on retreatment probabilities are only available for the surgical treatment alternatives. Figure 7.3, shows the probability for retreatment over 5 years following an initial intervention. The confidence intervals are rather wide, indicating a great degree of uncertainty for the treatment with α-blockers, 5α-reductase inhibitors, balloon dilation (this holds true also for all other investigational device treatments available today), and watchful waiting. Assessment of retreatment probability will have to be part of future clinical BPH studies to determine cost-effectiveness (e.g. pharmacoeconomic studies).

Other outcomes that are not presented in the balance sheet, but are widely used to measure the efficacy of therapeutic interventions for BPH, are the peak urinary flow rate (Q_{max}) and residual urine. The reason for their absence is the fact, that they represent biological or indirect health outcomes. Of relevance to patients in their attempt to make a treatment choice are only the direct health outcomes discussed above. The full guideline document discusses these outcomes in great detail. Both the probability for an improvement in peak flow rate as well as the absolute improvement in peak flow rate increase with increasing invasiveness of the intervention (Figure 7.4). Thus, those interventions, which are associated with more risks (=harm), hold greater promise not only with regard to improvements in direct but also with regard to this indirect or proxy outcome. With regard to residual urine volume, this relationship is less clear. In fact, the relative improvements (decrease) in residual urine volumes are rather simi-

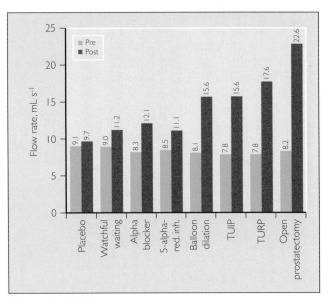

Figure 7.4 Combined mean pre-and posttreatment maximum flow rates for various treatment modalities

Source: Adapted from McConnell JD, Barry MJ, Bruskewitz RC *et al. Benign Prostatic Hyperplasia: Diagnosis and Treatment. Clinical Practice Guideline*, No. 8. AHCPR Publication No. 94–0582. Rockville, MD: Agency for Health Care Policy and Research, US Department of Health and Human Services 1994

lar for all analyzed treatment alternatives with the exception of watchful waiting, for which an increase in residual urine has been reported.

PATIENT PREFERENCES

In choosing treatments for a disease such as BPH, which principally affects the quality rather than the quantity of life and where the optimal decision may be dictated by personal values rather than scientific evidence, different patients may have different opinions concerning the benefits and harms of direct outcomes. Depending on how bothered a patient is by his symptoms, one patient may find the risks of surgery or of other treatments acceptable, given the potential benefit. Another patient may not find the risk of any therapy acceptable, because he is not bothered by his symptoms or because he is averse to any risk, or both. These differences in how individual patients weigh risks and benefits are clearly shown in studies of patient preferences.

Most patients with mild symptoms prefer watchful waiting, whereas there is a very wide range of preferences in patients with moderate symptoms. Although surgery is the most commonly elected therapy for those patients with severe symptoms, a significant number of patients elected watchful waiting or another alternative therapy.

It is clear from these studies that the majority of BPH patients with mild symptoms are not sufficiently bothered by their symptoms to accept the risks of therapy, including non-invasive therapies. In patients with moderate and severe symptoms, there is a wide range of preferences probably due to varying levels of "bothersomeness" and risk aversion among individual patients.

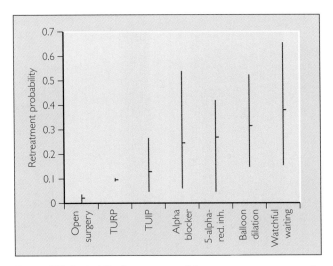

Figure 7.3 Probability for treatment failure or retreatment over 5 years from the time of initial treatment for seven different treatment modalities. Shown are the median probability (horizontal mark) and the 95% confidence interval (CI) calculated from data available in the literature. The wider the CI, the greater the uncertainty associated with the estimate

Given the variations in patient preferences, and because the physician's values (personal perceptions of benefits and harms) may be different from the patient's, it is important that the patient's values take precedence in determining choice of treatment. Although patients with severe symptoms are more likely to be bothered, and thus will be more likely to accept the risk of surgery, a considerable number of these patients will still prefer watchful waiting or other therapies.

It is also apparent that the "need" for therapy in patients with symptomatic BPH should, in most cases, be determined by the informed patient rather than by the physician. As made evident above, most patients with mild symptoms do not perceive a need for therapy even with non-invasive approaches. Patients with severe symptoms may choose surgery, but many will have a preference for non-surgical intervention.

However, an appreciable number of patients with moderate symptoms, after being fully informed, will also elect surgical intervention. Therefore, the concept that patients should only receive surgery if they have failed medical therapy is not appropriate. Some patients with moderate symptoms, and significantly bothered by their symptoms, view the potential benefits of surgery as clearly superior to other forms of therapy, and the risks as acceptable.

IMPLICATIONS AND APPLICATIONS OF THE GUIDELINES

Based on the population-based study of urinary symptoms in men in Olmsted County, MN, Jacobsen et al. made predictions regarding the number of patients who would be eligible for a discussion of treatment alternatives based on their symptom severity in the USA in the next decades.[140] While in 1995, 5.56 million Caucasian men between the ages of 50 and 79 are predicted to have an AUA-SI of >7 points and a peak flow rate of <15 mL s^{-1} (Table 7.7), this number is likely to increase to 11.1 million by the year 2030, based on the predicted aging of the population. The fact that about 300,000 TURPs are done yearly in the USA indicates that only a minority of the eligible 5.5 million men currently receive surgical therapy. Furthermore, only 13% of the men in Olmsted County with an AUA-SI of >7

points had consulted a physician about their condition. If primary care physicians administer the AUA-SI to patients in their practices, it is possible that we shall witness a tremendous increase in the number of men referred for LUTS, who will ultimately be eligible for one of the recommended treatment alternatives.

Patients who have selected treatment after a full discussion of the benefits and risks involved with each treatment as recommended in the guidelines adhere remarkably well to the initially chosen therapy. Kaplan et al.[141] followed 145 men with LUTS for 2 years, asking how likely patients were to adhere to their originally chosen treatment. Using the AUA-SI and the recommendation of the guidelines to place men with mild symptoms on watchful waiting, while offering treatment choices to men with moderate-to-severe symptoms, 111/145 (76%) were maintained on their original therapy at 1 year, and 99/145 (68%) at 2 years. An additional 31 (21%) patients switched to an alternative non-surgical treatment.

Such reports underline the soundness of the fundamental recommendations made in the guidelines regarding treatment choices, and make them an ideal tool to give to family physicians and general practitioners when dealing with the ever-increasing number of aging men with LUTS.

SUMMARY

The BPH guidelines provide a rational diagnostic and treatment algorithm for practitioners consulting with patients presenting with LUTS suggestive of BPH. They also serve several very important purposes:

- They represent the first attempt of a comprehensive review of the English-language literature regarding the evaluation and treatment of men presenting with symptoms of BPH.
- They are presented in a comprehensible and transparent fashion to the reader, inasmuch as each piece of supporting evidence is explicitly listed.
- A decision diagram is presented allowing health care providers to evaluate and treat patients with BPH in a rational fashion.

Age	US population base	% with AUA-SI >7	% with Q_{max} <15	% of population base	Number eligible
50–59	8,988,000	32	51	16.9	1,515,377
60–69	8,348,000	41	65	26.6	2,221,028
70–79	5,210,000	46	76	35.1	1,826,384
TOTAL					5,562,789

Table 7.7 Men eligible for treatment for BPH based on an AUA-SI of >7 points and a flow rate of <15 mL s^{-1} and on the population data from the Olmsted County study of urinary tract symptoms

Source: Adapted from Jacobsen SJ, Girman CJ, Guess HA et al. New diagnostic and treatment guidelines for benign prostatic hyperplasia. Potential impact in the United States. Arch Intern Med 1995; **155**(5): 477–81. © 1995, American Medical Association

- A balance sheet of treatment outcomes should help patients and health care providers in their shared decision making regarding treatment alternatives.
- They uncovered significant knowledge gaps and areas for future basic and clinical research.

As more treatment alternatives become available, it is estimated that the guidelines will be updated in the near future to reflect both the changing health care environment and the ever-expanding armamentarium of treatment choices.

REFERENCES

1 McPherson K, Wennberg JE, Hovind OB, Clifford P. Small area variations in the use of common surgical procedures: an international comparison of New England, England and Norway. *N Engl J Med* 1982; **307**: 1310–14.

2 Wennberg JE, Mullay AG Jr, Hanley D *et al.* Assessment of prostatectomy for benign urinary tract obstruction. Geographic variations and the evaluation of medical care outcomes. *JAMA* 1988; **259**(20): 3027–30.

3 Fowler FJ Jr, Wennberg JE, Timothy RP *et al.* Symptoms status and quality of life following prostatectomy. *JAMA* 1988; **259**(20): 3018–22.

4 Roos NP, Wennberg JE, Malenka DJ *et al.* Mortality and reoperation after open and transurethral resection of the prostate for benign prostatic hyperplasia. *N Engl J Med* 1989; **320**(17): 1120–4.

5 Malenka DJ, Roos N, Fisher ES *et al.* Further study of the increased mortality following transurethral prostatectomy: a chart-based analysis. *J Urol* 1990; **144**: 224–8.

6 Lepor H, Sypherd D, Machi G, Derus J. Randomized double-blind study comparing the effectiveness of balloon dilation of the prostate and cystoscopy for the treatment of symptomatic benign prostatic hyperplasia. *J Urol* 1992; **147**: 639–44.

7 McConnell JD, Barry MJ, Bruskewitz RC *et al. Benign Prostatic Hyperplasia: Diagnosis and Treatment. Clinical Practice Guidelines*, No. 8. AHCPR Publication No. 94–0582. Rockville, MD: Agency for Health Care Policy and Research, Public Health Service, US Department of Health and Human Services 1994.

8 Eddy DM. Clinical decision making: from theory to practice. The challenge. *JAMA* 1990; **263**: 287–90.

9 Eddy DM. Clinical decision making: from theory to practice. Anatomy of a decision. *JAMA* 1990; **263**: 441–3.

10 Eddy DM. Clinical decision making: from theory to practice. Practice policies – what are they? *JAMA* 1990; **263**: 877–80.

11 Eddy DM. Clinical decision making: from theory to practice. Practice policies: where do they come from? *JAMA* 1990; **263**: 1265–75.

12 Eddy DM. Clinical decision making: from theory to practice. Practice policies – guidelines for methods. *JAMA* 1990; **263**: 1839–41.

13 Eddy DM. Clinical decision making: from theory to practice. Guidelines for policy statements: the explicit approach. *JAMA* 1990; **263**: 2239–43.

14 Eddy DM. Clinical decision making: from theory to practice. Comparing benefits and harms: the balance sheet. *JAMA* 1990; **263**: 2493–505.

15 Eddy DM. Clinical decision making: from theory to practice. Designing a practice policy. Standards, guidelines and options. *JAMA* 1990; **263**: 3077–84.

16 Eddy DM. Clinical decision making: from theory to practice. Resolving conflicts in practice policies. *JAMA* 1990; **264**: 389–91.

17 Eddy DM. Clinical decision making: from theory to practice. Rationing by patient choice. *JAMA* 1991; **265**: 105–8.

18 Eddy DM. Clinical decision making: from theory to practice. What to do about costs? *JAMA* 1990; **264**: 1161–70.

19 Eddy DM. Clinical decision making: from theory to practice. Connecting value and costs. *JAMA* 1990; **264**: 1737–9.

20 Eddy DM. Clinical decision making: from theory to practice. The individual vs society. *JAMA* 1991; **265**: 2399–406.

21 Eddy DM. Clinical decision making: from theory to practice. What care is "essential"? What services are "basic"? *JAMA* 1991; **265**: 782–8.

22 Eddy DM. Clinical decision making: from theory to practice. Oregon's methods. Did cost-effectiveness analysis fail? *JAMA* 1991; **266**(15): 2135–41.

23 McConnell JD, Barry MJ, Bruskewitz RC *et al. Benign Prostatic Hyperplasia: Diagnosis and Treatment. Quick Reference Guide for Clinicians.* AHCPR Publication No. 95–0583. Rockville, MD: Agency for Health Care Policy and Research, Public Health Service, US Department of Health and Human Services 1994.

24 McConnell JD, Barry MJ, Bruskewitz RC *et al. Treating Your Enlarged Prostate. Patient Guide.* AHCPR Publication No. 94–0584. Rockville, MD: Agency for Health Care Policy and Research, Public Health Service, US Department of Health and Human Services 1994.

25 Thompson IM, Ernst JJ, Gangai MP. Adenocarcinoma of the prostate: results of routine urological screening. *J Urol* 1984; **132**: 690–2.

26 Chodak GW, Keller P, Schoenberg H. Routine screening for prostate cancer using the digital rectal examination. *Prog Clin Biol Res* 1988; **269**: 87–98.

27 Lee F, Littrup PJ, Torp-Pedersen ST. Prostate cancer: comparison of transrectal US and digital rectal examination for screening. *Radiology* 1988; **168**: 389–94.

28 Vihko P, Kontturi M, Lukkarinen O, Ervasti J, Vihko R. Screening for carcinoma of the prostate. Rectal examination, and enzymatic and radioimmunologic measurements of serum acid phosphatase compared. *Cancer* 1985; **56**(1): 173–7.

29 US Preventive Services Task Force. Screening for prostate cancer. An assessment of the effectiveness of 169 interventions. In: Fisher M, Eckhart C (eds) *Guide to Clinical Preventive Services*, 1st ed. Baltimore, MD: Williams & Wilkins 1989; 63–6.

30 Barry MJ, Cockett AT, Holtgrewe HL *et al.* Relationship of symptoms of prostatism to commonly used physiological and anatomical measures of the severity of benign prostatic hyperplasia. *J Urol* 1993; **150** (2 Pt 1): 351–8.

31 Chute CG, Guess HA, Panser LA *et al.* The non-relationship of urinary symptoms, prostate volume, and uroflow in a population based sample of men. *J Urol* 1993; **149**: 356A.

32 Mohr DN, Offord KP, Melton LJ. Isolated asymptomatic microhematuria: a cross sectional analysis of test-positive and test-negative patients. *J Gen Intern Med* 1987; **2**: 318–24.

33 Mohr DN, Offord KP, Owen RA. Asymptomatic microhematuria and urologic disease. *JAMA* 1986; **256**: 224–9.

34 Messing EM, Young TB, Hunt VB. The significance of asymptomatic microhematuria in men 50 or more years old: findings of a home screening study using urinary dipsticks. *J Urol* 1987; **137**: 919–22.

35 Mebust WK, Holtgrewe HL, Cockett ATK, Peters PC. Transurethral prostatectomy: immediate and postoperative complications. A cooperative study of 13 participating institutions evaluating 3885 patients. *J Urol* 1989; **141**: 243–7.

36 Holtgrewe HL, VAIK WL. Factors influencing the mortality and morbidity of transurethral prostatectomy: a study of 2015 cases. *J Urol* 1962; **87**: 450–9.

37 Melchior J, Valk WL, Foret JD, Mebust WK. Transurethral prostatectomy in the azotemic patient. *J Urol* 1974; **112**: 643–7.

38 Mukamel E, Nissenkorn I, Boner G, Servadio C. Occult progressive renal damage in the elderly male due to benign prostatic hypertrophy. *J Am Geriatr Soc* 1979; **27**(9): 403–6.

39 Hara M, Inorre T, Fukuyama T. Some physico-chemical characteristics of gamma-seminoprotein, an antigenic component specific for human seminal plasma. *Jpn J Legal Med* 1971; **25**: 322.

40 Wang MC, Valenzuela LA, Murphy GP, Chu TM. Purification of a human prostate specific antigen. *Invest Urol* 1979; **17**: 159.

41 Armitage TG, Cooper EH, Newling WW, Robinson MRG, Appleyard I. The value of the measurement of serum prostate specific antigen in patients with benign prostatic hyperplasia and untreated prostate cancer. *Br J Urol* 1988; **62**: 584.

42 Ercole CJ, Lange PH, Mathisen M *et al.* Prostate specific antigen and prostatic acid phosphatase in the monitoring and staging of patients with prostatic cancer. *J Urol* 1987; **138**: 1181.

43 Hudson MA, Bahnson RR, Catalona WJ. Clinical use of prostate specific antigen in patients with prostate cancer. *J Urol* 1989; **142**: 1011.

44 Oesterling JE, Chan DW, Epstein JI *et al.* Prostate specific antigen in the preoperative and postoperative evaluation of localized prostatic cancer treated with radical prostatectomy. *J Urol* 1988; **139**: 766–72.

45 Lange PH, Ercole CJ, Lightner DJ *et al.* The value of prostate specific antigen determinations before and after radical prostatectomy. *J Urol* 1989; **141**: 873–9.

46 Partin AW, Carter HB, Chan DW *et al.* Prostate specific antigen in the staging of localized prostate cancer: influence of tumor differentiation, tumor volume and benign hyperplasia. *J Urol* 1990; **143**: 747–52.

47 Sershon P, Barry MJ, Oesterling JE. Serum PSA values in men with histologically confirmed BPH versus patients with organ confined prostate cancer. *J Urol* 1993; **149**: 421A.

48 Monda JM, Barry MJ, Oesterling JE. Prostate specific antigen: its inability to decrease the prevalence of stage A prostate cancer. *J Urol* 1993; **149**: 421A.

49 Gormley GJ, Stoner E, Bruskewitz RC *et al.* The effect of finasteride in men with benign prostatic hyperplasia. The Finasteride Study Group [see comments]. *N Engl J Med* 1992; **327**(17): 1185–91.

50 Guess HA, Heyse JF, Gormely GJ *et al.* Effect of finasteride on serum PSA concentration in men with benign prostatic hyperplasia. Results from the North American phase III clinical trial. *Urol Clin North Am* 1993; **20**(4): 627–36.

51 Oesterling JE, Jacobsen SJ, Chute CG *et al.* The establishment of age specific reference ranges for prostate specific antigen. *J Urol* 1993; **149**: 510A.

52 Dalkin BL, Ahmann FR, Kopp JB *et al.* Derivation and application of upper limits for prostate specific antigen in men aged 50–74 years with no clinical evidence of prostatic carcinoma. *Br J Urol* 1995; **76**(3): 346–50.

53 Collins GN, Lee RJ, McKelvie GB *et al.* Relationship between prostate specific antigen, prostate volume and age in the benign prostate. *Br J Urol* 1993; **71**(4): 445–50.

54 McCormack RT, Rittenhouse HG, Finlay JA *et al.* Molecular forms of prostate-specific antigen and human kallikrein gene family: a new era. *Urology* 1995; **45**: 729–44.

55 Leinonen J, Lovgren T, Vornanen T, Stenman UH. Double-label time-resolved immunofluorometric assay of prostate-specific antigen and of its complex with alpha 1-antichymotrypsin. *Clin Chem* 1993; **39**(10): 2098–103.

56 Christensson A, Bjork T, Nilsson O *et al.* Serum prostate specific antigen complexed to alpha 1-antichymotrypsin as an indicator of prostate cancer. *J Urol* 1993; **150**(1): 100–5.

57 Catalona WJ, Smith DS, Wolfert RL *et al.* Increased specificity of PSA screening through measurement of percent free PSA in serum. *J Urol* 1995; **153**: 312A.

58 Partin AW, Kelly CA, Subong ENP *et al.* Measurement of the ratio of free PSA to total PSA improves prostate cancer detection for men with total PSA levels between 4.0 and 10.0 ng/ml. *J Urol* 1995; **153**: 295A.

59 Oesterling JE, Jacobsen SJ, Klee GG *et al.* Free, complexed and total serum prostate specific antigen: the establishment of appropriate reference ranges for their concentrations and ratios. *J Urol* 1995; **154**: 1090–5.

60 Britton JP, Dowell AC, Whelan P. Prevalence of urinary symptoms in men aged over 60. *Br J Urol* 1990; **66**: 175–6.

61 Beier-Holgersen R, Bruun J. Voiding pattern of men 60 to 70 years old: population study in an urban population. *J Urol* 1990; **143**: 531–2.

62 Diokno AC, Brown MB, Goldstein N, Herzog AR. Epidemiology of bladder emptying symptoms in elderly men. *J Urol* 1992; **148**(6): 1817–21.

63 Black N, Petticrew M, Ginzler M *et al.* Do doctors and patients agree? *Int J Technol Assess Health Care* 1991; **7**(4): 533–44.

64 Boyarsky S, Jones G, Paulson DF, Prout GR Jr. A new look at bladder neck obstruction by the Food and Drug Administration regulators: guidelines for investigation of benign prostatic hypertrophy. *Trans Am Assoc Genitourin Surg* 1976; **68**: 29–32.

65 Madsen P, Iversen P. A point system for selecting operative candidates. In: Hinman F (ed.) *Benign Prostatic Hypertrophy*. New York: Springer 1983: 763–5.

66 Barry MJ, Fowler FJ Jr, O'Leary MP, Bruskewitz RC, Holtgrewe HL, Mebust WK. Correlation of the American Urological Association symptom index with self-administered versions of the Madsen–Iversen, Boyarsky and Maine Medical Assessment Program symptom indexes. Measurement Committee of the American Urological Association. *J Urol* 1992; **148**(5): 1558–63; discussion 1564.

67 O'Leary MP, Barry MJ, Fowler FJ Jr. Hard measures of subjective outcomes validating symptom indexes in urology. *J Urol* 1992; **148**(5): 1546–8; discussion 1564.

68 Barry MJ, Fowler FJ Jr, O'Leary MP *et al.* The American Urological Association symptom index for benign prostatic hyperplasia *J Urol* 1992; **148**(5): 1549–57; discussion 1564.

69 Moon TD, Brannan W, Stone NN *et al.* Effect of age, educational status, ethnicity and geographic location on prostate symptom scores. *J Urol* 1994; **152**(5 Pt 1): 1498–1500.

70 Barry MJ, Williford WO, Chang YC *et al.* BPH-specific health status measures in clinical research: how much change in AUA Symptom Index and the BPH Impact Index is perceptible to patients? *J Urol* 1995; **154**: 1770–4.

71 Lepor H, Machi G. Comparison of AUA symptom index in unselected males and females between fifty-five and seventy-nine years of age. *Urology* 1993; **42**: 36–41.

72 Chancellor MB, Rivas DA. American Urological Association symptom index for women with voiding symptoms: lack of index specificity for benign prostatic hyperplasia. *J Urol* 1993; **150**: 1706–10.

73 Chai TC, Belville WD, McGuire EJ, Nyquist L. Specificity of American Urological Association voiding symptom index: comparison of unselected and selected samples of both sexes. *J Urol* 1993; **150**: 1710–14.

74 Jacobsen SJ, Girman CJ, Guess HA *et al.* Natural history of prostatism: factors associated with discordance between frequency and bother of urinary symptoms. *Urology* 1993; **42**(6): 663–71.

75 Barry MJ, Fowler JFJ, O'Leary MP *et al.* The Measurement

Committee of The American Urological Association. Measuring disease-specific health status in men with benign prostatic hyperplasia. *Med Care* 1995; **33**: AS145–55.

76 Guess HA, Chute CG, Garraway WM *et al*. Similar levels of urological symptoms have similar impact on Scottish and American men – although Scots report less symptoms. *J Urol* 1993; **150**(5 Pt2): 1701–5.

77 Roberts RO, Rhodes T, Panser LA *et al*. Natural history of prostatism: worry and embarrassment from urinary symptoms and health care-seeking behavior. *Urology* 1994; **43**(5): 621–8.

78 Hald T, Nordling J, Andersen JT *et al*. A patient weighted symptom score system in the evaluation of uncomplicated benign prostatic hyperplasia. *Scand J Urol Nephrol* 1991; **138** (Suppl): 59–62.

79 Epstein RS, Deverka PA, Chute CG *et al*. Urinary symptom and quality of life questions indicative of obstructive benign prostatic hyperplasia. Results of a pilot study. *Urology* 1991; **38**(1 Suppl): 20–6.

80 Bolognese JA, Kozloff RC, Kunitz SC *et al*. Validation of a symptoms questionnaire for benign prostatic hyperplasia. *Prostate* 1992; **21**(3): 247–54.

81 Eri LM, Tveter KJ. Measuring the quality of life of patients with benign prostatic hyperplasia. Assessment of the usefulness of a new quality of life questionnaire specially adapted to benign prostatic hyperplasia patients. *Eur Urol* 1992; **21**(4): 257–62.

82 Epstein RS, Deverka PA, Chute CG *et al*. Validation of a new quality of life questionnaire for benign prostatic hyperplasia. *J Clin Epidemiol* **45**(12): 1431–45.

83 Lukacs B, McCarthy C, Grange JC. Long-term quality of life in patients with benign prostatic hypertrophy: preliminary results of a cohort survey of 7,093 patients treated with an alpha-1-adrenergic blocker alfuzosin. QOL BPH Study Group in General Practice. *Eur Urol* 1993; **24**(Suppl 1): 34–40.

84 Lukacs B, Leplege A, MacCarthy C, Comet D. Construction and validation of a BPH specific health related quality of life scale including evaluation of sexuality. *J Urol* 1995; **153**: 320A.

85 O'Leary MP, Fowler FJ, Lenderking WR *et al*. A brief male sexual function inventory. *J Urol* 1995; **46**: 697–706.

86 Sagnier PP, Richard F, Botto H *et al*. [Adaptation and validation in the French language of the International Score of Symptoms of Benign Prostatic Hypertrophy] [French]. *Prog Urol* 1994; **4**(4): 532–8; discussion 539–40.

87 Hunter DJW, Berra-Unamuno A, Martin-Gordo A. Prevalence of urinary symptoms and other urological conditions in Spanish men aged 50 and over. *J Urol* 1996; **155**: 1965–70.

88 Cockett ATK, Khoury S, Aso Y *et al*. (eds) *The 2nd International Consultation on Benign Prostatic Hyperplasia (BPH), Paris, 1993, 27–30 June*. Jersey: Scientific Communication International 1993.

89 Sagnier PP, Girman CJ, Garraway M *et al*. International comparison of the community prevalence of symptoms of prostatism in four countries. *Eur Urol* 1996; **29**: 15–20.

90 Barry MJ, Mulley AG Jr, Fowler FJ, Wennberg JW. Watchful waiting vs immediate transurethral resection for symptomatic prostatism. The importance of patients' preferences. *JAMA* 1988; **259**(20): 3010–17.

91 Di Mare JR, Fish S, Harper JM, Politano VA. Residual urine in normal male subjects. *J Urol* 1963; **96**: 180–1.

92 Roehrborn CG, Peters PC. Can transabdominal ultrasound estimation of postvoiding residual (PVR) replace catheterization? *Urology* 1988; **31**: 445–9.

93 Hartnell GG, Kiely EA, Williams G. Real-time ultrasound measurement of bladder volume: a comparative study of three methods. *Br J Radiol* 1987; **60**: 1063–5.

94 Birch NC, Hurst G, Doyle PT. Serial residual urine volumes in men with prostatic hypertrophy. *Br J Urol* 1988; **62**: 571–5.

95 Bruskewitz RC, Iversen P, Madsen PO. Value of postvoid residual urine determination in evaluation of prostatism. *Urology* 1982; **20**: 602–4.

96 Jensen KM, Jorgensen JB, Mogensen P. Urodynamics in prostatism. III. Prognostic value of medium-fill water cystometry. *Scand J Urol Nephrol* 1988; **114**(Suppl): 78–83.

97 Guess HA, Girman CJ, Jacobsen SJ, Oesterling JE, Lieber MM. What levels of peak urinary flow and residual urine volume are associated with impaired renal function? *J Urol* 1995; **153**: 475A.

98 Rosier PFWM, DE Wildt MJAM, Wijkstra H *et al*. Residual urine and the correlation with detrusor contractility and bladder outlet obstruction in symptomatic BPH. *J Urol* 1995; **153**: 452A.

99 Wasson JH, Reda DJ, Bruskewitz RC *et al*. A comparison of transurethral surgery with watchful waiting for moderate symptoms of benign prostatic hyperplasia. The Veterans Affairs Cooperative Study Group on Transurethral Resection of the Prostate. *N Engl J Med* 1995; **332**(2): 75–9.

100 Riehmann M, Goetzman B, Langer E *et al*. Risk factors for bacteriuria in men. *Urology* 1994; **43**(5): 617–20.

101 Grino PB, Bruskewitz R, Blaivas JG *et al*. Maximum urinary flow rate by uroflowmetry: Automatic or visual interpretation. *J Urol* 1992; **149**: 339–41.

102 Golomb J, Lindner A, Siegel Y, Korczak D. Variability and circadian changes in home uroflowmetry in patients with benign prostatic hyperplasia compared to normal controls. *J Urol* 1992; **147**: 1044–7.

103 Reynard J, Lim C–S, Abrams P. The value of multiple free-flow studies in men with lower urinary tract symptoms (LUTS). *J Urol* 1995; **153**: 397A.

104 Barry MJ, Girman CJ, O'Leary MP *et al*. Using repeated measures of symptom score, uroflowmetry and prostate specific antigen in the clinical management of prostate disease. *J Urol* 1995; **153**: 99–103.

105 Girman CJ, Panser LA, Chute CG *et al*. Natural history of prostatism: urinary flow rates in a community-based study. *J Urol* 1993; **150**(3): 887–92.

106 Oesterling JE, Girman CJ, Panser LA *et al*. Correlation between urinary flow rate, voided volume, and patient age in a community-based population. *Prog Clin Biol Res* 1994; **386**: 125–39.

107 Chancellor MB, Blaivas JG, Kaplan SA, Axelrod S. Bladder outlet obstruction versus impaired detrusor contractility: the role of uroflow. *J Urol* 1991; **145**: 810–12.

108 Jensen KM-E, Andersen JT. Urodynamic implications of benign prostatic hyperplasia. *Urologe A* 1990; **29**: 1–4.

109 Krah J, Höfner K, Tan HK, Jonas U. The limitation of uroflow in BPH-patients with low and high Q_{max} values. *J Urol* 1995; **153**: 275A.

110 Abrams P. Objective evaluation of bladder outlet obstruction. *Br J Urol* 1995; **76**: 11–15.

111 Abrams PH, Griffiths DJ. The assessment of prostatic obstruction from urodynamic measurements and from residual urine. *Br J Urol* 1979; **51**: 129–34.

112 Abrams PH, Farrar DJ, Turner-Warwick RT *et al*. The results of prostatectomy: a symptomatic and urodynamic analysis of 152 patients. *J Urol* 1979; **121**(5): 640–2.

113 Schäfer W, Ruebben H, Noppeney R, Deutz F-J. Obstructed and unobstructed prostatic obstruction. *World J Urol* 1989; **6**: 198–203.

114 Schäfer W, Noppeney R, Ruebben H, Lutzeyer W. The value of free flow rate and pressure/flow-studies in the routine investigation of BPH patients. *Neurourol Urodyn* 1989; **7**: 219–21.

115 Spångberg A, Teriö H, Ask P, Engberg A. Pressure/flow studies preoperatively and postoperatively in patients with benign prostatic hypertrophy: estimation of the urethral pressure/flow relation and urethral elasticity. *Neurourol Urodyn* 1991; **10**: 139–67.

116 Rollema HJ, Kramer AEJL, Van den Ouden D. Improved selection and follow-up of prostatectomy patients by on line

assessment of uroflow classifications factors. *Neurourol Urodyn* 1987; **6**: 218.

117 Rollema HJ, van Mastrigt R. Objective analysis of prostatism: a clinical application of the computer program CLIM. *Neurourol Urodyn* 1991; **10**: 71–6.

118 Rollema HJ, Van Mastrigt R. Improved indication and followup in transurethral resection of the prostate using the computer program CLIM: a prospective study. *J Urol*; **148**(1): 111–5; discussion 15–16.

119 Rollema HJ, van Mastrigt R, Janknegt RA. Urodynamic assessment and quantification of prostatic obstruction before and after transurethral resection of the prostate: standardization with the aid of the computer program CLIM. *Urol Int* 1991; **47** (Suppl 1): 52–4.

120 Seaman EK, Jacobs BZ, Blaivas JG, Kaplan SA. Persistence or recurrence of symptoms after transurethral resection of the prostate: a urodynamic assessment. *J Urol* 1994; **152**(3): 935–7.

121 Wilkinson AG, Wild SR. Survey of urological centres and review of current practice in the pre-operative assessment of prostatism. *Br J Urol* 1992; **70**(1): 43–5.

122 Holtgrewe HL, Mebust WK, Dowd JB *et al*. Transurethral prostatectomy: practice aspects of the dominant operation in American urology. *J Urol* 1989; **141**(2): 248–53.

123 Christofferson I, Moller I. Excretory urography: a superfluous routine examination in patients with prostatic hypertrophy. *Eur Urol* 1981; **7**: 65–7.

124 Butler MR, Donnelly B, Komaranchat A. Intravenous urography in evaluation of acute retention. *Urology* 1978; **12**: 464–6.

125 Bauer DL, Garrison RW, McRoberts JW. The health and cost implications of routine excretory urography before transurethral prostatectomy. *J Urol* 1980; **123**(3) 386–9.

126 Wasserman NF, Lapointe S, Eckmann DR, Rosel PR. Assessment of prostatism: role of intravenous urography. *Radiology* 1987; **165**(3): 831–5.

127 Stavropoulos N, Christodoulou K, Chamilos E *et al*. Evaluation of patients with benign prostatic hypertrophy: IVU versus ultrasound. *J R Coll Surg Edinb* 1988; **33**(3): 140–2.

128 Solomon DJ, Van Niekerk JP. Ultrasonography should replace intravenous urography in the pre-operative evaluation of prostatism. *S Afr Med J* 1988; **74**(8): 407–8.

129 Lilienfeld RM, Berman M, Khedkar M, Sporer A. Comparative evaluation of intravenous urogram and ultrasound in prostatism. *Urology* 1985; **26**(3): 310–12.

130 Cascione CJ, Bartone FF, Hussain MB. Transabdominal ultrasound versus excretory urography in preoperative evaluation of patients with prostatism. *J Urol* 1987; **137**(5): 883–5.

131 Muzafer MH. Pre-prostatectomy intravenous urography – is it a must? *Int Urol Nephrol* 1986; **18**(1): 65–9.

132 Donker PJ, Kakiailatu F. Preoperative evaluation of patients with bladder outlet obstruction with particular regard to excretory urography. *J Urol* 1978; **120**: 685–6.

133 Pinck BD, Corrigan MJ, Jasper P. Pre-prostatectomy excretory urography: does it merit the expense? *J Urol* 1980; **123**(3): 390–1.

134 Wilkinson AG, Wild SR. Is pre-operative imaging of the urinary tract worthwhile in the assessment of prostatism? *Br J Urol* 1992; **70**(1): 53–7.

135 Böss HP, Knönagel H. Value of intravenous urography versus ultrasound in preoperative assessment of prostatic hyperplasia [in German]. *Ultraschall Med*; 1992; **13**(5): 228–33.

136 Berry SJ, Coffey DS, Walsh PC, Ewing LL. The development of human benign prostatic hyperplasia with age. *J Urol* 1984; **132**(3): 474–9.

137 Roberts RO, Rhodes T, Panser LA *et al*. Natural history of prostatism: worry and embarrassment from urinary symptoms and health care-seeking behavior. *Urology* 1994; **43**(5): 621–8.

138 Eddy D. The Confidence Profile Method: a Bayesian method for assessing health technologies. *Oper Res* 1989; **37**: 210–38.

139 Eddy DM, Hasselblad V (eds) *FAST*PRO. Software for Meta-Analysis by the Confidence Profile Method*, 1st edn. San Diego: Academic Press; Harcourt Brace Jovanovich 1992.

140 Jacobsen SJ, Girman CJ, Guess HA *et al*. New diagnostic and treatment guidelines for benign prostatic hyperplasia. Potential impact in the United States. *Arch Intern Med* 1995; **155**(5): 477–81.

141 Kaplan SA, Olsson CA, Te AE. The AUA symptom score in the evaluation of men with lower urinary tract symptoms: at two years follow up, does it work? *J Urol* 1996; **155**: 1971–4.

COMMENTARY

In this chapter, Dr Roehrborn has extensively discussed and eloquently updated the practical points from the practice guidelines published by the Agency for Health Care Policy and Research (AHCPR) of the US Department of Health and Human Services.

Management of BPH is affected by a multitude of factors, including disease severity, patient expectations, physician's preferences, treatment outcomes, and economic factors. Practice patterns vary significantly with regard to optimal evaluation protocol, treatment selection, and follow-up. There is an intense need to review existing literature with an analytical point of view and create a consensus guideline for BPH evaluation, treatment, and follow-up. This has been performed elegantly by the AHCPR Guidelines Committee including their formulated guidelines of BPH management based on peer-reviewed literature.

Even with the existence of guidelines, many urologists continue to perform diagnostic procedures and surgical treatments based on old biases and habits that are entrenched. As noted by Standaert and Denis in Chapter 4 ("Socioeconomics and Trends in Management of Benign Prostatic Hyperplasia: European Perspective") only 35% of urologists in Belgium even perform IPSS scores, despite its availability and recommendation by the Guidelines Committee. In a recent study in the USA, only 7.5% of patients treated by TURP were noted to have AUA symptom scores documented.[1] In the USA, and specifically in Florida, where the Editor practices, there are wide variations in practice patterns as seen in Figure 7.5.[2] This sort of variation has been noted not just in Florida but in every state and between states, again reiterating the point made by Dr Holtgrewe in Chapter 3 ("Socioeconomics and Trends in Management of Benign Prostatic Hyperplasia: United States Perspective") that, if urologists are to remain leaders in urologic disease management, they need critically to evaluate changing trends in urologic care with a view to performing those tests and procedures of proven benefit, based on both personal experience as well as

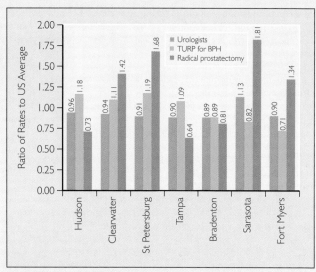

Figure 7.5 The Urological Surgical Signature Of Seven Southwest Florida Hospital Referral Regions (1994–95). The figure gives the ratio of rates of urologists and of prostate surgery relative to the national average. Although the member of urologists per 100,000 residents is nearly the same in each of the seven hospital referral regions, the amount and kind of prostate surgery varies substantially. The urologists treating patients who live in the Hudson hospital referral region perform surgery for benign prostatic hyperplasia ("TURP for BPH") at a rate 18% higher than the national average, but perform relatively little surgery (27% below the national average) for prostate cancer (radical prostatectomy). Urologists treating Medicare residents of the St Petersburg hospital referral region perform 2.6 times more radical prostate procedures per 1000 male Medicare enrollees than the urologists treating residents of the neighboring Tampa hospital referral region, who perform the surgery at a rate that is 36% below the national average. In the Bradenton hospital referral region, rates for both procedures are below the national average: in Sarasota, surgery for benign prostate disease is below the national average but rates of surgery for prostate cancer are 1.8 times the national average. The urologists serving Medicare residents of the Fort Myers hospital referral region perform more surgery for prostate cancer than the national average, but less surgery than the national average for benign prostate disease

Source: The Urological Surgical Signature of Seven Southwest Florida Hospital referral Regions (1994–95). *The Dartmouth Atlas of Health Care* 1998: **66**
© Trustees of Dartmouth College 1998.

peer-reviewed data. Having stated this, it is also clear that this task is more difficult with managed care and capitated care, wherein traditional fees for service insurance companies create layers of paperwork and bureaucracy, which prevents doctors from treating patients optimally. Hopefully, this is only a temporary transition period towards cost-effective care, which eventually will result in better outcomes for patients.

The AHCPR convened a multidisciplinary panel, which reviewed the entire published literature and followed the so-called explicit approach described by David Eddy to summarize the data. The practice guideline was targeted at patients over the age of 50 with LUTS suggestive of BPH. Patients with confounding comorbidities and diseases

known to offset BPH were excluded from these guidelines. These patients require individual in-depth evaluation based on their own comorbidities.

The recommended initial protocol for BPH evaluation included: focused urological and medical history, physical examination, and DRE, urinalysis, creatinine, and PSA test (optional). The panel also recommended the use of American Urological Association Symptom Score (or International Prostate Symptom Score – IPSS). Patients with clear-cut indications for surgery, such as refractory retention, UTI, hematuria, bladder stones, or renal insufficiency secondary to BPH, are offered surgical treatment including TURP, TUIP, as well as open surgery.

Patients who do not qualify for immediate surgical intervention are subsequently grouped on the basis of symptom severity and bother. Minimally symptomatic patients not bothered are offered watchful waiting, while all others are offered optimal diagnostic testing, such as uroflow, and postvoid residual urine estimation. Alternatively, they receive direct medical or minimally invasive treatments.

The selection of various treatment modalities is based upon the probability of positive and negative outcomes after treatment. If surgical treatment or minimally invasive treatment is planned, cystoscopy is included, depending upon the physician's preferences. Some of these recommendations on optimal testing and cystoscopy were deliberately left vague to accommodate varying physician and patient preferences.

The guidelines, however, clearly did not recommend the use of routine imaging of upper tracts in the evaluation of BPH without other complications or findings. However, any patient with hematuria, UTI, urinary retention, urolithasis, previous urological surgery, as well as patients with renal insufficiency were recommended to undergo imaging owing to this cohort having a high yield for positive findings.

The AHCPR guideline also evaluated the treatment outcomes of various treatments previously available up to 1994. The data on TURP, TUIP, and to some extent medical management is still relevant. Elsewhere, in this book the costs, benefits and risks of new procedures and medical agents are discussed in further detail.

Among medical treatments, we must be compelled to include uroselective α-blockers, which achieve significant symptom improvement with minimal cardiovascular side-effects. Newer data have also appeared regarding the risk for developing acute urinary retention and follow-up surgery after medical management (see Chapter 13, "Hormonal Therapy in Benign Prostatic Hyperplasia"). These studies have also shown that 5α-reductase inhibitors can reduce the risk of acute retention and surgery by 50%. Additionally, newer minimally invasive modalities such as microwave therapy, TUNA, and interstitial laser will undoubtedly figure in treatment options. Electrovaporization is emerging as a safe and effective alternative to TURP among invasive surgical procedures.

Overall, the practice guidelines is a major landmark, which has set the standard for further defining the costs and benefits of BPH evaluation and treatment modalities.

1 Hood H, Burgess P, Holtgrewe HL *et al*. Adherence to Agency for Health Care Policy and Research Guidelines for benign prostatic hyperplasia. *J Urol* 1997; **158**: 1417–21.

2 The Urological Surgical Signature of Seven Southwest Florida Hospital referral Regions (1994–95): *The Dartmouth Atlas of Health Care* 1998: **66**.

Urodynamics in the Evaluation of Benign Prostatic Hyperplasia[a]

8

R. D. Cespedes and E. J. McGuire

INTRODUCTION

The last two decades have seen a dramatic change in the way urologists think concerning benign prostatic hyperplasia (BPH) and the development of obstructive uropathy. The common belief that the symptom complex called "prostatism" is entirely due to bladder outlet obstruction and the inevitable clinical manifestation of BPH appears unfounded. Studies have shown that the relationship between bladder function, outlet obstruction, and abnormal voiding symptoms are much more complex than originally believed. It is clear that voiding symptoms may develop for reasons other than prostatic obstruction.

It is essential that one understands that the diagnosis of obstructive uropathy is not the same as that of BPH. Benign prostatic hyperplasia is a pathological diagnosis which may be entirely asymptomatic, requiring no therapy, whereas bladder outlet obstruction is a *urodynamic* diagnosis and generally does requires treatment. This is illustrated by the common scenario in which patients with large prostates secondary to BPH may have minimal voiding symptoms, while others with small or normal prostates may be severely obstructed.[1,2] Additionally, "silent" obstructive uropathy with severe upper tract damage may occur without significant voiding symptoms. Carefully performed studies have shown that between 25 and 50% of patients undergoing urodynamics for "prostatism" may not be urodynamically obstructed.[3-5] This is underscored by the results of a retrospective review of 787 patients with symptomatic prostatism evaluated with videourodynamics, in which 23% had isolated prostatic obstruction, and 39% had both bladder outlet obstruction and detrusor instability. Importantly, only 64% had any evidence of bladder outlet obstruction, 17% had impaired detrusor contractility, and 1% had sensory urgency.[6] These studies emphasize the concept that "prostatism" may include multiple conditions which may exist singly or together. These include (1) prostatic obstruction, (2) detrusor instability, (3) impaired detrusor contractility, (4) sensory urgency, and (5) primary bladder neck obstruction.[7-10] There is good evidence that the diagnosis of bladder outlet obstruction due to BPH cannot be made based on symptoms alone. For example, the American Urological Association (AUA) symptom score, while providing a reasonably reliable method of assessing voiding symptom severity and progression, cannot reliably differentiate between diseased and non-diseased states, nor the underlying reason for the diseased state.[11] Similar symptoms and worse AUA symptom scores are often found in elderly females in whom obstruction is not present.[12] An additional confounding problem in correlating symptoms to disease process is the documented waxing and waning of prostatism symptoms. Clark found that symptomatic improvement occurred in 25 of 36 patients with BPH when followed long-term, with improvement lasting a mean 1.9 years.[13] In a prospective study using subjective and objective criteria, Birkhoff and colleagues found that 8 of 26 patients with obstructive uropathy due to BPH were subjectively improved at 3 years and that 4 of 26 were objectively improved.[14] In another study of patients with prostatism evaluated with urodynamics, after 5 years only 20% of overtly obstructed patients had undergone surgery and, of the entire group, only 10% required surgery.[15]

The poor correlation between the patient's symptoms and objective evidence of obstruction has led to the use of urodynamic tests, including uroflowmetry and pressure-flow studies, which many believe are the tests of choice in this group of patients. Although the need for urodynamic tests in diagnosing and selecting patients for treatment of BPH may appear intuitively obvious, the role of urodynamics remains controversial. This is due in part to a difference in philosophy, in which some investigators believe that bothersome symptoms in and of themselves justify surgical treatment, whereas some investigators feel that obstruction should be documented in all cases, thereby avoiding surgery in unobstructed patients.[16,17] An important concern in these cost-conscious times is whether the unequivocal diagnosis of obstruction improves the outcome of treatment sufficiently to justify the increased cost and invasiveness of a urodynamic evaluation. Abrams found that including pressure-flow studies in the preoperative evaluation significantly reduced the symptomatic failure rate of transurethral resection of the prostate (TURP) from 28 to 12%.[18] Bruskewitz and colleagues[19] performed a prospective analysis on 46 patients with prostatism symptoms. Patients were urodynamically categorized as obstructed or unobstructed and then treated surgically to relieve the obstruction. Postoperatively, 89% of unobstructed patients had symptomatic

[a]The opinions or assertions contained herein are the private views of the authors and are not to be construed as reflecting the views of the Air Force or Department of Defense

improvement, whereas 92% of obstructed patients were subjectively improved. In a recent review of the English-language literature, a median 88% subjective improvement was found following TURP for prostatism symptoms (not urodynamically proven).[20] Based in part on these last two studies, the routine use of urodynamics in the preoperative assessment has been questioned.[16] Included in this argument are the inherent problems with interpreting urodynamic studies, such as the unclear objective diagnosis of obstruction ("even the experts don't agree"), the variable techniques used, different equipment utilized, differing treatment philosophy, patient population, and test reproducibility.[21,22] These arguments, unfortunately, ignore the fact that a large number of patients will improve spontaneously without treatment, and additionally, that TURP is a treatment for prostatic obstruction and not for unobstructed voiding symptoms. Nevertheless, the recently released BPH guidelines have classified pressure-flow studies as an optional study with necessity based on the physician's judgment.

The purpose of this chapter is to illustrate the notable lack of correlation between the patient's symptoms with known urodynamic parameters and to outline the importance and utility of the available studies in the diagnosis of bladder outlet obstruction.

VOIDING SYMPTOMS

Traditionally, voiding symptoms associated with BPH have been classified as "*irritative*," which includes dysuria, frequency, urgency, urge incontinence, and nocturia; or "*obstructive*," which includes dribbling, hesitancy, intermittency, straining, and weak force of stream. Although these symptoms are what usually bring the patient to the physician, most studies have shown that voiding symptoms and total symptom scores do not correlate with urodynamic signs of obstruction.[23-26] Prospective studies have demonstrated that the symptoms of prostatism wax and wane over time, and the incidence of symptoms vary with the patient's age and gender. Sommer and colleagues[27] found that, in a non-selected population, voiding symptoms increased progressively from the fifth to the seventh decades, and the incidence of voiding symptoms in the group diagnosed with prostatism was similar to asymptomatic patients in the sixth and seventh decades. The only symptoms more prevalent in prostatism patients were nocturia and urge incontinence. Correlating these results with a modified Madsen–Iversen score, the authors found that 20% of *asymptomatic* men in the sixth and seventh decades had symptom scores equal in severity to those men undergoing prostatectomy for BPH. More recently, Barry and colleagues[28] developed the seven-item AUA symptom index, which includes the symptoms of incomplete emptying, frequency, intermittency, urgency, weak stream, hesitancy, and nocturia, with an included measurement of bother symptoms. Patients were divided into mild (0–7), moderate (8–19), and severe (20–35), depending on the overall score. The AUA symptom score was found to be valid with respect to patient's

rating of the urinary difficulty and differentiating between BPH patients and normal controls. However, in patients with voiding symptoms, it has never been shown to be predictive of the underlying disease. Recently, Yalla and colleagues[29] demonstrated that the AUA symptom score could not distinguish between obstructed and non-obstructed voiding. Therefore, the AUA symptom score is not useful or recommended as a screening tool for BPH. However, it may be useful for measuring changes in symptoms over time and improvement after therapeutic interventions.

It is clear that patient symptom analysis and symptom scores by themselves cannot distinguish outflow obstruction due to BPH from other causes of voiding dysfunction, and further evaluation is necessary to ascertain the underlying cause.

PROSTATE SIZE AND CYSTOSCOPY IN DIAGNOSING BLADDER OUTLET OBSTRUCTION

Urologists have routinely used symptoms, prostate size, cystoscopy, radiologic imaging studies, and the measurement of postvoid residuals as means of diagnosing bladder outlet obstruction. If one believed that the voiding symptoms collectively called "prostatism" were due to an increase in prostate size, then it would be intuitively obvious that the larger the prostate became, the more severe the symptoms. This is, of course, incorrect, and most studies have shown that there is no correlation between resected prostate weight and the results of urodynamic studies.[30,31] Andersen and Nordling[32] did find a statistically significant *association* between prostatic weight at time of cystoscopy, maximal flow rate, detrusor opening pressure, and the calculated urethral resistance. However, these variables by themselves cannot distinguish obstructed from non-obstructed patients. Even if estimated prostatic size were correlated with obstruction, the common methods of assessing prostatic size would be relatively inaccurate. This is most pronounced on digital rectal exam (DRE); however, even measurement at the time of cystourethroscopy is relatively inaccurate.[33,34] Bissada and colleagues[35] measured prostatic size by DRE and cystourethroscopy, comparing it with the resected weight, and found a wide variation between preoperative estimation and the actual resected weight in glands of all sizes. Although an estimation of prostatic size may be important after the decision to operate has been made, cystoscopy is not useful as a method of diagnosing outlet obstruction from other causes of voiding symptoms, because it is a static, anatomic test, which appears to have little correlation with the dynamic act of voiding.

Another frequently utilized "sign" of obstruction is bladder trabeculation. Many urologists believe that the degree of obstruction is correlated with severity of bladder trabeculation. According to the theory of "bladder compensation", after prostatic obstruction occurs, trabeculation develops owing to muscular hypertrophy and is therefore an attribute of the obstructed bladder, compensated for the obstruction.

Studies have shown that there is little correlation between bladder trabeculation and the results of urodynamic studies or the severity of obstruction.[36] Additionally, the obstructed bladder is not always trabeculated, but the unstable, unobstructed bladder is frequently trabeculated and is present in both males and females.[37] Therefore, bladder trabeculation cannot be reliably equated with simple hypertrophy of muscle cells or increased strength of the bladder musculature, and cannot be automatically considered indicative of bladder outlet obstruction. A more reliable association instead exists with detrusor instability. This is further supported by Simonsen et al.,[38] who found a positive correlation between bladder trabeculation, age, and irritative symptoms, but not obstructive symptoms. Moreover, the absence of bladder trabeculation is not good evidence against obstruction.

There is good evidence that bladder outlet obstruction cannot be reliably diagnosed by prostate size, the clinical impression at time of cystoscopy, or bladder trabeculation, and further evaluation is necessary to determine whether the patient has prostatic obstruction.

POSTVOID RESIDUAL URINE VOLUME DETERMINATIONS

Again, according to the "theory of compensation," after outlet obstruction occurs, the bladder goes through certain phases of "compensation." Initially, the bladder is supposed to "compensate" by muscular hypertrophy, leading to trabeculation, which later yields to detrusor decompensation, which initially manifests itself as a progressively larger residual urine with endstage total decompensation leading ultimately to urinary retention. This cherished doctrine appears to be largely untrue, however.[39–41] What does appear to be true is that postvoid residuals *tend* to be lower in unobstructed men than in symptomatic men. However, such a great overlap exists that an abnormal value is difficult to establish. It has also been shown that the residual volume tends to decrease significantly in patients with prostatism treated with TURP.[40] In studies of normal males, mean residual urine volumes were determined to be between 12 and 28 mL.[42,43] However, two separate groups have shown large differences in intra-individual residual urine measured by catheterization, leading to further confusion of the issue.[19,44] Abrams and Griffiths[23] have theorized that residual urine reflects a dysfunction in detrusor musculature, as opposed to an indicator of bladder obstruction. However, Bruskewitz and colleagues[19] and Jensen and colleagues[45] were unable to correlate residual urine volumes with pressure parameters or postoperative outcomes. Finally, Andersen and colleagues[41] found that almost 25% of patients with severe obstruction had postvoid residuals less than 50 mL, while some patients who were unobstructed by urodynamics had an elevated postvoid residual. Most importantly, the postvoid residual volume cannot reliably predict urodynamic or symptomatic outcome after surgery.[46]

Therefore, large postvoid residuals may be causally related to bladder outlet obstruction and/or may be related to bladder dysfunction in the unobstructed patient, and are therefore unreliable as an indicator for the diagnosis of bladder outlet obstruction due to BPH. A patient with a large postvoid residual requires further diagnostic studies to determine the cause.

UROFLOWMETRY

The measurement of the urinary flow rate is probably the most commonly used screening procedure for diagnosing bladder outlet obstruction, owing to its simplicity and noninvasiveness. The parameters that can be easily measured include the average flow rate, peak flow rate, voided volume, time to maximum flow, and a graphic representation of the urinary flow pattern. A normal flow rate and voiding pattern is seen in Figure 8.1. Of all the various parameters of uroflowmetry, the most predictive parameter appears to the be the maximum urinary flow rate (Q_{max}), which has become the most widely used parameter for urodynamic evaluation of BPH throughout the world.[47] Also, because Q_{max} is easily measured and changes minimally with placebo treatments, the maximum flow rate has become an objective measurement of treatment outcomes in numerous studies.[48,49] A recent review by the Agency for Health Care Policy and Research (AHCPR) Committee[50] in 1992 found that the maximum urinary flow rate was used by 24 of 51 organizations as an indicator for the appropriate use of surgical therapy for BPH. As a result, the uroflow appears to have become the diagnostic "test of choice" for the diagnosis of BPH. However, in well-performed studies, does it really measure what it is proclaimed to measure?

Studies comparing patients with prostatism and asymptomatic men have shown a considerable overlap in the Q_{max} between the two groups.[24,51,52] Multiple investigators have attempted to construct nomograms to better define the "normal" Q_{max}. Perhaps the most widely used is the Siroky et al.[53,54] nomogram in which "normal" values were generated from 300 flow-rate measurements in 80 normal men. The nomogram was verified using both asymptomatic men

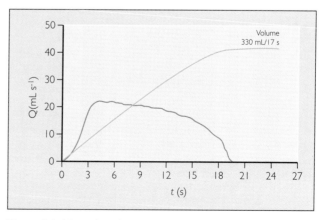

Figure 8.1 Normal uroflow in a minimally symptomatic 42-year-old man. The patient voided 330 mL in 17 s with a maximum flow rate (Q_{max}) of 24 mL s^{-1} (Q_{avg}, 19 mL s^{-1}; time to Q_{max}, 3.35 s)

and patients with obstruction, with "abnormal" defined as more than two standard deviations from the mean. Unfortunately, the diagnosis of obstruction was determined by clinical examination, which is insufficient. Schäfer and colleagues[55] found that only 75% of patients diagnosed with obstruction using this nomogram actually had outflow obstruction. Abrams and Griffiths[23] and later Andersen[24] proposed a classification system utilizing a Q_{max} of less than 10 mL s^{-1} as definitive proof of bladder outlet obstruction, while a Q_{max} of greater than or equal to 15 mL s^{-1} ruled out obstruction. Those patients in the 10–15 mL s^{-1} group were considered equivocal and required further urodynamic evaluation, such as a pressure-flow study.[23,24] An "equivocal" obstructive flow rate and pattern is seen in Figure 8.2. Although simplistic, this classification system was entirely empiric and not widely applicable to the diagnosis of obstruction.

Besides establishing a definition of a "normal" flow rate, other problems do exist. Age itself is a factor, as Girman *et al.* reported that only 29% of men over the age of 70 have a Q_{max} greater than 15 mL s^{-1}, and therefore age-standardized nomograms may be helpful.[56] Additionally, the maximum urinary flow rate is volume dependent, and the relationship between volume and flow is nonlinear, with a minimum volume of 150 mL necessary to determine maximum flow rate accurately. Rollema and colleagues[57] believe that a minimum of 250 mL is actually a more accurate figure. Further, artifacts may occur with machine vs. manually read maximum flow rates. Grino *et al.*[58] found that manually read Q_{max} values were approximately 1.5 mL lower than the machine-read uroflows, possibly owing to straining artifact, and suggested that an accurate Q_{max} lasts a minimum of 2 s. The reproducibility of the Q_{max} is also an issue. In patients followed in serial uroflowmetry studies, approximately 20% of patients had an episodic increase of approximately 4 mL s^{-1}.[28] Lastly, and perhaps most importantly, Q_{max} or any parameter of uroflowmetry has been questioned as an accurate parameter to define patients who have true bladder outlet obstruction. Several studies have demonstrated that a low flow rate could not distinguish between bladder outlet obstruction and impaired detrusor contractility.[59,60] Additionally, 7–25% of men with confirmed bladder outlet obstructions secondary to BPH have Q_{max} values considered to be within the normal range.[61,62] Further, no parameter of the uroflowmetry allows the distinction of the different types of obstruction, such as urethral stricture vs. true bladder outlet obstruction.[63,64]

As shown by its many limitations, the uroflow alone cannot be used to make a reliable diagnosis of bladder outlet obstruction. However, because it is inexpensive, non-invasive, and easy to perform, it may be helpful as a screening tool, which, if abnormal, prompts further study to clarify the etiology. If the study is normal, a watchful waiting attitude can be selected, with further investigation if symptoms do not resolve spontaneously without treatment.

CYSTOMETRY

The most commonly performed urodynamic study performed by the urologist is the cystometrogram (CMG). Filling cystometry, using a water media, is most commonly used and provides information on sensation, bladder capacity, detrusor stability, and detrusor compliance. Whereas the search for involuntary detrusor contractions using a filling CMG has little application in the diagnosis and treatment of BPH, the evaluation of detrusor compliance has ultimate importance in the diagnosis of obstructive uropathy. Often overlooked as a screening study, the diagnosis of poor compliance on a CMG mandates that surgical intervention be performed to relieve the bladder obstruction and avoid upper tract damage. Although poor compliance is uncommonly discovered, its importance should be emphasized.

The prognostic value of preoperative filling cystometry has also been investigated by prospective trials. These trials have shown that detrusor instability is present in up to 50% of patients with outlet obstruction, and yields little prognostic outcome information after prostatectomy.[65,66] The only significant prognostic sign is the failure of detrusor instability to resolve *postoperatively*, which portends a poor prognosis in terms of symptom resolution.

Therefore, the importance of a CMG in the evaluation for bladder outlet obstruction is to exclude poor detrusor compliance, not to demonstrate detrusor instability. If a pressure-flow study is performed, a CMG can be performed during bladder filling.

PRESSURE-FLOW STUDIES

A pressure-flow study is performed by placing a urodynamic catheter into the bladder to allow the simultaneous measurement of pressure and flow rate during voiding. The pressure-flow study allows the patient's voiding cycle to be measured dynamically and is the only reliable way of directly evaluating bladder outlet obstruction. Some investigators use a rectal catheter so that subtracted pressures

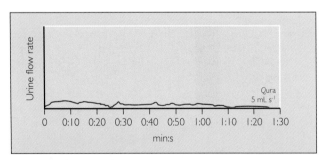

Figure 8.2 An "equivocal" uroflow in a 69-year-old man with a moderately elevated AUA symptom score of 18. The patient voids 404 mL with a maximum flow rate of 11.2 mL s^{-1}. The postvoid residual was abnormally elevated at 115 mL. The flow pattern is relatively flat, with a prolonged duration of flow and intermittent straining by the patient. A pressure-flow study documented bladder outlet obstruction. (Delay time, 0 s; voiding time, 1 min 24 s; flow time, 1 min 21 s; time to maximum flow, 0.07 s; average flow rate, 4.0 ml s^{-1})

can be measured to rule out an abdominal source for the intravesical pressure. If the procedure is carefully monitored by the physician or trained personnel, this catheter is rarely necessary. The principal uses of the pressure-flow study are to (1) verify a high-pressure, low-flow state; (2) identify patients with voiding symptoms and a low flow rate based on impaired detrusor contractility; (3) identify patients who have voiding symptoms and a normal flow rate but a high-pressure bladder consistent with obstruction; and (4) document a normal voiding pressure to avoid unnecessary surgery.

Controlled studies have shown a high degree of reproducibility in pressure-flow studies when groups of patients were retested at varying intervals after periods of either observation or placebo treatments.[67,68] Additionally, intraindividual variations appear to be small and are not clinically significant.[69] For its many good points, perhaps the biggest problem with pressure-flow data has been the interpretation of what constitutes an abnormally high pressure. A value of over 100 cmH$_2$O at Q$_{max}$ was proposed by Smith in 1968.[70] However, this value has fluctuated down to 45 cmH$_2$O as suggested by Griffiths.[71] A typical obstructive pressure-flow study is seen in Figure 8.3.

Early models of bladder outlet obstruction centered around urethral obstruction and were unfortunately based on a rigid tube system, which is inconsistent with the actual non-rigid hydrodynamics of voiding. Subsequent mathematical models such as the Abrams and Griffiths nomogram allow classification of pressure-flow data into obstructed, unobstructed, or equivocal voiding patterns.[23] An example of an obstructive pressure-flow study analyzed on the Abrams–Griffith nomogram is shown in Figure 8.4. Data plots that are in the equivocal area require further

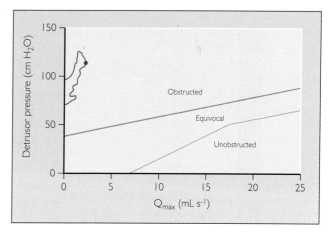

Figure 8.4 This severely obstructed pressure-flow study in a 65-year-old man is plotted on the Abrams–Griffiths nomogram. The detrusor pressure at Q$_{max}$ is plotted as a single point in the obstructive region of the nomogram

analysis. In the Abrams–Griffiths nomogram, the slope of the plot is indicative of the degree of obstruction; i.e. the steeper the slope, the more obstructed the patient. This is due to the higher pressure necessary to produce an increased flow rate. Therefore, if the slope of the pressure-flow curve is greater than 2 cmH$_2$O mL^{-1} s^{-1}, the patient is obstructed. Additionally, if the closing pressure (closing pressure is the detrusor pressure at the time when flow stops) is greater than approximately 40 cmH$_2$O, the patient is also categorized as obstructed.

Although the use of a nomogram to diagnose bladder outlet obstruction is useful, it is much more important to be able to predict the clinical outcome after relief of obstruction. In other words, what is the prognostic value of a pressure-flow study in predicting whether a patient will benefit from an operative procedure? Additionally, which urodynamic parameters are instrumental in predicting a good outcome? In 1979, Abrams[18] reported that using a pressure-flow study (and the Abrams–Griffiths nomogram) lowered the failure rate of TURP from 28% to 12%. In a prospective, blind study, Jensen et al.[72] found positive prognostic value for the Abrams–Griffiths nomogram with a 93% success rate in the obstructed group vs. 78% in the unobstructed group. Interestingly, the reason for the high success rate in the unobstructed patients is unknown, because the pressure-flow parameters were essentially unchanged postoperatively. This improvement may be partially due to a placebo effect, which appears to be quite strong in the treatment of BPH, and/or some other, unexplained factors. In another prospective study, Kuo and Tsai[73] found that patients with a Q$_{max}$ of less than 15 mL s^{-1} and those patients demonstrating high pressure with obstruction had the best subjective outcome after a prostatectomy. The worst outcomes were found in patients with a Q$_{max}$ of greater than 15 mL s^{-1} and those with a low pressure, no obstruction, preoperative urodynamic evaluation. Bruskewitz and colleagues[19] performed a prospective analysis on 46 patients with prostatism symptoms and found a lower rate of improvement using

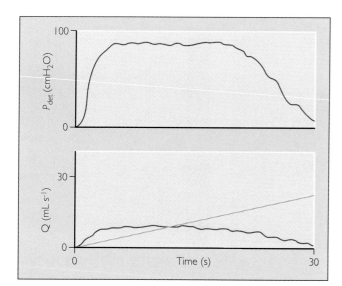

Figure 8.3 An obstructed pressure-flow study in a 73-year-old man. The patient voids an adequate volume (221 mL) at a maximum flow rate of 9 mL s^{-1} (Q$_{avg}$, 7 mL s^{-1}). The detrusor pressure at time of maximum flow is 90 cmH$_2$O, clearly demonstrating bladder outlet obstruction

preoperative urodynamic evaluation. Patients were evaluated with pressure studies, and categorized as obstructed or unobstructed. All patients were then treated surgically to relieve the obstruction. Postoperatively, 89% of unobstructed patients had symptomatic improvement, whereas 92% of obstructed patients were subjectively improved.

Another confounding problem in evaluating outcomes after surgical or medical therapy is the unknown positive predictive value for an individual patient, since other comparative groups are unavailable. For example, the true prevalence of patients with prostatism is unknown and no long-term follow-up of a large group of urodynamically obstructed, symptomatic patients who remain untreated currently exists. Additionally, the prevalence of asymptomatic, urodynamically obstructed males is unknown. Therefore, true predictive values for any of these parameters cannot be made.

Perhaps the best type of data includes the continuous plotting of pressure against urine flow for an entire voiding period. These data utilize computerized definitions of bladder outlet flow obstruction and are based on the urethra as a distensible tube with a proximal flow controlling area. Schäfer[74] described a relationship between the detrusor pressure and flow rate, which he termed the passive urethral resistance relation (PURR). "Linear PURR," a simplified version that does not require computer analysis, allows the categorization of the degree of prostatic obstruction by plotting the opening pressure and pressure at maximum flow on a specialized graph and connecting a line between them (Figure 8.5). Additionally, a categorization of the detrusor from very weak to strong can be made. More recently, Rollema and Mastrigt[75] developed a computer program "CLIM," in which continuous detrusor pressures and flow rates during voiding are stored in a computer and analyzed. In their CLIM study of 29 patients who underwent

TURP for symptomatic reasons, 34% were unobstructed by their definition. Of this group undergoing TURP for symptoms only, 70% had an unsatisfactory result compared with 20% of the obstructed group.

In comparison with Abrams and Griffiths' less complex nomogram, the computer models yield equivalent results. However, they do allow a quantitative number to be given to the degree of obstruction, whereas in the Abrams–Griffiths nomogram, only one of three categories is possible. A precise number may allow better correlation in future studies. Unfortunately, these complex nomograms and computerized systems are too complicated to be useful in the daily diagnosis and treatment of patients. However, they are important in the long-term analysis and study of outlet obstruction, especially when treatments other than transurethral resection are entertained.

The pressure-flow evaluation of patients with "prostatism" is important because it is clearly the test of choice for determining whether the detrusor is impaired and gives the most accurate assessment of whether bladder outlet obstruction is present. Although it is fundamentally impossible to define a sharp division between the obstructed and unobstructed state, the more sophisticated models do allow varying degrees of obstruction to be quantitated, making them useful for research purposes, whereas the Abrams–Griffiths nomogram is simpler to use, making it more clinically useful. At present, for treating patients with voiding symptoms and bladder outlet obstruction with a procedure designed to unobstruct the patient, a pressure-flow study is the most accurate test. Trepidation about the complexity of the methods used to analyze the data, the exact cut-off of what is considered obstruction ("even the experts disagree"), and the inability of the urologist to perform this test does not negate this basic fact.

It is also clear that the routine use of pressure-flow studies would improve the postoperative outcome of surgical therapy for bladder outlet obstruction. However, the exact magnitude is unknown at the present time. It is interesting that a prostatectomy performed in the unobstructed patient, which does not change the urodynamic parameters, appears symptomatically to improve approximately 60–75% of patients for reasons that have not been fully elucidated. Further study is needed in both of these areas.

VIDEOURODYNAMICS

Although pressure-flow studies allow the accurate assessment of bladder outlet obstruction, the exact site of obstruction is not always clear. The simultaneous recording of bladder and urethral pressure using fluoroscopy is the most precise method of determining whether obstruction exists and the exact site. Figure 8.6 reveals a normal videourodynamic study in a patient with typical prostatism symptoms. No treatment is necessary in this instance. Figures 8.7 and 8.8 illustrate the ability of a videourodynamic study to confirm poor detrusor compliance, prostatic obstruction, and good sphincteric relaxation during the

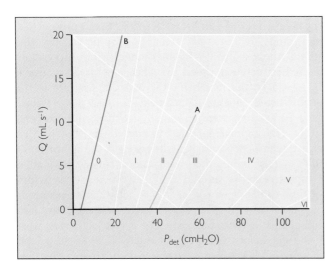

Figure 8.5 Linear PURR reveals mild–moderate bladder outlet obstruction and normal detrusor strength preoperatively (A) and unobstructed voiding with normal detrusor strength after TURP (B)

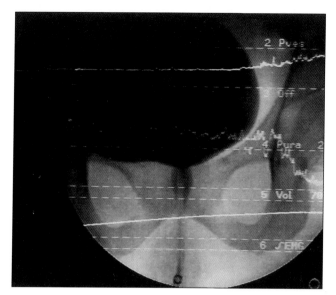

Figure 8.6 This is a videourodynamic study of a middle-aged man with moderate voiding symptoms and an AUA score of 12. The study shows good opening of the bladder neck, good relaxation of the external sphincter, and a voiding pressure of 30 cmH$_2$O. No treatment is necessary in this case

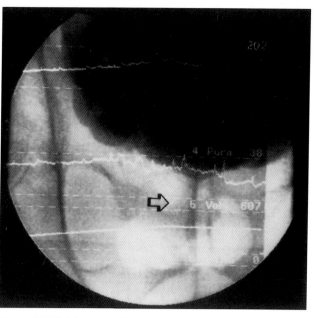

Figure 8.8 This is a magnified view of the prostatic urethra in an elderly gentleman with severe prostatic obstruction. The prostatic urethra does not open during voiding and the patient develops detrusor pressures over 150 cmH$_2$O. Note the heavily trabeculated bladder. This patient requires surgical therapy to relieve the obstruction

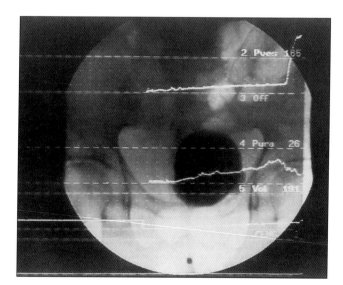

Figure 8.7 This is a 70-year-old man with severe voiding symptoms, including occasional urge incontinence. The videourodynamic study reveals poor compliance, very low functional capacity (note the bladder diverticulum), good sphincteric relaxation, and a voiding pressure over 100 cmH$_2$O. This patient requires surgical therapy to relieve the obstruction and avoid potential upper tract damage

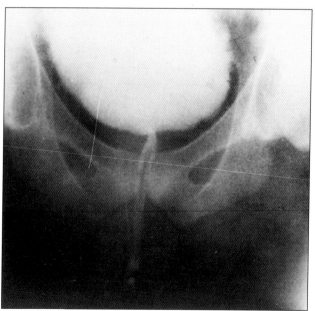

Figure 8.9 This is a voiding study in a 32-year-old man with significant voiding complaints. He failed medical therapy and desired further evaluation. The pressure-flow study (not included here) revealed a mildly obstructive pressure, and this voiding study demonstrated the point of obstruction at the bladder neck. A transurethral incision of the bladder neck gave excellent symptomatic relief

study. In Figure 8.9, a videourodynamic study demonstrates that the point of obstruction in this patient lies at the bladder neck, not the prostate.

In most cases, electromyography (EMG) is unnecessary as the continuous measurement of urethral pressure and documented normal neural status of the patient is generally all that is necessary for these studies. A simultaneous EMG may be helpful if the patient has known neurologic abnormalities. Another important parameter that is easily measured using videourodynamics is the degree of relaxation of the external sphincter, which allows one to categorize the study as adequate or not. In practice, videourodynamics allows one to distinguish between nonobstruction, detrusor impairment, obstruction at the bladder neck, and true prostatic obstruction. Typically, with the catheter moving in an out, one can define a pressure drop during the voiding cycle, which delineates the point of obstruction. In our urodynamics laboratory, we routinely use the fluoroscopic representation of the urethra, the voiding pressure, and the pressure drop across the prostatic urethra when the external urethra is maximally relaxed to diagnose obstruction. Because of the ability of videourodynamics to observe these phenomena, it is clearly superior to other methods of evaluation.

Although a videourodynamic study is certainly the most accurate study for determining obstruction and the point of obstruction, it is currently infrequently used owing to the higher cost, complexity, need for special training, and radiation exposure. Its main utility is for those equivocal cases in which a diagnosis cannot be made using simpler means.

CONCLUSIONS

The role of a urodynamic evaluation is to help the clinician determine whether a pathological process is at the heart of a patient's voiding complaints. The pressure-flow study will determine whether the detrusor or outlet is at fault, and videourodynamic evaluation can locate the site of obstruction, if required. The role of urodynamics in diagnosing whether BPH is responsible for bladder outlet obstruction appears to be complex and controversial. However, the role of urodynamics is actually quite simple. Before the application of operative procedures in which the relief of obstruction is the primary goal, it is paramount that the diagnosis of obstruction be made. Unfortunately, the clinical evaluation of patients with BPH, including symptom scores, cystoscopy, CMG, and even flow rates fail in a reliable manner to diagnose obstruction. The only reliable way of delineating obstructed from unobstructed voiding is a pressure-flow study with or without fluoroscopy. Although many complicated mathematical schemata and computer-aided models have been made, pressure-flow data applied to the Abrams–Griffiths nomogram appears to be adequate for the prognostic identification of patients who will do well after surgery. Although some would argue that a precise diagnosis of obstruction is not necessary and that symptom scores or flow rates are good enough, this is simply not valid when the treatment proposed is designed to unobstruct the patient. At present, when many new treatment modalities exist that minimize symptoms with minimal morbidity, the cost and morbidity of applying a relatively non-invasive study to avoid an invasive procedure or lifelong medical therapy is time and money well spent. Additionally, the empiric application of medical therapy, which will not relieve significant bladder outlet obstruction, may in time endanger the health of the truly obstructed patient. From a scientific viewpoint, without appropriate urodynamic studies, we have no idea of the initial disease that we are treating and therefore, when patients "fail" or "improve", we cannot be sure why this has occurred. The usage of urodynamics *only* when "things don't add up" makes little sense in this day and age.

REFERENCES

1 Ashley DJ. Observations on the epidemiology of prostatic hyperplasia in males. *Br J Urol* 1966; **38**: 567–9.

2 Christensen MM, Bruskewitz RC. Clinical manifestations of benign prostatic hyperplasia and indications for therapeutic intervention. *Urol Clin North Am* 1990; **17**: 509–16.

3 Coolsaet BRLA, Blok C. Detrusor properties related to prostatism. *Neurourol Urodyn* 1986; **5**: 435–9.

4 Dean GE, Kaplan SA, Blaivas JG. The differential diagnosis of prostatism. A urodynamic survey. *J Urol* 1991; **145**: 264A (abstract. 207).

5 Hellstrom P, Lukkarinen O, Kontturi M. Bladder neck incision or transurethral electroresection for the treatment of urinary obstruction caused by a small benign prostate? A randomized urodynamic study. *Scand J Urol Nephrol* 1986; **20**: 187–92.

6 Kaplan SA, Te AE. Uroflowmetry and urodynamics. *Urol Clin North Am* 1995; **22**: 309–20.

7 Abrams PH, Farrar DJ, Turner-Warwick RT *et al.* The results of prostatectomy: a symptomatic and urodynamic urinalysis of 142 patients. *J Urol* 1979; **121**: 640–2.

8 Andersen JT. Detrusor hyperreflexia in benign intravesical obstruction. *J Urol* 1976; **115**: 532–4.

9 Norlen LJ, Blaivas JG. Unsuspected proximal urethral obstruction in young and middle aged men. *J Urol* 1986; **135**: 972–6.

10 Kaplan SA, Te AE, Jacobs BZ. Urodynamic evidence of vesical neck obstruction in men with misdiagnosed chronic non-bacterial prostatitis and the therapeutic role of endoscopic incision of the bladder neck. *J Urol* 1994; **152**: 2063–65.

11 Lepor H, Machi G. Comparison of the AUA symptom index in unselected males and females between 55 and 79 years of age. *Urology* 1993; **42**: 36–40.

12 Chancellor MB, Rivas DA. The American Urological Association symptom index for women with voiding symptoms: lack of index specificity for benign prostatic hyperplasia. *J Urol* 1993; **150**: 1706–9.

13 Clark R. The prostate and the endocrine. A controlled series. *Br J Urol* 1937; **9**: 254–7.

14 Birkhoff TD, Widerhorn AR, Hamilton ML, Zinsser HH. Natural history of benign prostatic hypertrophy and urinary retention. *Urology* 1976; **7**: 48–52.

15 Bell AJ, Finnelly RCL, Abrams PH. The natural history of untreated "prostatism". *Br J Urol* 1981; **53**: 613–16.

16 McConnell JD. Why pressure flow studies should be optional and not mandatory studies for evaluating men with benign prostatic hyperplasia. *Urology* 1994; **44**: 156–8.

17 Abrams PH. In support of pressure flow studies for evaluating men with lower urinary tract symptoms. *Urology* 1994; **44**: 153–5.

18 Abrams PH. Prostatism and prostatectomy: the value of urine flow rate measurements in the preoperative assessment for operation. *J Urol* 1979; **117**: 70–1.

19 Bruskewitz R, Jensen KM, Iversen P, Madsen PO. The relevance of minimum urethral resistance in prostatism. *J Urol* 1983; **129**: 769–71.

20 McConnell JD, Barry MJ, Bruskewitz RC *et al. Benign Prostatic Hyperplasia: Diagnosis and Treatment. Clinical Practice Guidelines,* No. 8. AHCPR Publication No. 94–0582. Rockville, MD: Agency for Health Care Policy and Research, Public Health Service, US Department of Health and Human Services 1994: 1–17.

21 Donovan JL, Abrams P, Schäfer W. The International Continence Society Study on BPH: urodynamic quality control and data analysis. *J Urol* 1994; **151**: 294A (abstract 268).

22 Kirchner-Hermanns R, Thorner M, Schafer W *et al.* Reproducibility of urodynamic data in BPH: influence of patient and investigator on data quality and analysis. *J Urol* 1994; **151**: 295A (abstract 269).

23 Abrams PH, Griffiths BJ. The assessment of prostatic obstruction from urodynamic measurements and from residual urine. *Br J Urol* 1979; **151**: 129–34.

24 Andersen JT. Prostatism: clinical, radiological and urodynamic aspects. *Neurourol Urodyn* 1982; **1**: 241–93.

25 Coolsaet BRLA, Elbadawi A. Urodynamics in the management of benign prostatic hypertrophy. *World J Urol* 1989; **6**: 215–24.

26 McGuire EJ. The role of urodynamic investigation in the assessment of benign prostatic hypertrophy. *J Urol* 1992; **148**: 1133–6.

27 Sommer P, Nielsen KK, Bauer T, Kristensen ES *et al.* Voiding patterns in men evaluated by a questionnaire survey. *Br J Urol* 1990; **65**: 155–60.

28 Barry MJ, Fowler FJ, O'Leary MP *et al.* The American Urological Association symptom index for benign prostatic hyperplasia. *J Urol* 1992; **148**: 1549–57.

29 Yalla SV, Sullivan MP, Lecamwasam HF *et al.* Correlation of the American Urological Association symptom index with obstructive and non-obstructive prostatism. *J Urol* 1995; **153**: 674–80.

30 Scott FB, Cardus D, Quesada EM, Riles T. Uroflowmetry before and after prostatectomy. *South Med J* 1967; **60**: 948–52.

31 Jensen KME, Bruskewitz RC, Iversen P, Madsen PO. Significance of prostatic weight in prostatism. *Urol Int* 1983; **38**: 173–8.

32 Andersen JT, Nordling J. Prostatism II. The correlation between cystourethroscopic, cystometric and urodynamic findings. *Scan J Urol Nephrol* 1980; **14**: 23–7.

33 Meyerhoff HH, Hald T. Are doctors able to assess prostatic size? *Scan J Urol Nephrol* 1978; **12**: 219–21.

34 Meyerhoff HH, Ingemann L, Nordling J, Hald T. Accuracy in preoperative estimation of prostatic size. *Scan J Urol Nephrol* 1981; **15**: 45–51.

35 Bissada NK, Finkbeiner AE, Redman JF. Accuracy of preoperative estimation of resection weight in transurethral prostatectomy. *J Urol* 1978; **116**: 201–2.

36 Nielsen KK, Kristensen ES, Pedersen OS *et al.* Prostatectomy. Symptomatological, uroflowmetric and cystometric changes after operation and correlation between symptoms, cystometry, cystourethroscopy, and flow measurements. *Ugeskr Laeger* 1986; **148**: 70–4.

37 Elbadawi A. BPH associated voiding dysfunction: detrusor is pivotal. *Contemp Urol* 1994; **6**: 21–38.

38 Simonsen O, Moller-Madsen B, Dorflinger T *et al.* The significance of age on symptoms, urodynamic findings and cystoscopic findings in benign prostatic hypertrophy. *Urol Res* 1987; **15**: 355–8.

39 Griffiths HJL, Castro J. An evaluation of the importance of residual urine. *Br J Rad* 1970; **43**: 409–13.

40 Bruskewitz RC, Iversen P, Madsen PO. Value of post void residual urine determination in evaluation of prostatism. *Urology* 1982; **20**: 602–4.

41 Andersen JT, Nordling J, Walter S. Prostatism. I. The correlation between symptoms, cystometric and urodynamic findings. *Scand J Urol Nephrol* 1979; **13**: 229–36.

42 DiMare JR, Fish SR, Harper JM *et al.* Residual urine in normal male subjects. *J Urol* 1963; **96**: 180–1.

43 Andersen JT, Jacobsen O, Worm-Petersen J *et al.* Bladder function in healthy elderly males. *Scand J Urol Nephrol* 1978; **12**: 123–7.

44 Birch NC, Hurst G, Doyle PT. Serial residual volumes in men with prostatic hypertrophy. *Br J Urol* 1988; **62**: 571–5.

45 Jensen KME, Jorgensen JB, Mogensen P. Urodynamics in prostatism. III. Prognostic value of medium fill water cystometry. *Scand J Urol Nephrol* 1988; **114**: (Suppl) 78–83.

46 Neal DE, Ramsden PD, Sharples L *et al.* Outcome of elective prostatectomy. *Br J Urol* 1989; **299**: 762–7.

47 Layton TN, Drach GW. Selectivity of peak versus average male urinary flow rates. *J Urol* 1981; **125**: 839–41.

48 Kelly MJ, Roskamp D, Leach GE. Transurethral incision of the prostate: a preoperative and postoperative analysis of symptoms and urodynamic findings. *J Urol* 1989; **142**: 1507–9.

49 Barry MJ. Medical outcomes research and benign prostatic hyperplasia. *Prostate* 1990; **3**: 61–74.

50 McConnell JD, Barry MJ, Bruskewitz RC *et al. Benign Prostatic Hyperplasia: Diagnosis and Treatment. Clinical Practice Guidelines,* No. 8. AHCPR Publication 94–0582. Rockville, MD: Agency for Health Care Policy and Research, Public Health Service, US Department of Health and Human Services 1994.

51 Jensen KME, Jorgensen JB, Mogensen P. Urodynamics in prostatism. I. Prognostic value of uroflowmetry. *Scand J Urol Nephrol* 1988; **114**: (Suppl) 63–71.

52 Jensen KME, Jorgensen JB, Mogensen P, Bille-Brahe NE. Some clinical aspects of uroflowmetry in elderly males. *Scand J Urol Nephrol* 1986; **20**: 93–9.

53 Siroky MB, Olsson CA, Krane RJ. The flowrate nomogram. 1. Development. *J Urol* 1979; **122**: 665–8.

54 Siroky MB, Olsson CA, Krane RJ. The flowrate nomogram. 2. Clinical correlation. *J Urol* 1980; **123**: 208–10.

55 Schäfer W, Noppeney R, Rubben H, Lutzeyer W. The value of free flowrate and pressure flow studies in the routine investigation of BPH patients. *Neurourol Urodyn* 1988; **7**: 219–21.

56 Girman CJ, Panser LA, Chute CG *et al.* Natural history of prostatism: urinary flow rates in a community based study. *J Urol* 1993; **150**: 887–92.

57 Rollema HJ, Griffiths DJ, Van Duyl WA *et al.* Flow rate versus bladder volume: an alternative way of presenting some features of the micturition of healthy males. *Urol Int* 1977; **32**: 401–12.

58 Grino PB, Bruskewitz R, Blaivas JG *et al.* Maximum urinary flow rate by uroflowmetry: automatic or visual interpretation. *J Urol* 1993; **149**: 339–41.

59 Chancellor MB, Blaivas JG, Kaplan SA *et al.* Bladder outlet obstruction versus impaired detrusor contractility. The role of uroflow. *J Urol* 1991; **145**: 810–12.

60 Rollema HJ, Mastrigt R. Detrusor contractility before and after prostatectomy. *Neurourol Urodyn* 1987; **6**: 220–1.

61 Gerstenberg TC, Andersen JT, Klarskov P *et al.* High flow intravesical obstruction in men: symptomatology, urodynamics and the results of surgery. *J Urol* 1982; **127**: 943–5.

62 Iversen P, Bruskewitz RC, Jensen KME *et al.* Transurethral prostatic resection in the treatment of prostatism with high urinary flow. *J Urol* 1983; **129**: 995–7.

63 Jorgensen JB, Jensen KME, Mogensen P *et al.* Urinary flow curves and their prognostic value in males over the age of 50 years. *Neurourol Urodyn* 1992; **11**: 473–81.

64 Gleason DM, Bottaccini MR, Drach GW *et al.* Urinary flow velocity as an index of male voiding function. *J Urol* 1982; **128**: 1363–7.

65 Balslev-Jorgensen J, Jensen KME, Mogensen P. Significance of predominantly irritative symptomatology before a prostatic operation. *J Urol* 1990; **143**: 739–41.

66 Dorfling T, Frimodt-Moller PC, Bruskewitz RC et al. The significance of uninhibited detrusor contractions in prostatism. *J Urol* 1985; **133**: 819–21.

67 Nielsen KK, Kromann-Andersen B, Poulsen AL et al. Subjective and objective evaluation of patients with prostatism and infravesical obstruction treated with both intra prostatic spiral and transurethral prostatectomy. *Neurourol Urodyn* 1994; **13**: 13–19.

68 Tammela TLJ, Kontturi MJ. Urodynamic effects of finasteride in the treatment of bladder outlet obstruction due to benign prostatic hyperplasia. *J Urol* 1993; **149**: 342–4.

69 Rosier PFWM, deLa Rosette JJMCH, Koldewijn EL et al. Variability of pressure flow analysis parameters in repeated cystometry in patients with benign prostatic hyperplasia. *J Urol* 1995; **153**: 1520–5.

70 Smith JC. Urethral resistance to micturition. *Br J Urol* 1968; **40**: 125–56.

71 Griffiths DJ. Urethral resistance to flow: the urethral resistance relation. *Urol Int* 1975; **30**: 28–32.

72 Jensen KME, Jorgensen JB, Mogensen P. Urodynamics in prostatism. II. Prognostic value of pressure flow study combined with stop-flow tests. *Scand J Urol Nephrol* 1988; **144**(Suppl): 72–7.

73 Kuo HC, Tsai TC. The predictive value of urine flow rate and voiding pressure in the operative outcome of benign prostatic hypertrophy. *J Taiwan* 1988; **141**: 873–9.

74 Schäfer W. Principles and clinical application of advanced urodynamic analysis of voiding dysfunction. *Urol Clin N Am* 1990; **17**: 553–66.

75 Rollema HJ, Mastrigt RV. Improved indication and follow up in transurethral resection of the prostate using the computer program CLIM: a prospective study. *J Urol* 1992; **148**: 111–16.

COMMENTARY

In this chapter, Drs Cespedes and McGuire, who are world-renowned experts in urodynamic evaluation of patients, have extensively reviewed the relevant literature and reiterated herein the role of various urodynamic tests in evaluation of lower urinary tract dysfunction. As noted in other chapters on evaluation of BPH, this chapter reiterates the fact that BPH and urodynamic evidence of obstruction are not synonymous. In a large controlled study of urodynamics in patients with symptoms of prostatism, 23% of patients had prostatic obstruction, while 39% had a combination of both outlet obstruction and detrusor instability. Another confounding variable is that while the natural history of patients with symptoms suggests that 25% of them will undergo surgery, owing to progression of symptoms, it is unclear whether all of these patients have obstruction. Indeed, urodynamics studies have shown that only 20% of even clearly obstructed patients need surgery when followed by watchful waiting over 5 years. The question then arises whether urodynamics has any role in patients with BPH symptoms. In this regard, Abrams found that using pressure-flow studies in the preoperative evaluation significantly reduced the failure rate of TURP from 28% to 12%. However, it is also clear from review of TURP literature that across the board only 11–12% of patients fail from TURP, even when TURP is being done without urodynamic data and only for symptoms. Based on these data most urologists in the USA currently do not believe that an invasive urodynamic study is necessary prior to surgery for BPH.

Among common urodynamic parameters available for the evaluation of BPH, uroflow, and postvoid residual urine volume measurements are fraught with considerable variables that diminish their utility. So, also is the use of CMG. The major study of value in BPH appears to be pressure-flow cystometry which can:

(1) verify high pressure, low flow, and the presence of bladder outlet obstruction vs. low pressure, low flow, and the presence of impaired detrusor function;

(2) detect normal flow normal pressure states, which would indicate other reasons for symptoms and therefore obviate the need for surgery. Even this test has problems in interpretation, since it is unclear as to what is a normal voiding pressure, despite considerable effort by Abrams, Griffiths, and others in constructing nomograms and computer models to delineate limits of normal voiding pressure.

Videourodynamics is a more recent development and an extension of pressure-flow studies. Currently, it is the most accurate study available for determining obstruction. The study involves the simultaneous recording of bladder and urethral pressure using fluoroscopy, and allows not only the documentation of high pressure, low flow, and obstruction, but also the site of obstruction, thereby making available to the surgeon a good method of scientifically documenting the problem, which would allow a proper plan of therapy. Unfortunately, the use of videourodynamics involves considerable expense, irradiation, is invasive, and most patients would not want to undergo the procedure because of the discomforts and costs associated with it. In conclusion, however, as we strive towards a better definition of what constitutes BPH, LUTS, or BPO, we need a precise understanding of the pathophysiology of obstruction, and some form of simplified videourodynamic study may be useful in patients who fail to respond to initial trials of medical management. While realizing it is not cost effective, its importance can be better stated by a quote from Dr Elbadawi:

"Urodynamicists bear the responsibility for providing urologists with a long-overdue real consensus on simpler, less costly, more comprehensible and more practical, yet informative, means and parameters of evaluation. This could be a formidable endeavor since identifying the common ground would entail setting aside personal convictions and preferences, disagreements on the merits versus limitations of various approaches, and insistence on interjecting real or abstract ideas and concepts that may be inconsequential from the practical standpoint – despite their scientific validity and importance."[1]

1 Elbadawi A.K Voiding dysfunction in benign prostatic hyperplasia: trends, controversies and recent revelations. I. symptoms and urodynamics. *Urology* 1998; **51** (Suppl 5A): 62–70.

Transrectal Ultrasonography in the Evaluation of Benign Prostatic Hyperplasia

K. Shinohara

9

Transrectal ultrasonography (TRUS) was first introduced clinically for prostate imaging in 1968,[1] and since then has been used extensively to examine benign and malignant prostate conditions. TRUS gives information regarding prostate size, anatomy, and pathology. In conjunction with prostate biopsy, it is currently regarded as the standard for detecting prostate cancer. For evaluation of benign prostatic hyperplasia (BPH), TRUS has had a major role in determining the efficacy of hormonal manipulation or surgical intervention. The observed changes in prostate volume, shape, and appearance after these treatments may be used as objective indicators of outcome.

TRANSRECTAL ULTRASONOGRAPHY: EQUIPMENT AND PROCEDURE

EQUIPMENT

Generally, a 5–7.5-MHz transducer is used for transrectal prostate imaging. Depending on the manufacturer and model, an axial, sector, linear, or phased-array scanner is used. A biplane or endfiring probe is most common (Figure 9.1). Although each can produce both transverse and longitudinal images of the prostate, the images will differ slightly and sonographers must be familiar with these differences. A biplane probe gives a true transverse image, i.e. the section perpendicular to the probe axis. An endfiring probe gives the oblique frontal image, which is not truly perpendicular to the axis (Figure 9.2), but is almost parallel to the proximal part of the prostatic urethra. Thus, the image often creates a sectioning of the prostatic urethra from the verumontanum to the bladder neck, referred to as the "Eiffel tower sign" because of its shape (Figure 9.3).

Probe frequency

In the early years of TRUS, a 3.5-MHz probe was used. However, more recent equipment uses 6–7.5-MHz probes, because these generally provide images with better resolution and can visualize finer anatomic changes in the gland. On the down side, they lack deep sound-wave penetration. In a large prostate gland, a 7.5-MHz probe will not enable clear visualization of the anterior aspect. Current machines are often equipped with a multifrequency function, which allows the operator to select the ideal frequency for the individual gland without changing the probe.

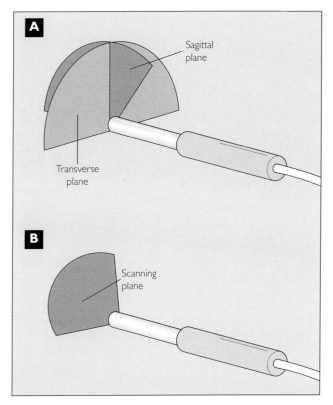

Figure 9.1 The two commonly used TRUS probes: (A) biplane probe; (B) endfiring probe

PROCEDURE

Before undergoing TRUS, patients should receive a Fleets enema to evacuate the rectal contents, as fecal material or gas in the rectum will cause artifacts and interfere with the examination. Placement in either the right or left decubitus position makes the procedure easier than placement in the lithotomy position. The patient's hip and knee should be bent at right angles, and the pelvis should be facing slightly downward. With this positioning, the operator can move the probe freely in any direction. The transducer is inserted through the anus, and images of the prostate, seminal vesicles, and bladder neck are obtained through the rectal wall. To obtain better images, a balloon with 30–50 mL of water is sometimes placed around the probe tip.

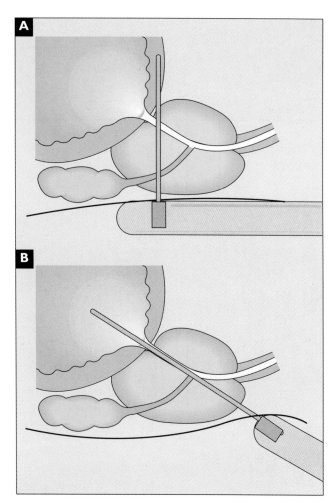

Figure 9.2 Transverse scanning plane with the biplane probe (A) perpendicular to the rectal wall; with the endfiring probe (B), the plane is almost parallel to the proximal part of the prostatic urethra

PROSTATE ANATOMY

To evaluate the prostate with TRUS, an understanding of the zonal anatomy of the gland as described by McNeal is essential (Figure 9.4).[2,3] The normal gland is divided into three zones: transition, peripheral, and central. In addition, the fibromuscular stroma is positioned anterior to the prostatic urethra.

The transition zone lies on both sides of the prostatic urethra. In the normal gland, this occupies only a small portion of the prostate, but it increases with age. This is the common finding in BPH. The central zone surrounds the ejaculatory ducts. At the gland's base, this zone occupies the greatest part of the cross-sectional image, but it diminishes at the level of the verumontanum where the ejaculatory ducts merge into the urethra. At the mid-portion and the apex, the peripheral zone constitutes the majority of the gland. In BPH, this zone is compressed posterolaterally by the enlarged transition zone and becomes the so-called surgical capsule.

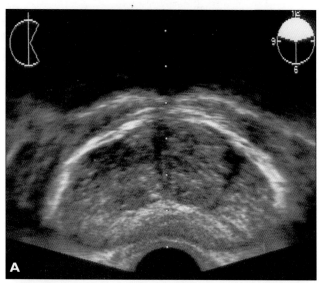

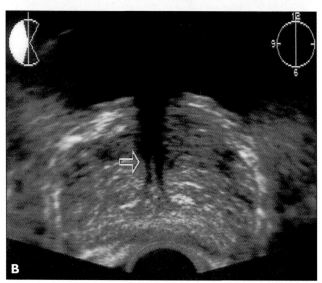

Figure 9.3 Transverse scan of the mid-prostate with (A) the biplane probe and (B) the endfiring probe. With the latter, sectioning of the verumontanum and the urethra forms the "Eiffel tower sign" (arrow)

A group of glands at the level of the bladder neck in the mid-line underneath the trigone may get hyperplasia and grow into the bladder lumen – the so-called median lobe seen on cystoscopy.[4] The prostatic urethra passes through the anterior half of the prostate and changes direction anteriorly about 45° at the level of the verumontanum. The ejaculatory ducts are the continuation of the ampullae of the vasa deferentia penetrating the prostate gland from the posterocranial aspect; they change direction anteriorly near the level of the verumontanum to open into the urethra. The ampullae of the vasa deferentia lie medial to the seminal vesicles in the mid-line.

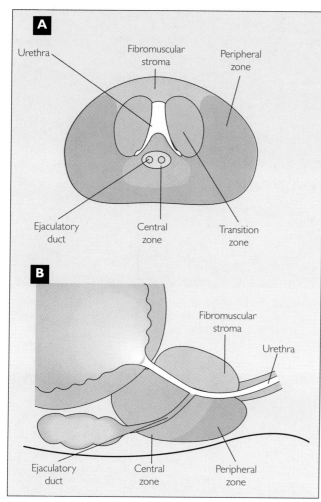

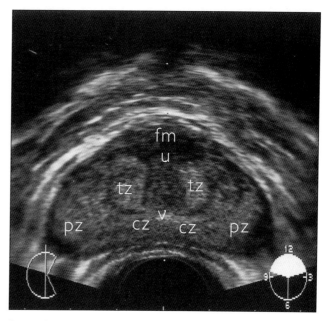

Figure 9.5 Transverse section at mid-gland. The transition zone (tz) is visible on both sides of the urethra. The verumontanum (v) is seen as an inverted V-shaped structure. The peripheral zone (pz) is the area with fine homogeneous echogenicity surrounding the transition zone. The central zone (cz) is the area surrounding the ejaculatory duct complex; however, it is not differentiated from the peripheral zone sonographically. The fibromuscular stroma (fm) is seen anterior to the urethra (u)

Figure 9.4 Zonal anatomy of the prostate gland. (A) Transverse view and (B) sagittal view at the mid-gland. The transition zone lies on both sides of the urethra. The central zone surrounds the ejaculatory duct complex. The peripheral zone extends from the apex of the gland to the posterior and lateral aspect of the central and transition zones. The fibromuscular stroma lies anterior to the urethra at the base

NORMAL PROSTATE

Transverse Plane

At the prostatic apex (below the verumontanum), the echogenic, relatively homogeneous peripheral zone surrounds the posterolateral aspect of the urethra. Above the verumontanum, the transition zone begins to be visualized as a relatively coarse area of lower echogenicity on both sides of the urethra. In the middle of the gland, the verumontanum is often seen as an inverted V-shaped structure (Figure 9.5). The ejaculatory duct complex (composed of the paired ejaculatory ducts and sometimes the utricle surrounded by a fibrous tissue layer) is seen in the mid-line posterior to the urethra as a small hypoechoic area. The peripheral and central zones are not clearly differentiated from each other on ultrasonography and are seen as a relatively fine, homogeneous, echogenic

area, surrounding the transition zone and the urethra. At the base of the gland, the fibromuscular stroma is seen as an area of very low echogenicity anterior to the urethra. The rest of the tissue surrounding the urethra is primarily the central zone, which exhibits relatively homogeneous, fine echogenicity.

The neurovascular bundle is seen at the posterolateral aspect of the gland on both sides. Anteriorly, the dorsal vein complex and Santorini's venous plexus are seen as anechoic fluid-filled structures. The vascular pedicle of the prostate is seen between the seminal vesicle and the base of the gland. Further outside, the levator ani, obturator internus, and pubic bone are seen. Posterior to the prostate are the adventitia and muscularis propria of the rectum. The ampullae of the vasa deferentia are seen behind the bladder trigone as two round hypoechoic structures. The seminal vesicles extend posterolaterally from the ampullae.

Sagittal Plane

In the mid-line image, the bladder neck, prostatic urethra, ejaculatory duct complex, and membranous urethra are visible. The tissue between the urethra and the ejaculatory duct complex is the central zone; the hypoechoic tissue anterior to the urethra is the anterior fibromuscular stroma; and the remainder of the tissue is the peripheral zone (Figure 9.6). In the mid-line image, the transition zone is not

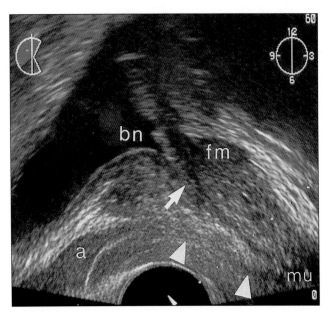

Figure 9.6 Longitudinal section of the normal prostate in the midline. The bladder neck (bn) and surrounding fibromuscular stroma (fm) are seen. The prostatic urethra and periurethral sphincter are seen as a parallel linear structure (arrow). The ejaculatory duct complex (arrowheads) is seen as a continuation of the ampullae (a). The membranous urethra (mu) is seen distal to the apex

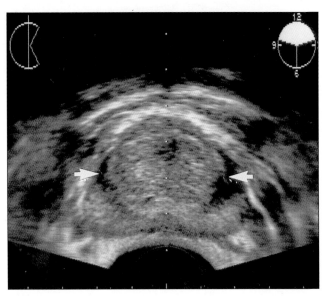

Figure 9.7 Transverse section of a gland with BPH. A hypoechoic fibrous tissue layer (arrows) separates the transition zone from the central and peripheral zones

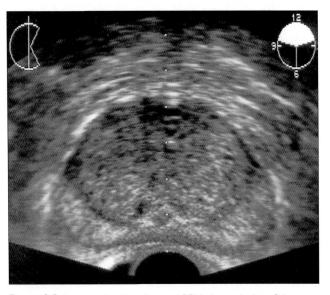

Figure 9.8 In a gland with advanced BPH, the majority of the gland is composed of transition zone. The peripheral and central zones are compressed to a thin layer posterolaterally

seen. At slightly off mid-line, the sagittal image shows the transition zone surrounded by the peripheral and central zones. Further laterally the sagittal section shows only the peripheral and central zones. The bladder trigone muscle and the ureteral orifices are often appreciated on this view.

At the apex, the dorsal vein complex is seen anterior to the membranous urethra. The corpus spongiosum is seen as a structure of low echogenicity, caudal to the apex of the prostate. The membranous urethra originates at the apex and enters the corpus spongiosum to become the bulbar urethra. The shape of the apex varies significantly among individuals: in some, apical tissue extends behind the membranous urethra; in others, the urethra runs behind the apical tissue.

ANATOMICAL CHANGES WITH BENIGN PROSTATIC HYPERPLASIA

TRANSVERSE VIEW

The anatomy of the prostate gland is usually altered significantly by various conditions associated with aging. The patient population for TRUS usually consists of elderly men whose prostates are rarely normal but are often enlarged or atrophied, containing calcifications or cystic degeneration. In a prostate with BPH, the transition zone is enlarged and the fibrous tissue dividing it from the peripheral zone is often clearly seen as a hypoechoic layer (Figure 9.7). In a large prostate with advanced BPH, the peripheral and central zones are compressed posterolaterally and become very thin (Figure 9.8). The transition zone is generally heterogeneous as it contains adenomas of varying

echogenicity and also appears coarser than the peripheral zone. The urethra, which is compressed bilaterally by the hypertrophied transition zone and elongated anteroposteriorly, is not readily delineated in either the transverse or the longitudinal view because of refraction artifacts created by the "kissing" transition zone in the mid-line (Figure 9.9). Occasionally, however, urine trapped around the verumontanum will delineate it. At the apex, the transition zone may no longer be seen and the peripheral zone and the urethra may be the sole structures visualized on TRUS. At the base,

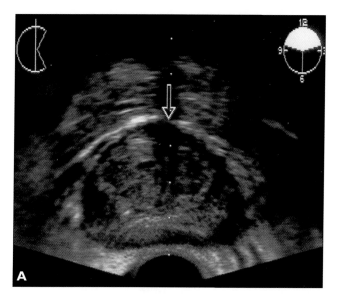

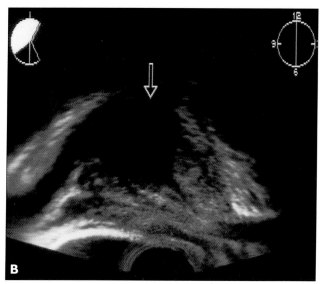

Figure 9.9 (A) In a gland with an enlarged transition zone, sound waves traversing the edge of the zone are reflected, creating an edge artifact that shadows the urethra in the mid-line (arrow). (B) On sagittal view, the urethra is shadowed at the base for the same reason

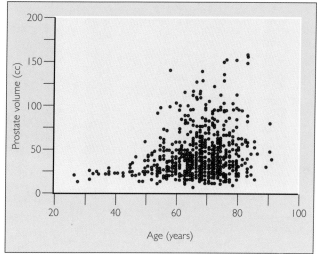

Figure 9.10 Prostate gland volume distribution as a function of age in 300 consecutive cases of TRUS. Individual gland size begins to vary after age 40

the transition zone dominates the gland and often protrudes into the bladder lumen.

PROSTATE VOLUME MEASUREMENT BY TRANSRECTAL ULTRASONOGRAPHY

Treatment decisions are often based on the severity of symptoms. Although prostate size does not correlate significantly with symptom severity or urinary flow rate,[5] men with an enlarged prostate have a higher risk of developing moderate-to-severe symptoms.[6] Digital examination is known to underestimate prostate size, especially if the gland is large.[7] Moreover, accurate prostate volume measurement is important for assessing treatment outcome and for selecting appropriate surgical treatment, such as microwave therapy, needle ablation, laser surgery, transurethral resection, or open prostatectomy.

Normal prostate volume is considered to be approximately 25–30 cm[3]. Individual differences are not significantly observed before age 40; thereafter, the size range widens, with some prostates beginning to increase significantly while others atrophy (Figure 9.10).

PLANIMETRIC METHOD

The first method described for prostate volume measurement was the planimetric technique with serial step-sectioning.[8] With this method, serial transverse images are obtained at 5-mm intervals from the base to the apex. The prostate boundary of each image is traced with a planimeter to calculate cross-sectional area, and the prostate volume is approximated by summing-up disks of each cross-sectional area with an 0.5-cm thickness (Figure 9.11). This method requires a device to move the TRUS probe accurately every 5 mm, and the patient must remain completely still. Because prostate movement longitudinally is quite significant during the procedure, the risk of error is high. The method is theoretically accurate, but in practice often lacks reproducibility and is time consuming.

PROLATED ELLIPSOID METHOD

Because of the limitations of the planimetric technique, the prolated ellipsoid method is now commonly used for prostate volume measurement.[9] This is generally easier and prostate movement is not a consideration. With this method, the prostate gland is approximated to a prolated ellipsoid body with the same width, height, and length (Figure 9.12). Prostate volume is calculated according to the following formula:

$$V = A \times B \times C \times \pi/6 \text{ (about 0.52)}$$

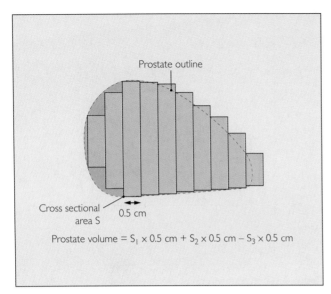

Figure 9.11 Planimetric volume measurement with step-sectioning. The prostate gland volume is approximated by summing up 0.5-cm-thick columns from each cross-sectional area of the gland

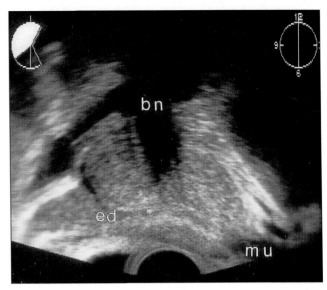

Figure 9.13 Sagittal section on the true mid-line should show three anatomical land marks: the membranous urethra (mu), ejaculatory duct (ed), and bladder neck (bn)

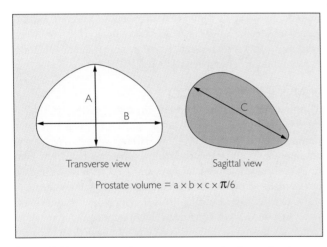

Figure 9.12 Prostate volume measurement by the prolated ellipsoid method. Three dimensions of the gland are measured, and the volume is calculated on the screen

view is not accurately perpendicular to the sagittal view plane (Figure 9.14).

In a model, in-vitro TRUS volume measurement by the prolated ellipsoid method reportedly neither over- nor underestimated gland size.[9]

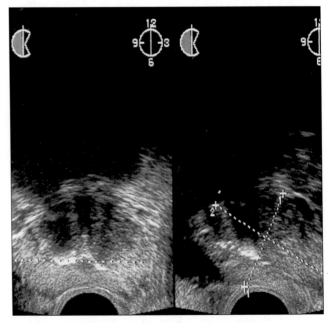

Figure 9.14 Prolated ellipsoid volume measurement with an end-firing probe. The anteroposterior diameter (height) is measured on the sagittal instead of the transverse view because the measurement may be exaggerated on the oblique transverse section obtained by this type of probe

where A is the transverse diameter, B is the anteroposterior diameter, and C is the superior–inferior diameter.

Transverse diameter (width) and anteroposterior diameter (height) are measured on the largest transverse section of the prostate. To measure the superior–inferior diameter (length) accurately, the mid-line sagittal section should be obtained. In this image, three landmarks – the membranous urethra, bladder neck, and ejaculatory duct – should be seen (Figure 9.13). If an endfiring probe is used, the height should be measured on the sagittal view, as the transverse

In the figure (Figure 9.11):

Prostate outline

Cross sectional area S   0.5 cm

Prostate volume = $S_1 \times 0.5$ cm + $S_2 \times 0.5$ cm − $S_3 \times 0.5$ cm

In the figure (Figure 9.12):

A

B

C

Transverse view   Sagittal view

Prostate volume = $a \times b \times c \times \pi/6$

Prolated ellipsoid measurement alternative

The superior–inferior diameter measurement can be technically difficult because the boundaries at the apex and base may not be clearly seen simultaneously. In this case, a formula of $V = A^2 \times B \times \pi/6$ can be used to estimate the volume.[10] As the transverse diameter (A) and length of the prostate (C) are often similar, this approximation can be close to the prolated ellipsoid method, although it often overestimates gland size.[9] Another, newer method with biplane planimetry has been reported.[11]

TRANSITION ZONE MEASUREMENT

Transition zone size can be estimated with the prolated ellipsoid method. On the transverse image, the width and height are measured at the level where the transition zone appears largest. On the sagittal view, the transition zone is not seen on the mid-line section and should be imaged slightly off the mid-line, where the length should then be measured (Figure 9.15). Transition zone volume is generally about 20 cm³ less than total prostate volume. However, significant transition zone hyperplasia may be seen in the normal-size prostate and, conversely, minimal hyperplasia may be seen in a 50-cm³ gland (Figure 9.16).

TRANSITION ZONE INDEX

As the transition zone is the zone most greatly affected, the ratio between transition zone volume and total prostate volume (TZ index) may correlate more significantly with symptoms than does prostate volume alone. This TZ index was found to be a significant factor in predicting improvement of flow rate after finasteride therapy.[12] It was also found to correlate with the risk of developing acute urinary retention.[13] However, other studies have reported that the TZ index added little to the evaluation of the BPH patient.[14, 15]

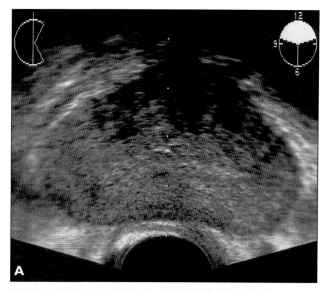

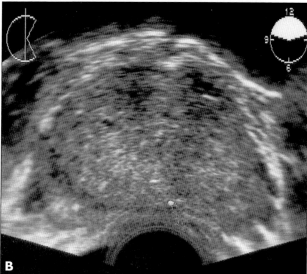

Figure 9.16 In (A), a 35-cm³ prostate gland, transition zone hyperplasia is minimal. In (B), a 36-cm³ prostate, the transition zone is significantly enlarged even though gland volume is about same as in (A)

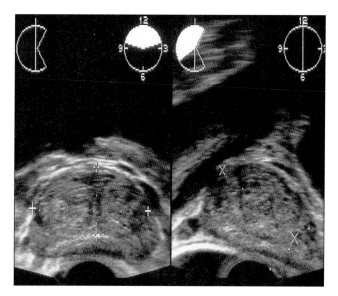

Figure 9.15 Transition zone volume measurement by the prolated ellipsoid method. The length of the zone is measured on the off-mid-line sagittal section

PRESUMED CIRCLE AREA RATIO

As the prostate enlarges, the gland shape more closely resembles a globe. The cross-sectional image is therefore closer to a circle. This roundness of the cross-sectional area, which may be related to intraprostatic pressure rather than to prostate size, is expressed by the presumed circle area ratio (PCAR). The PCAR is calculated as the ratio between the largest cross-sectional area of the gland and the smallest imaginary circle in which the section fits (Figure 9.17). One study showed that PCAR was more significantly correlated with urodynamic parameters than prostate size, transition zone size, or TZ index.[16]

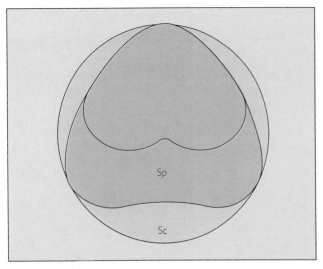

Figure 9.17 Presumed circle area ratio is calculated as the ratio between the largest cross-sectional area of the gland (Sp) and the area of a presumed circle that will include the cross-section (Sc)

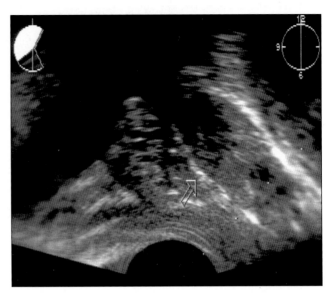

Figure 9.19 Calcifications along the floor of the urethra (arrow) delineating its course on the mid-line sagittal view

CONDITIONS ASSOCIATED WITH BENIGN PROSTATIC HYPERPLASIA

In the gland with BPH, not only is transition zone enlargement present but other conditions are frequently associated. Most common is calcification, usually at the posterior aspect of the transition zone. This is caused by a small calcified body in the terminal portion of the prostatic ducts. The shape is usually arcuate linear (Figure 9.18). Linear calcifications are also seen on the floor of the urethra, delineating its course in the longitudinal view (Figure 9.19). Sometimes diffuse calcifications are seen in the peripheral zone, suggesting a history of prostatic

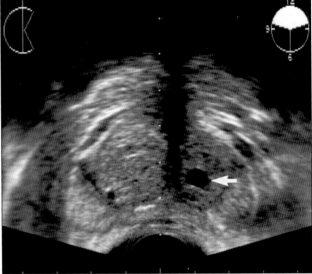

Figure 9.20 A small degenerative cyst is seen in the transition zone (arrow)

infection. Small degenerative cysts are also quite common with BPH (Figure 9.20). When the BPH is advanced, seminal vesicles are often thicker and shorter in the lateral direction, but the cause of this remains unknown.

TYPES OF BENIGN PROSTATIC HYPERPLASIA

ASYMMETRICAL BENIGN PROSTATIC HYPERPLASIA

Although transition zone hyperplasia is usually symmetrical, asymmetry is sometimes seen (Figure 9.21). In

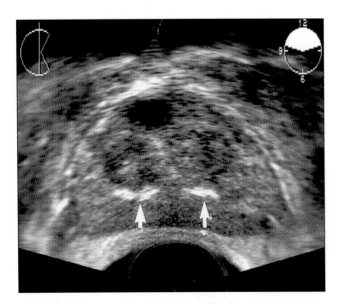

Figure 9.18 Common linear arcuate calcification at the posterior aspect of the transition zone in BPH (arrows)

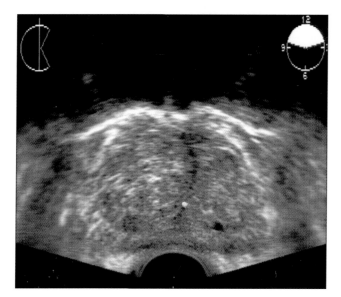

Figure 9.21 Asymmetrical transition zone hyperplasia. The right transition zone is significantly enlarged, pushing the urethra toward the left

extreme cases, one-sided transition zone hyperplasia may be encountered.

MEDIAN LOBE HYPERPLASIA

On cystoscopy, a hump behind the bladder neck characterizes median lobe hyperplasia. This tissue is completely separate from the transition zone and is considered to arise from the glandular tissue at the bladder neck under the trigone. On TRUS, this hyperplasia is seen as the round

prostatic tissue protruding into the bladder lumen from the posterior aspect of the bladder neck (Figure 9.22). Sometimes median lobe hyperplasia is as large as the body of the prostate, and the gland assumes an hour-glass shape. Transition zone hyperplasia can protrude into the bladder lumen, but this condition is distinct from median lobe hyperplasia.

EXOPHYTIC HYPERPLASIA

At the base of the prostate, a small hyperplastic nodule, often containing multiple cysts, is sometimes seen. This nodule protrudes exophytically from the prostate base and extends behind the bladder neck or between the seminal vesicles. It sometimes distorts the seminal vesicle configuration and is misdiagnosed as a malignancy (Figure 9.23). Because of the location of this exophytic adenoma, it

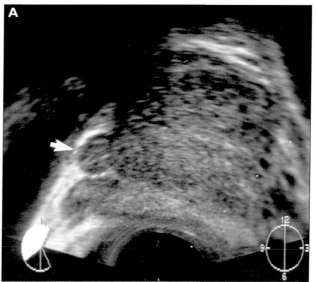

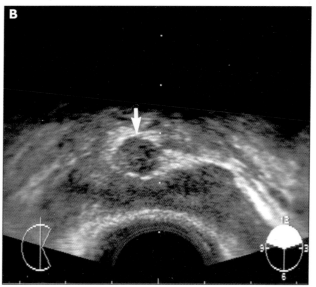

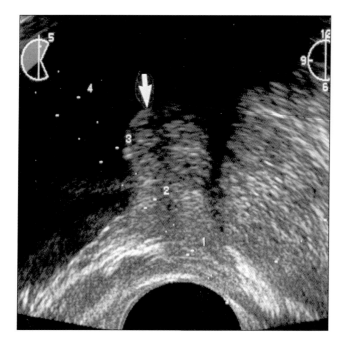

Figure 9.22 Median lobe hyperplasia protruding into the bladder lumen (arrow). Numbers 1–5 represent centimeter markings to measure the size of the median lobe

Figure 9.23 On sagittal section (A), an exophytic adenoma is seen protruding from the base of the gland (arrow). On the transverse view (B), the adenoma extends between the bladder neck and seminal vesicle, compressing the latter (arrow)

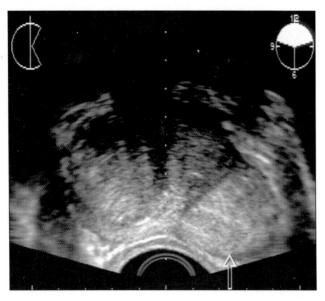

Figure 9.24 A hyperplastic adenoma is seen in the left peripheral zone protruding from the base of the prostate gland

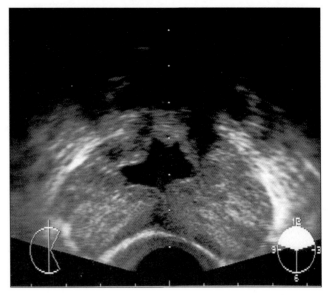

Figure 9.25 After open prostatectomy, a large defect is seen in the prostate gland

rarely causes bladder outlet obstruction. In very rare cases, a hyperplastic adenoma is seen in the peripheral zone that protrudes from the gland laterally or posteriorly (Figure 9.24).

CHANGES ON TRANSURETHRAL SONOGRAPHY AFTER SURGICAL TREATMENT

AFTER OPEN PROSTATECTOMY

Simple open prostatectomy removes all the hypertrophied transition zone from the prostate, and the TRUS image will often show a large defect in the middle of the gland (Figure 9.25).

AFTER TRANSURETHRAL RESECTION

After transurethral resection of the prostate (TURP), a common finding is a tissue defect in the middle of the prostate, especially at the bladder neck level. With extensive TURP, the transition zone can be completely resected, leaving a large defect from the bladder neck to the verumontanum, although in most cases residual transition zone is seen in the prostate (Figure 9.26). The tissue defect after TURP gradually decreases over time, and an area of extravasation can be seen on TRUS as a calcified line long after TURP. Narrowing of the defect at the bladder neck in a patient with urinary obstructive symptoms suggests bladder-neck contracture. Retrograde injection of saline from the external meatus during TRUS delineates this condition well.

AFTER LASER ABLATION

In the early postoperative stage, laser ablation often leaves a small defect surrounded by tissue with multiple cystic changes. The finding suggests ablated necrotic tissue in the prostatic urethra.[17]

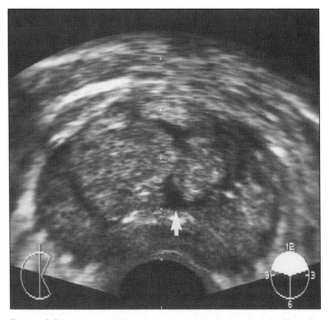

Figure 9.26 After TURP, a tissue defect is seen in the middle of the gland (arrow) on transverse section. Residual transition zone is seen in both lobes

CHANGES ON TRANSURETHRAL SONOGRAPHY AFTER MEDICAL TREATMENT

A number of studies have been published regarding changes in prostate volume after hormonal manipulation for BPH. The commonly used 5α-reductase inhibitor, finasteride,

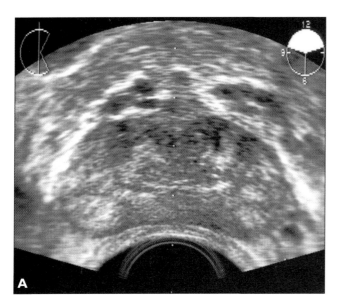
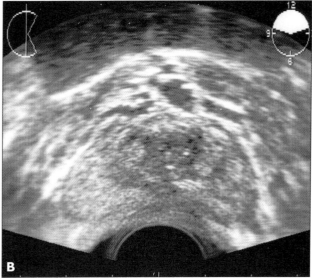

Figure 9.27 Transverse section of a BPH gland before and after hormone therapy. (A) BPH before administration of luteinizing-hormone-releasing hormone (LHRH) agonist. (B) Three months after LHRH treatment, the gland is significantly smaller (35% volume reduction)

showed an average 19% volume reduction in 12 months.[18] The antitestosterone, flutamide, showed a 23% volume reduction in 3 months.[19] A more potent testosterone inhibitor, gonadotropin-releasing hormone (GnRH) agonist,

has been used for BPH and showed a greater volume reduction ranging from 25% to 51% within 3–4 months of administration (Figure 9.27).[20–22] No data are available regarding specific zonal decreases after medical treatment for BPH.

REFERENCES

1 Watanabe H, Kato H, Kato T *et al*. Diagnostic application of ultrasonotomography to the prostate. *Jpn J Urol* 1968; **59**: 273–9.

2 McNeal JE. Regional morphology and pathology of the prostate. *Am J Clin Pathol* 1968; **49**: 347–57.

3 McNeal JE. The prostate and prostatic urethra: a morphologic study. *J Urol* 1972; **107**: 1008–16.

4 McNeal JE. Origin and evolution of benign prostatic enlargement. *Invest Urol* 1978; **15**: 340–5.

5 Barry MJ, Cockett AT, Holtgrewe HL *et al*. Relationship of symptoms of prostatism to commonly used physiological and anatomical measures of the severity of benign prostatic hyperplasia. *J Urol* 1993; **150**(2 Pt 1): 351–8.

6 Girman CJ, Jacobsen SJ, Guess HA *et al*. Natural history of prostatism: relationship among symptoms, prostate. volume and peak urinary flow rate. *J Urol* 1995; **153**: 1510–15.

7 Roehrbon CG, Girman CJ, Rhodes T *et al*. Correlation between prostate size estimated by digital rectal examination and measured by transrectal ultrasound. *Urology* 1997; **49**: 548–57.

8 Watanabe H, Igari D, Tanahashi Y, Harada K, Saito M. Measurement of size and weight of prostate by means of transrectal ultrasonotomography. *Tohoku J Exp Med* 1974; **114**: 277–85.

9 Littrup PJ, Williams CR, Egglin TK, Kane RA. Determination of prostate volume with transrectal US for cancer screening. Part II. Accuracy of in vitro and in vivo techniques. *Radiology* 1991; **52**: 49–53.

10 Terris MK, Stamey TA. Determination of prostate volume by transrectal ultrasound. *J Urol* 1991; **145**: 984–7.

11 Kimura A, Kurooka Y, Kitamura T, Kawabe K. Biplane planimetry as a new method for prostatic volume calculation in transrectal ultrasonography. *Int J Urol* 1997; **4**: 152–6.

12 Tewari A, Shinohara K, Narayan P. Transition zone volume and transition zone ratio: predictor of uroflow response to finasteride therapy in benign prostatic hyperplasia patients. *Urology* 1995; **45**: 258–64.

13 Kurita Y, Masuda H, Terada H *et al*. Transition zone index as a risk factor for acute urinary retention in benign prostatic hyperplasia. *Urology* 1998; **51**: 595–600.

14 Witjes WP, Aarnink RG, Ezz-el-Din K *et al*. The correlation between prostate volume, transition zone volume, transition zone index and clinical and urodynamic investigations in patients with lower urinary tract symptoms. *Br J Urol* 1997; **80**: 84–90.

15 Lepor H, Nieder A, Feser J, O'Connell C, Dixon C. Total prostate and transition zone volumes, and transition zone index are poorly correlated with objective measures of clinical benign prostatic hyperplasia. *J Urol* 1997; **158**: 85–8.

16 Kojima M, Ochiai A, Naya Y *et al*. Correlation of presumed circle area ratio with infravesical obstruction in men with lower urinary tract symptoms. *Urology* 1997; **50**: 548–55.

17 Narayan P, Leidich R, Fournier G *et al*. Transurethral evaporation of prostate (TUEP) with ND:YAG laser using a contact free beam technique: Results in 61 patients with benign prostate hyperplasia. *Urology* 1994; **43**: 813–20.

18 Gormley GJ, Stoner E, Bruskewitz RC *et al*. The effect of finasteride in men with benign prostatic hyperplasia. The Finasteride Study Group. *N Engl J Med* 1992; **327**: 1185–91.

19 Stone NN. Flutamide in treatment of benign prostatic hypertrophy. *Urology* 1989; **34**(4 Suppl): 64–8.

20 Eri LM, Tveter KJ. A prospective, placebo-controlled study of the luteinizing hormone-releasing hormone agonist leuprolide as treatment for patients with benign prostatic hyperplasia. *J Urol* 1993; **150**(2 Pt 1): 359–64.

21 Peters CA, Walsh PC. The effect of nafarelin acetate, a luteinizing-hormone-releasing hormone agonist, on benign prostatic hyperplasia. *N Engl J Med* 1987; **317**: 599–604.

22 Lukkarinen O. Effect of LH–RH analogue in patients with benign prostatic hyperplasia. *Urology* 1991; **37**: 92–4.

COMMENTARY

In this chapter, Dr Shinohara, who is a pioneer in TRUS assessment for prostatic disease, discusses the instrumentation and findings on TRUS-based anatomy of normal and abnormal prostates.

The use of TRUS has truly revolutionized the study of prostatic anatomy. Owing to the extensive experience gained over the last 30 years, TRUS-based anatomy of the normal and abnormal prostate is now clear, understandable, and useful for management of a variety of prostatic diseases.

For TRUS measurements, most urologists use a 5- or 7.5-MHz transducer with a biplane or endfiring probe. There are differences between each probe and, based on this, the images will vary slightly, and so the urologist should be familiar with these differences. However, both transducers provide reasonable measurements and except for very large prostates can provide most of the information necessary for assessment. For BPH, the TRUS is often unnecessary and the AHCPR guidelines do not recommend it as part of the work up for BPH (See Chapter 7 "AHCPR (US) Guidelines for the Diagnosis and Treatment of Benign Prostatic Hyperplasia"). However, a TRUS measurement is useful for properly biopsying patients who present with elevated PSA or prostatic nodules, for detecting median lobe hyperplasia, for assessing prostatic volume, and for determining rare abnormalities such as seminal vesicle cysts or other pathologies.

TRUS is unable to differentiate stromal from epithelial hyperplasia. TRUS, however, can be used as a guide to rule out BPH as a cause of lower urinary tract symptoms (LUTS) by noting lack of an enlarged prostate or a significant median lobe. Most urologists, however, prefer a cystoscopy to TRUS to assess median lobe or prostate size. A preoperative TRUS is mandatory for procedures such as the TUNA for determining the length of the needle to be placed in each lobe for treatment.

The reliability of TRUS-measured volume has been determined by several studies. In our own study, we found that TRUS-based volume estimation is reasonably accurate. We compared volumes determined by TRUS with magnetic resonance imaging (MRI) and TRUS-estimated weights with surgical specimen weights. We noted that TRUS and MRI measurement of prostate volumes were quite similar, and TRUS underestimated the prostate weight by 10% against a gold standard of prostatic weight as determined from the surgical specimens. We suggest multiplying the TRUS measurement by a factor of 1.10 to measure the prostatic volume correctly. We conclude that, since TRUS is inexpensive, user-friendly, non-invasive, and equally as accurate as MRI, it should be the preferred modality instead of MRI when an imaging study is desired in the evaluation and follow up of BPH.[1]

In a prior study we also evaluated the role of zonal prostatic volume estimation in prediction of response to finasteride therapy in another study. Twenty-three patients with symptomatic BPH who were treated with finasteride (5 mg day^{-1}) for 12 months underwent TRUS evaluation of total and transition zone (TZ) volume of prostate, as well as measurement of peak flow rate, and modified Boyarsky symptom score which was determined at baseline and 12 months. Statistical analysis was done by unpaired t, Mann–Whitney, and Spearman rank correlation tests among responders (more than 3 cm^3 s^{-1} improvement in peak flow rate) and non-responders (less than 3 cm^3 s^{-1} improvement in peak flow rate) to therapy. Responders had substantial reduction in TZ volume (44.8% vs. 16.05%; $P<0.03$) and TZ ratio (25% vs. 5% increase, $P<0.02$) compared with non-responders. Secondly, there was a significant correlation between reduction in TZ volume ($r=0.50$; $P<0.03$) and TZ ratio ($r=0.60$; $P<0.006$) with improvement in peak flow rates. No similar correlation was seen with total prostate volume changes. Finally, pretreatment TZ ratio helped in predicting peak-flow improvement following finasteride therapy ($r=0.52$; $P<0.01$) and there was a 2.5-fold increased chance of improvement if baseline TZ ratio was more than 0.51. The modified Boyarsky symptom score decreased by 3.1 (mean), but there was no correlation with changes in peak urinary flow rate, total prostate volume, TZ volume, and TZ ratio. TZ ratio did not have significant predictive value for improvement in symptom score. Results of this study suggested that prostatic zonal volume may be used prior to therapy to predict uroflow response to finasteride and similar agents.[2]

Boyle and associates evaluated the predictive value of prostatic volume measurement in patients receiving finasteride in six randomized clinical trials comparing 5 mg finasteride with placebo in the treatment of (BPH).[3]

The findings for the 2601 men in these trials provide an opportunity to investigate the heterogeneity of the effects seen in the individual studies and to identify pretreatment predictors of outcomes as expressed by symptoms or peak urinary flow rates. A formal meta-analysis using an Empirical Bayes approach employed data from all finasteride studies, which included the Phase III trials in North America and internationally, the Prospect, Early Intervention, and SCARP trials, and the Veterans Administration Cooperative Study, which compared terazosin, finasteride, and the combination of these two drugs. A pooled analysis was also undertaken on the combined dataset.

Results revealed that the effect of finasteride treatment on improvements in total symptom severity, frequency score, and peak urinary flow rate was consistent across all six trials and similar among men with similar prostate volumes at baseline. Symptom severity improved by 1.8 points (95% confidence interval (CI), 0.7–2.9) in men with prostate volumes of less than 20 cm^3 ($n=72$), while the improvement was 2.8 points (95% CI, 2.1–3.5) for men with volumes greater than 60 cm^3 ($n=272$) on the Quasi-IPSS Scale (range 0–30). Similarly, improvements in peak urinary flow rate ranged from 0.89 mL s^{-1} (95% CI, –0.05–1.83) for men with prostate volumes less than 20 cm^3 to 1.84 mL s^{-1} (95% CI, 1.37–2.30) in men with volumes greater than 60 cm^3. The difference in the magnitude of improvement between finasteride and placebo becomes significant (that is, no over-lap in 95% CI) for men with a baseline prostate volume assessed by either TRUS or MRI of greater than 40 cm³, which encompasses approximately 50% of the entire population. Baseline prostate volume was a key predictor of treatment outcomes: approximately 80% of the variation in the treatment effects noted between studies could be attributed to differences in mean prostate volumes at baseline. Variation in entry criteria results in large differences in baseline symptom severity status, prostate volume, and, consequently, apparent inconsistencies in the overall outcomes of these trials. This meta-analysis suggested that finasteride is most effective in men with large prostates.

Recently, some authors have also evaluated TRUS findings with urodynamic parameters. Witjes and associates attempted to determine whether, in patients with LUTS, measurement of the TZ of the prostate by TRUS and the ratio between the TZ volume and total prostate volume (TZ index) correlates better with clinical and urodynamic investigations than total prostate volume alone. One hundred and fifty consecutive patients with LUTS underwent a standardized screening program, including the International Prostate Symptom Score (IPSS), a physical examination, TRUS of the prostate, and urodynamic investigations with pressure-flow studies. The total prostate volume and TZ volume were assessed from TRUS, using the ellipsoid formula. Spearman's rank correlation coefficients were calculated between different prostate volume measurements and specific symptomatic and urodynamic variables. The relationships between specific IPSS symptoms, symptom scores, and the prostate volume measurements were not statistically significant except for one domain, nocturia, which appeared to be statistically significantly correlated with the TZ index ($r=0.25$). The correlations for free flow, pressure-flow variables, and prostate volume measurements were stronger, but only moderate at best. The highest correlations were between TZ volume and the linear passive urethral resistance obstruction category, urethral resistance factor, and detrusor pressure at maximum flow ($r=0.43$, 0.44, and 0.40, respectively). The differences between the correlations of prostate volume and TZ index and these variables were small ($r=0.39$, 0.38, and 0.37, respectively, for prostate volume, and $r=0.38$, 0.40, and 0.33, respectively, for TZ index). There were very small differences between the correlations of total prostate volume, TZ volume, and TZ index, and clinical and pressure-flow variables.[4]

All these studies in total suggest that TRUS may have a greater role in evaluation of BPH than heretofore believed. However, the role of TRUS in initial evaluation of BPH is still complementary to other assessments, such as symptom score and uroflow.

1 Tewari A, Indudhara R, Shinohara K *et al*. Comparison of transrectal ultrasound prostatic volume estimation with magnetic resonance imaging volume estimation and surgical specimen weight in patients with benign prostatic hyperplasia. *J Clin Ultrasound* 1996; **24**(4): 169–74.

2 Tewari A, Shinohara K, Narayan P. Transition zone volume and transition zone ratio: predictor of uroflow response to finasteride therapy in benign prostatic hyperplasia patients. *Urology* 1995, **45**(2): 258–64.

3 Boyle P, Gould AL, Roehrborn CG. Prostate volume predicts outcome of treatment of benign prostatic hyperplasia with finasteride: meta-analysis of randomized clinical trials. *Urology* 1996; **48**(3): 398–405.

4 Witjes WP, Aarnink RG, Ezz-el-Din K *et al*. The correlation between prostate volume, transition zone volume, transition zone index and clinical and urodynamic investigations in patients with lower urinary tract symptoms. *Br J Urol* 1997; **80**(1): 84–90.

Prostatic Obstruction and Effects on the Urinary Tract

10

M. Patel, A. Tewari, and J. Furman

INTRODUCTION

Bladder outlet obstruction in the male as a result of prostate disease can be due to inflammation, hyperplasia, or malignancy; of this, benign prostatic hyperplasia (BPH) is one of the most common urologic disorders afflicting the elderly male. The prevalence is greater than 50% among men over the age of 60 years and reaches approximately 90% at the age of 85 years; the mortality rate directly attributable to the obstruction produced by BPH is estimated at only 1.8 per 100,000.[1] The diagnosis and treatment of BPH relies heavily on the presenting symptoms and clinical findings. Unfortunately, these clinical findings correlate poorly with the severity of bladder outlet obstruction, and in some reports, it has been estimated that 25% of patients referred for urinary outlet obstruction due to prostate disease present with no obstructive symptoms.[2,3] Furthermore, there are patients with severe prostatic hyperplasia and urinary obstruction who present with renal insufficiency without any symptoms of prostatic obstruction.[4,5]

The majority of the patients with bladder outlet obstruction due to prostatic disease do present with a constellation of voiding symptoms referred to as "prostatism," which includes symptoms of irritative and obstructive voiding. The irritative symptoms consist of frequency, nocturia, urgency, and urge incontinence; these presenting signs may be due to a decrease in effective bladder volume, to elevated residual volume with urinary stasis, or to local irritation factors, possibly caused by the growing prostatic adenoma. The nocturia symptom has been postulated to be caused by a reversal in the circadian rhythm of urine production seen in elderly men, some of whom may excrete as much as two-thirds of their daily urine volume at night.[6] The symptoms of obstruction include decreased force of stream, intermittent urinary flow, difficulty in initiating the urine stream, straining upon urination, prolonged urination, postvoidal dripping, and a sensation of incomplete bladder emptying with urinary retention. Once again, these obstructive symptoms are not absolute; it has been shown that only 20% of patients with BPH will experience urinary retention.[7] Another presenting sign is gross hematuria; if present in men over the age of 60 years, it is most commonly due to BPH. It is believed that the blood originates from the dilated veins in the prostatic urethra caused by compression from the enlarging

adenoma. However, this assumption should not be made, and a thorough work-up should be done, especially for malignancy. It should be noted that these symptoms of irritative and obstructive patterns are not diagnostic for prostatism; they are present in cases of urinary/bladder infection, bladder malignancy, neurogenic voiding dysfunction, impaired detrusor contractility, detrusor instability, and sensory urgency.

Numerous studies[8-10] have shown that the symptoms of prostatism can fluctuate considerably over the course of time. In addition, Ball and associates have shown that these symptoms not only stabilize, but also substantially improve over time without any pharmacological or surgical intervention. This has lead to a variation in diagnostic and treatment options in the management of BPH amongst urologists throughout the country. The indications for treatment to relieve infravesical obstruction are not straightforward except in patients with complications such as upper urinary tract obstruction/dilatation, detrusor decompensation, urinary retention, recurrent infection, bleeding, and stones.[11] Fortunately, the Agency for Health Care Policy and Research (AHCPR) established guidelines in 1994 for the initial evaluation of all patients presenting with prostatism.[1] It recommends that the initial evaluation should include a detailed history, American Urological Association (AUA) Symptom Index, physical examination with DRE, and a focused neurologic exam, urinalysis, and creatinine serum levels in all patients. Although routine screening for prostate-specific antigen (PSA) remains controversial, the AHCPR has included the test as optional, along with uroflow studies. Any other urodynamic tests or imaging studies are optional on the basis of the findings of the initial evaluation. An elevated serum creatinine level warrants upper tract imaging. Pressure-flow studies are necessary if the patient's history and physical exam are suggestive of a primary bladder disorder. High residual urine volumes (>30% of bladder volume) suggest altered bladder contractility and warrants a pressure-flow study. High bladder pressures with low urinary flow rates are diagnostic of obstruction; whereas, low pressures and flows indicate poor bladder contractility. These tests and several others that are not recommended by the AHCPR as routine exams upon initial evaluation of a patient are discussed herein.

Most BPH patients with bladder outlet obstruction without symptoms do not require treatment. Patients who do present with "prostatism" symptoms (obstructive or irritative) should be encouraged to participate in various treatment options. These options vary from non-invasive treatment such as medical management with α-blockers to highly invasive treatment of surgical intervention. Patient preference for the less invasive alternatives, increasing patient awareness of BPH, and an increasing range of available treatments is likely to add momentum to this shift from highly invasive surgical therapy to minimally (or non-) invasive medical management. These various treatments are discussed in other chapters.

Watchful waiting is a good conservative approach to the treatment of BPH, but should not be overly used. Watchful waiting is appropriate in patients with minimal symptoms, but periodic re-evaluations are necessary to ensure that prostatic disease progression does not occur. Watchful waiting in some patients with BPH may result in complications such as overflow incontinence, bladder decompensation and obstructive uropathy that may advance to chronic renal failure, urinary tract infection, or bladder stones. As the prostate enlarges and narrows the lumen of the prostatic urethra, this increase in bladder outlet resistance causes the bladder to respond by increasing its force of contraction to void the urine. By developing this increased intravesical voiding pressure, the bladder is able to maintain flow; this additional work exerted by the muscular bladder wall to overcome the outlet resistance will result in detrusor hypertrophy, hyperplasia, and the deposition of collagen within the bladder wall. The latter results in the thickening of the bladder wall – the wall loses its compliance and its elasticity properties. This loss of compliance causes the intravesical pressures to rise greatly with small changes in volume, leading to a decrease in the functional capacity of the bladder. This, in turn, will lead to the development of detrusor instability and loss of normal control over the reflex detrusor response. Early in the course of obstruction, the bladder is able to compensate; but if untreated for extended periods of time, urge incontinence or possibly hydronephrosis may result. To avoid these unwanted circumstances, watchful waiting should be done under careful consideration and monitored closely in patients with mild BPH symptoms (AUA score ≤ 7).

BPH is the most common form of urinary outlet obstruction in men of elderly age; however, there are other disorders that can cause obstruction at any age. Pelvic lipomatosis, retroperitoneal fibrosis, prostatic carcinoma, foreign body, ureteral stones, chronic prostatitis with fibrosis, bladder neck fibrosis/contracture, urethral strictures (secondary to infection/injury) and meatal stenosis (either acquired (Tb, radiation) or congenital), ureteroceles, lower urinary tract malignancy (of the urethra or bladder neck), local extension of cancer into the bladder base, and fibrosis of the urethral or ureter due to scarring from irradiation are other potential causes of urinary obstruction in the male.

THE PATHOPHYSIOLOGY OF OUTLET OBSTRUCTION

Obstruction to urine flow can occur anywhere within the urinary tract, but is more common at the prostatic urethra location in elderly men. Proximal to the obstruction, pressures within the bladder, collecting system, and renal tubules will rise. Ultimately, renal injury will result because of cellular atrophy and necrosis if the obstruction to urine flow is not relieved within 6 weeks. After this period, irreversible changes will occur, which will eventually lead to renal failure. Acute prostatic obstruction will produce distention of the bladder, ureter, and renal pelvis that is associated with pain. On the other hand, a slow progressing (chronic) obstruction, as found in cases of BPH, will cause massive dilatation of the bladder and the collecting system with or without any associated pain (dull, aching flank discomfort) or clinical symptoms. This so-called "silent" obstruction can lead to hydronephrosis and to renal insufficiency. Elevated hydrostatic pressure in the urethra proximal to the obstruction site will cause urethral dilation with thinning of the wall; this may develop into a diverticulum. Furthermore, urine stasis in this outpouching may get infected, causing pyelonephrosis, sepsis, periurethral abscess, or other localized infection.

In cases of BPH, compression of the urethra causes the bladder to undergo several changes, some of which are irreversible if obstruction is not promptly relieved. During the early stages of obstruction (called the compensation stage), the bladder smooth muscle wall undergoes hypertrophy, and the wall thickens by two to four times its normal size (Figures 10.1A and B and 10.2A and B). This compensation allows the bladder to contract more forcefully to ensure complete emptying of the bladder. However, this hypertrophy does have its price. The hypertrophied muscular wall is usually superimposed with an infection. Microscopic examination of the wall reveals submucosal edema with plasma cell, lymphocyte, and polymorphonuclear (PMN) cell infiltration. Further examination reveals that the inner surface of the bladder wall, which is normally smooth, develops trabeculae. With hypertrophy, the individual smooth muscle bundles of a distended bladder become taut, giving a coarsely interwoven appearance to the mucosal surface. During the compensation stage, the inner surface of the trigonal smooth muscle and the interureteric ridge, which normally are slightly raised above its surrounding tissue, undergoes hypertrophy. The ridge then becomes prominent. This trigone hypertrophy causes increased resistance to urine flow in the intravesical ureteral segments due to the accentuated downward pull on them.[12] This mechanism is believed to be the cause of functional obstruction of the ureterovesical junctions, resulting in elevated pressures that radiate retrogradely to the kidney, causing hydroureteronephrosis. In the presence of significant residual urine volume, there is further stretching of the ureterotrigonal complex, and the obstruction increases. It is recommended that this additional obstruction should be

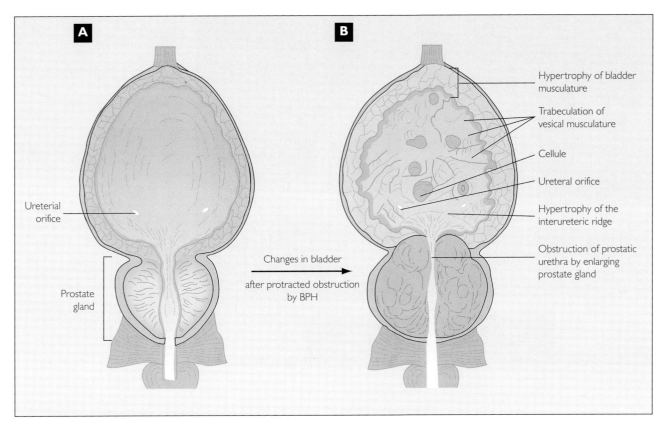

Figure 10.1 Chronic changes in urinary bladder due to protracted obstruction of prostatic urethra

eliminated by either passing a urethral catheter or doing a prostatectomy as early as possible. The latter treatment leads to permanent release of the ureterotrigonal stretch, causing gradual softening of the trigone hypertrophy with relief of the obstruction.[12]

If the prostatic urethra is not opened up to alleviate the elevated bladder pressure, several complications, such as cellules and diverticula, can begin to form. Normal intra-vesical pressure is approximately 30 cm of water at the beginning of micturition. Pressures two to four times as great may be reached by a hypertrophic (trabeculated) bladder during the compensation stage to force urine past the obstruction. This increased pressure tends to push the bladder mucosa between the superficial smooth muscle bundles, causing the formation of small outpouchings called cellules. If these cellules force their way entirely through the musculature of the bladder wall, they become saccules, then eventually diverticula. Diverticula have no muscle wall and are therefore unable to expel their contents into the bladder efficiently even after the obstructed prostatic ure-thra is alleviated. When a superimposed infection occurs in the diverticula, it is difficult to eradicate the infectious organism; thus, surgical intervention to remove the divertic-ula will be needed.[12] If a diverticulum pushes through the bladder wall to impinge on the anterior surface of the ureter, the ureterovesical junction will become incompe-tent, leading to retrograde movement of urine up the ureters to the kidneys. This will present with further complications such as pyelonephritis, sepsis, and/or kidney scarring with renal insufficiency.

In the face of progressive urethral obstruction, possibly aggravated by prostatic infection with edema the detrusor muscle will fail (decompensation stage), result-ing in the presence of residual urine after voiding.[12] The increased thickness of the bladder wall that develops during the compensation stage causes a decrease in compliance of the bladder wall; there is abnormal increase in intravesical pressures for small changes in volume. This loss of compliance leads to a decrease in the functional capacity of the bladder. This, in turn, will lead to the development of detrusor instability and loss of normal control over the reflex detrusor response. Eventually, this leads to decompensation and incomplete emptying of the bladder contents.

THE EFFECTS OF PROSTATIC URETHRAL OBSTRUCTION ON THE UPPER URINARY TRACT

During the early compensation stage, the pressure in the bladder is normal while it fills with urine. This pressure increases upon voiding as the walls of the bladder contract. The pressure is not transmitted to the ureters, renal pelvises, calyces, and kidney because of the ureterovesical valves that prevent the retrograde flow of urine upon bladder contraction. However, in the presence of trigonal

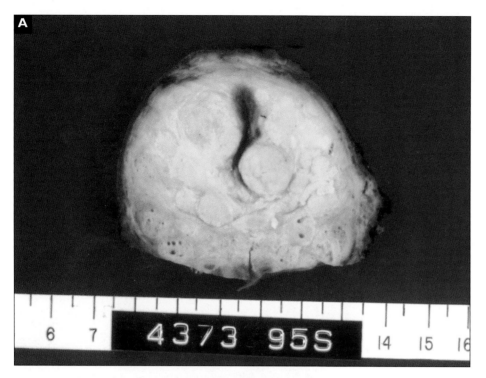

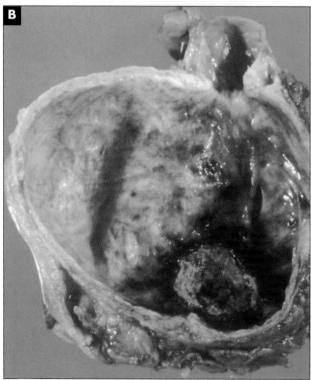

Figure 10.2 (A) Prostate with BPH nodule next to urethra compressing and distorting urethral lumen. (B) Bladder with hypertrophy, trabeculation, and diverticula secondary to BPH

hypertrophy, the increased resistance to urine flow in the intravesical ureteral segments causes a back-pressure on the ureter and kidney, resulting in hydroureteronephrosis (dilatation of the renal pelvis and calyces beyond the normal capacity of 3–10 mL and associated with progressive atrophy of the kidney due to obstruction to the outflow of urine). Figures 10.3A–C and 10.4A–C. Furthermore,

during the decompensation stage in the presence of residual urine, there is an added stretch on the already hypertrophic ureterotrigonal complex. This increased tension in the trigone area increases the resistance to urine flow at the terminal end of the ureter, causing damage to the dilated ureter and kidney. With decompensation of the uretero-trigonal complex, the ureterovesical valve competence is

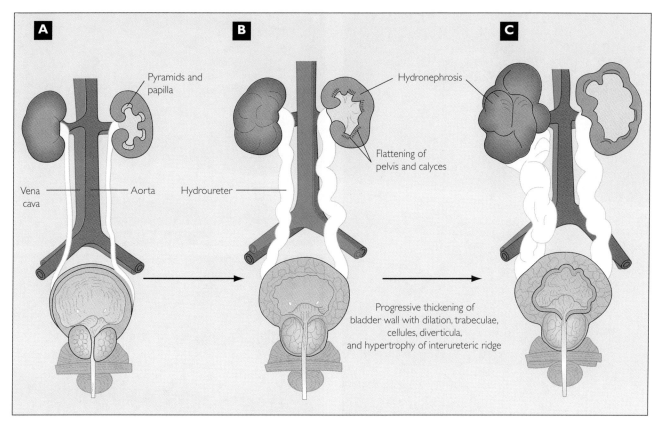

Figure 10.3 Progressive bilateral hydronephrosis due to prostatic outlet obstruction. Note the progressive changes in the pyramids in the kidney, from the normal concave shape to flattening of the papilla, and eventually concavity (A) Early stage. (B) Partly compensated stage. (C) Decompensated stage

lost and vesicoureteral reflux occurs. Due to this reflux, the intravesical pressure is transmitted directly to the renal pelvis, aggravating the degree of hydroureteronephrosis.[12] From the resulting retrograde pressure due to either reflux or obstruction (from the stretched trigone), the smooth muscle layers of the ureter wall undergoes hypertrophy in an attempt to force the urine downward by increased peristaltic activity. Ureter dilation and wall hypertrophy elongate the ureter, and eventually, fibrous bands develop, which angulates the ureter to form kinks, leading to tortuosity of the ureter. Upon peristaltic contractions, the fibrous bands further angulate the ureter, causing secondary ureteral obstruction.[12] During the decompensation stage of the ureter, the ureteral wall loses its contractile ability and becomes atonic, resulting in further dilation.

In the absence of prostatic obstruction, the pressure within the renal pelvis is zero. This pressure increases in the presence of stretched trigone hypertrophy or vesicoureteral reflux; the elevated pressure causes dilation of the renal pelvis and calyces. The degree of hydronephrosis that develops depends on the duration, degree, and site of the obstruction.[12] The higher the obstruction in the urinary tract, the greater the effect on the kidney. If the renal pelvis is entirely intrarenal and the obstruction is at the ureteropelvic junction, all the pressure will be exerted on the renal tissue. If the renal pelvis is extrarenal (embedded

in fat), only a portion of the pressure is exerted on the kidney, because the extrarenal kidney resting in adipose tissue allows it to dilate more readily, decreasing the applied pressure.

The development of hydronephrosis is first visibly evident in the calyces. Normally, the calyces are concave in shape with the papilla projecting into it. With elevated intrapelvic pressure, the kidney, grossly, will appear enlarged with simple dilatation of the pelvis and calyces, at the earliest stage of hydronephrosis. Histologically, the kidney will reveal cortical tubular atrophy with interstitial fibrosis. With progression of the disease, there will be blunting of the apices of the pyramids, followed by flattening of the papilla, and eventually the papilla become convex-shaped (cupped). These changes are due to two activities: first, there is compression atrophy of the kidney from an increase in intrapelvic pressure; and secondly, ischemic atrophy from hemodynamic changes, mainly manifested in arcuate vessels that run at the base of the pyramids parallel to the kidney outline, these vessels are more vulnerable to compression between the renal capsule and the centrally increasing intrapelvic pressure.[12] In this latter form of atrophy, the kidney is not uniformly atrophic: rather, it is spotty depending on the blood supply. The arterioles are "end arteries"; therefore, ischemia is most marked in the areas farthest from the interlobular arteries.

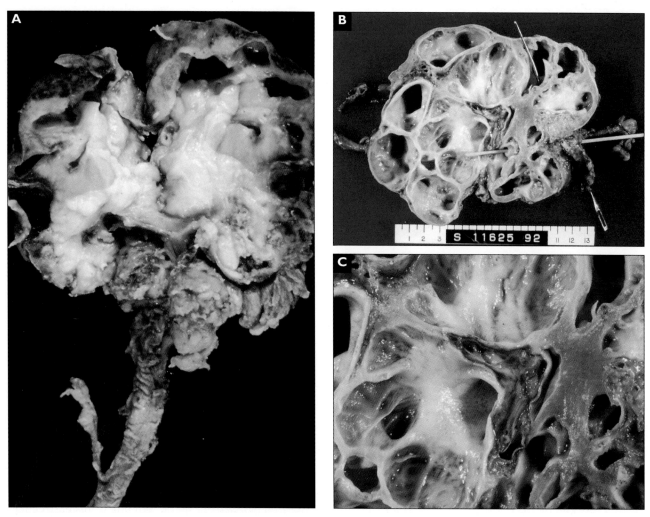

Figure 10.4 (A) Hydronephrosis and cortical atrophy of kidney in a patient with renal failure and death due to BPH. (B) Hydronephrosis and end stage kidney in patient with long-standing BPH. (C) Higher power view of hydronephrotic kidney

As the retrograde pressure increases, hydronephrosis progresses, with the cells nearest the main arteries exhibiting the greatest resistance.[12] This increased pressure is transmitted up the tubules, leading to dilation of the tubules; and finally the tubule cells atrophy from ischemia and compression. In far-advanced cases, the kidney may become transformed from a bean-shaped solid structure to a thin-walled cystic structure, filled with water, electrolytes, red blood cells, and white blood cells (if there is a superimposed infection). The kidney may enlarge to a diameter of 15–20 cm in size, but contain atrophic renal parenchyma with thinning of the cortex and total obliteration of the pyramids.

Even with complete obstruction of the prostatic urethra, glomerular filtration persists for some time because the filtrate subsequently diffuses back into the renal interstitium and perirenal spaces, where it ultimately returns to the systemic circulation via the lymphatic and venous systems. Because of this continued filtration, the affected calyces and pelvis become dilated. The high pressure in the pelvis is transmitted back through the collecting ducts into the

cortex, causing renal (pressure) atrophy, but it also compresses the renal vasculature of the medulla, causing decreased plasma flow in the inner medulla, resulting in renal (ischemic) atrophy. Even though medullary vascular disturbances can be reversed in the face of protracted obstruction, the same cannot be said of the medullary function disturbances. The initial functional alterations are largely due to damage of tubule cells, which is manifested primarily by impaired concentrating ability. Only later does the glomerular filtration rate (GFR) begin to diminish. When the outlet obstruction is acute in nature and complete, the reduction of the glomerular filtration usually leads to mild dilation of the pelvis and calyces with occasional incidence of renal parenchyma atrophy. On the other hand, when the obstruction is chronic in nature and incomplete, the glomerular filtration is not suppressed, and will continue to progressively dilate the kidney.

During the development of hydronephrosis, the closer the intrapelvic pressure approaches the glomerular filtration pressure (6–12 mmHg), the less urine will be made and secreted. As the GFR and the renal plasma flow are reduced, the concentrating power of the renal tubules is gradually lost due to ischemic necrosis of the cells, resulting in an elevated blood urea nitrogen and creatinine concentrations.[12] As hydronephrosis develops, urine is excreted into the renal pelvis, and the fluid and soluble substances have been shown to be reabsorbed through the tubules and lymphatics. This has been demonstrated by injecting phenolsulfonphthalein (PSP) into the obstructed unilateral renal pelvis; the PSP gets absorbed in a few hours and is excreted by the contralateral (unobstructed) kidney. Furthermore, it has been shown that if the intrapelvic pressure in the hydronephrotic kidney rapidly increases to a level approaching filtration pressure (resulting in cessation of filtration), a safety mechanism is activated that produces a break in the surface lining of the collecting structure at the weakest point – the fornices.[12] This leads to escape and extravasation of urine from the renal pelvis into the surrounding renal interstitium (also known as pyelointerstitial backflow). This extravasated fluid is absorbed by the renal lymphatics, and the pressure in the renal pelvis drops, allowing further filtration of urine.[12] This explains the process by which a severely marked hydronephrotic kidney continues to function in the face of outlet obstruction.

CLINICAL SYMPTOMS PRESENT IN BLADDER OUTLET OBSTRUCTION

Normally, contraction of the detrusor muscle and the trigone pulls the bladder neck open to form a funnel-shaped structure through which urine is expelled out of the prostatic urethra. The intravesical pressure generated during micturition varies between 20 and 40 cm of water. With bladder outlet obstruction due to BPH, the bladder musculature undergoes hypertrophy in order to develop intravesical pressures of 50–100 cm of water or more, to overcome the increased outlet resistance. Despite this compensation, the encroaching prostate appears to interfere with the mechanism that ordinarily opens the internal orifice. Furthermore, the contraction of the bladder wall does not last long enough to empty out all the volume, resulting in residual volume. After the refractory phase of the bladder muscle wall is completed and muscle has time to recover, voiding can be initiated once again by increasing the intravesical pressures. This leads to symptoms of increased frequency of urination with the feeling of incomplete emptying of the bladder.

During the early stages of outlet obstruction when the vesical muscle begins to hypertrophy, the force and size of the urine stream remain normal because the expelling power of the hypertrophic bladder wall is much greater than the urethral resistance, allowing normal micturition. During this phase (of compensation), the bladder appears to be hypersensitive. As the bladder is distended, the need to void is felt. In patients with a normal bladder, these early urges can be suppressed, and the bladder relaxes and distends further to receive more urine. However, in patients with a hypertrophic detrusor, the contractions of the detrusor muscle are so strong that it produces a series of

contractions, called spasms, producing the symptoms of an irritable bladder.[12] The earliest symptoms of bladder outlet obstruction are urgency and frequency. Along with these symptoms, the patient will also experience hesitancy in initiating urination, while the vesical muscle develops contraction strong enough to overcome resistance at the prostatic urethra. Eventually, there is some loss in compensation as the obstruction persists. If vesical tone becomes impaired or if urethral resistance exceeds detrusor power, some degree of decompensation will occur. The high obstructive resistance causes some loss in the force and size of the urinary stream, and the stream becomes slower as resistance increases. Once outlet resistance force is greater than the hypertrophic detrusor force, there is not enough strength that can be generated by the vesical wall to expel the urine out of the bladder, resulting in the accumulation of residual urine.

During prolonged periods of outlet obstruction without relief, the tone of the compensated bladder muscle can be temporarily flaccid when there is rapid filling of the bladder or by overstretching of the detrusor muscle. This will cause increased difficulty in urination, since the vesical wall does respond with contraction when stimulated by overstretching of the transitional epithelium. In addition to difficulty in urination, the patient will present with marked hesitancy and the need for straining to initiate urination; there will be a weak stream of urine that will prematurely terminate before the bladder completely empties.

As the degree of obstruction increases, there is a gradual increase in the urethra resistance compared with the power of the bladder musculature. Therefore, it becomes increasingly difficult to expel all the urine during the contraction phase of the detrusor. The symptoms of obstruction become more marked. The amount of residual urine gradually increases, and this diminishes the functional capacity of the bladder.[12] Progressive frequency of urination is also noted. On occasion, as the bladder decompensates, it becomes overstretched and attenuated; it may contain as much as 1000–3000 mL of urine. Due to the flaccid state of the bladder musculature (due to the overstretching), it loses its power of contraction, and overflow (paradoxical) incontinence results.

Overflow (paradoxical) incontinence arises from the accumulation of large amounts of residual urine in the bladder, secondary to outlet obstruction via BPH at the prostatic urethra. The clinical symptoms of overflow incontinence are nocturia, hesitancy in starting urination, straining to urinate with terminal dribbling, and reduced size and force of the urinary stream. With chronic overflow incontinence, patients can develop hydronephrosis and impaired renal function (renal insufficiency). These patients will present with a dilated, overdistended, palpable bladder; pain in the flank area, radiating to the umbilicus (along the course of the ureter); and fever, chills, burning sensation upon urination, hematuria, and cloudy urine when obstruction is superimposed with an infection. With prolonged outflow obstruction, these patients can control micturition, but lose their sensory awareness of bladder filling, especially in patients with diabetic neuropathy (which is very popular in the elderly population). Nausea, vomiting, weight loss, weakness, and pallor may be present in patents with uremia secondary to prolonged bilateral hydronephrosis. Outlet obstruction due to BPH encroachment on the prostatic urethra is surgically treated. Postoperatively, if the bladder has become adynamic because of prolonged overfilling and overstretching, bethanechol chloride (50–100 mg day^{-1}) can be given to help facilitate bladder emptying.

In bilateral partial obstruction, the earliest clinical signs evident are those of inability to concentrate urine by the distal convoluted tubules; this is reflected by symptoms of polyuria and nocturia. Some patients do present with distal tubular acidosis, renal salt wasting, and tubulointerstitial nephritis with scarring and atrophy of the papilla and medulla. Hypertension is common in such patients. In patients with complete bilateral obstruction, they present with oliguria or anuria may be present which is incompatible with long survival unless the obstruction is relieved.

After relieving outlet obstruction, three types of diuresis can occur in any patient with protracted obstruction of the prostatic urethra. The most common, urea diuresis, occurs secondary to the accumulation of osmotically active urea in the renal medulla during the obstruction. The excretion of the retained urea along with water is self-limiting (lasting 24–48 h), and requires little attention. Salt diuresis, the second most common form, is the excretion of excess extracellular fluid (total body water and salt) that has accumulated during the period of obstruction; this process is called "unloading". This type of diuresis is also self-limiting until a normovolemic state is reached, at which time, it may continue beyond the normal fluid balance to a pathological state of an imbalance of electrolytes. Therefore, in this type of diuresis, careful monitoring of the patient is extremely important along with aggressive IV fluid and electrolyte replacement, to avoid severe dehydration and salt depletion. Finally, the third type of diuresis, water diuresis, occurs due to impaired response of the collecting tubules to antidiuretic hormone (ADH).[13] It acts as a self-limiting nephrogenic diabetes insipidus disorder; in order words, there is end-organ resistance of the nephrogenic tubules to the circulating ADH. Water diuresis is believed to occur rarely.

Regardless of complete or incomplete chronic obstruction, the patients are usually asymptomatic and present with non-specific complaints, such as an increase in abdominal circumference (i.e. my pants no longer fit me), ankle edema, anorexia headaches, generalized malaise, fatigue, shortness of breath, and weight gain. Most of these men with obstructive uropathy are in a volume-expanded state, and will present with azotemia (uremia). Additional uremia-related symptoms may be evident: mental status changes, tremors (resting and intentional), and gastrointestinal bleeding. In cases of acute outlet obstruction, which is rarely caused by BPH, the patient usually presents with sharp flank pain that radiates to the groin or ipsilateral thigh. In addition, these men will commonly present with nausea, vomiting, chills, and fever. If acute bilateral obstruction occurs, the patient also may experience a sudden onset of anuria. When chronic outlet obstruction is the predominant clinical picture, the urinary diagnostic indices are most often similar to those seen with acute tubular necrosis, such as increased urinary sodium concentration, decreased urine osmolality, and decreased urine/plasma creatinine ratio.[14]

ASSESSMENT OF RENAL FUNCTION AFTER PROLONGED BLADDER OUTLET OBSTRUCTION

Under normal physiologic conditions, the kidney has the ability to concentrate urine in the distal convoluted tubules (DCT) and collecting ducts. The ascending and descending limbs of the loop of Henle are impermeable to water and possess active transport mechanisms to reabsorb sodium chloride into the interstitium space; hence, NaCl is reabsorbed without water. As a result, the tubular fluid sodium concentration and osmolarity decrease below that of plasma, and increases the osmolarity of the surrounding interstitium to produce a hypo-osmolar tubular fluid entering the distal tubule and collecting ducts. The permeability of the distal tubules and collecting ducts to NaCl and water is tightly regulated by aldosterone and vasopressin, respectively. Normally, the DCT and collecting ducts reabsorb 12% of the filtered NaCl; this amount increases to 14% in the presence of aldosterone, making the tubular fluid more dilute. Therefore, it is the responsibility of ADH to determine the final tubule fluid (urine) osmolarity. ADH is secreted from the supraoptic nuclei of the hypothalamus in response to an increase in serum osmolality or a decrease in blood volume. The presence of ADH on the principal cells in the late distal tubules and the collecting ducts will result in the reabsorption of (free) water via the formation of H_2O channels in the luminal membrane. Free water is the remaining H_2O present in the diluting segments of the kidney after all possible solutes are reabsorbed. The amount of free water necessary to be excreted to maintain a urine osmolality equal to plasma is called the free water clearance, which is used to estimate the ability of the nephron to concentrate or dilute the urine. In the absence of ADH, this free water is excreted as dilute urine; thus, free water clearance (C_{H_2O}) is positive (urine is hyposmotic to plasma). Vice versa, in the presence of ADH, the free water is not excreted but is reabsorbed by the distal tubules and collecting ducts, creating a negative free water clearance (urine is hyperosmotic to plasma). To determine the C_{H_2O}, the osmolar clearance must first be determined by using this formula:

$$C_{osm} = (U_{osm} \times V)/P_{osm}$$

where C_{osm} is the osmolar clearance (mL min^{-1}), U_{osm} is the urine osmolality (mosm kg^{-1}), and V is the urine volume flow (mL min^{-1}). The determined C_{osm} can now be used to calculate the free water clearance (C_{H_2O}) by using the formula: $C_{H_2O} = \dot{V} - C_{osm}$, where $\dot{V}$ is urine flow rate. These formulae may be of value when trying to determine the etiology of a polyuria, such as a solute diuresis, a water diuresis, or a combination of water–solute diuresis.

Another tool that can be used to assess the state of renal function in these BPH obstructed patients is the specific gravity of their urine. There is some correlation between the specific gravity of the urine and the urine osmolality, as evident from the following results obtained by Reiser and Porush:[15] a specific gravity (sp) of 1.0 corresponds to 50 mosm kg^{-1} H$_2$O; sp=1.01 corresponds to 300 mosm kg^{-1} H$_2$O; and sp=1.02 corresponds to 800 mosm kg^{-1} H$_2$O. If the urine osmolality or specific gravity is greater than 800 mosm kg^{-1} H$_2$O or 1.020, respectively, in the absence of proteinuria and glycosuria, then it can be assumed that the kidney's ability to concentrate urine is intact. The normal patient will have a urine osmolality greater than 900 mosm kg^{-1} H$_2$O. However, to assess properly the cause of a patient's polyuria, a water-deprivation test with the use of vasopressin should be performed. See Table 10.1 for a summary of the test.

As mentioned previously, postobstructive diuresis can result in a water diuresis, solute diuresis, or a combination of both (mixed water–solute diuresis). Solute diuresis occurs secondary to (1) an impaired medullary solute gradient as a result of a decreased sodium and urea reabsorption in the ascending limb of the loop of Henle and the collecting ducts, respectively; (2) a washout of the medullary solute gradient as a result of increased medullary blood flow; and (3) decreased utilization of the medullary solute gradient because of increased distal nephron urine flow and solute concentration.[16] If C$_{osm}$ is the amount of urine required to excrete a given load of urinary solute isosmotically (300 mosm L^{-1}), the electrolyte osmolality clearance (C$_{osm(E)}$) can be derived from the following formula: C$_{osm(E)}=V[2(U_{Na} + U_K)]/(2P_{Na})$, where V is the urine volume, U_{Na} is the urine sodium concentration, and U_K is the urine potassium concentration. The difference of C$_{osm}$ – C$_{osm(E)}$ will give the non-electrolyte component (for example, urea, protein, and glucose) of a solute diuresis.[17]

In the case of water diuresis, urine is excreted in a very dilute form; urine osmolality will be less than 150 mosm kg^{-1} H$_2$O, and the ratio of U_{osm}/P_{osm} will be less than 0.9. During solute diuresis, the U_{osm} will be greater than 250 mosm kg^{-1} H$_2$O, and the U_{osm}/P_{osm} ratio will be >0.9. However, if the U_{osm} is ≥ 250 mosm kg^{-1} H$_2$O and the U_{osm}/P_{osm} ratio is <0.9, then a mixed water–solute diuresis is present.[17]

Calculation of the C$_{osm}$/C$_{cr}$ ratio (where C$_{cr}$ is the creatinine clearance) can also give insight into the type of postobstructive diuresis a patient may have. An elevated C$_{osm}$/C$_{cr}$ ratio above 3% is consistent with a solute or a mixed water–solute diuresis; however, in the latter case, the elevated C$_{osm}$/C$_{cr}$ ratio is usually coexisting with a U_{osm}/P_{osm} ratio of less than 0.9. A low C$_{osm}$/C$_{cr}$ ratio is consistent with a water diuresis.[17]

MANAGEMENT OF PATIENT WITH POST-OBSTRUCTIVE DIURESIS

Most patients with chronic bladder outlet obstruction are in a volume-expanded state due to accumulation of solutes and water; hence, their postobstructive diuresis may be a normal physiologic response to this volume-expanded state.[18] This diuresis and natriuresis is secondary to retained amounts of urea, sodium, and water during the protracted obstruction; impaired concentrating ability and sodium reabsorption ability due to damage to the distal convoluted tubules and collecting ducts; and possibly circulating hormones.[16] The term postobstructive diuresis (urine output >200 mL h^{-1} for 24 h) refers to the increased polyuria and natriuresis that the patient experiences after the alleviation of bilateral ureteral obstruction. This certainly does not mean that a urologist should wait for 24 h to see if the patient has urinated more than 4.8 L in order to diagnosis postobstructive diuresis. A patient who presents with complaints and symptoms of bladder outlet obstruction and whose laboratory data reveals azotemia requires immediate attention, rather than waiting for 24 h. The diagnosis of postoperative diuresis should be concluded from the patient's history, physical examination, and the evidence of azotemia in the laboratory data (Figure 10.5).

The most important initial treatment in any patient with urinary tract obstruction, especially with laboratory data of

	Urine osmolality after dehydration (mosm kg^{-1} H$_2$O)	Change in urine volume and osmolality following vasopressin given after dehydration
Normal	>900	No further change
Central diabetes insipidus		
Complete	<200	Urine volume is reduced and osmolality increased markedly, but does not approach normal maximal osmolality
Partial	<500	Urine volume is reduced and osmolality is increased by 20–30%
Nephrogenic diabetes insipidus (present in patients with BPH)	<300	Urine volume unchanged; osmolality remains low
Compulsive water drinking	600–800	Osmolality may rise but by less than 10%. No further change in urine volume

Table 10.1 Water-deprivation test: anticipated response to fluid deprivation followed by vasopressin in patients with hypotonic polyuria

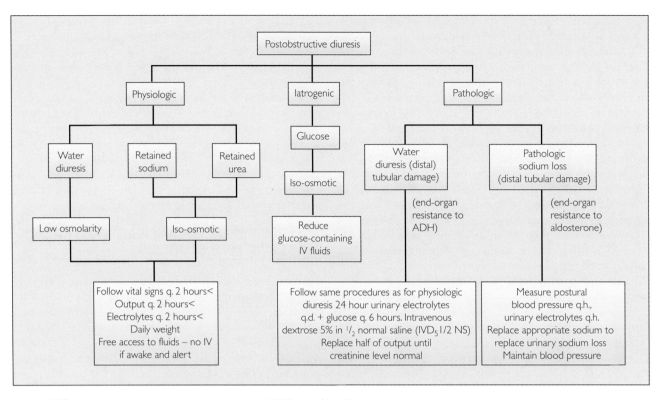

Figure 10.5 Management of post-obstructive diuresis (>200 mL h^{-1} for 24 h)

Source: Gulmi FA, Felson D, Vaughan ED Jr. Pathophysiology of urinary tract obstruction. In: 1998 *Campbell's Urology*, 7th edn, Vol. 1. London: WB Saunders 1998

azotemia, is to clear the obstruction by placing a Foley catheter. It has been noted that a patient's urine may turn bloody immediately after placing the catheter; this is not hemorrhagic cystitis. The gross hematuria is secondary to rapid refilling of the venous system with a possible rupture of a vein in the lining of the bladder mucosa.

The rationale for immediate relief of obstruction is based on the physiology of fluid reabsorption during obstruction. Despite the presence of outlet obstruction, the renal function is intact and continues to filtrate the plasma, leading to increased intrapelvic pressure; this results in pyelolymphatic and pyelovenous urine backflow as well as possible fornix rupture and extravasation.[19,20] This is particularly important, especially when the patient develops an elevated temperature and leukocytosis; this complication suggests that there is direct movement of urine and bacteria back into the vascular system during the obstruction. These patients can rapidly enter into septic shock, which is a life-threatening condition. Thus, the obstruction must be relieved before any severe complications occur.

After the patient's obstruction is alleviated, the potential occurrence of postobstructive diuresis needs to be considered and evaluated in the patient. These patients can be started on IV fluids (0.4% NaCl) at a 2 hourly rate equal to half the previous 2 h of urine output. However, if the patient is in congestive heart failure (fluid overload), then IV fluid must be withdrawn allowing the patient to diurese

until the congestive heart failure resolves.[17] During this period, it is necessary to monitor the serum and urine electrolytes every 6–12 h to replace appropriately the sodium and potassium, preventing any occurence of hyponatremia and hypokalemia. Providing D5W intravenously is usually not necessary; the patient should be encouraged to take food orally. If this is not possible, D5W should be given intravenously.[17] According to Gulmi and associates, it is recommended that IV fluids should be given to replace the urine output mL for mL every 2 h in addition to oral intake until the patient's serum BUN and creatinine come down to baseline levels. Once the patient's BUN and creatinine have normalized, oral IV fluids can be stopped.[17]

REVERSIBILITY OF OBSTRUCTION AND ITS EFFECT ON RENAL FUNCTION

The return of function in previously outlet obstructed kidneys is remarkable, yet unpredictable. Several experimental studies have shown recovery of renal function after alleviating outlet obstruction of 4 weeks' duration. At least two patient studies have shown that renal function was recovered after alleviating outlet obstruction of 56 and 69 days' duration.[12] Contrin has stated that serious irreversible damage occurs after about 3 weeks of complete obstruction and 3 months of incomplete obstruction.[21] However, it has also been documented that irreversible loss of renal function can begin as early as 7 days. The extent of recovery of kidney function after outlet obstruction is difficult to determine, especially preoperatively.

Surgical correction of bilateral hydronephrosis secondary to BPH outlet obstruction is successful in most cases when infection can be controlled and renal function has been preserved. Surgery (usually TURP) must relieve the outlet obstruction in order to eliminate urine stasis and vesicoureteral reflux; and infection must be treated, and normal intraluminal pressure gradients must be preserved to ensure stabilization of renal function.

CONCLUSION

Chronic obstruction of the prostatic urethra by BPH or prostatic adenocarcinoma can initiate a series of events leading to renal insufficiency. Obstructed urinary flow causes urinary stasis and increased urinary intraluminal pressure in the bladder. The former predisposes to the formation of stones and urinary tract infections; whereas, the latter consequence leads to hydroureteronephrosis. It should be noted that the presenting signs and symptoms depend on the nature, duration, and level of the obstruction.

Chronic dilatation of the renal pelvis causes muscular atony, fibrosis, and loss of peristaltic activity. Since urine is normally excreted at extremely low pressures, prolonged and severe hydronephrosis ultimately results in pressure atrophy of the renal parenchyma; this, in turn, affects the collecting tubules and medullary interstitium initially, and then the proximal tubules, cortical interstitium, and glomeruli, with gradual loss of renal function.

REFERENCES

1 McConnell JD, Barry MJ, Bruskewitz RC *et al. Benign Prostatic Hyperplasia: Diagnosis and Treatment. Clinical Practice Guidelines.* No. 8. AHCPR Publication No. 94–0582. Rockville, MD: Agency for Health Care Policy and Research, Public Health Services, US Department of Health and Human Services 1994: 29–34.

2 Coolsaet BL. Ventrodorsal vesical repair of complicated vesicovaginal and vesicorectal fistulas. *J Urol* 1984; **131**(1): 116–7.

3 Abrams PH, Feneley RCL. The significance of the symptoms associated with bladder outflow obstruction. *Urol Int* 1978; **33**: 171.

4 Sarmina I, Resnick MI. Obstructive uropathy in patients with benign prostatic hyperplasia. *J Urol* 1989; **141**: 866.

5 Berry SJ. The development of human benign prostatic hyperplasia with age. *J Urol* 1994; **132**: 474.

6 Kirkland JL, Lye M, Levy DW, Banerjee AK. Pattern of urine flow and electrolyte excretion in healthy elderly people. *Br Med J* 1983: **287**(6406): 1665–7.

7 Boyarsky S, Jones G, Paulson DF, Proust GR Jr. A new look at bladder neck obstruction by the Food and Drug Administration regulators: guidelines for investigation of benign prostatic hypertrophy. *Trans Am Assoc Genitourin Surg* 1977; **68**: 29.

8 Birkoff JD, Wiederhorn AR, Hamilton ML, Zinsser HH. Natural history of benign prostatic hypertrophy and acute urinary retention. *Urology* 1976; **7**: 48–52.

9 Craigen AA, Hickling JB, Saunders CRG, Carpenter RG. Natural history of prostatic obstruction. *JR Coll Gen Practice* 1969; **18**: 226–32.

10 Ball AJ, Feneley RCL, Abrams PH. The natural history of prostatism. *Br J Urol* 1971; **53**: 613–16.

11 Resnick MI, Older RA. *Diagnosis of Genitourinary Diseases*, 2nd edn. New York and Stuttgart: Thieme Medical Publishers 1997; 337.

12 Tanagho EA, McAninch JN. *Smith's General Urology*, 14th edn. East Norwalk, Connecticut: Appleton and Lange 1995; 173–80.

13 Klaar S. *et al.* Urinary tract obstruction. In: Brenner BM, Rector F (eds) *The Kidney*, 3rd edn. Philadelphia: WB Saunders 1986; 1443–90.

14 Gulmi FA, Felsen D, Vaughan ED Jr. *Management of Post-Obstructive Diuresis – AUA Update Series*, Vol. XVII. Lesson 23. American Urologic Association 1998: 178–83.

15 Reiser IW, Porush JG. Evaluation of renal function. In: Massry SG, Glassock RL (eds) *Textbook of Nephrology*, 3rd edn, Chap. 98. Baltimore, MD: Williams & Wilkins 1995; 780.

16 Gonzalez JM, Suki WN. Polyuria and nocturia. In: Massry SG, Glassock RL (eds) *Textbook of Nephrology*, 3rd edn. Baltimore MD: Williams & Wilkins 1995; 547–52.

17 Gulmi FA, Felson D, Vaughan ED Jr. Pathophysiology of urinary tract obstruction. In: *Campbell's Urology*, 7th edn, Vol. 1. London: WB Saunders 1998; 342–85.

18 Loo MH, Vaughan ED Jr. *Obstructive Nephropathy and Post-Obstructive Diuresis – AUA Update Series*, Vol. IV, Lesson 9. American Urological Association 1985.

19 Narath PA. The hydromechanics of the calyx renalis. *Int Urol* 1940; **43**: 145–176.

20 Stenberg A, Olsen L, Josephson S. Partial ureteric obstruction in weanling rats. *Scand J Urol Nephrol* 1985; **19**: 139.

21 Contrin K. *Robbins: Pathologic Basis of Diseases*, 5th edn. Philadelphia: WB Saunders 1994; 1025–26.

COMMENTARY

In this chapter Drs Patel, Tewari, and Furman discuss the changes that occur in the urinary system with obstruction due to prostatic disease. They discuss the pathophysiology of obstruction and the mechanisms involved in bladder decompensation and renal failure. Bladder outlet obstruction as a result of prostatic disease can result in progressive and irreversible changes in the urinary system. Mechanical or functional obstruction can cause pathologic changes in the bladder and subsequently in the upper tracts that result in progressive renal dysfunction. While the AHCPR guidelines recommend the routine use of serum creatinine to determine whether there is upper tract dysfunction, significant elevation of serum creatinine occurs only late in the course of the disease, and it may not be a sufficiently sensitive indicator for silent obstruction. In this regard it has also been noted in a recent study that medical renal disease and hypertension along with increasing age was a factor in elevation of creatinine in up to 11% of patients seen for BPH symptoms.[1] Therefore, to prevent patients with silent obstruction and renal failure from being missed, it is important to follow all patients over the age of 50 with periodic assessment of symptoms and to intervene and perform tests when symptoms changes. This should be done more to determine lack of renal decompensation and bladder decompensation rather than to treat the patient who is minimally symptomatic. Again, one has to reconcile the fact that, in medicine, cost effectiveness does not always equate with good patient care.

With regard to detrusor function in BPH, the recent observations by Dr Elbadawi are very relevant.[2] He notes that trabeculation just denotes an impaired function rather than obstruction; the presence of collagen infiltration in detrusor muscle is related to obstruction; and ultrastructural studies of detrusor muscle have further confirmed the findings of myohypertrophy in obstruction. Superimposed on this is a series of changes that are variable, depending on whether the obstructed detrusor is stable or decompensated. These studies have redefined the role of the detrusor muscle as a major component in outlet obstruction and may explain many of the associated abnormalities of bladder behavior noted in patients with BPH. As such the "detrusor is not a passive responder but an active contributor to dysfunction associated with BPH." In this regard, the recent data reported by Gray is also important.[3] Their investigations noted in an experimental study that partial obstruction to the bladder caused an immediate increase in residual bladder volume, which diminished as bladder wall compliance increased. However, 89% of obstructed animals had hyperactive detrusor contractions compared with 12% of controls. The voiding pressures always continued to be high for the entire period of observation. These observations of Conner and associates are provocative and support the hypothesis that, in some patients at least, watchful waiting may eventually lead to detrusor dysfunction with decompensation and silent renal failure.

Even in the absence of renal failure watchful waiting may be harmful in some patients, who eventually will end up with bladder decompensation. Data supporting this fact have recently become available from a study by Drs Djavan and associates.[4] In their findings, patients – age 80 and above, with acute urinary retention, residual urine volumes greater than 1500 cm^3, with no evidence of detrusor insta-

bilities and maximal detrusor pressure less than 28 cm of water – should not be offered surgery for BPH, since the surgery failed and patients were unable to void. These studies have added further impetus to the hypothesis that the bladder is a central player in patients with lower urinary tract symptoms.

It has been noted by Robbins and Kumar that renal injury will result because of cellular atrophy and necrosis if the obstruction to urine flow is not relieved within 6 weeks. However, this relates more to acute obstruction rather than chronic obstruction – which BPH induces. Bladder hypertrophy is one of the early consequences of outlet obstruction and a hypertrophied bladder is susceptible both to infection as well as inflammation. Trigonal hypertrophy may also cause increased resistance to urine flow – which then increases the functional obstruction. With decompensation of the bladder, there is a loss of compliance, which results in rapid increases in intravesical pressure with small changes in volume. This leads to a decrease in the functional capacity of the bladder. Patients with BPH often present with frequency and voided volumes that are less than 125 cm.[3] This may be related in part both to partial emptying of the bladder as well as changes in bladder capacity secondary to decompensation. Increased bladder pressure may also be transmitted as increased tension in the trigone area, which then causes increased ureteral pressure and vesicoureteral reflux. In the absence of prostatic obstruction, the pressure in the renal pelvis is zero. It is important, therefore, that in patients who have upper-tract dysfunction, secondary to prostatic obstruction, a period of stabilization be provided with a Foley catheter, if necessary, as a temporizing measure prior to definitive surgical therapy.

Finally, in evaluating patients with BPH it is always important in the history and physical exam to look for signs of upper tract dysfunction and symptoms such as nausea, vomiting, weight loss, weakness, and pallor, which may be the presenting symptoms of patients with uremia. One of the features of a BPH patient who presents with acute urinary retention is the possibility of postobstructive diuresis occurring after the retention is relieved. In this regard, it is important to admit the patient and treat him appropriately, as these patients may end up as a urologic emergency. The types of diuresis and a treatment algorithm have been discussed in detail in this chapter by Drs Patel, Tewari, and Furman.

1 Gerber GS, Goldfischer ER, Karrison TG, Bales GT. Serum creatinine measurements in men with lower urinary tract symptoms secondary to benign prostatic hyperplasia. *Urology* 1997; **49**(5): 697–702.

2 Elbadawi A. Voiding dysfunction in benign prostatic hyperplasia: trends, controversies and recent revelations. ii pathology and pathophysiology. *Urology* 1998; **51**(5A): 73–82.

3 Gray M. Progressive changes in detrusor function with bladder outlet obstruction. *J Urol*, 1997; **158**: 318.

4 Djavan B, Madersbacher S, Klinger C, Marberger M. Urodynamic assessment of patients with acute urinary retention: is treatment failure after prostatectomy predictable? *J Urol* 1997; **158**: 1829–33.

Section III

MEDICAL TREATMENT

MEDICAL TREATMENT

P. Narayan

One of the most dramatic changes that has occurred in the management of BPH over the last few years has been the advent of medical therapy. The symptoms of prostatism are thought to arise secondary to outlet obstruction either due to the mechanical mass of an enlarged prostate or because of spasm of smooth muscles of the prostatic capsule and urethra. More recently, there is evidence that the symptoms of lower urinary tract dysfunction may substantially be influenced by bladder function. The process of micturition is initiated in the micturition center located below the pons and is heavily influenced by cortical connections. The medial pontine micturition center, through this connection with the sacral spinal center, sends either excitatory or inhibitory impulses to regulate the micturition reflex. Evidence has shown that electrical or chemical stimulation of the medial pontine micturition center results in the contraction of the detrusor muscles and relaxation of the external sphincter, causing outflow of urine. Disruptions of positive control, as evident in spinal cord lesions, have been shown to cause detrusor contraction without sphincter relaxation, resulting in dyssynergia. Apart from the autonomic nervous system, micturition is also under voluntary control from the suprapontine cerebral centers, which can influence the lower extremities to assist in the urination process.

The basic voiding reflex is mediated at the level of the sacral spinal cord, and the upper tract influences are mostly inhibitory. Fibers in the pelvic nerves are the afferent limb of the voiding reflex, while the parasympathetic fibers to the bladder constitute the efferent limb. Furthermore, the bladder smooth muscle has some inherent contractile activity. There are no somatic motor nerves that control these stretch receptors in the bladder wall. Instead, these stretch receptors initiate a reflex contraction that is lower in threshold than the inherent contractile response of the muscle; this threshold for bladder wall contraction is adjusted by the activity of facilitatory and inhibitory centers in the brainstem. There is a facilitatory area in the pontine region and an inhibitory area in the midbrain. In addition to these regulatory mechanisms, there is another facilitatory area in the posterior hypothalamus.

A variety of diseases, medications, and aging may influence the inhibitory reflexes from higher centers causing the bladder to become somewhat autonomous, resulting in no voluntary control of the voiding reflex, leading to involuntary voiding. There is also evidence that there is "cross-talk" between neurotransmitters of the prostatic urethra, bladder, and spinal cord, which influences the behavior of not only the prostatic urethra but also bladder contractions. Established older data, however, suggest that up to 40% of urethral pressure is caused by smooth muscle contraction, mediated by α-1 adrenergic receptors. Current nomenclature also allows for the alignment of subtypes of α-1 adrenergic receptors, and it has been determined that in the prostate nearly 70% of the α-1 receptors are of the α1-a subtype. This data has provided the rationale for the use of α-1a adrenergic receptor antagonists to treat symptoms of prostatism. There is also evidence that α-1a receptors may be subdivided further into four subgroups (see chapter 11). Currently α-blockers as a class are used in 80% of patients receiving initial management for BPH. While non-selective α-blockers such as phenoxybenzamine were used initially, more recently, long-acting, once-a-day, second-generation α-blockers, such as terazosin and doxazosin, have been approved for use in BPH based on their efficacy in improving symptoms and uroflow in comparison with placebo in double-blind, randomized clinical trials. The downside of these agents is that they are also approved for use in the treatment of hypertension, and therefore, there is an incidence of postural hypotension of 2.7–8.3% as well as other related side-effects such as headache, asthenia, dizziness, flu-like syndrome, and syncope. They also have additional disadvantages in that they need to be titrated up to the optimal dose over a period of 3–5 weeks. While most α-blockers do not lower the blood pressure to a greater degree in patients who are controlled hypertensives, there is a fear of this event occurring, and therefore, concomitant use of other antihypertensive agents need to be watched while patients are on α-blockers. In order to nullify these side effects, a subtype selective α-1a blocker has been recently introduced. This agent is tamsulosin hydrochloride, which in several preclinical studies has been shown to bind preferentially with 13 times more efficacy to prostatic smooth muscles compared with vascular smooth muscles. Tamsulosin also has a 10–12 times higher selectivity for prostatic receptor subtypes. In several placebo-controlled, randomized clinical studies of tamsulosin vs. placebo, tamsulosin, at a dose of 0.4 mg, has been shown to cause a significant improvement in symptom scores as well as uroflow in comparison with placebo. Furthermore, the incidence of adverse events, such as postural hypotension and other cardiovascular-associated side effects were low. Additionally, patients who are on other antihypertensives, such as calcium channel blockers, ACE inhibitors, and β-blockers, did not need to be titrated or withdrawn from their antihypertensive medication since tamsulosin does not treat hypertension. Two side effects of tamsulosin that were significant were abnormal ejaculation and dizziness. It is thought that the dizziness is probably related to effects on the central baroreceptors or blockade of α-receptors in the central nervous system. The occurrence of dizziness as a side effect demonstrates the fact that tamsulosin is not exclusively directed towards the prostate, indicating that α-1a receptors are found in other areas besides the prostate gland. Abnormal ejaculation appears to be related to the blockade of sympathetic adrenoreceptors of the vas deferens and seminal vesicles, although this has yet to be further studied. In addition to having minimal influence on the cardiovascular system, the benefit of tamsulosin's once-a-day dosing schedule is that it does not need dose-titrating and the optimal dose can be started on day 1, providing faster relief of symptoms.

Another class of medical agents that have been popular in Europe and now in the USA are phytotherapeutic agents. Two groups of plant extracts that have been studied for phytotherapeutic management of BPH are lignans and isoflavonoids. These extracts are similar in structure to steroids found in the human body, especially sex steroids. The main sources of lignans are sesame seeds, cereals, fruits, and vegetables, while the main source of isoflavonoids is from soybean and other legumes. Of the many commercially available phyto-agents used for BPH, the most common are plant extracts of Saw palmetto berries, *Pygeum africanum*, β-sitosterol, and rye pollen. Many different mechanisms of action of these plant extracts have been proposed due to their mixed molecular composition. Among their breakdown products are daidzein and genistein, and these compounds may be involved in inhibition of steroid metabolism, lowering of cholesterol, stimulation of sex hormone binding globulins, inhibition of aromatase, and inhibition of 5α-reductase. They have also been postulated to have beneficial effects on inhibiting tumorigenesis, tyrosine kinase activity, topoisomerase and angiogenesis in experimental studies. Several clinical trials have been conducted on the use of these agents compared with placebo. These studies have shown that these agents have a benefit in decreasing BPH symptoms and improving uroflow compared with placebo. However there have also been contradictory reports on the degree of their efficacy compared to placebo. Their side effects have been minimal in the range of less than 5%. The precise mode of action is still unclear, since their active ingredient is unknown.

In summary, it may be stated that medical agents do provide an alternative treatment for BPH, especially in comparison with surgery, which has many drawbacks. Treatment for BPH is typically based on the severity of the symptoms and the patient's preferences. The most common surgical procedure for BPH is TURP, which provides relief from urinary symptoms, but is also associated with some morbidity, and high initial costs. With today's growing technological advances, the development of newer agents specifically targeted to block growth factor autocrine loops or mediate "cross-talk" of neurotransmitters between the prostatic urethra and bladder appears promising.

Alpha-blockers in Clinical Management

P. Narayan and A. Tewari

11

INTRODUCTION

Benign prostatic hyperplasia (BPH) is a common disease that affects all men with aging. Patients develop symptoms usually after age 50. Ninety per cent of men in their 80s exhibit histological evidence of disease,[1] 50% will experience symptoms due to BPH,[2] and 10% will develop acute urinary retention. The aging of the population also increases the number of men at risk for BPH. In the past year, more than 1.7 million men have made an office visit to the urologist,[3,4] and this number keeps increasing.

In the last decade, there has been a recognition that BPH is not an inevitable feature of aging. BPH is currently considered more a disease that affects the quality of life and, therefore, treatments are currently designed to relieve symptoms and reduce side effects. Patients who have symptoms of BPH are currently initially managing with medical agents. It has also been well established that patients with mild symptoms (International Prostate Symptom Score, IPSS<7) do not need therapy, since a majority of the normal population aged over 50 years will have mild symptoms. Additionally, there are adequate clinical data that medical management options can alleviate symptoms for up to 5 years in long-term trials, with excellent patient satisfaction and low incidence of long-term complications. Finally, the use of medical agents has allowed primary care physicians to manage patients with BPH.

In recent years α-blockers have become the most commonly prescribed initial medication for BPH. Approximately 80% of the patients receiving medical management are prescribed α-blockers by their primary care physician.[5] This chapter will discuss the current status of α-blockers in management of BPH.

PHARMACOPHYSIOLOGICAL RATIONALE FOR THE USE OF α-BLOCKER DRUGS IN THE MANAGEMENT OF BENIGN PROSTATIC HYPERPLASIA

During fetal development, the prostate gland is often referred to as being composed of five distinct lobes – anterior, posterior, median, and two lateral lobes. In the adult prostate with hyperplasia the periurethral glands enlarge and the prostate essentially has 2 concentric layers:

the outer layer (the external prostate gland proper) and the two inner layers (the periurethral glands). Prostate cancer occurs mostly in the peripheral outer layer while BPH occurs in the inner layer.

BPH arises from a combination of fibrous, stromal, and glandular proliferation. The ratio of glandular and fibrous components are variable. However, in most instances the stromal to glandular ratio is 2–5 times higher in patients with hyperplasia. The glands and stroma involved in causing symptoms of BPH arise from the mesenchyme around the proximal urethra. Glands that grow cranially into the lumen cause median lobe enlargement. Glands that enlarge laterally cause lateral lobe enlargement. This periurethral tissue causes both compressible and spastic effects on the urethra and forms the basis for current therapeutic strategies. Median lobe enlargement causes a ball valve obstruction of the bladder resulting in high residual urine in addition to obstructive symptoms. Lateral lobe enlargement results in elongation, narrowing, and compression of the prostatic urethra. Both types of enlargement also give rise to complications such as hematuria, infection, calculi, and renal failure.

Pathophysiology of this disease is still evolving. There is no cause and effect relationship between symptoms and obstruction either on the basis of urodynamic studies or objective measurements of prostate size. Also studies on natural history of BPH have found that many patients with symptoms get better spontaneously, with no treatment.

While the obstructive features are predominant in the cause of BPH symptoms, the irritative symptoms can occur without the obstructive symptoms. There are several related conditions of the bladder, sphincter, and urethra that cause symptoms similar to BPH. Many urologists now prefer to use the term "lower urinary tract symptoms" (LUTS), rather than prostatism, for the condition. LUTS comprises not only patients with BPH but also those with chronic non-bacterial prostatitis, bladder dysfunction, sphincter dysfunction, symptoms due to age-related changes, and symptoms related to multiple medications, among others. Recent data that women have IPSS scores similar to men also suggest that the bladder and urethra may be an additional cause of symptoms in patients with BPH. Several innovative studies are currently in progress in the field of bladder physiology as a contributor to BPH symptoms.

Several lines of evidence suggest that α-blockers have a scientific basis for relieving urinary obstruction secondary to BPH. The scientific rational for using α-blocker therapy for BPH is based on the following observations: a) prostatic smooth muscle contraction is the result of α-receptor mediated sympathetic stimulation; b) contraction of smooth muscles in the prostatic capsule, adenoma, and bladder neck results in decreased bladder outflow; c) several drugs are now available that can block α-receptor activity to cause relaxation of the prostatic smooth muscle. Finally, there is evidence that α receptors present in the anterior horn of the spinal cord may modulate both autonomic and somatic nerve response in the lower urinary tract.

Marco Caine[6] in the 1970s demonstrated using isometric measurements on tissue strips, that human prostatic smooth muscles contract under the influence of sympathetic innervation and that their effects were mediated through the α-adrenergic receptors. Several authors have since reported that BPH patients with predominant stromal component have a greater degree of dynamic obstruction.[7] The additional observation that 40% of the area density of BPH tissue is smooth muscle provides further evidence that prostate smooth muscle is likely to be an important factor in the development of clinical BPH.[8,9]

Evidence that α-blockers bind to prostatic tissue and mediate contractile response of prostatic smooth muscles has been demonstrated in animal and human studies.[7,10]

Table 11.1 provides a summary of the common α-blockers in clinical use along with recommended doses, side effects, and pharmacokinetics. While some of these agents are nonspecific, drugs such as tamsulosin have relatively specific binding characteristics that are preferential for prostatic tissue.

To further investigate the role of prostatic tissue components involved in α receptor blockade, Lepor and associates compared prostatic tissue specimens derived from men undergoing transurethral resection of the prostate (TURP) for clinical BPH (symptomatic BPH) with prostatic tissue from men undergoing cystoprostatectomy for bladder cancer (asymptomatic BPH). Preoperatively, symptom scores, peak flow rate, and prostate volumes were routinely measured. The α-1 receptor density was observed to be equivalent in tissue specimens obtained from men both with symptomatic and with asymptomatic BPH.[10] The contractile response to α-1 agonists was also similar between these groups.[11] These studies suggested that the development of clinical BPH was not due to upregulation of the α receptors or increased responsiveness of prostate smooth muscle to α-1 agonists. While other investigators have reported that the α receptors are upregulated in men with BPH, these studies compared tissues from different regions of the prostate and not just the periurethral gland tissue from men with and without clinical BPH. In Lepor's studies, the stromal–epithelial ratio was greater in the men with symptomatic BPH, suggesting that the cellular composition

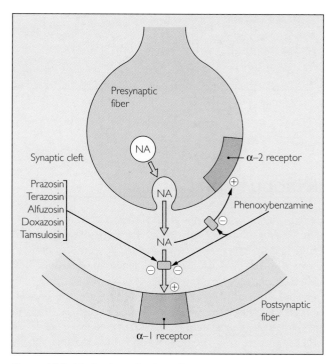

Figure 11.1 Mechanism of action of α-receptor antagonists at the synaptic junction. NA = norepinephrine.

of the inner gland (transitional zone) may represent an important factor contributing to the pathophysiology of clinical BPH.[12] Since the neurotransmitter for the α-1 receptor is norepinephrine, another plausible mechanism contributing to the pathophysiology of clinical BPH is increased adrenergic innervation. Spitsbergen has reported that the frequency of micturition in the spontaneous hypertensive rat is greater than in controls, implying that the increased levels of norepinephrine may mediate voiding dysfunction.[13] In 1990, Gup *et al.*[11] reported an inverse relationship between the American Urological Association (AUA) symptom score vs. catecholamine level in consecutive men undergoing prostatic biopsy for an elevated prostate-specific antigen (PSA) or abnormal digital rectal examination, who had no evidence of prostate. This observation strongly suggests that the pathophysiology of clinical BPH is not due to increased adrenergic innervation.

In another study, 26 men with clinical BPH who were candidates for medical management completed the Boyarsky symptom score and underwent uroflowmetry and transrectal ultrasonography (TRUS)-guided biopsy of the prostate before initiating therapy with the α-1-blocker terazosin.[14] The mean percent of smooth muscle was quantified from the biopsy specimens. Also quantified were the pairwise relationships between percent smooth muscle; baseline peak flow rate vs. baseline total symptom score; percent change in peak flow rate, and percent change in the symptom score demonstrated a statistically and clinically significant relationship between the baseline peak flow rate and the percent smooth muscle. Furthermore, there was no significant relationship between the baseline total symptom score and per cent smooth muscle.

These observations suggest that the amount of prostate smooth muscle does contribute to BOO and not symptomatology. These observations provide further evidence that LUTS and BOO are not causally related. The relationship between the increase in peak flow rate and the percent smooth muscle was highly significant, suggesting that the improvement in BOO secondary to terazosin treatment can be related to relaxation of the prostatic smooth muscle. A very weak and statistically insignificant relationship was observed between the percent changes in the total symptom score and the percent smooth muscle, suggesting that the symptom improvement associated with terazosin therapy is not likely to be mediated via relaxation of prostate smooth muscle. An important implication of these findings is that other α-1-mediated mechanisms other than relaxation of smooth muscles may account for the symptom improvement elicited by α-1-blockers in men with BPH. In summary, prostate smooth muscle density contributes to the severity of BOO and accounts for the α-1-blockade-mediated reduction of BOO in men with clinical BPH. Prostate smooth muscle density does not appear to be a major factor contributing to the severity of LUTS or of

the α-mediated improvements in symptomatology in men with clinical BPH (see Figure 11.1).

α-ADRENERGIC RECEPTORS: STRUCTURE AND CLASSIFICATION

Adrenergic receptors are classified as α and β based on their structure, binding characteristics, and tissue distribution. Beta receptors are found in the heart, juxtaglomerular renal cells, pancreatic β-cells, and smooth muscle cells of vascular, respiratory, and uterine organs among others. Alpha receptors are present in the brain, spinal cord, vascular smooth cells, cardiac muscle, and prostatic tissue among others. Both types of receptors are transmembrane proteins made up of seven helices, which are structurally arranged to form an extracellular domain (the site of the norepinephrine–receptor complex) and an intracellular domain (the site of the G-protein) (Figure 11.2).

The α receptors are further subdivided as α-1 and α-2 subtypes. Alpha-2 receptors are presynaptic in location and serve to regulate the amount of neurotransmitter transmission across the synapse. Norepinephrine is the primary neurotransmitter and stimulation of α-2 receptors results in feedback inhibition of norepinephrine release. Because of their wide distribution, blockade of α-2 receptors results in significant systemic and cardiac effects. Similar to α-1 receptors, α-2 receptors are transmembrane proteins linked to a G-inhibitory protein on the intra-

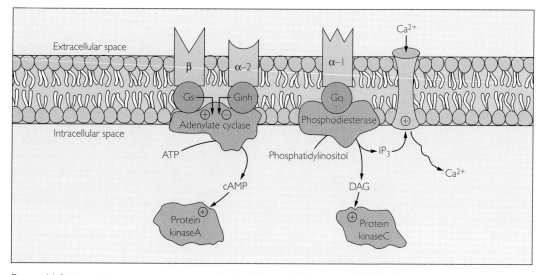

Figure 11.2 Second messenger system associated with α and β receptors. DAG=diacylglycerol; IP$_3$=inositol-1,4,5-triphosphate; Gs, Ginh, Gq=proteins.

cellular surface. Activation of the α-2 receptor causes activation of the Gs protein, which, in turn, leads to deactivation of adenyl cyclase system and decreased production of cyclic AMP.

The α-1 receptors are mediated primarily by the G coupling protein Gq, which leads to the stimulation of phospholipase C-β resulting in mobilization of calcium from intracellular stores. This in turn activates the protein kinase enzyme to bring about an intracellular response, leading to smooth muscle relaxation.

CDNAs encoding for human α-1 adrenergic receptors (α1ARs) have been cloned and characterized pharmacologically. These include α1a, α1b and α1d. The nomenclature of α, ARs were changed in 1995.[15] In older literature α1a was referred to as an α1c or α1a/d. More recently in addition to the wild type α1a-1 three other carboxy terminal splice variants of α1a (α1a-2, α1a-3, and α1a-4) have also been cloned.[16,17]

These studies have also shown that α1a-1 AR (wild type) predominates (85–95%) in human heart and prostate followed by α1a-4AR (10–15%). Recent data also suggest that the α1 AR postulated by Muramatsu in 1994 may have detected only a low affinity state of α1aAR and not another distinct 1AR subtype.[18,19] The role of α antagonists that are subtype selective for 1AR is somewhat complicated by several recent observations. These include data that small blood vessels in humans express α1a receptors; this implies that some potential vascular side effects can occur even with subtype selective α1aAR antagonists; it has been noted that human detrusor muscle expresses 1d more than 1a and no 1b. This implies that bladder irritability, which may be a substantial part of LUTS, may be mediated by other ARs than prostate; therefore the pure 1a subtype receptors may be limited in effectiveness with regards to irritative symptoms. An agent such as tamsulosin however, which has both 1a and 1d subtype antagonism may be more effective than newer pure 1a subtype antagonists.

α-1-ADRENOCEPTOR ANTAGONISTS

Development of α-Adrenergic Blocking Agents: Shotgun to Telescopic Site

Phenoxybenzamine

Phenoxybenzamine at a dose of 10–20 mg was one of the early agents used in the management of BPH; however, it was a non-selective α-1 and α-2 receptor antagonist, which produced many side effects including tiredness, nasal stuffiness, postural hypotension and anejaculation in up to 30% of patients. It has also been shown to have teratogenic properties in animal studies.[20,21] Therefore, this drug is no longer used in the management of BPH.

The next agents developed were more selective α-1 receptor antagonists. While agents such as prasozin and alfusozin are short acting agents, others such as terazosin and doxazosin are long acting and can be given once per day. Prazosin had fewer side effects and patients responded better than phenoxybenzamine. The main side effects of prazosin are its first-dose effect and vascular side effects during the morning dosage. In long-term studies, more than 32% of patients discontinued the use of prazosin owing to various adverse effects. However, because it is a generic drug in many countries, it is one of the least expensive α-blockers when price is a consideration.

Currently available once-a-day agents include terazosin, doxazosin, and tamsulosin. Indoramin and alfusozin are not available in the USA. Relative α-receptor sensitivity and the pharmacological properties of these drugs are summarized in Table 11.1.

Short-Acting Antagonists

Prazosin

There are not many recent studies on prazosin. Prazosin is not approved for BPH in the USA. In 1983, Hedlund and co-workers published results of a double-blinded, placebo-controlled, crossover study with prazosin for the treatment of BPH.[22] The study was small and included only 20 patients. Predominant improvement was in obstructive symptoms.

In 1987, Kirby and associates performed a double-blind, placebo-controlled study using prazosin. The study included 50 patients and results revealed a significant improvement in symptom scores and uroflow compared to placebo. However, there was a significant drop rate of 25%. Other double-blind, placebo-controlled studies evaluating prazosin have shown statistically significant increases in both symptom score and uroflow.[24–26]

Alfuzosin

Alfuzosin is a quinazoline derivative and is also a selective α-1 antagonist. The agent is used orally at a dose of 2.5 mg three times a day. Ramsey and coworkers reported on a study of 31 patients. Symptom scores improved over placebo, but uroflow rates were not significantly improved.[27] Jardin and associates[28–30] reported a community based, randomized study of 518 men treated with alfuzosin for BPH. There was a significant decrease in obstructive and irritative symptoms, a significant increase in mean urinary flow rate, and a decrease in postvoid residual urine volume. Study drawbacks included the fact that 55% of the men entered the study without a urinary flow rate evaluation, and only 39% of the patients were evaluated with regard to postvoid urine volume.

The pharmacokinetics of alfuzosin suggest three times a day daily dosing for optimal effects. However, other dosages may be effective. In a recent study, Kaplan et al.[31] examined the potential of intermittent dosing of alfuzosin. This prospective open-label, parallel, randomized trial involved two phases. The first involved 111 men taking 2.5 mg three times daily for 3 months. After this 3-month period, patients who responded to alfuzosin (defined as a

Drug agent	Mechanism of action	Pharmacokinetics	Dosing/administration	Adverse reactions
Phenoxybenzamine	• α-1 and α-2 adrenoceptor antagonist • Short acting • Irreversible antagonist • Increases blood flow to skin, mucosa, and abdominal viscera	• IV T½–24 hours • Duration of action = 3–4 days, and the effects of daily administration are cumulative for nearly 1 week • Hepatic metabolism	• 5–10 mg b.i.d. orally • Requires dose titration when initiating therapy	Postural hypotension, inhibited ejaculation with retrograde ejaculation, nasal congestion, nausea/vomiting, tachycardia, miosis
Prazosin	• α-1 adrenoceptor antagonist • Short acting • Reversible antagonist • Severely decreases diasystolic BP	• High first-pass hepatic metabolism with bile excretion • After oral administration, peak plasma concentration is reached in 3 hours • T½ = 2–3 hours	• 1–5 mg b.i.d. orally • Requires dose titration when initiating therapy	Syncope, postural hypotension, dizziness, nasal congestion, fluid retention
Alfuzosin	• α-1 adrenoceptor antagonist • Reversible antagonist • Short acting	• Elimination metabolic peak plasma effects noted in 1–2 hours • T½ = 2–3 hours	• 3–4 mg t.i.d. orally • Requires dose titration when initiating therapy	Syncope, postural hypotension, dizziness, nasal congestion, fluid retention
Terazosin	• α-1 adrenoceptor antagonist • Reversible antagonist • Long acting	• Hepatic metabolism with metabolite excreted in urine (40%) and bile/feces (60%). • Minimal first-pass effect • After oral administration, peak plasma concentration is reached in 40 minutes • T½ = 12 hours	• 2–10 mg q.d. orally • Requires dose titration when initiating therapy • Treatment should be initiated with a 1 mg dose given at bedtime	Syncope, postural hypotension, dizziness, asthenia, impotence, flu-like syndrome, headache
Doxazosin	• α-1 adrenoceptor antagonist • Reversible antagonist • Long acting	• High first-pass hepatic metabolism with enterohepatic recycling • After oral dose, peak plasma concentration is reached in 2–3 hours • T½ = 22 hours	• 4–8 mg q.d. orally • Requires dose titration when initiating therapy	Syncope, postural hypotension, dizziness, headache
Tamsulosin	• α-1A adrenoceptor antagonist • Reversible antagonist • Long acting	• Hepatic metabolism with metabolite excreted in urine • After oral administration, peak plasma concentration is reached in 5 days • T½ = 9–13 hours	• 0.4 mg or 0.8 mg q.d. orally • Should be given ½ hour after breakfast	Postural hypotension, syncope, dizziness, abnormal ejaculation (includes ejaculation failure, ejaculation disorder, retrograde ejaculation, and ejaculation decrease)

Table 11.1 Summary of α-adrenergic antagonists. All of the α-blockers require 2–4 weeks of treatment before therapeutic effects can be seen

40% decrease in the IPSS and a 30% increase in Q_{max}) were enrolled into a 6-month Phase II study. These Phase II participants were then randomized into one of three groups: group 1 continued alfuzosin 2.5 mg t.i.d. every day; group 2 received alfuzosin 2.5 mg t.i.d. every other day; and group 3 discontinued alfuzosin. Measurement of uroflow (Q_{max}) and completion of the IPSS were used to evaluate efficacy. Results during the Phase II trial revealed: the IPSS was 7.1 and 6.5 for group 1; 6.5 and 6.7 for the group taking alfuzosin every other day (group 2); and 11.4 and 12.3 for group 3 at 3 months and 6 months, respectively. The Q_{max} was 12.7 mL s^{-1} and 11.7 mL s^{-1} for group 1; 12.2 mL s^{-1} and

11.9 mL s^{-1} for group 2; and 9.7 mL s^{-1} and 9.3 mL s^{-1} for group 3 at 3 months and 6 months, respectively. There were no differences among group 1, patients taking alfuzosin everyday, and group 2, patients taking alfuzosin every other day (*P*=0.43). However, groups 1 and 2 performed better than group 3 (*P*<0.02 and *P*<0.015, respectively). The data clearly indicate that patients who took alfuzosin daily (group 1) did no better than men who took alfuzosin every other day.[31] Patients who discontinued the drug, however, developed recurrence of symptoms.

Long-Acting Antagonists

Terazosin

Terazosin, is a selective α-1-adrenergic antagonist. The drug is used at a dose of 5–20 mg once-a-day and is indicated for the treatment of both BPH and hypertension. Lepor and associates in 1992 published the first randomized placebo-controlled, Phase II trial of terazosin for treatment of BPH in 1992.[32,33] This study included 285 men with symptomatic BPH who were randomly assigned in equal proportions to receive placebo, 2 mg, 5 mg, or 10 mg of terazosin administered once daily. All terazosin-treatment groups exhibited a significantly greater decrease in total Boyarsky symptoms score compared with the placebo cohort (*P*<0.001). The increase in peak urinary flow rate for the 10 mg group was 3.0 mL s^{-1}, which was a significant change compared with baseline (*P*<0.001). This change was also significant compared with the placebo group (*P*<0.009). The improvements in symptom scores and urinary flow rates did not reach a plateau during the trial. This suggests that doses higher than 10 mg may further improve symptom scores. The adverse effects of using terazosin were acceptable.[32-34] In the 2, 5, and 10 mg study groups, the incidence of postural hypotension was 2.7%, 8.3%, and 5.7%, respectively. The 8.3% for the 5 mg group was the only measurement statistically different from the placebo cohort. Other reported events include headache (5.8%), asthenia (2.9%), dizziness (2.9%), flu syndrome (1.4%), UTI (1.4%), and syncope (1.4%).

Other Phase II studies have shown similar results. One was a randomized, placebo-controlled, double-blind study of dosing of terazosin (10 mg day^{-1}) in 30 patients with symptomatic BPH.[35] Fabricius and associates[36] demonstrated peak urinary flow rate increased 54%, mean flow rate increased 55%, and residual volume decreased 56%. The mean obstructive symptom score, irritative symptom score, and physician global assessment score improved by 68%, 34%, and 27%, respectively. All of these changes were significant when compared with the baseline placebo group. Long-term studies of terazosin have revealed that the efficacy and safety of the drug is maintained. In a study of 494 men from 23 centers, terazosin was started at a dose of 1 mg and titrated to a maximum of 20 mg per day. The duration of the study was 4 years. At all follow up intervals there was a significant decrease in symptom scores and increases in uroflow rates as compared to baseline. The

symptom score duration of at least 302 was noted in 62–77% of patients, while uroflow improvement of at least 30% was noted in 40–59% of patients. Of those that withdrew (43%), 11% did so for failure, 19% for adverse events and 13% for other reasons. Side effects include dizziness (6.7%), asthenia (3.8%), and somnolence (2%).[36] The most frequent adverse events in this study were headache, asthenia, and hypotension.

Not all studies suggest that terazosin is effective for BPH at the 5 and 10 mg doses. In a study from Italy conducted by Di Silverio and co-workers[37] terazosin was used in 137 patients who were randomized to receive placebo or 2 mg, 5 mg, or 10 mg of terazosin. There were statistically significant differences between the placebo and active treatment groups when using the least-squares method (*P*=0.012); however, there were no statistically significant differences when percent changes from baseline were compared.[37]

In another study by Lloyd *et al* in the UK, 86 patients with symptomatic BOO were randomized to receive terazosin or placebo. No statistically significant differences were noted between terazosin and placebo patients either in symptom score improvement or uroflow measurements. These studies however have been criticized for lack of adequate numbers and for other drawbacks.[38]

Doxazosin

Several studies have documented the utility of doxazosin as a treatment for BPH. Holme and associates[39] studied 91 patients in a double-blind, placebo-controlled study. Forty-seven patients who received 4 mg of doxazosin daily for 9 weeks and 44 patients received placebo. Reduction in irritative symptoms was 80% for the treatment group and 45% for the placebo group (*P*<0.05). Obstructive symptoms decreased by 63% for the treatment group and 31% for the placebo group (*P*<0.05). Subjectively, 81% of the treatment group felt considerably better compared with 39% of the placebo group. The peak urinary flow rate increased by 25% in the doxazosin group, but there was no change in the placebo cohort (*P*=0.07).[39] Very few side effects occurred in either groups, and no patient dropped out because of untoward events.

Chapple and associates[40] reported the results of a double blind randomized study of 133 patients, 67% of whom received doxazosin 4 mg daily, and 68 who received a placebo. Patients treated with doxazosin experienced a statistically significant improvement in nearly all symptoms compared with placebo: frequency, 44% vs. 27% (*P*=0.06); nocturia 39% vs. 19% (*P*=0.02); urgency, 60% vs. 38% (*P*=0.004); and premicturition delay, 56% vs. 26% (*P*=0.003).[40] The increase in peak urinary flow rate was 2.6 mL s^{-1} in the treatment group, compared with 1.1 mL s^{-1} for the placebo cohort. This improvement was not statistically significant (*P*=0.09). There was, however, a statistically significant improvement in the mean urinary flow rate (1 mL s^{-1} for the treatment group vs. 0.2 mL s^{-1} for the placebo cohort (*P*=0.04)).[40]

In 1995, Fawzy and associates[41] conducted a 16-week, double-blind, placebo-controlled study of 100 normotensive men to evaluate the role of doxazosin in the treatment of BPH. In this study, the subjects were titrated to a maximally efficacious or tolerated dose of 8 mg; 87.8% of the participants tolerated up to 8 mg. Patients taking doxazosin showed a significant improvement in maximum urinary flow rate as early as week 2 and was sustained throughout the study. The proportion of patients with a clinically meaningful increase in peak flow rate of at least 3 mL s^{-1} was significantly greater in the doxazosin group (39%) than in the placebo group (17%).[41]

Gillenwater *et al.*[42] reported on another multicenter, double-blind, placebo-controlled, dose-response study of 248 hypertensive men with BPH; 161 of these patients completed the study and were randomized to receive placebo, 2 mg, 4 mg, 8 mg, or 12 mg of doxazosin. This study revealed that the maximum flow rate increased significantly in the doxazosin groups by up to 3.6 mL s^{-1} compared with an increase of 0.1 mL s^{-1} in the placebo group. The proportion of patients with a 3 mL s^{-1} or greater increase in peak flow rate was significantly larger in the 8 mg and 12 mg doxazosin groups compared with the placebo group; there was less of a change in peak flow rate in patients taking 2 mg or 4 mg of doxazosin compared with placebo, but a rate of least 3 mL s^{-1} was noted. In the end-point analysis of symptoms, 4 mg of doxazosin was superior to placebo in decreasing the severity of the obstructive symptoms, irritative symptoms, and total symptoms.[42] The severity of total and obstructive symptoms also decreased significantly with 8 mg of doxazosin. Adverse events were reported by 48% of the men taking doxazosin and 35% of the placebo-treated patients. The side effects most frequently reported were dizziness, headache, and fatigue. Only 2.5% of the doxazosin-treated men experienced hypotension. The incidence of adverse events did not increase with increasing dose or duration of treatment.[42]

Long-Term Results for Terazosin and Doxazosin

The efficacy of both doxazosin and terazosin seems to be sustained over long-term treatment in non-comparative studies; published data are available from open studies of up to 45–48 months with doxazosin and 42 months with terazosin.[43,44] Data from 450 patients entering a long-term extension study with doxazosin also showed sustained statistically significant improvements in maximum urinary flow (mean improvement at endpoint analysis is 1.9 mL s^{-1}, $P<0.01$). Statistically significant and sustained improvements from baseline in severity and bother scores for total, obstructive, and irritative BPH symptoms also occurred with doxazosin treatment ($P<0.001$ in all cases). Premature discontinuation rates were 17% due to adverse events, 9% for insufficient clinical response, and 25% for administrative reasons. The most common adverse events resulting in discontinuation from the doxazosin study were dizziness (3.3%), fatigue (2.0%), headache (1.3%), and edema (1.3%). In the terazosin study (494 patients

enrolled), peak urinary flow rates were significantly higher than baseline at all assessments throughout the 42 months; these flow rates increased throughout the study, ranging from 1.0 to 4.0 mL s^{-1}. Furthermore, the Boyarsky symptom scores were also significantly improved throughout the long-term study, with the mean total score improving by at least 4 points (40%) at all visits beyond 3 months. Withdrawal rates were similar to those recorded in the long-term doxazosin study. Premature discontinuation rates were 19% due to adverse events, 11% for therapeutic failure, and 13% for administrative reasons. The most common adverse events resulting in premature termination from the study were dizziness (6.7%), asthenia (3.8%), and somnolence (2.0%).

The long-term data for doxazosin and terazosin presented in the preceding paragraph are compromised by the lack of a placebo control, and the criticism that the data reflect a "responder subgroup" of patients.

α-1A Subtype Selective α-Adrenergic Antagonist

Tamsulosin

Tamsulosin is a (–)-S-[2-[[2-(o-ethoxyphenoxy) ethyl] amino] propyl]-2-methoxybenzenesulfonamide HCl, a sulfamoylphenethylamine derivative which possesses potent and selective α-1A receptor antagonism. The structure of tamsulosin differs from alfusozin, terazosin, and doxazosin all of which are quinazoline derivatives. In preclinical trials, tamsulosin has been shown to have 13 times more efficacy for prostatic smooth muscle compared with vascular smooth muscles. Other studies have revealed a 10–12 times higher affinity for prostatic receptors as opposed to vascular and extraprostatic tissue. Recent changes in nomenclature of α-blockers reveal the α-1a receptors predominate in the prostate, while α-1b receptors predominate in the vascular smooth muscle. Tamsulosin belongs to a class of α-1a receptor antagonist that has preferred selectivity for prostatic smooth muscle, although it does have some binding to vascular smooth muscle receptors. It may also have some effects on the bladder secondary to its α-1d binding effects. Tamsulosin is available as a slow modified release capsule which allows for a once-a-day dosing. Tamsulosin binding is remarkable for its significantly lower degree of non-specific binding compared with other α-receptor antagonists.[45–58]

Tamsulosin was recently approved in the USA as Flomax (Boerhringer Ignelheim Pharmaceuticals, Inc., Ridgefield, CT) for treatment of BPH. The recommended dose is 0.4 mg once-a-day half an hour after a meal. The administration after food allows for reduction in peaks and troughs of drug levels in the serum and thereby reduces side effects. There were three multicenter studies undertaken in the USA with identical protocols. Two were of short duration (13 weeks) one was an extension (40 weeks) and one was a one year long-term study that included patients completing the other 2 trials as well as new patients who were eligible.[57–59] Eligibility was limited to patients with baseline AUA scores of 13, peak flow rates of 4–15 mL s^{-1} and residual urine volume of < 300 cc. Both short-term studies had a lead in placebo period of 4 weeks followed by a period of 9 weeks during which the patients were randomized in equal thirds to placebo, 0.4 mg or 0.8 mg of tamsulosin. Patients on 0.8 mg took 0.4 mg during the first week of the randomization.

Results of one study of 745 patients was reported by Narayan, Tewari and the tamsulosin investigator group.[57] Results revealed that patients taking 0.4 and 0.8 mg tamsulosin had a statistically significant improvement in symptom score of 28.4 and 31.9% compared to 18.8% with placebo ($P<0.5$). The percentage and number of patients who showed an improvement or reduction in the total AUA symptom score that was >25% from baseline to endpoint was 56% (134/238, 55% (133/244), and 40% (95/235) in the groups of 0.8 mg q.d., 0.4 mg q.d., and placebo, respectively ($P<0.05$).

In another study, Lepor and associates reporting for the tamsulosin investigator group analyzed the results of 755 patients. Improvements in symptom score for the 0.4 and 0.8 mg groups were 42 and 48% compared to 28% for placebo ($P<0.5$). Uroflow improvement was noted by week one and was maintained through the study; 40% of patients had a noticeable decrease of >25% in symptom scores by first assessment at week one and 70 and 74% achieved that response by study endpoint.

Two 12-week, double-blind, placebo-controlled studies of tamsulosin 0.4 mg once daily have been conducted in Europe.[57,58] More than 300 patients with symptomatic BPH were enrolled into each study. A meta-analysis of data from 575 patients (tamsulosin 382, placebo 193) was recently reported; the results showed a small improvement in peak flow rate with tamsulosin ($+1.6$ mL s^{-1}) which was statistically significant compared with placebo ($+0.6$ mL s^{-1}, $P=0.002$).[47] Tamsulosin also significantly improved the mean total Boyarsky symptom score compared with the placebo (-3.3 and -2.2 points; $P=0.002$). Long-term, open-labeled follow-up of these studies showed that about 70% of the patients receiving tamsulosin achieved a clinically significant improvement in BPH symptoms and the benefits were maintained over 12 months.[55] Although tamsulosin is reported to have modest uroselectivity,[46] dizziness was noted in 5% of patients.

In both studies the effects of tamsulosin treatment were observed soon after the initiation of therapy. Significant differences vs. placebo in the total AUA symptom score were apparent after 1 week of treatment with 0.4 mg day^{-1} tamsulosin. Changes in uroflow demonstrated that tamsulosin has rapid onset of action. A statistically significant difference relative to baseline was observed after the first dose of 0.4 mg day^{-1} tamsulosin vs. placebo ($P<0.001$). Furthermore, the mean change from baseline to endpoint was statistically significantly greater in both tamsulosin treatment groups than in the placebo ($P<0.001$). Additionally, statistically significant differences in uroflow compared with placebo occurred within 4–8 h after a single dose of tamsulosin 0.4 mg day.[60]

Overall, tamsulosin was well tolerated at doses of 0.4 and 0.8 mg day^{-1}. Adverse events that occurred more frequently in tamsulosin-treated patients included rhinitis, abnormal ejaculation, infection, and dizziness. The incidence and severity of abnormal ejaculation were shown to be dose dependent. There was a higher overall incidence of discontinuation due to adverse events in the 0.8 mg day^{-1} tamsulosin group (13%) relative to the 0.4 mg day^{-1} tamsulosin group and placebo group (7% and 9%, respectively; $P=0.115$).[60]

A 40 week extension study of the 13 week study was conducted to determine the long-term safety of tamsulosin and to identify whether response to tamsulosin was sustained, during maintenance therapy. Of the 618 patients from the 13-week initial study, 418 (68%) continued into the extension phase of the same double-blind medication and dose.[61] Statistically significant improvements were observed in all treatment groups ($P<0.001$). However, the improvements in the AUA symptom scores were greater in each of the tamsulosin groups (0.4 and 0.8 mg day^{-1}) than in the placebo group, and were comparable in the two tamsulosin treatment groups. A total of 78% (103/132) of the patients treated with tamsulosin 0.8 mg day^{-1} demonstrated a decrease in total AUA symptom score of 25% or more from baseline; 81% (111/137) of patients in the 0.4 mg day^{-1} tamsulosin group responded accordingly; and 59% (72/123) of the patients in the placebo group responded accordingly. The mean changes in maximum urinary flow relative to baseline within the two tamsulosin groups were statistically significant ($P<0.001$); the placebo group did not achieve a change in statistical significance. In the 0.8 mg day^{-1} tamsulosin group, 38% of the patients had a 30% or more increase in Q_{max} from baseline; 40% achieved the same in the 0.4 mg day^{-1} tamsulosin group; and 22% achieved the same in the placebo group.[61]

It was also noted that in the tamsulosin 0.4 mg day^{-1} group, the percentage of non-responders (patients who had less than 25% decrease in the total AUA symptom score from baseline) who became responders (patients who had demonstrated a decrease in the total AUA symptom score of 25% or more from baseline) was 43%; this was significantly higher than that for responders who became non-responders (6%). In contrast, in the placebo group, the percentage of non-responders at the end of the Phase III trial who became responders (21%) at the end of the extension phase was lower than the percentage of responders who became non-responders (23%).[61]

There was an overall higher incidence of adverse events in the tamsulosin 0.8 mg day^{-1} group than in the 0.4 mg day^{-1} tamsulosin and placebo groups. The overall incidence of adverse events in the 0.4 mg day^{-1} tamsulosin and placebo groups was similar. The most commonly reported treatment-emergent side effect for all three groups was infection (colds and upper respiratory infections). The overall incidence of cardiovascular side effects was indistinguishable between the three groups: 14%, 10%, and 14% for the placebo group, 0.4 mg day^{-1} tamsulosin group, and 0.8 mg day^{-1} tamsulosin group, respectively. Another adverse event, abnormal ejaculation occurred in 26% of the 0.8 mg day^{-1} tamsulosin group compared with 10% and 0% in the 0.4 mg day⁻¹ tamsulosin group and placebo group, respectively.[61] From these data, it can be concluded that continued exposure to tamsulosin beyond the initial 13 weeks is not accompanied by enhanced risk for adverse events; the adverse events seen at the end of the 53-week trial period were similar to those seen at the end of the initial 13-week trial period.

Adverse Events of α-1-Adrenergic Antagonists

Cardiovascular Effects

A major untoward effect of α-blockers in patients with BPH is the incidence of postural hypotension and syncopal attacks. Patients with BPH are often elderly, have cardiac disease and may be dehydrated. Cardiovascular side effects of α-blockers are exaggerated in such patients. Alpha-blockers such as terazosin and doxazosin were developed for treating hypertension and have been approved for lowering blood pressure in hypertensive patients. In patients who have both hypertension and BPH, α-blockers may solve two problems with one treatment. However, it is precisely in this group of patients that risks for postural hypotension are also higher. Many patients with hypertension have cardiac disease and may be on other antihypertensive medications. Addition of α-blockers may enhance side effects in such patients. The Joint National Commission on Hypertension recommends life-style modifications, diuretics, calcium-channel blockers, ACE (Angiotensin Converting Enzyme) Inhibitors, and β-blockers as the first line management for hypertension.[62,63] The rationale for this is the fact that these agents have proven efficacy in reducing the risk of myocardial infarction, cerebrovascular accidents, and TIA in such patients. Alpha-blockers for hypertension are used mostly as an additional, rather than as a primary agent for treatment of hypertension. The second major objection to using α-blockers is the spontaneous incidence of postural hypotension in men with aging. The Shep Study, for example, reported the incidence of spontaneous postural hypotension (a fall in systolic BP of ≥ 20 mmHg after 1 minute of quiet standing); it was reported that 20% of patients older than 65 years have postural hypotension, of which one-half are symptomatic.[64] This study further concluded that the incidence of postural hypotension in the elderly increases with prolonged standing; 10.4% experienced hypotension after 1 minute of standing, 12% at 1–3 minutes of standing, and 17.3% at 3 minutes. A major cause of morbidity in elderly patients is falls and hip fractures due to spontaneous postural hypotension. Adding an α-blocker causes this problem to worsen; this does not happen when elderly patients are given Ca-channel blockers or ACE inhibitors. Finally, patients already on antihypertensives may need to be watched more carefully when α-blockers are added. With constraints on time, the urologist would rather treat BPH than have to counsel patients on the risks of postural hypotension. Therefore, many urologists prefer α-1 receptor subtype selective agents which do not need to be coordinated with other antihypertensive medications.

There are however, some benefits to α-blockers. In patients with both hypertension and BPH α-blockers may be more cost effective. Additionally hypertension often coexists with other risk factors for coronary heart disease; for example, abnormal lipid profile and insulin resistance/glucose intolerance. Proponents in favor of α-blockers to treat both diseases cite favorable effects of drugs such as doxazosin on these metabolic variables.[64,65] Benefits include reduction in high blood pressure and serum lipids, an increase in fibrinolysis, inhibition of platelet aggregation, attenuation of the adverse hemodynamic and homeostatic effects of smoking, and regression of cardiac hypertrophy. Alpha-blockers are also reported to improve insulin sensitivity and glucose intolerance, both in hypertensive patients with insulin resistance and in non-insulin-dependent diabetic patients.[66] Such benefits provide a further rationale for choosing α-1 adrenoceptor blockade for the treatment of men with BPH who have one or more of these risk factors. Alpha-blockers do not appear to lower blood pressure substantially in patients with normal blood pressure. Kaplan *et al* investigated the effects of doxazosin on the blood pressures of 32 pharmacologically normotensive (in other words, blood pressure controlled by antihypertensive medication) patients with BPH and 31 physiologically normotensive patients with BPH.[68] The results showed that doxazosin-induced reductions in blood pressure were small and clinically insignificant in both groups (no differences between groups). Further evidence is available from the Hytrin Community Assessment Trial (HYCAT), a community-based, double-blinded, randomized trial of the treatment of symptomatic BPH with terazosin versus placebo; 524 of the patients enrolled (274 were given terazosin and 250 were given placebo) were also treated with concurrent single or combination antihypertensive therapy.[69] There were no significant differences between the terazosin and placebo patients in the incidence of blood pressure-related adverse events. These studies indicate the doxazosin or terazosin may be introduced for the treatment of BPH in hypertensive men whose blood pressure is already adequately controlled by other antihypertensive agents, without the fear of a further clinical reduction in blood pressure. However, monitoring of blood pressure is recommended, at least initially, when α-blockers are given in addition to any other existing antihypertensive medication.

In the US tamsulosin studies, dizziness occurred in a small percentage of patients (8-mg dosage caused dizziness in 23% of patients; 4-mg, 20%; and placebo, 15%; $P=0.039$ between 0.8-mg and placebo). Since dizziness was not associated with postural hypotension, it could be due to the binding of drug to baroreceptors in the central or peripheral nervous system. This incidence of dizziness, however, is comparable with terazosin and doxazosin studies.[42,45,58,68,69,70–76] The lack of significant cardiovascular effects and hypotension with tamsulosin was also noted in the European studies. In the meta-analysis of the European trial, treatment-emergent adverse effects occurred in 36% of the tamsulosin group and 32% of the placebo group ($P=0.802$). During the 60 weeks

Side effect	Terazosin[1]			Doxazosin[2]			Tamsulosin[3]		
	Percentage with terazozin	Percent with placebo	P value	Percentage with doxazosin	Percent with placebo	P value	Percentage with tamsulosin	Percent with placebo	P value
Asthenia/fatigue	7.4%	3.3%	<0.05	8.0%	1.7%	<0.05	11%	9.0%	NS
Postural hypotension	3.9%	0.8%	<0.05	–	–	–	1%	1.0%	NS
Dizziness	9.1%	4.2%	<0.05	15.6%	9.0%	<0.05	20%	15.0%	NS
Discontinued due to side effects	20%	1.2%	NS	12%	4.0%	NS	9%	8%	NS

[1] From the package drug insert of terazosin
[2] From the package drug insert of doxazosin
[3] Data from the use of FDA approved dose of tamsulosin (0.4 mg in US93.01 Study)

Table 11.2 Comparative table for cardiovascular side effects with the use of terazosin, doxazosin, and tamsulosin in the USA

of tamsulosin treatment, 60% of the patients experienced at least one treatment-emergent adverse event. Fifty-one (21%) of the patients experienced adverse events considered by the investigator to be probably or possibly related to tamsulosin.[47,54,55,58,77] Tables 11.1 and 11.2 provide a summary of α-antagonists and their incidence of adverse events caused at doses used for the treatment of BPH.

CLINICAL RELEVANCE OF α-1 SELECTIVITY

Several studies have been performed to study both the α-1 preferential selectivity of tamsulosin as well as to determine the clinical relevance of this effect.[78–80] One study compared tamsulosin (0.4 mg) to terazosin (5 mg) in order to determine which drug caused more suppression of phenylephrine induced increase in blood pressure. This study was performed in 10 human volunteers each of whom received placebo, tamsulosin (0.4 mg) or terazosin (5 mg) each for 3 days at least 1 week apart. On each day an IV infusion of phenylephrine was given in incremental doses. Both plasma drug levels and patient vital signs were monitored continuously. Results revealed that phenylephrine suppressed blood pressure in patients on placebo. While blood pressure suppression was noted with tamsulosin at low doses of phenylephrine (up to 1 µg/kg/min) it was not noted at higher doses. Blood pressure suppression was complete with terazosin at all doses (from 0.25–4 µg/kg/min). When the plasma of patients was analyzed for drug concentration it was found that tamsulosin was maximally bound to α-1a receptors slowly over 5 hours. Binding was four-fold lower to α-1b and 1d receptors. Terazosin binding to α-1a was rapid in one hour and binding to 1a was similar to 1d. Alpha-1b binding of terazosin was higher than that of tamsulosin and also the effects lasted longer (23.5 hours). Rapid receptor blockade may force the body to enhance counter regulation mechanisms which would be a major factor in the side-effect profile of terazosin and other similar α-blockers. Studies on orthostatic hypotensive episodes in patients randomized

between tamsulosin and terazosin have also revealed statistically significant higher rates of orthostatic events in patients on terazosin. These studies collectively suggest that α-1a receptor preferential binding of tamsulosin may have clinical relevance in not reducing blood pressure in normotensive men and by reducing incidence of orthostatic events.

PATIENT SELECTION

One of the more frustrating questions facing urologists is how to determine which patients will respond best to which type of therapy (i.e. how to predict outcome). It has been shown in one small study that the clinical response to α-blockade in BPH is related to the peak urinary flow rate and AUA symptom score.[62] As the onset of symptomatic improvement with α-1-adrenoceptor antagonists is rapid (within 1–3 weeks), it may be appropriate to give men with symptoms of BPH a trial therapy of α-blockade, assuming the patient does not require immediate surgery. If the patient does not respond within 3–4 months, alternative therapy should be considered. Patients with a history of orthostatic hypotension should not be treated with α-blockers.

While watchful waiting is currently recommended for patients with mild BPH symptoms (AUA score ≤ 7), those with moderate-to-severe symptoms (AUA score ≥ 8) should be given information on the risks and benefits of watchful waiting, medical therapies, and surgery.[7] A trial of medical therapy should not be restricted to patients presenting with milder symptoms; as seen in clinical studies with doxazosin and terazosin, α-blockade has been reported to be most effective in patients presenting with more severe symptoms prior to treatment.[63,64,70] Although some studies suggest that patients with severe symptoms generally prefer a surgical rather than a medical approach, recent experience in clinical practice has shown that many patients prefer a therapy less invasive than TURP (but more aggressive than watchful waiting), even if their symptoms are relatively severe (AUA score >19). Furthermore, most patients (85%) remain satisfied with their initial choice of therapy 12 months after its inception.[71] Patient preference for the less-invasive alternatives, increasing patient awareness of BPH, and an increasing range of available treatments is likely to add momentum to this shift from highly invasive surgical therapy to minimally (or non-) invasive medical management.

Watchful waiting is a good conservative approach to the treatment of BPH, but should not be overly used. If watchful waiting is excessively performed in some patients with BPH, extended complications resulting from increased bladder outlet resistance, such as urinary incontinence, may result. As the prostate enlarges and narrows the lumen of the prostatic urethra, this increase in bladder outlet resistance causes the bladder to respond by increasing its force of contraction to void the urine. By developing this increased intravesical voiding pressure, the bladder is able to maintain flow; this additional work exerted by the muscular bladder wall to overcome the outlet resistance will result in detrusor hypertrophy, hyperplasia, and the deposition of collagen within the bladder wall. The latter results in the thickening of the bladder wall – the wall loses its compliance and its elastic properties. This loss of compliance causes the intravesical pressures to rise greatly with small changes in volume, leading to a decrease in the functional capacity of the bladder. This, in turn, will lead to the development of detrusor instability and loss of normal control over the reflex detrusor response. Early in the course of obstruction, the bladder is able to compensate; but if watchful waiting is performed for extended periods of time, urge and overflow incontinence may result. To avoid these unwanted circumstances, watchful waiting should be done under careful consideration and monitored closely in patients with mild BPH symptoms (AUA score ≤7).

COMBINATION OF α-BLOCKADE WITH FINASTERIDE

There is a rationale for combining α-blockade agents with 5α-reductase inhibitors. While α-blockers reduce the dynamic component of obstruction by reducing prostatic smooth muscle tone, 5α-reductase inhibitors act on the fixed element of obstruction; they reduce the enlarged prostate by inhibiting 5α-reductase enzyme, which is responsible for the conversion of testosterone to dihydrotestosterone (DHT), the hormone responsible for promoting the growth of the prostatic adenoma. As such, treatment with a 5α-reductase inhibitor (such as finasteride) can significantly decrease the symptoms of obstruction, increase urinary flow, and decrease prostatic volume. Although some practicing urologists may already use this combined medical approach of an α-blocker plus a 5α-reductase inhibitor, there are currently no data available to support this theoretical synergism. The VA Cooperative study, in which patients were treated for 1 year with combined terazosin

and finasteride, recently confirmed the safety and efficacy of terazosin for the treatment of clinical BPH, but failed to confirm the effectiveness of finasteride.[73] This study failed to show any advantage of terazosin/finasteride combination therapy over terazosin monotherapy; however, the mean prostate volume of the study group was small at 27cc which may have biased the study against the 5α-reductase inhibitor. The results of two further studies to investigate doxazosin/finasteride combination therapy (the PRIDICT study and the US NIH-sponsored Medical Therapy of Prostatic Symptoms [MTOPS] study) in which patients with larger prostates were included, are still pending. In particular, the MTOPS study, a long-term (4–6 year) protocol with a similar design to the VA Cooperative study, is expected to give more definitive answers to questions concerning the effects of these two drugs on the microscopic and clinical progression of the disease.

CONCLUSIONS

The ideal medical agent for treatment of BPH must a) improve quality-of-life by relieving symptoms, b) have minimal side-effects, c) be cost effective, and d) eventually cause a regression of the disease process. Currently available agents do not meet several of these criteria. Alpha-blockers currently must be used continuously although many physicians and patients find intermittent therapy is quite reasonable. There are studies that suggest that alternate day regimens are effective. The waxing and waning of BPH symptoms and results of studies of watchful waiting suggest that many men may remain stable for years without using therapy. Currently used agents also have side-effects and costs are significant. In this regard it is important to determine which patients are candidates for a trial of medical therapy for BPH. Any patient who is suffering from clinically significant BPH symptoms and is not in urinary retention is a potential beneficiary from treatment with an α-1-adrenergic blocker or 5α-reductase inhibitor (which is discussed in the following chapters). These therapies are not limited to the poor surgical candidate but can be useful for any patient with bothersome symptoms. Even in patients with moderate-to-severe symptoms, 85% remain satisfied with α-blocker therapy for up to a period of 1 year after treatment.[75,77,81] Symptoms of a more severe nature and urinary retention, however, are contraindications to medical therapy. Patients with a history of orthostatic hypotension should not be treated with α-blockers.

With regard to finasteride, a major advantage is that it is an oral medication that can be given once a day. It also has few known side effects. There are, however, disadvantages associated with finasteride. Since this medication must be taken indefinitely, the expense is a concern. Cost to the patient for a 1-month supply of finasteride is US$60.68, making the annual expense of US$728.16. (These costs were determined from data collected from randomly chosen pharmacies in the Midwestern USA.) In addition, it may take 6–12 months to achieve the maximum therapeutic effect from finasteride. Another concern is that finasteride decreases the serum PSA by approximately 50%. This may alter the usefulness of serum PSA for detecting clinically significant prostate cancer at an early, potentially curable stage.

The α-1-adrenergic antagonists have several advantages. The long-acting drugs allow for once-a-day dosing. The therapeutic effect, as indicated by a greater than 30% increase in peak urinary flow rate, is realized in more than 50% of the patients receiving the therapy. The beneficial effect from treatment is realized as early as 1 week with tamsulosin or 2–3 weeks after reaching the maximum dose with other agents. The major disadvantage of these medications for the treatment of BPH includes the 10%

incidence of untoward effects related to the cardiovascular system as well as titration to achieve maximum benefit. Some of these disadvantages have been solved by the use of subtype selective α-1A-blockers. As with the 5α-reductase inhibitors, the α-1 adrenergic antagonists must be taken indefinitely to maintain the therapeutic effect. Irrespective of the dose, the monthly expense to the patient on terazosin therapy is US\$45.83, or an annual cost of US\$549.96. The monthly expense for a patient on doxazosin is as high as US\$31.97, depending on the dosage prescribed. Furthermore, the new subtype selective α-1A-blocker, tamsulosin, costs US\$39.91 per month, with an annual cost of US\$478.92.

REFERENCES

1 Berry SJ, Coffey DS, Walsh PC, Ewing LL. The development of human benign prostate hyperplasia with aging. *J Urol* 1984; **132**(3): 474–9.

2 Girman CJ, Jacobsen SJ, Guess HA *et al*. Natural history of prostatism: relationship among symptoms, prostate volume and peak urinary flow. *J Urol* 1995; **153**: 1510–15.

3 Barry MJ, Fowler FJ Jr, Bin L, Oesterling JE. A nationwide survey of practicing urologists: current management of benign prostatic hyperplasia and clinically localized prostate cancer. *J Urol* 1997; **158**: 488–91.

4 Barry MJ, Roehrborn C. Management of benign prostate hyperplasia. *Annu Rev Med* 1997; **48**: 177–89.

5 Collins MM, Barry MJ, Bin L *et al*. Diagnosis and treatment of benign prostate hyperplasia: practice patterns of primary care physicians. *J Gen Intern Med* 1997; **12**: 224–9.

6 Caine M, Raz S. Some clinical implications of adrenergic receptors in the urinary tract. *Arch Surg* 1975; **110**: 247–50.

7 Shapiro E, Hartanto V, Lepor H. The response of alpha blockers in benign prostate hyperplasia is related to the percent area density of prostate smooth muscle. *Prostate* 1992; **21**: 297–307.

8 Furuya S, Kumamoto Y, Yokoyama E *et al*. Alpha-adrenergic activity and urethral pressure in prostatic zone in benign prostate hypertrophy. *J Urol* 1982; **128**: 836–9.

9 Chapple CR, Aubry ML, James S *et al*. Characterization of human prostate adrenoreceptors using pharmacology receptor binding localization. *Br J Urol* 1989; **63**: 487–96.

10 Gup DI, Shapiro E, Baumann M, Lepor H. Contractile properties of human prostate adenomas and the development of infravesical obstruction. *Prostate* 1989; **15**(2): 105–14.

11 Gup DI, Shapiro E, Baumann M, Lepor H. Autonomic receptors in human prostate adenomas. *J Urol* 1990; **143**(1): 179–85.

12 Shapiro E, Becich MJ, Hartanto V, Lepor H. The relative proportion of stromal and epithelial hyperplasia is related to the development of symptomatic benign prostate hyperplasia. *J Urol* 1992; **147**(5): 1293–7.

13 Spitsbergen JM, Clemow DB, McCarty R *et al*. Neurally mediated hyperactive voiding in spontaneously hypertensive rats. *Brain Res* 1998; **790**(1–2): 151–9.

14 Shapiro E, Hartanto V, Lepor H. The response to alpha blockade in benign prostatic hyperplasia is related to the percent area density of prostate smooth muscle. *Prostate* 1992; **21**(4): 297–307.

15 Hieble U, Bylund D, Clarke D *et al*. International union of pharmacology. Recommendation for nomenclature of alpha

1-adrenoceptors: consensus update. *Pharmacol Rev* 1995; **47**: 267–70.

16 Hirasawa A, Shibata K, Horie K *et al*. Cloning functional expression and tissue distribution of human alpha 1c-adrenoceptor splice variants. *FEBS Lett* 1995; **363**: 226–56.

17 Chang D, Chang T, Yamanishi S *et al*. Molecular cloning genomic characterization and expression of novel human alpha 1a-adrenoceptor isoforms. *FEBS Lett* 1998; **422**: 279–83.

18 Muramatsu I, Oshita M, Ohmura T *et al*. Pharmacological characterization of alpha 1-adrenoceptor subtypes in the human prostate: functional and binding studies. *Br J Urol* 1994; **74**: 572–78.

19 Ford A, Daniels D, Chang D *et al*. Pharmacological pleiotropism of the human recombinant alpha 1-adrenoceptor classification. *Br J Pharmacol* 1997; **121**: 1127–35.

20 Abrams PH, Shah PJR, Stone R, Choa RG. Bladder outflow obstruction treated with phenoxybenzamine. *Br J Urol* 1982; **54**: 527–30.

21 Caine M, Perlberg S, Shapiro A. Phenoxybenzamine for benign prostate obstruction: review of 200 cases. *Urology* 1981; **17**: 542–6.

22 Hedlund H, Andersson KE, Ek A. Effects of prazosin in patients with benign prostatic obstruction. *J Urol* 1983; **130**: 275–8.

23 Kirby RS, Coppinger SW, Corcoran MO *et al*. Prazosin in the treatment of prostatic obstruction: a placebo-controlled study. *Br J Urol* 1987; **60**: 136–42.

24 Shapiro A, Mazouz B, Caine M. The alpha-adrenergic blocking effect of prazosin on the human prostate. *Urol Res* 1981; **9**: 17–20.

25 Dutkiewicz S, Filipek M. Prazosin concentration monitoring in the treatment of prostatic adenoma. *Int Urol Nephrol* 1991; **23**: 143–50.

26 Chapple CR, Noble JG, Milroy EJ. Comparative study of selective alpha-1 adrenoceptor blockade versus surgery in the treatment of prostatic obstruction. *Br J Urol* 1993; **72**: 822–5.

27 Ramsay JW, Scott GI, Whitfield HN. A double-blind controlled trial of a new alpha-1 blocking drug in the treatment of bladder outflow obstruction. *Br J Urol* 1985; **57**: 657–9.

28 Jardin A. Efficacy of an alpha-blocker, alfuzosin, on urinary disorders in men with prostatic adenoma: intermediate results of a European multicenter study. *Ann Urol Paris* 1988; **22**: 333–40.

29 Jardin A, Bensadoun H, Delauche Cavallier MC, Attali P. Alfuzosin for treatment of benign prostatic hypertrophy: the BPH–ALF Group. *Lancet* 1991; **337**: 1457–61.

30 Jardin A, Bensadoun H, Delauche Cavallier MC *et al*. Long-term treatment of benign prostatic hyperplasia with alfuzosin: a 24–30 month survey, BPH–ALF Group. *Br J Urol* 1994; **74**: 579–84.

31 Kaplan SA, Reis RB, Cologna A *et al*. Intermittent alpha-blocker therapy in the treatment of men with lower urinary tract symptoms. *Urology* 1998; **52**: 12–16.

32 Lepor H, Auerbach S, Puras Baez A *et al*. A randomized, placebo-controlled multicenter study of the efficacy and safety of terazosin in the treatment of benign prostatic hyperplasia. *J Urol* 1992; **148**: 1467–74.

33 Lepor H. Long-term efficacy and safety of terazosin in patients with benign prostatic hyperplasia: Terazosin Research Group. *Urology* 1995; **45**: 406–13.

34 Lepor H, Henry D, Laddu AR. The efficacy and safety of terazosin for the treatment of symptomatic BPH. *Prostate* 1991; **18**: 345–55.

35 Lepor H. Terazosin in treatment of BPH: In: Kirby R, McConnell J *et al*. (eds) *Textbook of Benign Prostatic Hyperplasia*. Oxford: ISIS Medical Media 1996.

36 Fabricius PG, Hannaford JM. Placebo-controlled study of terazosin in the treatment of benign prostatic hyperplasia with 2-year follow-up. *Br J Urol* 1992; **70** (Suppl 1): 10–16.

37 Di Silverio F. Use of terazosin in the medical treatment of benign prostatic hyperplasia: experience in Italy. *Br J Urol* 1992; **70** (Suppl 1): 22–6.

38 Lloyd SN, Buckley JF, Chilton CP *et al*. Terazosin in the treatment of benign prostatic hyperplasia: a multicentre, placebo-controlled trial. *Br J Urol* 1992; **70** (Suppl 1): 17–21.

39 Holme JB, Christensen MM, Rasmussen PC. 29-weeks doxazosin treatment in patients with symptomatic benign prostatic hyperplasia. *Scand J Urol Nephrol* 1994; **28**: 77–82.

40 Chapple CR, Carter P, Christmas TJ. A three-month, double-blind study of doxazosin as treatment for benign prostatic bladder outlet obstruction. *Br J Urol* 1994; **74**: 50–6.

41 Fawzy A, Braun K, Lewis GP *et al*. Doxazosin in the treatment of benign prostatic hyperplasia in normotensive patients: a multicenter study. *J Urol* 1995; **154**: 105–9.

42 Gillenwater JY, Conn RL, Chrysant SG *et al*. for the Multicenter Study Group. Doxazosin for the treatment of benign prostatic hyperplasia in patients with mild to moderate essential hypertension: a double-blind, placebo-controlled, dose-response multicenter study. *J Urol* 1995; **154**: 110–15.

43 Lepor H. Terazosin in treatment of BPH: In: Kirby R, McConnell J *et al*. (eds) *Textbook of Benign Prostatic Hyperplasia*. Oxford: ISIS Medical Media 1996.

44 Herbert L, Kaplan SA, Mobley DF *et al*. Doxazosin for benign prostatic hyperplasia: long-term efficacy and safety in hypertensive and normotensive patients. *J Urol* 1997; **157**: 525–30.

45 Yamada S, Tanaka C, Kimura R, Kawabe K. Alpha-1-adrenoceptors in human prostate: Characterization and binding characteristics of alpha-1 antagonists. *Life Sci* 1994; **54**: 1845–54.

46 Yamada S, Tanaka C, Ohkura T *et al*. High-affinity specific (3H) tamsulosin binding to alpha-1-adrenoceptors in human prostates with benign prostatic hypertrophy. *Urol Res* 1994; **22**: 273–8.

47 Chapple CR, Wyndaele JJ, Nordling J *et al*. for the European Tamsulosin Study Group. Tamsulosin, the first prostate-selective alpha-1A-adrenoceptor antagonist: a meta-analysis of two randomized, placebo-controlled, multicenter studies in patients with benign prostatic obstruction (symptomatic BPH). *Eur Urol* 1996; **29**: 155–67.

48 Wilde MI, McTavish D. Tamsulosin – a review of its pharmacological properties and therapeutic potential in the management of symptomatic benign prostatic hyperplasia. *Drugs* 1996; **52**: 883–98.

49 Taguchi K, Saitoh M, Sato S. Effects of tamsulosin metabolites at alpha-1 adrenoceptor subtypes. *J Pharmacol Exp Ther* 1997; **280**: 1–5.

50 Garcia Sainz JA, Romero Avila MT, Villalobos Molina R, Minneman KP. Alpha-1-adrenoceptor subtype selectivity of tamsulosin: studies using livers from different species. *Eur J Pharmacol* 1995; **289**: 1–7.

51 Takenaka T, Fujikura T, Honda K. Discovery and development of tamsulosin hydrochloride, a new alpha-1-adrenoceptor antagonist. *Yakugaku Zasshi* 1995; **155**: 773–89.

52 Soeishi Y, Matsushima H, Watanabe T. Absorption, metabolism, and excretion of tamsulosin hydrochloride in man. *Xenobiotica* 1996; **26**: 637–45.

53 Soeishi Y, Matsushima H, Teraya Y. Metabolism of tamsulosin in rat and dog. *Xenobiotica* 1996; **26**: 355–65.

54 Chapple CR. Selective alpha-1-adrenoceptor antagonists in benign prostatic hyperplasia: rationale and clinical experience. *Eur Urol* 1996; **29**: 129–44.

55 Schulman CC, Cortvriend J, Jonas U *et al*. for the European Tamsulosin Study Group. Tamsulosin, the first prostate-selective alpha-1A-adrenoceptor antagonist: analysis of a multinational, multicenter, open-label study assessing the long-term efficacy and safety in patients with benign prostatic obstruction (symptomatic BPH). *Eur Urol* 1996; **29**: 145–54.

56 Leonardi A, Hieble JP, Guarneri L *et al*. Pharmacological characterization of the uroselective alpha-1-antagonist Rec 15/2739 (SB 216469): role of the α-1L-adrenoceptor in tissue selectivity, part I. *J Pharmacol Exp Ther* 1997; **281**: 1272–83.

57 Abrams P, Schulman CC, Vaage S. Tamsulosin, a selective alpha-1c-adrenoceptor antagonist: a randomized, controlled trial I patients with benign prostatic "obstruction" (symptomatic BPH): the European Tamsulosin Study Group. *Br J Urol* 1995; **76**: 325–36.

58 Kawabe K. Efficacy and safety of tamsulosin in the treatment of benign prostatic hyperplasia. *Br J Urol* 1995; **76**(Suppl 1): 63–7.

59 Narayan P, Tewari A for the Tamsulosin Investigator Group. Phase III multicenter placebo-controlled study of tamsulosin in benign prostatic hyperplasia. *J Urol* 1998; **160**: 1701–6.

60 Lepor H for the Tamsulosin Investigator Group. Phase III multicenter placebo-controlled study of tamsulosin in benign prostatic hyperplasia. *Urology* 1998; **51**: 892–900.

61 Lepor H for the Tamsulosin Investigator Group. Long-term evaluation of tamsulosin in benign prostatic hyperplasia: placebo-controlled, double-blind extension of phase III trial. *Urology* 1998; **51**: 901–6.

62 Chalmers J. The place of combination therapy in the treatment of hypertension in 1993. *J Clin Exp Hypertens* 1993; **15**(6): 1299–1313.

63 Jerome M, Xakellis GC, Angstman C, Patchin W. Initial medication selection for treatment of hypertension in an open-panel HMO. *J Am Board Fam Pract* 1995; **8**(1): 1–6.

64 Labarthe DR, Blaufox MD, Smith WM *et al*. Systolic Hypertension in the Elderly Program (SHEP). Part 5: Baseline blood pressure and pulse rate measurements. *Hypertension* 1991; **17** (3 Suppl): 1162–76.

65 Pool JL. Effects of doxazosin on serum lipids: a review of the clinical data and molecular basis for altered lipid metabolism. *Am Heart J* 1991; **121**: 251–60.

66 Pool JL. Effects of doxazosin on coronary heart disease risk factors in the hypertensive patient. *Br J Clin Pract* 1994; **74**: 8–12.

67 Fulton B, Wagstaff AJ, Sorkin EG. Doxazosin, an update of its clinical pharmacology and therapeutic applications in hypertension and benign prostatic hyperplasia. *Drugs* 1995; **49**: 295–320.

68 Kaplan SA, Meade D, Alisera P *et al*. Doxazosin in physiologically and pharmacologically normotensive men with benign prostatic hyperplasia. *Urology* 1995; **46**: 512–17.

69 Roehrborn CG, Oesterling JE, Auerbach S *et al*. for the HYCAT Investigator Group: The Hytrin Community Assessment Trial study: a one-year study of terazosin versus placebo in the treatment of men with symptomatic benign prostatic hyperplasia. *Urology* 1996; **47**: 159–168.

70 Witjes WP, Rosier PF, Caris CT *et al*. Urodynamic and clinical effects of terazosin therapy in symptomatic patients with and without bladder outlet obstruction: a stratified analysis. *Urology* 1997; **49**: 197–205.

71 Frankel S. Measures of proscar, hytrin and cardura side effects. *Neurourol Urodyn* 1997; **16**: 63–6.

72 Lepor H, Nieder A, Feser J *et al*. Effect of terazosin on prostatism in men with normal and abnormal peak urinary flow rates. *Urology* 1997; **49**: 476–80.

73 Lepor H, Kaplan SA, Klimberg I *et al*. Doxazosin for benign prostatic hyperplasia: long-term efficacy and safety in hypertensive and normotensive patients. *J Urol* 1997; **157**: 525–30.

74 Kawachi I, Barry MJ, Giovanucci E *et al*. The impact of different therapies on symptoms of benign prostatic hyperplasia: a prospective study. *Clin Ther* 1996; **18**(6): 1118–27.

75 Debruyne FM, Witjes WP, Fitzpatrick J *et al*. The international terazosin trial: a multicentre study of the long-term efficacy and safety of terazosin in the treatment of benign prostatic hyperplasia – The ITT Group. *Eur Urol* 1996; **30**: 369–76.

76 Lepor H, Williford WO, Barry MJ *et al*. for the VA Cooperative Studies Benign Prostatic Hyperplasia Study Group. The efficacy of terazosin, finasteride, or both in benign prostatic hyperplasia. *N Engl J Med* 1996; **335**(8): 533–9.

77 Okada H, Kawaida N, Ogawa T *et al*. Tamsulosin and chlormadinone for the treatment of benign prostatic hyperplasia – The Kobe University YM617 Study Group. *Scand J Urol Nephrol* 1996; **30**: 379–85.

78 Schafers RF, Fokuhl B, Wasmuth A *et al*. Differential vascular alpha 1-adrenoceptor antagonism by Tamsulosin and terazosin. *Br J Clin Pharmacol* 1999; **47**: 67–74.

79 Taguchi K, Schafers RF, Michel MC. Radioreceptor assay analysis of tamsulosin and terazosin pharmacokinetics. *Br J Clin Pharmacol* 1998; **45**: 49–55.

80 de Mey C, Micel MC, McEwen J *et al*. A double-blind comparison of terazosin and Tamsulosin on their differential effects on ambulatory blood pressure and nocturnal orthostatic stress testing. *Eur Urol* 1998; **33**: 481–88.

81 Kaplan SA, Goluboff ET, Olsson CA *et al*. Effect of demographic factors, urinary peak flow rates, and Boyarsky symptom scores on patient treatment choice in benign prostatic hyperplasia. *Urology* 1995; **45**: 398–405.

COMMENTARY

Alpha-blockers as a class, are the most commonly used first-line agents in management of symptomatic BPH. Approximately 80% of patients receiving medical management are prescribed α-blockers by their primary care physician or urologist. Pathophysiology of BPH is unclear. It is thought that a significant portion (up to 40% in some series) of measured urethral pressure is contributed by outflow resistance secondary to spasm of the prostatic urethral muscles. The scientific rationale for using α-blocker therapy is based on the fact that (1) prostatic smooth muscle contracts with α receptor sympathetic stimulation, (2) contraction of smooth muscles in the prostate capsule and bladder neck results in decreased bladder outflow, (3) Several drugs are now available that can block α-receptor activity and relax the smooth muscles, (4) there are α receptors in the anterior horn of the spinal cord, which may modulate both autonomic and somatic nerve response in the lower urinary tract by means of "cross-talk". The initial studies of α-receptor activity in prostate comes from Marco Caine. Extensive studies have shown that approximately 40% of bladder outlet obstruction may be the result of smooth muscle contraction and that several drugs such as phenoxybenzamine, prazosin, terazosin, doxazosin, alfuzosin, and tamsulosin, combined extensively to prostatic α receptors and relieve smooth muscle contractions (Figure 11.1). It has also been noted that the stromal–epithelial ratio is higher in men with symptomatic BPH. The stromal tissue rather than epithelial mass contributes to bulk of obstruction in BPH. The neurotransmitter for the α-1 receptor is norepinephrine. It has been found that, in rats, the frequency of micturition is greater in hypertensive rats, implying that the increased levels of norepinephrine may mediate voiding dysfunction. Adrenergic receptors are classified as α and β receptors on the basis of their distribution, structure and mechanism of action as well as effect on target organs. The α receptors are further subdivided into two groups – α-1 and α-2. Alpha-1 receptors are postsynaptic in location and mediate contractions of smooth muscles in the prostate. Recently it has been shown that the α-1A, a subtype of the α-1 receptor, is predominant in the prostatic smooth muscles and forms 70% of these receptors. Phenoxybenzamine was one of the initial α-adrenergic blocking drugs used for the management of BPH. Because it was non-selective, it produced many side effects. Subsequently, prazosin was used, but since it is a short-acting antagonist, it must be given three times per day. Long-acting agents approved for US use include terazosin and doxazosin. Both these agents cause significant improvement in symptoms in uroflow compared with placebo in many clinical trials. However the side effects of these agents include an incidence of postural hypotension of 2.7–8.3% as well as headache, asthenia, dizziness, flu syndrome, and rarely syncope. They also have additional disadvantages in that they need to be titrated up to the optimal dose over a period of 3–5 weeks. While most α-blockers do not lower the blood pressure further in patients who are normotensive, there is a fear of this event occurring and therefore titration of other anti-hypertensives needs to be watched while patients are on α-blockers. These disadvantages have been somewhat nullified by the development of a new α-blocker, tamsu-losin hydrochloride, discussed further in Chapter 12, which has the same efficacy as doxazosin and terazosin without similar cardiovascular side effects.

Tamsulosin: Role in the Management of Benign Prostatic Hyperplasia

12

P. Narayan and A. Tewari

INTRODUCTION

Symptomatic benign prostatic hyperplasia (BPH) is a major health care issue. The pathophysiology of symptoms in patients with BPH is not completely clear. Several lines of evidence suggest that prostatic smooth muscle spasm may be a contributory mechanism. The contraction of prostate and urethral smooth muscle is mediated by receptors and they are present in varying amounts at the bladder neck, prostatic urethra, capsule, and stroma of prostate. Marco Caine in 1973 was one of the earliest investigators to advocate the use of α-receptor antagonists to treat patients with symptoms of BPH.[1-11] Currently, there are two selective long-acting α-1-receptor antagonists, terazosin and doxazosin, that are approved for treatment of BPH in the USA.[12-20] Although both of these agents have several advantages over non-selective α-blockers such as phenoxybenzamine, they still cause significant side effects in 15–19% of patients.[12-28] Tamsulosin hydrochloride (Flomax, Boehringer Ingelheim Pharmaceuticals, Inc., Ridgefield, CT) is a new class of sulfonyl derivative, which has preferential selectivity for the 1A-adrenergic receptor subtype. The 1A-receptor subtype is predominant in prostatic smooth muscles. In several preclinical studies, tamsulosin has been shown to bind preferentially to prostatic smooth muscles as compared with vascular smooth muscles.[27-37] Tamsulosin also exhibited a higher selectivity for prostatic receptor subtypes when compared with terazosin, alfuzosin, and doxazosin.[27-37] This review is focused on tamsulosin, which is a uroselective α-adrenergic blocker.

SCIENTIFIC RATIONALE

The source of symptoms in a patient with BPH appears to be either from an obstructing adenoma (static or mechanical component) or spasmodic contractions of smooth muscles under α-receptor-mediated sympathetic stimulation (dynamic component). In many patients (especially those with large prostates) both mechanisms play a role. Currently, there are two major classes of drugs used in the management of BPH. Static or mechanical obstruction is due to the growth of acinar and stromal tissue under androgenic stimulation by testosterone and dihydrotestosterone. Antiandrogenic drugs such as 5α-reductase inhibitors are used to counteract mechanical enlargement. The dynamic component is a function of an increase in smooth muscle tone of the prostate and bladder neck leading to constriction of the bladder outlet. Smooth muscle tone is mediated by adrenergic receptors. Blockade of these adrenoreceptors can cause these smooth muscles to relax, resulting in an improvement in urine flow rate and a reduction in symptoms of BPH. Recent evidence also suggests that a blockade of adrenergic receptors may have central nervous system effects that may cause dizziness and other side effects.[2-6,10,11,13,14,16,17,21,25,26,28,38-56]

α-ADRENERGIC RECEPTORS: STRUCTURE AND CLASSIFICATION

Adrenergic receptors are classified as α and β receptors on the basis of their distribution, structure, and mechanism of action, and effects on the target organ.[2-6,10,11,13,14,16,17,21,25,26,28,38-56] Beta-receptors are present in vessels, heart, lungs, and other endocrine structures. Essentially, both types of receptors are *transmembrane proteins* made up of seven helices, an *extracellular domain*, and an *intracellular domain*. The extracellular domain acts as a site for the attachment of norepinephrine, while the intracellular domain is linked with a *G protein*, which activates the *adenyl cyclase system*, resulting in the formation of *cyclic AMP* (second messenger). The *cyclic AMP* in turn activates *protein kinase* to bring about an intracellular response.

Alpha receptors are grouped as α-1 and α-2 receptors. α-1 receptors are *postjunctional* in location and mediate contractions of smooth muscles in the prostate; α-2 receptors are widely distributed, *presynaptic* in location and serve as control mechanisms during synaptic and neuromuscular junction transmission. Alpha-2 receptor blockade results in a variety of systemic and cardiovascular effects due to their wide distribution.

Structurally, α-2 receptors are similar to β-receptors in being transmembrane proteins linked to the G protein system. Alpha-2 receptors involve *inhibitory G protein* (Gs) to cause deactivation of the adenyl cyclase systems and cyclic-AMP production. Alpha-1 receptors are also structurally similar but involve a *G protein–G plc* (G protein for phospholipase c) to activate intracellular calcium release while another intermediary-DAG (diacylglycerol) activates a protein kinase C. Both of these reactions result in smooth muscle contractions.

α-1 RECEPTOR SUBTYPES

Various studies have demonstrated that α-1 receptors predominate in the normal prostate. Since α-1 receptors are also present in various non-prostatic smooth muscles, they are not entirely uroselective. The prostate-specific subtype of the α-1a receptor is termed α-1 and contributes to 70% of all prostatic α-1 receptors. Alpha receptors can either be native (denoted by capital suffix) or cloned (denoted by lower case suffix). The true native α receptors are called α1a, α1b, and α1d in recent classifications proposed by the International Union of Pharmacology (IUPHAR). Their cloned counterparts are termed as α-1a, α-1b, and α-1d. In the older classification cloned 1A was called 1c, 1a/1b. Recently in addition to the wild type α1a, three other carboxyl terminal splice variants of α1a have also been cloned (see chapter 11). The significance of this receptor is still unknown.[17,25,28,47,49,51–53,56–73]

THERAPEUTIC IMPLICATIONS OF VARIOUS α-RECEPTOR SUBTYPES

Recognition of cloned prostate-specific, smooth muscle-specific adrenergic receptors (1a, previously called 1c) have major therapeutic implications, since their blockade spares other subtypes of adrenergic receptors. As reviewed in other chapters, several drugs have been used as α-blockers for the management of BPH. They vary in their receptor specificity, duration of action, dosing schedule, clinical response, and safety profiles.[17,25,28,47,49,51–53,56–73]

CLINICAL PHARMACOLOGY OF TAMSULOSIN

Tamsulosin hydrochloride is an antagonist of α-1 adrenoreceptors in the prostate. Tamsulosin [(–)-S-[2-[[2-(o-ethoxyphenoxy) ethyl]amino] propyl]-2-methoxybenzene-sulfonamide HCl] is a sulfamoylphenethylamine derivative that is a potent and selective α-1A-receptor antagonist. Tamsulosin hydrochloride appears as white crystals that are sparingly soluble in water and insoluble in ether. The molecular weight is 444.98. Each capsule for oral administration contains 0.4 mg of the active agent. In preclinical trials, tamsulosin has been shown to have 13 times more efficacy for prostatic smooth muscle compared with urethral smooth muscles. Other studies have revealed that tamsulosin has 10 to 12 times higher affinity for prostatic receptors as opposed to vascular and extra prostatic tissue. Recent changes in nomenclature of α-blockers reveal that α-1a receptors predominate in the prostate, while α-1b and α-1d receptors predominate in the vascular smooth muscle. There is also data that the bladder has 1-d receptors (see chapter 11).Tamsulosin belongs to a class of α-1A-receptor antagonists that has preferred selectivity for prostatic smooth muscle, although it does have some binding to vascular smooth muscle receptors also. Tamsulosin binding is remarkable for its significantly lower degree of nonspecific binding compared with other receptor antagonists.[27–30,32,34,35,47,52,62,63,65, 69–72,74–93]

Recently, Kurimoto and associates[94] attempted to evaluate the histological structure of BPH and its relationship with the density of α-1 adrenoceptors in smooth muscle. Specimens from hyperplastic tissues obtained from 14 patients with BPH were evaluated for the density of α-1 adrenoceptors in smooth muscle using autoradiography, Mallory–Azan staining, and computer-assisted image analyses. The binding of [3H] tamsulosin (a selective α-1-blocker) and the ratio of smooth muscle area was calculated, and the density of α-1 adrenoceptors per area of smooth muscle determined by dividing the degree of binding by the ratio of smooth muscle to total area. There was a significant difference between the ratio of smooth muscle area in the hyperplastic acinar nodule and the surrounding stroma ($P < 0.01$). The density of α-1 adrenoceptor per smooth muscle area was significantly higher in the hyperplastic acinar nodule than in the surrounding stroma ($P < 0.05$). There was no correlation between prostatic weight and the ratio of smooth muscle area or the density of α-adrenoceptors in each region.[94]

PHARMACOKINETICS

Absorption of tamsulosin from tamsulosin 0.4-mg capsules is essentially complete (over 90%) following oral administration under fasting conditions. Tamsulosin exhibits linear kinetics following single and multiple dosing, achieving steady-state concentrations by the fifth day of once-a-day dosing. The time of maximum concentration (C_{max}) is reached by 4–5 h under fasting conditions and by 6–7 h when tamsulosin is administered with food. Taking tamsulosin under fasting conditions results in a 30% increase in bioavailability and a 40–70% increase in peak concentrations. Tamsulosin is widely distributed to most tissues, including kidney, prostate, liver, gallbladder, heart, aorta, and brown fat, and is minimally distributed in the brain, spinal cord, and testes. Tamsulosin is extensively bound to human plasma proteins (94–99%), primarily α-1 acid glycoprotein (AAG) with linear binding over a wide concentration range (20–600 ng ml^{-1}).[27–30,32,34,35,47,52,62,63,65,69–72,74–93]

There is no enantiometric bioconversion from tamsulosin [R(–) isomer] to the S(+) isomer in humans. Tamsulosin is extensively metabolized by cytochrome P-450 enzymes in the liver, and less than 10% of the dose is excreted in urine unchanged. However, the pharmacokinetics profile of the metabolites in humans has not been established. Additionally, the cytochrome P-450 enzymes that primarily catalyze the Phase 1 metabolism of tamsulosin have not been conclusively identified. Therefore, possible interactions with other cytochrome P-450 metabolized compounds cannot be discerned with current information. The metabolites of tamsulosin undergo extensive conjugation to glucuronide or sulfate prior to renal excretion.[27–30,32,34,35,47,52,62,63,65,69–72,74–93]

Incubations with human liver microsomes showed no evidence of clinically significant metabolic interactions between tamsulosin and amitriptyline, albuterol (β-agonist), glyburide (glibenclamide), and finasteride (5α-reductase inhibitor for treatment of BPH). However, results of the testing *in vitro* of the tamsulosin interaction with diclofenac and warfarin were equivocal. On administration of the radiolabeled dose of tamsulosin to four healthy volunteers, 97% of the administered radioactivity was recovered, with urine (76%), representing the primary route of excretion compared with feces (21%) over 168 h. Following intravenous or oral administration of an immediate-release formulation, the elimination half-life of tamsulosin in plasma ranges from 5 to 7 h.[27–30,32,34,35,47,52,62,63,65,69–72,74–93]

The pharmacokinetics of tamsulosin have been compared in six subjects with mild–moderate ($30<CL_{cr}<70$ mL min^{-1} per 1.73 m^2) or moderate–severe ($10<CL_{cr}<30$ mL min^{-1} per 1.73 m^2) renal impairment and six normal subjects ($CL_{cr}<90$ mL min^{-1} per 1.73 m^2). Although a change in the overall plasma concentration of tamsulosin was observed as a result of altered binding to AAG, the unbound (active) concentration of tamsulosin, as well as the intrinsic clearance, remained relatively constant. Therefore, patients with renal impairment do not require an adjustment in tamsulosin dosing. However, patients with end-stage renal disease ($Cl_{cr}<10$ mL min^{-1} per 1.73 m^2) have not been studied.[27–30,32, 34,35,47,52,62,63,65,69–72,74–93]

The pharmacokinetics of tamsulosin have been compared in eight subjects with moderate hepatic dysfunction (Child–Pugh's classification: grades A and B) and eight normal subjects. While a change in the overall plasma concentration of tamsulosin was observed as the result of altered binding to AAG, the unbound (active) concentration of tamsulosin does not change significantly, with only a modest (32%) change in intrinsic clearance of unbound tamsulosin. Therefore, patients with moderate hepatic dysfunction do not require an adjustment in tamsulosin dosage.[27–30,32,34,35,47,52,62,63,65, 69–72,74–93]

In a recent study, Taguchi and associates[95] performed a pharmacokinetic analysis of tamsulosin and terazosin. Following ingestion of tamsulosin, median peak plasma levels of 16 ng mL^{-1} were reached after 5 h and declined to 2 ng mL^{-1} at 23.5 h. The time course in the radioreceptor assay was similar and, at most time points, binding to α-1a adrenoceptors was significantly greater than to α-1b and α-1d adrenoceptors. Following ingestion of terazosin, median peak plasma levels of 91 ng mL^{-1} were reached after 1 h and declined to 11 ng mL^{-1} at 23.5 h. In the radioreceptor assay, binding also peaked at 1 h and declined thereafter, but even after 23.5 h considerable binding activity remained detectable at all three subtypes. At most time points, binding to the α-1a and α-1d adrenoceptor was significantly greater than to the α-1b adrenoceptor. Authors concluded that the discordance between terazosin blood levels as determined by h.p.l.c. and radioreceptor assay at late time points indicates the possible involvement of metabolites on terazosin effects *in vivo*.

DRUG–DRUG INTERACTIONS

NIFEDIPINE, ATENOLOL, ENALAPRIL, WARFARIN, THEOPHYLLINE, CIMETIDE

In three studies in hypertensive subjects (age range 47–79 years) whose blood pressure was controlled with stable doses of Procardia XL, atenolol, or enalapril for at least 3 months, tamsulosin 0.4 mg for 7 days followed by tamsulosin 0.8 mg for another 7 days ($n=8$ per study) resulted in no clinically significant effects on blood pressure and pulse rate compared with placebo ($n=4$ per study). Therefore, dosage adjustments of these medications are unnecessary when tamsulosin is administered concomitantly. A definitive drug–drug interaction study between tamsulosin and warfarin was not conducted. Therefore, caution should be exercised with concomitant administration of warfarin and tamsulosin. In two studies in healthy volunteers ($n = 10$ per study; age range 19–39 years) receiving tamsulosin 0.4 mg day^{-1} for 2 days, followed by tamsulosin 0.8 mg day^{-1} for 5–8 days, single intravenous doses of digoxin 0.5 mg or theophylline did not result in any side effects.[30]

The pharmacokinetics and pharmacodynamic interaction between tamsulosin 0.8 mg day^{-1} (steady state) and furosemide 20 mg intravenously (single dose) was evaluated in 10 healthy volunteers (age range 21–40 years). Tamsulosin had no effect on the pharmacodynamics (excretion of electrolytes) of furosemide. While furosemide produced an 11–12% reduction in tamsulosin C_{max} and AUC, these changes are expected to be clinically insignificant and do not require adjustment of the tamsulosin dosage.[30]

The effects of cimetidine at the highest recommended dose (400 mg every 6 h for 6 days) on the pharmacokinetics of a single tamsulosin 0.4 mg dose were investigated in 10 healthy volunteers (age range 21–38 years). Treatment with cimetidine resulted in a significant decrease (26%) in the clearance of tamsulosin, which resulted in a moderate increase in tamsulosin AUC (44%). Therefore, tamsulosin should be used with caution in combination with cimetidine, particularly at doses higher than 0.4 mg.[30]

No laboratory test interactions with tamsulosin are known. Treatment with tamsulosin for up to 12 months had no significant effect on prostate-specific antigen.[30]

TAMSULOSIN AND CARCINOGENESIS

Male rats administered doses of up to 43 mg kg^{-1} day^{-1} and female rats administered 52 mg kg^{-1} day^{-1} had no increases in tumor incidence with the exception of a modest increase in the frequency of mammary gland fibroadenomas in female rats receiving doses >5.4 mg kg^{-1} ($P < 0.015$). The highest doses of tamsulosin evaluated in the rat carcinogenicity study were systemic exposures (AUC) in rats that were three times the exposures in men receiving the maximum therapeutic dose of 0.8 mg day^{-1}.[30]

Mice were administered doses up to 127 mg kg^{-1} day^{-1} in males and 158 mg kg^{-1} day^{-1} in females. There were no significant tumor findings in male mice. Female mice treated for 2 years with the two highest doses of 45 and 158 mg kg^{-1} day^{-1} had statistically significant increases in the incidence of mammary gland fibroadenomas ($P < 0.0001$) and adenocarcinomas ($P < 0.0075$). The highest dose levels of tamsulosin evaluated in the mice carcinogenicity study produced systemic exposures (AUC) in mice that were eight times the exposures in men receiving the maximum therapeutic dose of 0.8 mg day[-1].[30]

The increased incidences of mammary gland neoplasms in female rats and mice were considered secondary to tamsulosin-induced hyperprolactinemia. It is not known whether tamsulosin elevates prolactin in humans. The relevance for human risk of the findings of prolactin-mediated endocrine tumors in rodents is not known.[30]

Tamsulosin produced no evidence of mutagenic potential *in vitro* in the Ames reverse mutation test, mouse lymphoma thymidine kinase assay, unscheduled DNA repair synthesis assay, and chromosomal aberration assays in Chinese hamster ovary cells or human lymphocytes. There were no mutagenic effects in the in vivo sister chromatic exchange and mouse micronucleus assay.[30]

Studies in rats revealed significantly reduced fertility in males dosed with single or multiple daily doses of 300 mg kg[-1] day[-1] of tamsulosin (AUC exposure in rats about 50 times the human exposure with the maximum therapeutic dose). The mechanism of decreased fertility in male rats is considered to be an effect on the compound on the vaginal plug formation, possibly due to changes of semen content or impairment of ejaculation. The effects on fertility were reversible, showing improvement by 3 days after a single dose and 4 weeks after multiple dosing. Effects on fertility in males were completely reversed within 9 weeks of discontinuation of multiple dosing. Multiple doses of 10 and 100 mg kg[-1] day[-1] tamsulosin (1/5 and 16 times the anticipated human AUC exposure) did not significantly alter fertility in male rats. Effects of tamsulosin on sperm counts or sperm function have not been evaluated.[27,28,31,33,36,74,96,97]

Studies in female rats revealed significant reductions in fertility after single or multiple dosing with 300 mg kg[-1] day[-1] of the *R*-isomer or racemic mixture of tamsulosin, respectively. In female rats, the reductions in fertility after single doses were considered to be associated with impairments in fertilization. Multiple dosing with 10 or 100 mg kg[-1] day[-1] of the racemic mixture did not significantly alter fertility in female rats.[84]

ADVERSE REACTIONS

The incidence of treatment-emergent adverse events has been ascertained from six short-term US and European placebo-controlled clinical trials in which daily doses of 0.1–0.8 mg tamsulosin were used. These studies evaluated safety in 1783 patients treated with tamsulosin and 798 patients administered placebo. Table 12.1 summarizes the treatment-emergent adverse events that occurred in >2% of patients receiving either tamsulosin 0.4 mg, or 0.8 mg and at an incidence numerically higher than that in the placebo group during two 13-week US trials (US92-03A and US93-01) conducted in 1486 men.

In the two US studies, symptomatic postural hypotension was reported by 0.2% of patients (1 of 502) in the 0.4 mg group, 0.4% of patients (2 of 492) in the 0.8 mg group, and by no patients in the placebo group. Syncope

was reported by 0.2% of patients (1 of 502) in the 0.4 mg group, 0.4% of patients (2 of 492) in the 0.8 mg group, and by 0.6% of patients (3 of 493) in the placebo group.

In a recent study, de Mey and associates[98] compared orthostatic effects of tamsulosin with terazosin in 50 elderly normotensive male volunteers (mean age 68 years, range 61–78; 27 men with LUTS). The baseline blood pressure values were slightly higher in the tamsulosin (TAM) group, but under treatment there was little difference between the treatments with regard to circadian changes in ambulatory blood pressure and heart rate. Under terazosin (TER), there were 10 incidents of symptomatic hypotensive episodes in 9 subjects (2 with syncope); furthermore, there were 24 events of asymptomatic exaggerated ($\geq$ 20 mmHg) decrease in systolic blood pressure in 12 subjects. With TAM in contrast, there was only 1 subject who experienced symptomatic hypotensive episode on three occasions (this subject had a previous history of vertigo and ought not to have been included); 7 subjects on TAM showed 16 incidents of asymptomatic hypotensive episodes. The difference between TER and TAM was statistically significant for the number of subjects with positive symptomatic Orthostatic hypertension (P = 0.011). The authors concluded that once-daily dosing of TAM after breakfast at a fixed dose level (0.4 mg) offered a more efficient protection against undesired cardiovascular extension effects in the normotensive elderly treated for LUTS than with terazosin with step-up doses (1–5 mg) administered at night.

Abnormal ejaculation was associated with tamsulosin administration and was dose-related in the US studies. Withdrawal from these clinical studies because of abnormal ejaculation was also dose-dependent, with 8 of 492 patients (1.6%) in the 0.8 mg group and no patients in the 0.4 mg or placebo groups discontinuing treatment due to abnormal ejaculation.[27,28,30,31,33,36,74,96,97]

CLINICAL STUDIES

A total of 2296 patients were enrolled in four placebo-controlled clinical studies and one active-controlled clinical study (1003 received tamsulosin 0.4 mg once daily, 491 received tamsulosin 0.8 mg once daily, and 803 were control patients) in the US and Europe.[27,28,30,31,33,36,74,96,97]

In the two placebo-controlled, double-blind, 13 week, multicenter studies in the USA (Study 1 (US92-03A) and Study 2 (US93-01)), 1486 men with the signs and symptoms of BPH were enrolled. In both studies, patients were randomized to placebo, tamsulosin 0.4 mg once daily, or tamsulosin 0.8 mg once daily. Patients in the tamsulosin 0.8 mg once-daily treatment groups received a dose of 0.4 mg once daily for 1 week before increasing to the 0.8 mg once-daily dose. The primary efficacy assessments included (1) total American Urological Association (AUA) symptom score questionnaire, which evaluated irritative (frequency, urgency, and nocturia), and obstructive (hesitancy, incomplete emptying, intermittency, and weak stream) symptoms, where a decrease in score is consistent with improvement in

Drug agent	Mechanism of action	Pharmacokinetics	Dosing/administration	Adverse reactions
Phenoxybenzamine	• α-1 and α-2 adrenoceptor antagonist • Short acting • Irreversible antagonist • Increases blood flow to skin, mucosa, and abdominal viscera	• IV T½–24 h • Duration of action = 3–4 days, and the effects of daily administration are cumulative for nearly 1 week • Hepatic metabolism	• 5–10 mg b.i.d. orally • Requires dose titration when initiating therapy	Postural hypotension, inhibited ejaculation with retrograde ejaculation, nasal congestion, nausea/vomiting, tachycardia, miosis
Prazosin	• α-1 adrenoceptor antagonist • Short acting • Reversible antagonist • Severely decreases diasystolic BP	• High first-pass hepatic metabolism with bile excretion • After oral administration, peak plasma concentration is reached in 3 hours • T½ = 2–3 h	• 1–5 mg b.i.d. orally • Requires dose titration when initiating therapy	Syncope, postural hypotension, dizziness, nasal congestion, fluid retention
Alfuzosin	• α-1 adrenoceptor antagonist • Reversible antagonist • Short acting	• Elimination metabolic peak plasma effects noted in1–2 hours • T½ = 2–3 hours	• 3–4 mg t.i.d. orally • Requires dose titration when initiating therapy	Syncope, postural hypotension, dizziness, nasal congestion, fluid retention
Terazosin	• α-1 adrenoceptor antagonist • Reversible antagonist • Long acting	• Hepatic metabolism with metabolite excreted in urine (40%) and bile/feces (60%) • Minimal first-pass effect • After oral administration, peak plasma concentration is reached in 40 min • T½ = 12 h	• 2–10 mg q.d. orally • Requires dose titration when initiating therapy • Treatment should be initiated with a 1 mg dose given at bedtime	Syncope, postural hypotension, dizziness, asthenia, impotence, flu-like syndrome, headache
Doxazosin	• α-1 adrenoceptor antagonist • Reversible antagonist • Long acting	• High first-pass hepatic metabolism with enterohepatic recycling • After oral dose, peak plasma concentration is reached in 2–3 h • T½ = 22 h	• 4–8 mg q.d. orally • Requires dose titration when initiating therapy	Syncope, postural hypotension, dizziness, headache
Tamsulosin	• α-1A adrenoceptor antagonist • Reversible antagonist • Long acting	• Hepatic metabolism with metabolite excreted in urine • After oral administration, peak plasma concentration is reached in 5 days • T½ = 9–13 h	• 0.4 mg or 0.8 mg q.d. orally • Should be given half hour after breakfast	Postural hypotension, syncope, dizziness, abnormal ejaculation (includes ejaculation failure, ejaculation disorder, retrograde ejaculation, and ejaculation decrease)

Table 12.1 Summary of α-adrenergic antagonists. All of the α-blockers (except α1a specific subtype blockers) require 2–4 weeks of treatment before therapeutic effects can be seen

symptoms; and (2) peak urine flow rate, where an increased peak urine flow rate value over baseline is consistent with decreased urinary obstruction. Mean changes from baseline to week 13 in total AUA symptom score were significantly greater for groups treated with tamsulosin 0.4 mg and 0.8 mg once daily compared with placebo in both US studies (Table 12.2). The changes from baseline to week 13 in peak urine flow rate were also significantly greater for the tamsulosin 0.4 mg and 0.8 mg once-daily groups compared with placebo in Study 1 and for the tamsulosin 0.8 mg once-daily group in Study 2 (Table 12.2). Overall there were no significant differences in improvement observed in total AUA symptom scores or peak urine flow rates between the 0.4 mg and the 0.8 mg dose groups, with the exception that the 0.8 mg dose in Study 1 had a significantly greater improvement in total AUA symptom score compared with

Side effect	Terazosin[a]			Doxazosin[b]			Tamsulosin[c]		
	Terazozin (%)	Placebo (%)	P value	Doxazosin (%)	Placebo (%)	P value	Tamsulosin (%)	Placebo (%)	P value
1. Asthenia/fatigue	7.4	3.3	<0.05	8.0	1.7	<0.05	11	9.0	NS
2. Postural hypotension	3.9	0.8	<0.05	–	–	–	1	1.0	NS
3. Dizziness	9.1	4.2	<0.05	15.6	9.0	<0.05	20	15.0	NS
4. Discontinued due to side effects	20	1.2	NS	12	4.0	NS	9	8	NS

[a] From the package drug insert of terazosin
[b] From the package drug insert of doxazosin
[c] Data from the use of FDA approved dose of tamsulosin (0.4 mg in US93.01 Study)

Table 12.2 Comparative table for cardiovascular side effects with the use of terazosin, doxazosin, and tamsulosin in the USA

the 0.4 mg dose (data in file with Boehringer Ingelheim Pharmaceuticals, Inc., Ridgefield, CT).

In the meta-analysis of two European studies, Chapple[27] evaluated the efficacy and safety of modified-release tamsulosin 0.4 mg once daily compared with placebo in patients with benign prostatic enlargement, lower urinary tract symptoms, and prostatic obstruction. Patients entered a 2-week placebo run-in period, followed by randomization to treatment with tamsulosin (382 patients) or placebo (193 patients) once daily for 12 weeks. Maximum urinary flow rate improved to a greater extent in the tamsulosin group (1.6 mL s^{-1}, 16%) than the placebo group (0.6 mL s^{-1}, 6%) ($P = 0.002$). Total Boyarsky symptom score also improved to a greater extent in the tamsulosin group (3.3 points, 35.1% reduction) than the placebo group (2.4 points, 25.5% reduction) ($P = 0.002$). Significantly more tamsulosin patients (66%) than placebo patients (49%) had an $\geq 25\%$ decrease in total symptom score at the endpoint ($P < 0.001$). Twelve weeks of treatment with tamsulosin also produced significant improvements in the average urinary flow rate ($P = 0.005$) and voiding or "obstructive" ($P = 0.008$) and storage or "irritative" ($P = 0.017$) symptom scores. The incidence of drug-related adverse events was comparable for the tamsulosin and placebo groups (13 and 12%, respectively; $P = 0.802$). The same applies to the incidence of adverse events commonly attributed to α-1-adrenoceptor antagonists, such as dizziness, headache, postural hypotension, syncope, asthenia, somnolence, and rhinitis. There were no clinically significant changes in blood pressure or pulse rate in tamsulosin patients compared with placebo patients in either hypertensive or normotensive BPH patients.

In the other open-label extension study, Schulman and associates[33] evaluated the efficacy and safety of tamsulosin (0.4 mg as a modified-release formulation) once daily in patients with benign prostatic enlargement, lower urinary tract symptoms, and benign prostatic obstruction (symptomatic BPH) for up to 60 weeks. Patients were enrolled from two European, 12-week, placebo-controlled trials. This 60-week interim analysis included the patients ($n = 244$) randomized to tamsulosin in the two placebo-controlled trials. The significant improvements in the primary efficacy parameters, maximum urinary flow rate, and total Boyarsky symptom score that were observed during the placebo-controlled trials were sustained throughout the long-term extension study. Mean Q_{max} improved from baseline (before initiation of tamsulosin) to endpoint by 13.7% ($P < 0.001$) and remained between 11.5 and 12 mL s^{-1} during the entire follow-up period. Total Boyarsky symptom score improved by 36.2% from baseline to endpoint ($P < 0.001$). Similarly, the percentage of treatment responders, defined as an increase in Q_{max} of $\geq 30\%$ or a decrease in total symptom score of $\geq 25\%$, remained constant throughout the 60-week period. At endpoint, 69% of patients demonstrated this clinically significant total Boyarsky symptom score response. During the 60-week study period, 51 patients (21%) experienced an adverse event considered to be possibly or probably related to study medication, the most common of which were dizziness and abnormal ejaculation, both occurring in 5% of patients. There were no clinically significant changes in blood pressure or pulse rate during the study.[33]

Lepor[99] recently updated on a 40-week extension data of a Phase III multicenter placebo-controlled, double-blind outpatient trial involving 618 patients. Four hundred and eighteen patients (68%) continued into the extension phase on the same double-blind medication and dose. The mean changes in AUA symptom score from baseline to endpoint were statistically significant in all groups ($P < 0.001$). Significant improvements were observed in Q_{max} for both tamsulosin groups but not for the placebo group. The statistically significant improvements from baseline in efficacy parameters were maintained during the long-term extension phase. Tamsulosin at both dosages was well tolerated as maintenance therapy. Clinically significant orthostatic hypotension was not observed. Vital sign changes in either hypertensive or normotensive patients were not clinically significantly different across the three groups. Tamsulosin once daily at 0.4 or 0.8 mg was shown to be effective, safe, and well tolerated in the target BPH population during long-term use. The clinical relevance of $\alpha 1$ selectivity was recently addressed in several studies (see chapter 11). These studies collectively suggest that $\alpha 1a$ receptor preferential binding of tamsulosin may have clinical relevance in not reducing blood pressure in normotensive men and by reducing incidence of orthostatic events.

Overall, tamsulosin has several advantages: its long action allows for once-a-day dosing. Its therapeutic effect, as indicated by improvements in symptoms score is realised as early as one week after treatment. This is because the optimal dose is started from day 1. Additional advantages include the lack of side effects, even in patients at risk of postural hypotension such as the elderly and those on multiple cardiac medication; patients who have comorbid conditions such as diabetes and cardiac disease. Finally, the lower side effect profile of tamsulosin may also allow its use in combination with other relaxants and newer agents in the treatment of LUTS.

REFERENCES

1 Isaacs JT, Coffey DS. Etiology and disease process of benign prostatic hyperplasia. *Prostate Suppl* 1989; **2**: 33–50.

2 Caine M, Raz S. Some clinical implications of adrenergic receptors in the urinary tract. *Arch Surg* 1975; **110**: 247–50.

3 Caine M, Raz S, Zeigler M. Adrenergic and cholinergic receptors in the human prostate, prostatic capsule and bladder neck. *Br J Urol* 1975; **47**: 193–202.

4 Caine M, Pfau A, Perlberg S. The use of alpha-adrenergic blockers in benign prostatic obstruction. *Br J Urol* 1976; **48**: 255–63.

5 Caine M. The importance of adrenergic receptors in disorders of micturition. *Eur Urol* 1977; **3**: 1–6.

6 Caine M, Perlberg S. Dynamics of acute retention in prostatic patient and role of adrenergic receptors. *Urology* 1977; **9**: 399–403.

7 Caine M, Perlberg S, Meretyk S. A placebo-controlled double-blind study of the effect of phenoxybenzamine in benign prostatic obstruction. *Br J Urol* 1978; **50**: 551–4.

8 Caine M. Phenoxybenzamine for benign prostatic hypertrophy. *Compr Ther* 1979; **5**: 7–11.

9 Caine M, Perlberg S, Shapiro A. Phenoxybenzamine for benign prostatic obstruction. Review of 200 cases. *Urology* 1981; **17**: 542–6.

10 Caine M. Alpha-adrenergic mechanisms in dynamics of benign prostatic hypertrophy. *Urology* 1988; **32**: 16–20.

11 Caine M. Alpha-adrenergic blockers for the treatment of benign prostatic hyperplasia. *Urol Clin North Am* 1990; **17**: 641–9.

12 Hatano A, Tang R, Walden PD, Lepor H. The alpha-adrenoceptor antagonist properties of the enantiomers of doxazosin in the human prostate. *Eur J Pharmacol* 1996; **313**: 135–43.

13 Lepor H. The emerging role of alpha antagonists in the therapy of benign prostatic hyperplasia. *J Androl* 1991; **12**: 389–94.

14 Lepor H, Gup DI, Baumann M, Shapiro E. Comparison of alpha 1 adrenoceptors in the prostate capsule of men with symptomatic and asymptomatic benign prostatic hyperplasia. *Br J Urol* 1991; **67**: 493–8.

15 Lepor H, Henry D, Laddu AR. The efficacy and safety of terazosin for the treatment of symptomatic BPH. *Prostate* 1991; **18**: 345–55.

16 Lepor H, Shapiro E. Prostatic alpha adrenoceptors. *Prog Clin Biol Res* 1994; **386**: 271–7.

17 Lepor H, Tang R, Kobayashi S et al. Localization of the alpha 1A-adrenoceptor in the human prostate. *J Urol* 1995; **154**: 2096–9.

18 Jonler M, Riehmann M, Brinkmann R, Bruskewitz RC. Benign prostatic hyperplasia. *Endocrinol Metab Clin North Am* 1994; **23**: 795–807.

19 Jonler M, Riehmann M, Bruskewitz RC. Benign prostatic hyperplasia. Current pharmacological treatment. *Drugs* 1994; **47**: 66–81.

20 Kaplan SA, Meade DAP, Quinones S, Soldo KA. Doxazosin in physiologically and pharmacologically normotensive men with benign prostatic hyperplasia. *Urology* 1995; **46**: 512–7.

21 Chapple CR, Aubry ML, James S et al. Characterisation of human prostatic adrenoceptors using pharmacology receptor binding and localisation. *Br J Urol* 1989; **63**: 487–96.

22 Chapple CR. Alfuzosin for benign prostatic hypertrophy. *Lancet* 1991; **338**: 182.

23 Chapple CR, Noble JG, Milroy EJ. Comparative study of selective alpha 1-adrenoceptor blockade versus surgery in the treatment of prostatic obstruction. *Br J Urol* 1993; **72**: 822–5.

24 Chapple CR, Carter P, Christmas TJ et al. A three month double-blind study of doxazosin as treatment for benign prostatic bladder outlet obstruction. *Br J Urol* 1994; **74**: 50–6.

25 Chapple CR, Burt RP, Andersson PO et al. Alpha 1-adrenoceptor subtypes in the human prostate. *Br J Urol* 1994; **74**: 585–9.

26 Chapple CR. Alpha-adrenergic blocking drugs in bladder outflow obstruction: what potential has alpha 1-adrenoceptor selectivity? *Br J Urol* 1995; **76** (Suppl 1): 47–55.

27 Chapple CR, Wyndaele JJ, Nordling J et al. Tamsulosin, the first prostate-selective alpha 1A-adrenoceptor antagonist. A meta-analysis of two randomized, placebo-controlled, multicentre studies in patients with benign prostatic obstruction (symptomatic BPH). European Tamsulosin Study Group. *Eur Urol* 1996; **29**: 155–67.

28 Chapple CR. Selective alpha 1-adrenoceptor antagonists in benign prostatic hyperplasia: rationale and clinical experience. *Eur Urol* 1996; **29**: 129–44.

29 Andersson KE, Lepor H, Wyllie MG. Prostatic alpha 1-adrenoceptors and uroselectivity. *Prostate* 1997; **30**: 202–15.

30 Boehringer Ingelheim Pharmaceuticals, Inc., Ridgefield, CT 06877. *Tamsulosin Hydrochloride*, In Drug Package Insert, 1998.

31 Kawabe K. Efficacy and safety of tamsulosin in the treatment of benign prostatic hyperplasia. *Br J Urol* 1995; **76**(Suppl 1): 63–7.

32 Koiso K, Akaza H, Kikuchi K et al. Pharmacokinetics of tamsulosin hydrochloride in patients with renal impairment: effects of alpha 1-acid glycoprotein. *J Clin Pharmacol* 1996; **36**: 1029–38.

33 Schulman CC, Cortvriend J, Jonas U, Lock TM, Vaage S, Speakman MJ. Tamsulosin, the first prostate-selective alpha 1A-adrenoceptor antagonist. Analysis of a multinational, multicentre, open-label study assessing the long-term efficacy and safety in patients with benign prostatic obstruction (symptomatic BPH). European Tamsulosin Study Group. *Eur Urol* 1996; **29**: 145–54.

34 Sudoh K, Tanaka H, Inagaki O et al. Effect of tamsulosin, a novel alpha 1-adrenoceptor antagonist, on urethral pressure profile in anaesthetized dogs. *J Auton Pharmacol* 1996; **16**: 147–54.

35 Taguchi K, Saitoh M, Sato S et al. Effects of tamsulosin metabolites at alpha-1 adrenoceptor subtypes. *J Pharmacol Exp Ther* 1997; **280**: 1–5.

36 Wilde MI, McTavish D. Tamsulosin. A review of its pharmacological properties and therapeutic potential in the management of symptomatic benign prostatic hyperplasia. *Drugs* 1996; **52**: 883–98.

37 Narayan P, Tewari A. Overview of alpha-blocker therapy of BPH. *Urology* 1998; **51**(4A Suppl): 38–45.

38 Abrams P. Objective evaluation of bladder outlet obstruction. *Br J Urol* 1995; **76**(Suppl 1): 11–15.

39 Abrams P, Donovan JL, de la Rosette JJ, Schafer W. International Continence Society "Benign Prostatic Hyperplasia" Study: background, aims, and methodology. *Neurourol Urodyn* 1997; **16**: 79–91.

40 Abrams P. Urodynamic effects of doxazosin in men with lower urinary tract symptoms and benign prostatic obstruction. Results from three double-blind placebo-controlled studies. *Eur Urol* 1997; **32**: 39–46.

41 Andersson KE. Prostatic and extraprostatic alpha-adrenoceptors – contributions to the lower urinary tract symptoms in benign prostatic hyperplasia. *Scand J Urol Nephrol* 1996; **179**(Suppl): 105–11.

42 Appell RA. Pathogenesis and medical management of benign prostatic hyperplasia. *Semin Nephrol* 1994; **14**: 531–43.

43 Barry MJ, Cockett AT, Holtgrewe HL et al. Relationship of symptoms of prostatism to commonly used physiological and anatomical measures of the severity of benign prostatic hyperplasia. *J Urol* 1993; **150**: 351–8.

44 Barry MJ, O'Leary MP. Advances in benign prostatic hyperplasia. The developmental and clinical utility of symptom scores. *Urol Clin North Am* 1995; **22**: 299–307.

45 Boyarsky S, Jones G, Paulson DF, Prout GR Jr. A new look at bladder neck obstruction by the Food and Drug Administration regulators: guidelines for investigation of benign prostatic hypertrophy. *Trans Am Assoc Genitourin Surg* 1977; **68**: 29–32.

46 Boyle P. New insights into the epidemiology and natural history of benign prostatic hyperplasia. *Prog Clin Biol Res* 1994; **386**: 3–18.

47 Brune ME, Katwala SP, Milicic I et al. Effects of selective and nonselective alpha-1-adrenoceptor antagonists on intraurethral and arterial pressures in intact conscious dogs. *Pharmacology* 1996; **53**: 356–68.

48 Bruskewitz RC. Benign prostatic hyperplasia: drug and nondrug therapies. *Geriatrics* 1992; **47**: 39–42, 45.

49 Daly CJ, McGrath JC, Wilson VG. Pharmacological analysis of postjunctional alpha-adrenoceptors mediating contractions to (–)-noradrenaline in the rabbit isolated lateral saphenous vein can be explained by interacting responses to simultaneous activation of alpha 1- and alpha 2-adrenoceptors. *Br J Pharmacol* 1988; **95**: 485–500.

50 Daly CJ, McGrath JC, Wilson VG. Evidence that the population of postjunctional-adrenoceptors mediating contraction of smooth muscle in the rabbit isolated ear vein is predominantly alpha 2. *Br J Pharmacol* 1988; **94**: 1085–90.

51 Furukawa K, Chess Williams R, Uchiyama T. Alpha 1B-adrenoceptor subtype mediating the phenylephrine-induced contractile response in rabbit corpus cavernosum penis. *Jpn J Pharmacol* 1996; **71**: 325–31.

52 Garcia Sainz JA, Romero Avila MT, Villalobos Molina R, Minneman KP. Alpha 1-adrenoceptor subtype selectivity of tamsulosin: studies using livers from different species. *Eur J Pharmacol* 1995; **289**: 1–7.

53 Furukawa K, Rosario DJ, Smith DJ, Chapple CR, Uchiyama T, Chess Williams R. Alpha 1A-adrenoceptor-mediated contractile responses of the human vas deferens. *Br J Pharmacol* 1995; **116**: 1605–10.

54 Hanft G, Gross G, Beckeringh JJ, Korstanje C. Alpha 1-adrenoceptors: the ability of various agonists and antagonists to discriminate between two distinct [3H]prazosin binding sites. *J Pharm Pharmacol* 1989; **41**: 714–6.

55 Kawabe K, Moriyama N, Yamada S, Taniguchi N. Rationale for the use of alpha-blockers in the treatment of benign prostatic hyperplasia (BPH). *Int J Urol* 1994; **1**: 203–11.

56 Lepor H, Tang R, Shapiro E. The alpha-adrenoceptor subtype mediating the tension of human prostatic smooth muscle. *Prostate* 1993; **22**: 301–7.

57 Eltze M. Functional evidence for an alpha 1B-adrenoceptor mediating contraction of the mouse spleen. *Eur J Pharmacol* 1996; **311**: 187–98.

58 Hieble JP, Ruffolo RR Jr. The use of alpha-adrenoceptor antagonists in the pharmacological management of benign prostatic hypertrophy: an overview. *Pharmacol Res* 1996; **33**: 145–60.

59 Honda K, Miyata-Osawa A, Takenaka T. Alpha 1-adrenoceptor subtype mediating contraction of the smooth muscle in the lower urinary tract and prostate of rabbits. *Naunyn Schmiedebergs Arch Pharmacol* 1985; **330**: 16–21.

60 Lepor H, Nieder A, Feser J et al. Effect of terazosin on prostatism in men with normal and abnormal peak urinary flow rates. *Urology* 1997; **49**(3): 476–80.

61 Kenny BA, Naylor AM, Carter AJ et al. Effect of alpha 1 adrenoceptor antagonists on prostatic pressure and blood pressure in the anesthetized dog. *Urology* 1994; **44**: 52–7.

62 Yamada S, Tanaka C, Kimura R, Kawabe K. Alpha 1-adrenoceptors in human prostate: characterization and binding characteristics of alpha 1-antagonists. *Life Sci* 1994; **54**: 1845–54.

63 Van der Graaf PH, Shankley NP, Black JW. Analysis of the effects of alpha 1-adrenoceptor antagonists on noradrenaline-mediated contraction of rat small mesenteric artery. *Br J Pharmacol* 1996; **118**: 1308–16.

64 Tseng-Crank J, Kost T, Goetz A et al. The alpha 1C-adrenoceptor in human prostate: cloning, functional expression, and localization to specific prostatic cell types. *Br J Pharmacol* 1995; **115**: 1475–85.

65 Testa R, Guarneri L, Taddei C et al. Functional antagonistic activity of Rec 15/2739, a novel alpha-1 antagonist selective for the lower urinary tract, on noradrenaline-induced contraction of human prostate and mesenteric artery. *J Pharmacol Exp Ther* 1996; **277**: 1237–46.

66 Takeda M, Hatano A, Komeyama T et al. Alpha-1 adrenoceptor subtypes (high, low) in human benign prostatic hypertrophy tissue according to the affinities for prazosin. *Prostate* 1997; **31**: 216–22.

67 Pool JL. Role of the sympathetic nervous system in hypertension and benign prostatic hyperplasia. *Br J Clin Pract Symp Suppl* 1994; **74**: 13–7.

68 Michel MC, Buscher R, Kerker J et al. Alpha 1-adrenoceptor subtype affinities of drugs for the treatment of prostatic hypertrophy. Evidence for heterogeneity of chloroethylclonidine-resistant rat renal alpha 1-adrenoceptor. *Naunyn Schmiedebergs Arch Pharmacol* 1993; **348**: 385–95.

69 Maruyama K, Fukutomi J, Chiba T et al. Two district alpha(1)-adrenoceptor subtypes in the human prostate: assessment by radioligand binding assay using 3H-prazosin. *Gen Pharmacol* 1996; **27**: 1377–81.

70 Martin DJ, Lluel P, Guillot E et al. Comparative alpha-1 adrenoceptor subtype selectivity and functional uroselectivity of alpha-1 adrenoceptor antagonists. *J Pharmacol Exp Ther* 1997; **282**: 228–35.

71 Leonardi A, Hieble JP, Guarneri L et al. Pharmacological characterization of the uroselective alpha-1 antagonist Rec 15/2739 (SB 216469): role of the alpha-1L adrenoceptor in tissue selectivity, part I. *J Pharmacol Exp Ther* 1997; **281**: 1272–83.

72 Lachnit WG, Tran AM, Clarke DE, Ford AP. Pharmacological characterization of an alpha 1A-adrenoceptor mediating contractile responses to noradrenaline in isolated caudal artery of rat. *Br J Pharmacol* 1997; **120**: 819–26.

73 Kenny BA, Miller AM, Williamson IJ et al. Evaluation of the pharmacological selectivity profile of alpha 1 adrenoceptor antagonists at prostatic alpha 1 adrenoceptors: binding, functional and in vivo studies. *Br J Pharmacol* 1996; **118**: 871–8.

74 Abrams P, Schulman CC, Vaage S. Tamsulosin, a selective alpha 1c-adrenoceptor antagonist: a randomized, controlled trial in patients with benign prostatic "obstruction" (symptomatic BPH). The European Tamsulosin Study Group. *Br J Urol* 1995; **76**: 325–36.

75 Chueh SC, Guh JH, Chen J et al. Inhibition by tamsulosin of tension responses of human hyperplastic prostate to electrical field stimulation. *Eur J Pharmacol* 1996; **305**: 177–80.

76 Harada K, Ohmori M, Fujimura A. Comparison of the antagonistic activity of tamsulosin and doxazosin at vascular alpha 1-adrenoceptors in humans. *Naunyn Schmiedebergs Arch Pharmacol* 1996; **354**: 557–61.

77 Kurimoto S, Moriyama N, Hamada K et al. Quantitative autoradiography of alpha 1 adrenoceptors with [3H]tamsulosin in

human hypertrophied prostate using computerized image analysis. *Histochem J* 1995; **27**: 1007–13.

78 Michel MC, Hanft G, Gross G. Functional studies on alpha 1-adrenoceptor subtypes mediating inotropic effects in rat right ventricle. *Br J Pharmacol* 1994; **111**: 539–46.

79 Michel MC, Insel PA. Comparison of cloned and pharmacologically defined rat tissue alpha 1-adrenoceptor subtypes. *Naunyn Schmiedebergs Arch Pharmacol* 1994; **350**: 136–42.

80 Miyatake R, Park YC, Koike H et al. [Urodynamic evaluation of alpha-1 blocker tamsulosin on benign prostatic hyperplasia using pressure-flow study]. *Nippon Hinyokika Gakkai Zasshi* 1996; **87**: 1048–55.

81 Morita M, Numahata K, Ogata Y, Suzuki K. [The concentration of tamsulosin hydrochloride in the blood and prostatic tissue of the patients in benign prostatic hyperplasia]. *Nippon Hinyokika Gakkai Zasshi* 1997; **88**: 535–40.

82 Moriyama N, Akiyama K, Murata S et al. KMD-3213, a novel alpha1 A-adrenoceptor antagonist, potently inhibits the functional alpha1-adrenoceptor in human prostate. *Eur J Pharmacol* 1997; **331**: 39–42.

83 Noble AJ, Chess Williams R, Couldwell C et al. The effects of tamsulosin, a high affinity antagonist at functional alpha 1A- and alpha 1D-adrenoceptor subtypes. *Br J Pharmacol* 1997; **120**: 231–8.

84 Ratnasooriya WD, Wadsworth RM. Tamsulosin, a selective alpha 1-adrenoceptor antagonist, inhibits fertility of male rats. *Andrologia* 1994; **26**: 107–10.

85 Richardson CD, Donatucci CF, Page SO et al. Pharmacology of tamsulosin: saturation-binding isotherms and competition analysis using cloned alpha 1-adrenergic receptor subtypes. *Prostate* 1997; **33**: 55–9.

86 Schmidbauer CP, Madersbacher S. [Current drug therapy of benign prostatic hyperplasia]. *Wien Med Wochenschr* 1996; **146**: 161–4.

87 Soeishi Y, Matsushima H, Watanabe T et al. Absorption, metabolism and excretion of tamsulosin hydrochloride in man. *Xenobiotica* 1996; **26**: 637–45.

88 Soeishi Y, Matsushima H, Teraya Y et al. Metabolism of tamsulosin in rat and dog. *Xenobiotica* 1996; **26**: 355–65.

89 Takenaka T, Fujikura T, Honda K et al. Discovery and development of tamsulosin hydrochloride, a new alpha 1-adrenoceptor antagonist. *Yakugaku Zasshi* 1995; **115**: 773–89.

90 Yamada S, Tanaka C, Ohkura T et al. High-affinity specific [3H]tamsulosin binding to alpha 1-adrenoceptors in human prostates with benign prostatic hypertrophy. *Urol Res* 1994; **22**: 273–8.

91 Yamada S, Tanaka C, Suzuki M et al. Determination of alpha 1-adrenoceptor antagonists in plasma by radioreceptor assay. *J Pharm Biomed Anal* 1996; **14**: 289–94.

92 Yamagishi R, Akiyama K, Nakamura S et al. Effect of KMD-3213, an alpha 1a-adrenoceptor-selective antagonist, on the contractions of rabbit prostate and rabbit and rat aorta. *Eur J Pharmacol* 1996; **315**: 73–9.

93 Yang HT, Endoh M. (+/–)-tamsulosin, an alpha 1A-adrenoceptor antagonist, inhibits the positive inotropic effect but not the accumulation of inositol phosphates in rabbit heart. *Eur J Pharmacol* 1996; **312**: 281–91.

94 Kurimoto S, Moriyama N, Hamada K, Kawabe K. Evaluation of histological structure and its effect on the distribution of alpha1-adrenoceptors in human benign prostatic hyperplasia. *Br J Urol* 1998; **81**(3): 388–93.

95 Taguchi K, Schafers RF, Michel MC. Radioreceptor assay analysis of tamsulosin and terazosin pharmacokinetics. *Br J Clin Pharmacol* 1998; **45**(1): 49–55.

96 Sciarra A, Di Silverio F. Safety profile of selective alpha-1 adrenoceptor antagonists in the treatment of benign prostatic hyperplasia. *Minerva Urol Nefrol* 1997; **49**: 21–8.

97 Shibata K et al. Alpha 1a-adrenoceptor polymorphism: pharmacological characterization and association with benign prostatic hypertrophy. *Br J Pharmacol* 1996; **118**: 1403–8.

98 de Mey C, Michel MC, McEwen J, Moreland T. A double-blind comparison of terazosin and tamsulosin on their differential effects on ambulatory blood pressure and nocturnal orthostatic stress testing. *Eur Urol* 1998; **33**(5): 81–8.

99 Lepor H. Long-term evaluation of tamsulosin in benign prostatic hyperplasia: placebo-controlled, double blind extension of phase III trial. Tamsulosin Investigator Group. *Urology* 1998; **51**(6): 901–6.

COMMENTARY

Tamsulosin hydrochloride is a new class of sulfonyl derivative, which has preferential selectivity for the α-1A-adrenergic receptor subtype. The 1A-receptor subtype is predominant in prostatic smooth muscles. In several preclinical studies, tamsulosin has been shown to bind preferentially with 13 times more efficacy to prostatic smooth muscles compared with vascular smooth muscles. Tamsulosin also exhibits a higher selectivity for prostatic receptor subtypes (10–12 times higher affinity) when compared with terazosin, alfuzosin, and doxazosin. One of the mechanisms by which patients with prostatism or LUTS manifest is by spasm of prostatic smooth muscles which is predominant in the 1A-subtype of α receptors. Blockade of these receptors selectively can theoretically cause relief of symptoms without side effects on the cardiovascular system. In clinical trials in the USA, Europe, and Japan, tamsulosin has been found to cause relief of prostatism without significant effects on blood pressure. Four placebo-controlled clinical studies and one active controlled clinical study of tamsulosin was done in the USA and Europe. In the USA, at doses of 0.4 mg day^{-1}, there was a 9.6 point decrease in the AUA symptom score in one study and a 5.8 point decrease in another study. There was also improvement in uroflow rates, and all these changes, when compared to placebo, were not only statistically significant, but clinically significant as well.

Tamsulosin is administered in capsules of 0.4 mg half an hour after breakfast, and over 90% of absorption is complete following oral administration. It is given in once-a-day dosing. It is metabolized by the cytochrome P-450 enzymes in the liver and less than 10% is excreted in urine unchanged. Patients with renal impairment or hepatic impairment do not require adjustments in tamsulosin dosage. In three studies of hypertensive subjects of ages between 47 and 79, blood pressure was controlled with stable doses of procardia, atenolol, or enalapril for at least 3 months. Tamsulosin administration in these patients resulted in no clinically significant effects on blood pressure compared with placebo. Treatment with cimetidine can cause a decrease in clearance of tamsulosin, so it should be used with caution in patients on cimetidine. The treatment-related adverse events, as ascertained from both the US and European trials, reveal that symptomatic postural hypotension is reported by 0.2% of patients given 4 mg, and 0.4% of patients given 0.8 mg. Abnormal ejaculation was associated with tamsulosin administration and was dose dependent in US studies. In terms of orthostatic blood pressure changes, the effects of tamsulosin on the vital signs in the US trials showed a mean systolic blood pressure change from a decrease of 0.4 mmHg to an increase of 1.8 mmHg. The mean diastolic blood pressure change was from an increase of 1 mmHg to an increase of 2.4 mmHg in comparison with placebo. The heart rate also increased (6.5 min^{-1}) but it was not significant in comparison to the placebo effect (4.6 min^{-1}). Other trials showed similar results with no first-dose decrease in blood pressure. Furthermore, there were no statistically or clinically significant differences observed between the sitting systolic blood pressure and diastolic blood pressure.

In summary, the clinical effects of tamsulosin are evident within 1 week after initiating tamsulosin therapy. This is important in patients who need immediate relief from symptoms. Furthermore, there is no need for titration when starting a patient on tamsulosin, which allows optimal dose to be administered on day one. Finally, the cardiovascular adverse events are minimized and the incidence of syncope and orthostatic hypotension are only 0.2%, which enables safe use in elderly patients.

Hormonal Therapy in Benign Prostatic Hyperplasia

A. Tewari

13

INTRODUCTION

It is a known fact that the prostate gland is dependent on androgenic stimulation and attempts to deprive the prostate of its testosterone support is an established treatment for benign prostatic hyperplasia (BPH).

Testosterone is converted to dihydrotesterone (DHT) within the prostatic stromal and basal cells facilitated by 5α-reductase enzyme. DHT levels do not increase with age although there is a decrease in plasma testosterone.[1,4] The action of DHT is to bind to the androgen receptors, forming a complex that sets off a cascade of events resulting in growth, differentiation, or both in the prostate (see Chapter 1 also). In hyperplastic tissues, it is believed that there is a defect in the normal processes that causes differentiation rather than uncontrolled growth. There is also evidence that there is down regulation of the androgen receptor complex levels in certain target tissues after puberty thus controlling growth by this mechanism.

5α-REDUCTASE

Two 5α-reductase isoenzymes have been described.[2-4] The predominant enzyme in skin and liver is Type 1, 5α-reductase, while type II is expressed in the prostate.

The role of the Type 1 form of the enzyme in prostatic growth is unclear.[5] The Type 2 enzyme is the predominant enzyme involved in conversion of testosterone to DHT in prostate and is therefore important in both normal and abnormal prostate growth. This isoenzyme is primarily located within stromal cells and basal cells of the prostate. Acinar epithelial cells uniformly lack Type 2 enzyme activity.

Among evolving concepts of androgen activity in relation to prostatic hyperplasia, the role of the stromal and basal cells in prostatic tissue have become more significant recently. Type 2 isozyme secreted in the basal and stromal cells may act in a paracrine manner on androgen-dependent luminal epithelial cells stimulating growth. Type 1 isozyme-induced DHT from skin and liver may act in an endocrine manner, also stimulating epithelial cell growth. Type 2 isozyme expression has also been found in stromal cells of seminal vesicles and epithelial cells of epididymis.

Isolated deficiency in 5α-reductase was first observed in the Dominican Republic in the late 1960s. Patients with this deficiency presented at birth with ambiguous genitalia (pseudovaginal perineoscrotal hypospadias) a 46, XY karyotype, normally differentiated testes, and male internal ducts. Virilization and penile development proceeded normally at puberty but the prostate was rudimentary or absent. Walsh et al.[6] and Imperato-McGinley et al.[7] described two groups of patients with this inherited form of male pseudohermaphroditism due to deficient DHT production. A genetic mutation in the Type 2 isozyme gene was detected that resulted in defective or deficient 5α-reductase enzyme activity.[8] At puberty in these patients, the increase in gonadotropins stimulates a significant rise in testosterone levels, which allows the production of external virilization. As Type 1 5α-reductase is normal, plasma DHT is detectable, suggesting that circulating DHT may have a true endocrine effect on androgen-dependent tissues. Adult men with this disorder have normal muscular development and male sexuality, and other organ systems function normally.

Based on these observations from this rare genetic disorder, a hypothesis was developed that an inhibitor of 5α-reductase could reduce prostatic growth without affecting sexual function or breast growth, as seen with other androgen withdrawal therapies. In addition, as the enzyme's only activity is to convert testosterone to DHT, it was hypothesized that blockade of the enzyme should not lead to significant adverse effects, since testosterone levels would be normal.

DEVELOPMENT OF FINASTERIDE

Merck & Co. (Rahway, NJ) synthesized a 4-azasteroid 5α-reductase inhibitors that lacked affinity for the androgen receptor. One of these agents significantly decreased DHT levels in the hyperplastic canine prostate and also reduced the prostatic volume by up to 64%.[9] Further studies showed that it was a potent, reversible inhibitor of isotype 2 of 5α-reductase that can suppress plasma DHT levels (by approximately 80–90%) without affecting testosterone levels.[10-13] This fact was important in terms of maintaining normal libido and sexual function. Intraprostatic testosterone levels, however, are elevated after finasteride therapy and may affect treatment efficacy. Type 1 enzyme levels are normal, and this may explain the failure of finasteride to decrease serum and prostatic DHT levels to zero.[14]

Clinical trials aimed at determining the safety and efficacy of finasteride in men with BPH have been extensive. At 6 months, initial placebo-controlled Phase II studies of finasteride in a limited number of patients with BPH resulted in a 30% decrease in prostatic size and statistically significant improvement in urinary flow rate; these results are comparable with those of androgen withdrawal therapies.[15]

SCANDINAVIAN STUDY (SCARP)[16–19]

To study the long-term efficacy and safety of finasteride for BPH, the Scandinavian Open-Extension study was reported by Ekman on behalf of the *Scandinavian Finasteride Study Group*. The *SCARP Study* enrolled 182 patients into a double-blind randomized multicenter trial. The first phase of this study consisted of a 6-month double-blind, placebo-controlled multicenter trial, where 182 patients were randomized to receive either placebo or 5 mg finasteride. This was followed by a 66-month open-extension during which all subjects were treated with finasteride. During the first 6 months of the study, the finasteride group showed a 28% reduction in the prostatic volume in comparison with the placebo group; however, the placebo group did show a similar reduction in prostate size after 12 months of placebo treatment. As for the uroflow measurements, both groups showed an improvement in the peak urinary flow rates by over 1 mL s^{-1} during the first 3 months of the study. However, the peak urinary flow rates increased by the amount of 2.4 mL s^{-1} in the finasteride group at the 6-month period; the placebo showed no change at this time. But, at the 12-month point of the study, the placebo group was now prescribed finasteride (5 mg), instead of placebo. These "ex-placebo" subjects showed an immediate increase in the peak urinary flow rate by 2.8 mL s^{-1} At the end of study after 6 years of finasteride therapy, the peak urinary flow rates for all treated patients (treatment group + "ex-placebo" group) was improved by 2.2 mL s^{-1}. At the 6-month period, the total symptom score in the finasteride group improved by 3.4 points and remained at that level throughout the remainder of the 6-year trial. The placebo group also showed a 2.6 point improvement in the symptom score. As a mean, both groups showed an improvement in total symptom score by 30% from baseline. From these results, the author claims that the maximum effect of finasteride on the prostatic volume, total symptom score, and PSA reduction occurred within the first 3 months of treatment, and this improvement in urinary obstructive symptoms was maintained throughout the 6-year trial period. These results differ from the findings obtained by Moore and associates who reported a 5-year finasteride study.[20] Moore reported that prostate size and peak urinary flow rates continued to improve beyond the initial 1-year period and continued throughout their 5-year trial period. Nonetheless, this study reported by Ekman and associates demonstrates that finasteride reduces the prostate size by approximately 25% within the first 6 months of therapy, and this resulting improvement is sustained. Symptoms are improved by

approximately 30%, and any deterioration is not seen as long as the patient is on active finasteride treatment.[21]

In this 6-year study, 14 patients dropped out after the first 6-month open-extension period: only 1 in the placebo group, but 6 from the finasteride group due to unspecified adverse events. During the second phase of the trial, 14 subjects discontinued the study during the first 6 months, followed by 55 patients over the next 60 months; a total of 54.5% of the patients completed the study. Besides stating "adverse events", the author did not elaborate on the reasons why these patients discontinued the study. However, it was briefly stated that withdrawals from the study were "mainly related to cardiovascular problems, as would be expected from men in this age group." The incidence of adverse sexual events was 0.6–1.7%.

EUROPEAN STUDIES

On behalf of the *PROWESS Study Group*, Marberger reported the long-term effects of 5 mg day^{-1} of finasteride in patients with enlarged prostates and moderate symptoms of BPH over a 2-year period.[22] This double-blind, randomized, placebo-controlled multicenter study (consisting of 285 centers in 42 different countries) assessed the efficacy and safety of finasteride via several parameters, such as the modified Boyarsky score, obstructive symptom score, peak urinary flow rate, and prostatic volume. Of the 3270 men enrolled, 3168 contributed data to the safety analysis, and 2902 to the efficacy evaluation. The study consisted of a baseline period, which was subdivided into the initial screening period (lasting 1–1.5 months), followed by the placebo run-in period (lasting 1 month). After the placebo period, the subjects were randomly placed into one of two groups, either the finasteride (treatment) group or placebo (control) group. At 12 months into the trial, there was a significant improvement in the Boyarsky score in the finasteride group (2.9 point reduction) in comparison with the placebo (1.9 point reduction) group ($P<0.01$); this initial difference increased as the study progressed, leading to a 3.2 point reduction in the Boyarsky score in the treated group as compared to the 1.5 point reduction in the placebo group ($P<0.001$) at the end of the study. The initial improvement in the symptom score in the placebo group remained constant until 1 year, and then decreased as the study progressed to its conclusion. In contrast, the finasteride-treated group showed an initial improvement, which was followed by a greater improvement as the study continued through its 2 years. A similar trend was noticed in the obstructive symptom score. The obstructive symptoms in the finasteride group decreased 1.9 points at 12 months and 2.1 points at the end of 24 months. The placebo group showed a 1.3 point reduction at 12 months and a 1.1 point reduction at the end of the study (both showed a statistical difference, $P<0.001$). The peak urinary flow rate also showed significant improvement in the finasteride group in comparison with the placebo group ($P<0.002$); the flow rate in the finasteride group increased from the baseline value of 11.2 mL s^{-1} to 12.6 mL s^{-1} (Δ=1.4) at 2 years in contrast to the placebo group, which showed an increase from 10.9 mL s^{-1} to 11.7 mL s^{-1} (Δ=0.8) after 2 years. The prostate volume decreased 14.2% and 15.3% after 1 and 2 years of finasteride treatment, respectively; the placebo group surprisingly also showed a reduction of 5.4% and 8.9% after 1 year and 2 years, respectively. This was a significant statistical difference compared with baseline after 12 (P<0.01) and 24 months (P<0.001) of finasteride treatment. Furthermore, the investigators also concluded that there was a greater improvement in placebo-adjusted Boyarsky score in men with large prostates (>40 cm^3) than in men with small prostates (<40 cm^3); however, this was not a significant difference (P=0.053). As for other urologic endpoints, 15 of 1450 men (1.0%) in the finasteride group experienced an acute retention episode, compared with 37 of 1452 (2.5%) in the placebo group, and the corresponding figures for BPH-related surgical intervention were 51 of 1450 (3.0%) and 86 of 1452 (5.9%), respectively. The hazard occurrence rate decreased 57% for acute urinary retention and by 40% for surgical intervention by finasteride therapy compared with placebo.[22]

In terms of efficacy, this *PROWESS study* demonstrated that finasteride does improve symptom score, increase peak urinary flow, decrease prostatic volume, and reduce clinical endpoints, such as acute urinary retention (AUR) by 57% and BPH-related surgery by 40%. These events were statistically better than seen in the placebo group. In addition, this study showed that the benefits of finasteride were not only evident initially but also continued over the course of 2 years. This conclusion is consistent with other published material.[16,20,23] In another interesting finding, the authors concluded that men with enlarged prostates greater than 40 cm^3 experienced greater symptomatic improvement with finasteride than did patients with prostates less then 40 cm^3. The investigators felt that the baseline prostate volume was a key predictor of treatment outcome. Men with not only enlarged prostates but also with increased risk of having AUR and surgery are the patients who will benefit the most from finasteride treatment. Men with smaller prostates and mild urinary obstructive symptoms may not respond well to an agent that reduces prostatic volume; these patients are not good candidates for finasteride treatment for BPH.

In terms of safety, the author stated that finasteride was well tolerated throughout the study, and exhibited a similar profile to placebo with one exception – sexually related adverse events. The incidence of impotence, abnormal ejaculation, and decreased libido was 6.6%, 2.1%, and 4.0%, respectively, in the finasteride group in contrast to 4.7%, 0.6%, and 2.8%, respectively, in the placebo group. There were a high percentage of patients taking finasteride who experienced hypertension (3.0%) and myocardial infarctions (1.5%). However, 40% of these patients had a past history of cardiovascular disease prior to entering the study. In this study, acute MI was reported in 23 of 1577 patients taking finasteride compared with 8 of 1591 (0.5%) patients taking placebo.

There has been much debate over the contribution of the enlarged prostate to the symptomatic presentation of BPH. There have been investigators who part on both sides of this issue. The authors of the *PROWESS study* believe that the continued symptomatic improvement of finasteride-treated patients over the 2 years might be explained by the accompanying reduction in prostatic volume, thereby linking the clinical benefits of finasteride with its effect on increased prostate size. Even though this study is consistent with this theory, more research at the molecular level using finasteride must be done.

CANADIAN PROSPECT STUDY

In the Canadian *PROSPECT Study Group* reported by Nickel,[23] 613 patients (aged from 45 to 80 years) with symptomatic BPH were enrolled from 28 centers across Canada. All the enrolled subjects initially received placebo for a 1-month period and were then randomly assigned to receive either finasteride (5 mg) or placebo for a period of 2 years. The parameters used to assess the effects of finasteride were the Boyarsky symptom score, urinary peak flow rate, and prostatic volume (as determined by postvoid transurethral ultrasonography (TRUS)). Of the 303 patients randomized to the placebo group, 226 (74.6%) patients completed the study. In this placebo group, there was a statistically significant improvement in the Boyarsky score (P<0.001) from the initial baseline values for the entire 25-month study period. The symptom score decreased by 3.2 points during the first 9 months of placebo therapy, during which the first 2 months showed the greatest improvement. However, after 8 months of treatment, there was a decline in symptom improvement. At the end, the total symptom score did show a 2.3-point improvement from baseline values. The peak urinary flow rate showed a significant improvement over baseline during the 25-month study (P<0.001), with the greatest improvement (Δ=+1.4 mL s^{-1}) occurring during the first 5 months of placebo therapy. Once again, this improvement deteriorated over the course of the study, but at the end, the peak urinary flow rate was 1.0 mL s^{-1} better than the initial baseline values. Even though the placebo therapy caused a visible improvement in symptoms, as seen from the above results, it did not have any effect on the prostate gland itself. Prostate volume increased progressively throughout the study, resulting in a mean volume of 8.4% greater than baseline measurements. Similarly, the PSA levels in the placebo group increased over the course of the trial, showing a mean increase above baseline of 5.5% (at 12 months) and of 13.3% (at 25 months). According to Nickel,[23] the extent of the placebo response for symptoms (P=0.180) and peak urinary flow rate (P=0.550) was independent of age, but the response correlated with the initial severity of symptoms (P<0.001) and initial peak urinary flow rates (P=0.023) It was also noted by the investigator that patients with a prostate size of less than 40 cc had a clinically more important placebo response than those with a prostate greater than 40 cc. Furthermore, patients with small prostate glands (<40 cc), more severe symptoms, and a lower baseline peak urinary flow rate had the most significant response to placebo therapy over the course of 25 months. However, placebo therapy is not entirely without risks; 81.2% of the patents taking placebo experienced an adverse event, mostly urogenital complaints (40.3%). Of these, 13.2% discontinued the placebo therapy. (The investigator did not specify the exact urogenital adverse event reported by the placebo-treated patient.) From these findings, Nickel claims that placebo not only produces a rapid and significant improvement in peak flow rates and BPH symptoms (similar to finasteride and α-blockers), but also clinically important adverse events. Overall finasteride has shown significant improvement in uroflow and reduction in size and symptoms in patients with BPH (Figure 13.2).

PRIMARY CARE STUDY

On behalf of the *Primary Care Study Group*, Tenover

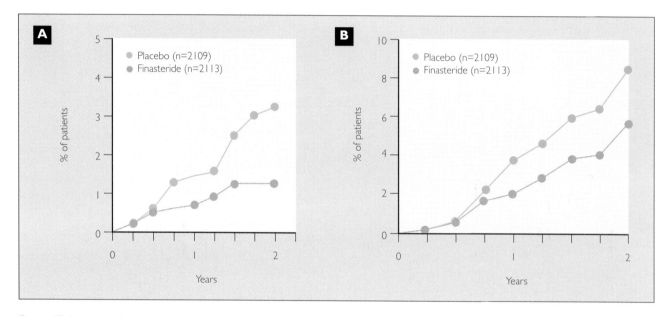

Figure 13.1 Acute urinary retention and BPH-related surgery. Pooled analysis of three, 2 year studies. (A) Acute urinary retention. (B) BPH-related surgery.

Source: PLESS study, with permission from Merck Inc.

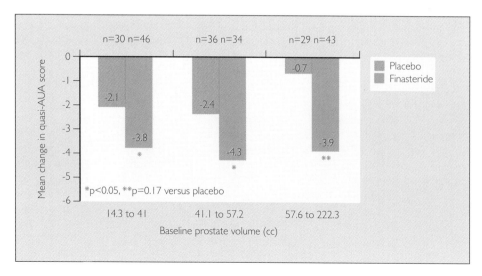

Figure 13.2 Symptom score response based on baseline prostate volume.

Source: PLESS study, with permission from Merck Inc.

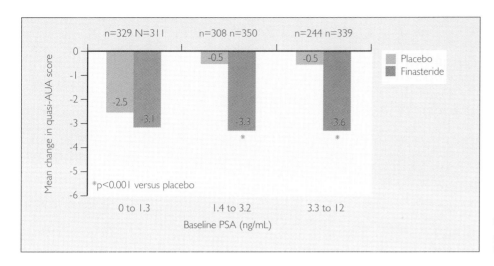

Figure 13.3 Symptom score response based on baseline PSA.

Source: PLESS study, with permission from Merck Inc.

reported the study of 2112 men with symptomatic BPH. Because increasing numbers of men are seeking treatment for BPH from primary care physicians, Tenover and associates examined the efficacy and tolerability of finasteride in the primary care setting. In this double-blind study, the subjects were randomized to receive either finasteride (5 mg) or placebo over a period of 12 months. The parameters used were the American Urological Association (AUA) symptom score and the BPH Impact Index; the latter is used for assessing bother, worry, physical discomfort, and restriction in physical activity. These parameters were monitored at 3, 6, 9, and 12 months after starting finasteride therapy. Patients treated with finasteride had a statistically significant mean decrease in the AUA symptom score in comparison with the placebo-treated patients; this was clearly evident at the beginning of month 6 and this improvement was maintained throughout the remaining course of the study. At the end of the trial, the mean decrease in the AUA symptom score was 4.96 for the finasteride group compared with 3.71 for the placebo group. Similarly, there was a statistically significant difference between the finasteride group and placebo group with regard to the BPH Impact Index, noted at months 9 and 12; the finasteride showed a much superior score. Overall assessments by the patient and investigator showed a greater improvement in the finasteride group than the placebo, as early as the sixth month. The incidence of drug-related adverse sexual events was significantly greater in finasteride-treated patients; however, only 2.2% of these men felt that the side effects were bothersome enough to withdraw from the study. Based on its favorable tolerability profile, and improvement in symptoms and quality of life, the investigators conclude that finasteride should be considered by primary care physicians for management of symptomatic BPH.

FINASTERIDE: ACUTE URINARY RETENTION AND NEED FOR SURGERY
(Figures 13.1–13.5)

There is some suggestion that finasteride reduces the risk for surgery and acute urinary retention. This issue was addressed in a recent double-blind, placebo-controlled multicenter (95 centers) trial.[24] On behalf of the *Finasteride Long-term Efficacy and Safety* group, (PLESS), McConnell reported this study involving 3040 men with symptomatic BPH. After a 1-month single-blind run-in period during which all men were treated with placebo, the patients were randomized to receive either 5 mg finasteride ($n=1524$) or placebo ($n=1516$) for the course of 4 years. The primary endpoint of this trial was the AUA symptom score report, with the incidence of surgery for BPH and the occurrence of AUR being the secondary endpoints. According to the investigators, 299 men required either surgery or catheterization for AUR throughout the 4-year period; in detail, 199 men (13%) were from the placebo group and 100 men (7%) were from the finasteride group. This shows a 51% reduction in the risk for surgery and catheterization for AUR with finasteride treatment ($P<0.001$). It was noted that the difference in the rates of these secondary endpoints was evident within the first 4 months of initiating finasteride treatment; this divergence continued throughout the 4-year trial period. It was determined that the probability of undergoing a transurethral resection of the prostate (TURP) procedure was 49% lower in the finasteride-treated treated group compared with the placebo group. This was concluded by the data showing 152 men (10%) in the placebo group and 69 men (5%) in the treatment group underwent a surgical procedure for BPH; this is a 55% reduction in the risk of transurethral prostatectomy with finasteride treatment

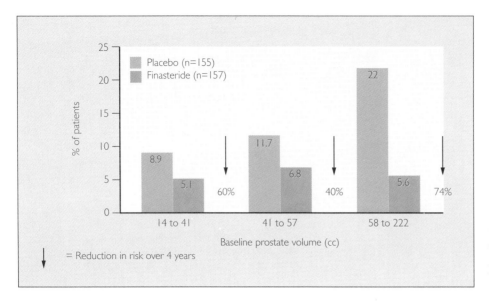

Figure 13.4 BPH-related surgery or acute urinary retention.

Source: Roehrborn et al, Urology 1999; 53(3): 473–480, Adapted with permission from Elsevier Science.

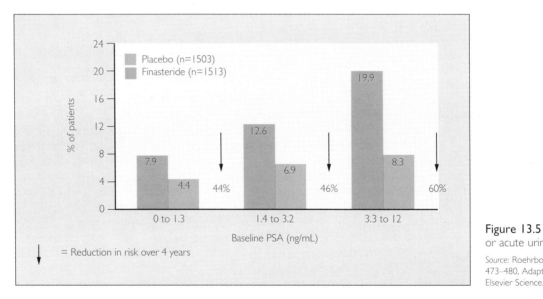

Figure 13.5 BPH-related surgery or acute urinary retention.

Source: Roehrborn et al, Urology 1999; 53(3): 473–480, Adapted with permission from Elsevier Science.

($P<0.001$). AUR developed in 99 men (7%) taking placebo compared with 42 men (3%) of men taking finasteride; this shows a 57% reduction in the risk of AUR with finasteride treatment ($P<0.001$). Furthermore, finasteride significantly decreased the risk of both spontaneous and precipitated acute urinary retention in relation to the control group ($P<0.001$ for both).

The AUA symptom scores decreased in both groups during the first 8 months of the study; however, over the course of the remaining period, finasteride showed continued improvement, while the placebo group did not. The mean symptom score decreased by 3.3 points in the finasteride group in comparison with 1.3 points in the placebo group, resulting in a mean difference of 2.1

($P<0.001$). Similarly, the mean prostatic volume decreased in the finasteride group, especially during the first year of treatment, with no further reduction seen thereafter. In contrast, the prostatic volume in the placebo group increased continuously with time. Statistically, there was an 18% reduction in volume in the finasteride group, as compared with a 14% enlargement seen in the placebo group; the mean difference between the groups is 32% ($P<0.001$). During the first 4 months of the study, it was evident that finasteride had a much greater influence on the peak urinary flow rate than did placebo. There was a 1.9 mL s^{-1} increase in the flow rate in the finasteride group vs. a 0.2 mL s^{-1} increase in terms of reducing morbidity that is associated with transurethral prostatectomy. The important finding here was that finasteride in comparison with placebo decreased the need for prostate surgery and the risk of AUR. Moreover, the differences were seen within the first 4 months of initiating the finasteride therapy, and it continued throughout the course of the 4-year trial period. This will have important economic and public health implications because TURP is one of the most common surgical procedures in elderly men of this age group. Besides finasteride, no other form of treatment, including α-blockers, has been reported to decrease the risk of BPH-related surgery and acute urinary retention. Over the course of the 4 years, 524 men (34%) from the finasteride-treated group discontinued the study owing to adverse events, compared with 633 men (42%) from the placebo group ($P<0.001$). The most common reasons for withdrawal were adverse drug effects or treatment failures. More men in the placebo group discontinued treatment because of lack of improvement or worsening of disease. However, more men from the finasteride group complained of adverse sexual events, such as sexual dysfunction (decreased libido and impotence), breast enlargement or tenderness, and rashes.

Andersen *et al.*[16] analyzed the combined sum of patients from the *SCARP*, *PROSPECT*, and *PROWESS* studies to show that finasteride significantly reduces AUR and the need for BPH-related surgery endpoints in patients with symptomatic BPH. In each study, the number of AUR occurrences recorded was consistently lower in the finasteride group than the placebo group (1.7% vs. 4.2% in *SCARP*; 0.9% vs. 1.6% in *PROSPECT*; 1.0% vs. 2.5% in *PROWESS*). This clearly shows that there is a lower risk of experiencing AUR with finasteride than with placebo ($P<0.001$) over the 2-year study period. In addition, there is an overall 57% decrease in the hazard rate for occurrence of AUR with finasteride compared with placebo. The hazard ratio was consistent in all of the three studies. As for the surgical intervention, a total of 227 patients had undergone a surgical procedure for BPH over the 2-year study period: 89 of 2113 (4.2%) in the finasteride group and 138 of 2109 (6.5%) in the placebo group. Again, the number of surgical procedures was consistently lower in the finasteride group than the placebo group for each study (5.9% vs. 7.3% in *SCARP*; 5.5% vs. 8.6% in *PROSPECT*; 3.5% vs. 5.9% in *PROWESS*). The hazard ratio demonstrates a clear treatment effect overall ($P<0.002$), with a 34% reduction in the hazard rate for occurrences of surgery with finasteride compared with placebo. The results of each of the three individual study analyses were again very similar. Of the 227 surgical procedures reported, 70 of the 89 (78.6%) in the finasteride group and 103 of 138 (74.6%) in the placebo group were TURPs. In each study, a consistently lower incidence of BPH-related endpoints was seen in the finasteride group than in the placebo group (7.4% vs. 9.6% in *SCARP*; 5.8% vs. 9.6% in *PROSPECT*; 4.1% vs. 6.6% in *PROWESS*). The estimated hazard ratio showed a 35% reduction in either BPH-related endpoint in the

finasteride group compared with the placebo group, indicating a clear overall treatment effect ($P<0.001$). This pooled analysis clearly indicates that 2 years of treatment with finasteride significantly decreases the occurrence of AUR and surgical intervention relative to placebo in patients with moderate symptomatic BPH. Furthermore, this report by Andersen clearly showed the rationale for using pharmacologic rather than surgical treatment in the management of patients with BPH.[4] This reversal in disease progression stems from an ability of finasteride to reduce prostate volume, thereby relieving urinary obstruction, and to decrease symptoms and increase urinary flow.

These data in combination suggest that one long-term effect of finasteride may be to reduce incidence of AUR and need for surgery. Indeed, if BPH causes bladder dysfunction over a prolonged period of time, it makes sense to reduce prostate size and decrease outflow resistance to prevent bladder deterioration. It is also possible that the human bladder can tolerate a certain amount of increased resistance, but with aging the ability to compensate is lost, which leads to patients presenting with acute retention and need for surgery.

Several questions remain at this time, however: (1) will these patients eventually fail medical treatment and need surgery to reduce bladder outlet obstruction and bladder decompensation? (2) What is the ideal duration of medical therapy? Would symptom improvement continue with longer therapy? (3) As the total number of patients benefited are small (1.5% in the *PROWESS Study* and 5% in the *US trial*), is it justified to place over 95% of patients on the drug for 4 years with a 6% incidence of side effects, in addition to cost, to avoid retention in 1.5–5% of patients? Selection of the patients is crucial to attain the maximum possible cost effective benefit from the pharmacological agent.

Tewari *et al.*[25] reported that transitional zone (TZ) volume and TZ ratio (TZ volume/total prostate volume) are more important than total prostate volume in the assessment of uroflow response to finasteride treatment. Primary reduction in prostate volume occurs in the TZ, and changes in this zone have a more pronounced effect on the relief of prostate urethral compression. Measurement of the TZ ratio will take into account variations in proportions of TZ vs. peripheral zones and thus simplify the monitoring of BPH patients on finasteride therapy. Furthermore, Tewari *et al.*[25] feel this will help identify uroflow responders and non-responders to finasteride therapy. Additionally, Roehrborn reviewed and analyzed six finasteride trials using meta-analysis.[26] The six trials used in this analysis were a clinical trial from North America (FN-3), a trial conducted internationally (FN-5), the *Scandinavian Reduction of the Prostate* (SCARP) study (FN-1), the *Proscar Safety Plus Efficacy Canadian Two-year (PROSPECT) study* (FN-4), the *Early Intervention trials* conducted in North America and Canada (FN-2), and the *VA Cooperative Study Group* (FN-6). The total number of participants was 2601 men who were given either placebo or finasteride. Using meta-analysis, he evaluated the average age, prostate volume, peak flow rate, and IPSS. The analysis showed that, depending on the prostatic volume, there was an improvement in both symptom score and peak flow rates in patients treated with finasteride vs. patients treated with placebo. Men with baseline prostate volumes greater than 40 cm^3 responded better to finasteride treatment than patients with less enlarged glands. From his results, he concluded that even though finasteride has been shown to be beneficial in the treatment of BPH from previous studies, it may not be appropriate for all men. According to the analysis, finasteride has been shown to be an effective treatment in symptomatic men with prostatic volumes of greater than 40 cm.^{3}

Thus, in conclusion, prostate volume can be an effective predictor of response to finasteride, and it may be used to identify which patients will respond to finasteride treatment.

COMBINATION THERAPY

Until the turn of this decade, watchful waiting and surgery were the only two widely accepted treatment options available for a man with symptomatic BPH. But, recent advances in the medical treatment for BPH, especially finasteride and α-blockers, have proven these agents to be safe with considerably less morbidity than surgery, making medical therapy a highly attractive alternative to the management of BPH. However, there were no studies comparing the combination use of finasteride and α-blockers in men with BPH. This was until Lepor on behalf of the *VA Cooperative Study Group* reported the safety and efficacy of placebo, terazosin (10 mg daily), finasteride (5 mg daily), and the combination of both drugs in 1229 men (between the ages of 45 and 80) with benign prostatic hyperplasia.[27] In this study, subjects were randomized into one of four groups: placebo ($n=305$), finasteride ($n=310$), terazosin ($n=305$), and combination (finasteride and terazosin) group ($n=309$).

There was a significant statistical difference in the AUA symptom scores in the terazosin and combination (terazosin plus finasteride) therapy group in comparison with baseline, and especially placebo and finasteride groups ($P<0.001$). However, there was no difference between the combination therapy group and the terazosin group ($P=1.0$). The symptom scores in the combination therapy and terazosin groups reached their respective lowest points at week 13 of the 52-week trial, and this was maintained throughout the remainder of the study. At the conclusion of the study period, the mean changes in the symptom score were significantly different in the combination therapy (6.2 point reduction) and terazosin (6.1 point reduction) groups in comparison with the placebo (2.6 point reduction) and finasteride (3.2 point reduction) groups. Similarly, the peak urinary flow rates were significantly higher in the combination therapy and terazosin groups compared with the placebo and finas-

teride groups ($P<0.001$). These changes were noted as early as the fourth week of the study, where the mean absolute changes between the combination therapy group and terazosin group were insignificant ($P=0.15$). At the end of the study, the peak urinary flow rates improved the most in the combination therapy group ($\delta=3.2$ mL s^{-1}), followed by the terazosin group ($\delta=2.7$ mL s^{-1}), finasteride group ($\delta=1.6$ mL s^{-1}), and placebo group ($\delta=1.4$ mL s^{-1}).

The mean change in the prostatic volume was the greatest in the finasteride and combination therapy groups, where both groups showed a significant difference in comparison to the placebo and terazosin groups ($P<0.001$). The mean change in prostatic volume observed at the end of the study showed that the combination therapy group had the highest reduction of 7.0 cm^3, followed by the finasteride group (6.1 cm^3 reduction), and the terazosin and placebo groups (0.5 cm^3 increase). The maximum reductions in prostate volume in the combination therapy and finasteride groups were observed during week 26. Similarly, the combination therapy and finasteride groups also showed a significant decrease in the PSA levels compared with the placebo and terazosin groups ($P<0.001$). The finasteride and combination therapy groups showed an equal decrease in the PSA level (0.9 mg mL^{-1} increase), followed by the terazosin and placebo groups, which showed a PSA decrease of 0.4 ng mL^{-1} and 0.1 ng mL^{-1}, respectively.

As for the side effects, patients taking either terazosin or combination therapy experienced postural hypotension and dizziness more than any other group ($P<0.001$). Patients taking finasteride or combination therapy experienced adverse sexual events (such as impotence and decreased libido) more than any other group ($P=0.05$). The men in the combination therapy group had significantly more ejaculatory abnormalities than men in any other group ($P<0.001$). During the trial period, several patients required dose reduction of the medication, especially in the terazosin and combination therapy groups. At the conclusion of the study, 80% of the men in the terazosin group were taking 10 mg of terazosin, 11% were taking reduced doses, and 9% were receiving none. In the combination therapy group, 80% were taking 10 mg of terazosin, 11% were receiving 5 mg, and 9% did not receive the drug.

There was also another recent study which evaluated the combination of finasteride and Dibenzyline (an α-blocker) in a prospective study in 190 men suffering from severe prostatism.[28] They were assessed by IPSS symptom score, digital rectal examination, TRUS, uroflowmetry and residual urine. The patients were randomly selected for medical treatment with Dibenzyline 10 mg b.i.d. ($n=71$), finasteride 5 mg q.d. ($n=54$), and a combination ($n=65$). Clinical assessments were carried out before treatment and 3 and 6 months after starting treatment. Patients who could not complete the treatment and those with prostatic cancer were excluded from the final statistics. The quality of life after 6 months of treatment and side effects were also assessed. A total of 172 patients completed the treatment course and 153 patients completed the periodic clinical assessments. Improvement in IPSS was noted in all three groups of patients at both 3 and 6 months. The prostatic volume was found to decrease in the finasteride group and the combination group at 6 months by 24.3 and 10.5%, respectively. Maximal flow rate (Q_{max}) was significantly improved in the Dibenzyline and combination groups but not in the finasteride group at 3 months. At 6 months a significant increase in Q_{max} was noted in all groups with a mean increase of 1.4–1.8 mL s^{-1}. The quality of life after treatment was satisfactory in 71.9% of the Dibenzyline group, 70.4% of the finasteride group, and 83.1% of the combination group. Side effects were higher in the Dibenzyline than the finasteride or combination group. The drop-out rate was higher in the Dibenzyline group (15.5%) than in the finasteride (7.5%) and combination (4.6%) groups. After 6 months of treatment, some of the patients discontinued medication and symptom relapse was noted in 92.6% of the Dibenzyline group, 57.6% of the finasteride group, and 71% of the combination group.[28]

The results of two further studies to investigate doxazosin/finasteride combination therapy, the *PRIDICT study* and the US NIH-sponsored *Medical Therapy of Prostatic Symptoms* (MTOPS study) in which patients with larger prostates were included, are still pending. In particular, the MTOPS study, a long-term (4–6 year) protocol with a similar design to the *VA Cooperative study*, is expected to give more definitive answers to questions concerning the effects of these two drugs on the microscopic and clinical progression of the disease.

COMPOSITION OF PROSTATE – RESPONSE TO FINASTERIDE

In a study of 40 subjects with BPH, Marks and co-workers[29] examined the prostatic tissue composition of patients taking finasteride for a 6-month period. Of the 40 men, 26 of them were given finasteride, while the others were given placebo. Compared with pretreatment biopsies, the finasteride group had a 55% decrease in inner gland epithelium ($P<0.01$) with little effect on the stroma and lumina. There also was a linear correlation between pretreatment inner gland epithelial content and prostate volume decrease induced by finasteride ($P<0.01$). By using TRUS on all men before and after treatment, it was determined that prostate volume decreased from an average of 37 cm^3 to 29 cm^3 as a result of the 6-month finasteride therapy; this 21% decrease is statistically significant ($P<0.01$). Furthermore, in this same group via the use of MRI, the mean prostate volume before treatment was 49 cm^3 and the TZ volume was 28 cm^3 (which represents 57% of the total gland volume). After 6 months of treatment, the mean prostate volume decreased to 41 cm^3 and the TZ volume decreased to 24 cm^3 (which represents 59% of the total gland volume). Both of the decreases are statistically significant ($P<0.05$). However, interestingly

enough, the ratio of the TZ to that of the mean prostate volume showed no difference; the prostate volume decrease between the inner and outer zones was proportionately distributed. After the 6-month treatment, no statistically significant changes were seen in the overall prostate tissue composition. However, in the inner gland, finasteride treatment caused a major change in the percent epithelium, causing a decrease from 13.5% (during pretreatment) to 6.0% after 6 months ($P<0.01$). In addition, in the TZ, the stroma-to-epithelial ratio increased from 4.4 to 10.3 after 6 months of finasteride treatment ($P<0.01$). There was no statistically significant change in the outer gland or the overall prostate. The three major findings obtained from this study are (1) a pronounced (yet selective) suppression of the epithelium is seen; (2) a more dramatic epithelial suppression of the inner prostate than the outer prostate; and (3) a prostate volume reduction that is correlated with pretreatment epithelial content of the inner but not outer prostate.

PROSTATE-SPECIFIC ANTIGEN AND FINASTERIDE (Figure 13.6)

Biological variability of serum PSA and its relationship with finasteride was recently evaluated. Percent change and crossover of PSA levels between the low (1.0–3.9 ng mL^{-1}) and high (4.0–10.0 ng mL^{-1}) ranges were evaluated in 72 men with BPH and 77 men with both BPH and prostate cancer (PCa) treated with finasteride or placebo for 6 months. Patients with PCa were studied as a model for evaluating the effects on PSA levels in patients with BPH and latent PCa. As recommended on the product label, PSA levels for finasteride-treated patients were doubled for interpretation. In patients with BPH, most placebo- and finasteride-treated patients had low PSA levels at baseline had subsequent PSA levels below 4.0 ng mL^{-1} throughout the study. Among patients with high baseline PSA levels, only 1 of 17 finasteride-treated patients, compared with 8 of 13 placebo-treated patients, crossed into the low range. In the *BPH/PCa study*, most placebo-treated patients maintained PSA levels in the same range (15 of 19 less than 4.0 ng mL^{-1}; 14 of 16 greater than 4.0 ng mL^{-1}). Almost one-third of finasteride-treated patients with low PSA levels at baseline crossed into the high range (8 of 22), whereas most patients with high PSA levels at baseline were not masked with treatment, with PSA levels remaining high (12 of 15). PSA levels cross between the low and high PSA ranges in both finasteride- and placebo-treated patients with BPH and those with both BPH and PCa. Doubling the PSA levels in finasteride-treated patients allows appropriate interpretation of PSA values and does not mask the detection of PCa.[30] In a study by Keetch *et al.*,[31] the effects of finasteride and terazosin on the PSA levels in 69 men with symptomatic BPH were examined. Of the 69 men, 33 subjects in the study took 5 mg day^{-1}, 14 were given terazosin (2–5 mg day^{-1}), and the others ($n=22$) were given no

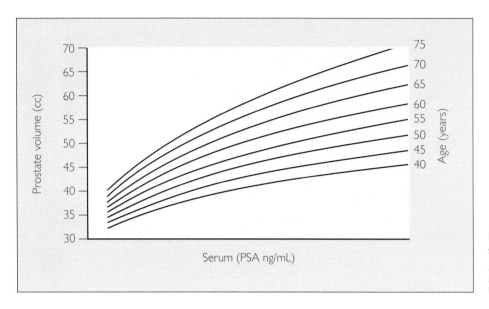

Figure 13.6 Relationship between serum PSA and prostate volume.

Source: Roehrborn et al, Urology 1999; 53(3): 581–589, Adapted with permission from Elsevier Science.

therapy (watchful waiting).[31] These investigators revealed that finasteride appears to lower total and free PSA levels equally in men taking 5 mg day[-1]; hence, it does not change the free/total ratio of serum PSA. On the other hand, terazosin does not appear to alter the total of free PSA levels in men with BPH. Only the finasteride group had significantly lower post-treatment total serum PSA levels compared with pretreatment levels. The median post-treatment free PSA levels were significantly lower in the finasteride group (0.26) compared with the terazosin (0.54) and watchful waiting (0.85) groups (*P*=0.0015). However, the median percent free PSA was not significantly different in the finasteride (23), terazosin (22), and watchful waiting (25) groups (*P*=0.66). Even though other prospective studies are needed, this study did conclude that the percent of free PSA (free/total) could potentially be used to screen for prostate cancer in men taking finasteride.

OTHER HORMONAL TREATMENTS

Apart from finasteride, other types of hormonal therapy have been tested in patients with BPH. GnRH agonists, such as leuprolide, can be used to decrease the release of trophic hormones (LH and FSH) from the anterior pituitary by desensitizing the GnRH receptor on gonadotropic cells. When given in pulsatile fashion, it stimulates gonadotropin release. However, if given in a steady, continuous dose, it causes a marked inhibition of gonadotropin (LH and FSH) release – in effect, a medical castration. Leuprolide and other GnRH agonists (nafarelin, buserelin) are administered as a long-acting depot preparation to sup-

press LH release, causing a reduction in testosterone and DHT. A drop in DHT levels will "starve" the hyperplastic prostate and decrease its size. Initial injections of leuprolide (*Lupron*) will cause a rise in LH and FSH levels, but with continued administration, these levels will be suppressed. Thus, testosterone will increase during the first week of administration, but will be reduced below baseline levels by the end of the second week of treatment. As for the side effects, most of them are related to the physiologic effect of decreased testosterone, such as hot flushes, decreased testicular size, impotence, and gynecomastia or breast tenderness.

Eri *et al.*[32,33,34] examined the effects of long-term use of leuprolide in patients with BPH. In this randomized placebo-controlled study consisting of 50 men, 26 of them received 3.75 mg leuprolide IM every 28 days for 24 weeks and 24 received placebo. Serum LH levels decreased by 90% and FSH levels decreased by 55% from initial baseline values. Serum testosterone levels decreased by 96% and DHT decreased by 90%. The adrenal-derived androgens, dehydroepiandrosterone and androstenedione, decreased by 24% and 48%, respectively. Another study noted that prostatic 5α-reductase activity and androgen receptor content decreased with leuprolide therapy.[35] As for the estrogens, estradiol decreased to non-detectable levels and estrone decreased by 35%. There were no statistical and significant changes noted in the prolactin levels and the sex hormone-binding globulin in comparison with the placebo group. These similar results were obtained by Salerno and associates in 1988.[36] They reported that prostatic DHT decreased by 90% and testosterone decreased by 75% from baseline after 3 months of GnRH agonist therapy.

In 1993, leuprolide was investigated in a double-blind, placebo-controlled study, where 50 men with BPH were randomized to receive 3.75 mg leuprolide depot IM every 28 days for 24 weeks or placebo.[33] The parameters measured were prostate volume, maximum urinary flow rate, symptom scores, and detrusor pressure during micturition. The prostate volume decreased by 34.5% in the leuprolide-treated group vs. 2.6% in the placebo group; urinary flow rates increase by 32% over the placebo group, and detrusor pressure upon micturition decreased by 24% in the leuprolide group in comparison with the placebo group. The latter two measurements imply that there was a decrease in the bladder outlet resistance. Symptom scores improved significantly in both groups compared with their respective baseline values. According to the investigators, leuprolide treatment was well tolerated by the experimental group, and the most common adverse events experienced were flushing and decreased sexual function.

In another study, the same authors examined the side effects of leuprolide in a double-blind, placebo-controlled study of 50 men with BPH.[32] All the men in the group taking 3.75 mg leuprolide depot IM every 28 days for 24 weeks experienced hot flushes, erectile dysfunction, and decreased libido. Despite the loss of interest in sexual activity, these leuprolide-treated patients were generally satisfied with their sexual life during treatment. Even though the adverse events were bothersome in the treated patients, 73% of them (at the conclusion of the study) expressed that they would repeat or continue leuprolide treatment. Five of the 26 men receiving leuprolide had a weight gain of >3 kg. Flutamide and other androgen receptor inhibitors (cyproterone, zanoterone) are steroidal competitive inhibitors of testosterone at its cytoplasmic receptor site. As a note, cyproterone also possesses progestational activity that provides negative feedback to the pituitary, causing a decrease in LH release. In animal studies, flutamide demonstrated anti-androgenic effects by inhibiting androgen uptake and/or by inhibiting nuclear binding of androgen in target tissue or both. However, elevations of plasma testosterone and estradiol levels have been noted following flutamide administration. A study by Monti et al. showed that flutamide did not change DHT levels in the prostate gland; however, the EGF was decreased in the total prostatic tissue, especially in the periurethral zone. The authors speculate that flutamide through the influence on growth factors (EGF) may cause shrinkage in the periurethral tissue, alleviating outlet obstruction and symptoms.[37]

In a double-blind, randomized trial using flutamide 750 mg day^{-1} for a 6-month period, 22 patients with BPH were enrolled to determine the effect of flutamide on the prostatic volume, PSA level, and serum testosterone levels.[38] Eleven patients were randomized to take flutamide and the other 11 to take placebo. After 6 months of therapy, the prostate volume decreased by 35% and the serum PSA decreased by 65% in comparison to the placebo ($P<0.001$). These changes occurred despite a 58.3% increase in the serum testosterone levels ($P<0.01$). According to the investigators, the patients treated with flutamide experienced very minimal adverse events, and concluded that it was an effective and safe therapy for BPH. However, this was contradicted by a more recent study done by the author and his associates in 1996.

In a study conducted by Narayan and associates, flutamide was used for a period of 24 weeks in a clinical trial to evaluate efficacy, safety, and dose–response profiles of flutamide at 32 centers (14 centers in the USA and 18 international centers).[39] A total of 372 patients were enrolled and randomized to receive one of the following five treatment regimens: placebo capsule, flutamide capsules 125 mg b.i.d., 250 mg q.d., 250 mg b.i.d., and 250 mg t.i.d. Patients were then evaluated throughout the study and also 8 weeks after the end of treatment (32 weeks). The parameters measured were peak urine flow rate, residual urine volume, symptom score, prostate volume, and PSA level. Baseline peak urinary flow rate and percent change from baseline in maximum flow rate showed a dose-related increase at 4 and 6 weeks; this increase was significant in the flutamide group taking 250 mg three times daily. At later time points, no significant differences between the flutamide and placebo groups were observed. At 4 and 6 weeks, 25% of patients taking flutamide 250 mg three times daily had more than a 3 mL s^{-1} increase in uroflow compared with about 10% of placebo patients ($P<0.05$). All flutamide-treated groups had a significant decrease in prostate volume from baseline to the last treatment visit compared with placebo, and this reduction was dose related (in comparison with placebo: $P<0.05$ for 125 mg twice daily and $P<0.001$ for all other treatment arms). The average decrease in the prostatic volume for the flutamide-treated groups ranged from 6% to 23% at 12 weeks and from 14% to 29% at 24 weeks. All treatment groups showed a subsequent increase in prostate volume after treatment was stopped. Furthermore, there was a significant reduction in residual urine volume at 24 weeks only in the flutamide 250 mg t.i.d. group. It increased following cessation of therapy. Urinary symptoms at 6, 12, 18, and 24 weeks did not show any significant difference between placebo and any of the flutamide dose groups. The investigators conclude that flutamide reduced the prostate volume in a dose-related fashion. Moreover, there was an improvement in the urinary flow rate at 4 weeks (3% for the 250 mg t.i.d. group, $P<0.05$), but the early positive effects did not maintain statistical significance owing to an increasing number of drop-outs due to adverse events. Similarly, there was a reduction in the postvoid residual volume, but it was only observed at the highest dose and at 24 weeks (median reduction, 23 mL, $P<0.05$). Irrespective of these findings, there were no significant differences in urinary symptoms among the placebo and flutamide groups.

The investigators concluded that the higher incidences of diarrhea, breast tenderness, and gynecomastia, however, were the main limiting factors in this study and until these problems are overcome, the role of flutamide in the management of BPH remains investigational. The most common adverse events experienced by the participants were nipple and breast tenderness (42–52%), diarrhea (29–34%), and gynecomastia (14–19%). Each of these adverse events had a significantly higher incidence in all flutamide dose groups compared with placebo, but none appeared to occur in a dose-related fashion. A total of 1–3% of the patients withdrew from the study owing to abnormal liver enzymes or impotence.

CONCLUSIONS

The benefit of finasteride over placebo in the treatment of BPH has been demonstrated in randomized, placebo-controlled trials. Approximately one-third to one-half of patients have clinically significant improvements, while modest benefits overall were seen in the study population. Uncontrolled studies suggest that the response to therapy may be sustained for up to 6 years, although it is yet to be determined whether the progression of BPH with time can be prevented. Given its minimal side effects, finasteride should be considered an acceptable treatment option for select group of patients with BPH. Recent data from several studies suggest that the ideal patient for finasteride therapy is someone who has a prostate gland greater than 40 cm³ in size. Secondly, there appears to be a benefit to finasteride in

reducing the incidence of AUR and BPH-related surgical interventions by up nearly 50% when used chronically for over 2 years. With regard to prostate cancer, patients should be informed of the effect that finasteride has in lowering serum PSA levels and the potential impact this may have on the detection of prostate cancer.

Flutamide treatment for BPH has shown promise in some clinical trials, However, the high incidence of adverse events has caused many of the participants in these studies to drop out, causing skewed results at the conclusion of the study. These adverse events, such as diarrhea, breast tenderness, and gynecomastia, were the limiting factors in this study and, until these problems are overcome, flutamide will remain an investigational drug. As for leuprolide, it has shown significant decreases in testosterone, DHT, LH, and FSH levels. Clinically, it has been shown to improve symptom scores and urinary flow rates, but it also produces adverse events related to decreased testosterone levels, such as hot flushes, decreased testicular size, impotence, and gynecomastia. However, several studies have shown that these side effects were not severe enough to cause the participants of the study to withdraw. Moreover, Eri and associates[22–24] reported that 73% of the participants of their leuprolide clinical trial expressed that they would repeat or continue leuprolide treatment if the option was given.

REFERENCES

1. Walsh PC, Hutchins GM, Ewing LL. Tissue content of dihydrotestosterone in human prostatic hyperplasia is not supranormal. *J Clin Invest* 1983; **72**: 1772–1777.

2. Finasteride Study Group. Finasteride (MK-906) in the treatment of benign prostatic hyperplasia. *Prostate* 1993; **22**: 291–299.

3. Kirby RS, Bryan J, Eardley I, *et al.* Finasteride in the treatment of benign prostatic hyperplasia: a urodynamic evaluation. *Br J Urol* 1992; **70**: 65–72.

4. Tammela TLJ, Kontturi MJ. Urodynamic effects of finasteride in the treatment of bladder outlet obstruction due to benign prostatic hyperplasia. *J Urol* 1993; **149**: 342–344.

5. Silver RI, Wiley EL, Davis DL, *et al.* Expression and regulation of steroid 5 alpha-reductase 2 in prostate disease. *J Urol* 1994; **152**: 433–437.

6. Walsh PC, Madden JD, Harrod MJ, *et al.* Familial incomplete male pseudohermaphroditism, Type 2: decreased dihydrotestosterone formation in pseudovaginal perineoscrotal hypospadias. *New Eng J Med* 1974; **291**: 944–949.

7. Imperato-McGinley J, Guerrero L, *et al.* Steroid 5 alpha-reductase deficiency in man: an inherited form of male pseudohermaphroditism. *Science* 1974; **186**: 1213–1215.

8. Thigpen AE, Davis DL, Milatovich A, *et al.* Molecular genetics of steroid 5 alpha-reductase 2 deficiency. *J Clin Invest* 1992; **90**: 799–809.

9. Brooks JR, Berman C, Garnes D, *et al.* Prostatic effects induced in dogs by chronic or acute oral administration of 5 alpha-reductase inhibitors. *Prostate* 1986; **9**: 65–75.

10. Rittmaster RS, Stoner E, Thompson DL, *et al.* Effect of MK-906, a specific 5 alpha-reductase inhibitor, on serum androgens and androgen conjugates in normal men. *J Androl* 1989; **10**: 259–262.

11. Vermeulen A, Giagulli VA, Schepper PD, *et al.* Hormonal effects of an orally active 4-azasteroid inhibitor or 5 alpha-reductase in humans. *Prostate* 1989; **14**: 45–53.

12. McConnell JD, Wilson JD, George FW, *et al.* Finasteride, an inhibitor of 5 alpha-reductase, suppresses prostatic dihydrotestosterone in men with benign prostatic hyperplasia. *J Clin Endocrinol Metab* 1992; **74**: 505–508.

13. Norman RW, Coakes KE, Wright AS, *et al.* Androgen metabolism in men receiving finasteride before prostatectomy. *J Urol* 1993; **150**: 1736–1739.

14. Thigpen AE, Silver RI, Guileyardo JM, *et al.* Tissue distribution and ontogeny of steroid 5 alpha-reductase isozyme expression. *J Clin Invest* 1993; **92**: 903–910.

15. Stoner E and the Finasteride Study Group. The clinical effects of a 5 alpha-reductase inhibitor, finasteride on benign prostatic hyperplasia. *J Urol* 1992; **147**: 1298–1302.

16. Anderson JT, Ekman P, Wolf H, *et al.* Can finasteride reverse the progress of BPH ? A two year placebo controlled study. *Urology* 1995; **46**(5): 631–637.

17. Bolognese JA, Kozloff RC, Kunik SC, *et al.* Validation of a symptoms questionnaire for benign prostatic hyperplasia. *Prostate* 1992; **21**: 247–254.

18. Byrnes CA, Morton AS, Liss CL, *et al.* Efficacy, tolerability and effect on health-related quality of life of finasteride compared to placebo in men with symptomatic benign prostatic hyperplasia: the community-based urology study of Proscar. *Clin Ther* 1995; **17**(5): 956–969.

19. Girman CJ, Kolman C, Liss CL, *et al.* Effects of finasteride on health-related quality of life in men with benign prostatic hyperplasia. (Submitted).

20. Moore E, Bracken B, Brenner W, *et al.* Proscar: five-year

experience [published erratum appears in *Eur Urol* 1996; **29**(2): 234]. *Eur Urol* 1995; **28**(4): 304–9.

21. Ekman P. Maximum efficacy of finasteride is obtained within 6 months and maintained over 6 years; follow-up of the Scandinavian Open-Extension study. *Eur Urol* 1998; **33**: 312–17.

22. Marberger ML. PROWESS Study Group. Long-term effects of finasteride in patients with benign prostatic hyperplasia: a double-blind, placebo-controlled, multicenter study. *Urology* 1998; **51**: 677–86.

23. Nickel JC. Long-term implications of medical therapy on benign prostatic hyperplasia end points. *Urology* 1998; **51** (Suppl 4A): 50–7.

24. McConnell JD, Bruskewitz R *et al*. The effect of finasteride on the risk of acute urinary retention and the need for surgical treatment among men with benign prostatic hyperplasia; the Finasteride Long-term Efficacy and Safety study group. *N Eng J Med* 1998; **338**: 557–63.

25. Tewari A, Shinohara K, Narayan P. Transition zone volume and transition zone ratio: predictor of uroflow response to finasteride therapy in benign prostatic hyperplasia patients. *Urology* 1995; **45**(2): 258–64; discussion 265.

26. Roehrborn CG. Meta-analysis of randomized clinical trials of finasteride. *Urology* 1998; **51**(Suppl 4A): 46–9.

27. Lepor H, Williford WO, Barry MJ, *et al*. The efficacy of terazosin, finasteride, or both in benign prostatic hyperplasia. *Veterans Affairs Cooperative Studies Benign Prostatic Hyperplasia Study Group. N Engl J Med* 1996; **335**(8): 533–9.

28. Kuo HC. Comparative study of therapeutic effects of dibenzyline, finasteride, and combination drugs for symptomatic benign prostatic hyperplasia. *Urol Int* 1998; **60**(2): 85–91.

29. Marks LS, Partin AW, Gormley GJ, *et al*. Prostate tissue composition and response to finasteride in men with symptomatic benign prostatic hyperplasia. *J Urol* 1997; **157**(6): 2171–8.

30. Oesterling JE, Roy J, Agha A, *et al*. Biologic variability of prostate specific antigen and its usefulness as a marker for prostate cancer: effects of finasteride. The Finasteride PSA Study Group. *J Urol* 1997; **50**(1): 13–18.

31. Keetch DW, Andriole GL, Ratliff TL, *et al*. Comparison of percent free prostate-specific antigen levels in men with BPH treated with finasteride, terazosin, or watchful waiting. *Urology* 1997; **50**: 901–5.

32. Eri LM, Tveter KJ. Safety, side effects and patient acceptance of the luteinizing hormone-releasing hormone agonist leuprolide in treatment of benign prostatic hyperplasia. *J Urol* 1994; **152**(2 Pt 1): 448–52.

33. Eri LM, Tveter KJ. A prospective, placebo-controlled study of the luteinizing hormone-releasing hormone agonist leuprolide in treatment for patients with benign prostatic hyperplasia. *J Urol* 1993; **150**(2 Pt 1): 359–64.

34. Eri LM, Haug E, Tveter KJ. Effects on the endocrine system of long-term treatment with the luteinizing hormone-releasing hormone against leuprolide in patients with benign prostatic hyperplasia. *Scand J Clin Lab Invest* 1996; **56**(4): 319–25.

35. Forti G, Salerno R, Moneti G, *et al*. Three months' treatment with a long acting gonadotropin releasing hormone agonist of patients with benign prostatic hyperplasia: effects of tissue androgen concentration, 5 alpha reductase activity and androgen receptor contents. *J Clin Endocrinol* 1989; **68**: 461–468.

36. Salerno R, Moneti G, Forti G, *et al*. Simultaneous determination of testosterone, dihydrotestosterone and 5 alpha-androstan-3-alpha-17-beta-diol by isotopic dilution mass spectrometry in plasma and prostatic tissue of patients affected by benign prostatic hyperplasia: effects of a 3-month treatment with a GnRH analog. *J Androl* 1988; **9**: 234.

37. Monti S, Sciarra F, Adamo MV, *et al*. Prevalent decrease of the EGF content in the periurethral zone of BPH tissue induced by treatment with finasteride or flutamide. *J Androl* 1997; **18**(5): 488–94.

38. Stone NN, Clejan SJ. Response of prostate volume, prostate specific antigen, and testosterone to flutamide in men with benign prostatic hyperplasia. *J Androl* 1991; **12**(6): 376–80.

39. Narayan P, Trachtenberg J, Lepor H, *et al*. A dose–response study of the effect of flutamide on benign prostatic hyperplasia: results of a multicenter study. *Urology* 1996; **47**(4): 497–504.

COMMENTARY

The prostate gland is androgen dependent and requires testosterone for its growth and development. For BPH to develop, two factors are necessary – androgens and aging. The mechanism by which testosterone causes prostatic growth is by its conversion to DHT within the prostatic stromal and basal cells. This is facilitated by the enzyme 5α-reductase. Two isotypes of 5α-reductase enzymes have been identified, each coded by a separate gene. The predominate enzyme in skin and liver is Type 1, whereas Type 2 is predominantly expressed in prostatic tissues. The role of the Type 1 enzyme in prostatic growth is not clear. However, Type 2 is involved in the conversion of testosterone to DHT and is therefore important in both normal and abnormal prostatic growth. Type 2 is primarily located within stromal cells and basal cells. Acinar epithelial cells uniformly lack Type 2 enzyme activity. Among evolving concepts of androgen action in relation to prostatic hyperplasia, the significant role of stromal and basal cells in prostatic tissue has become more evident recently. Type 2 isoenzyme secretions in the stromal and basal cells may act in a paracrine manner on androgen-dependent luminal epithelial cells stimulating growth. Type 1 enzyme may induce DHT from skin and liver to act in an endocrine manner to stimulate prostatic epithelial growth. Based on the fact that individuals with congenital defects in 5α-reductase enzyme develop deficient prostates while retaining normal testosterone and external virilization, Merck (Rahway, NJ) embarked on a program to synthesize 5α-reductase inhibitors that may mimic this situation.[1-4]

By blocking the activity of 5α-reductase, the androgenic stimulation of the prostate gland can be significantly reduced. The first drug with such capacity to be introduced on the market was finasteride. Following the administration of this drug to men, serum DHT levels were reduced by approximately 80–90% without effecting testosterone levels.

Several large Phase III trials have demonstrated the efficacy of finasteride in treating BPH. Clinical trials of this drug have been conducted in North America, Europe, Scandinavia, and other countries, and demonstrated uniformly that there was a 70–80% reduction in serum DHT with a mean reduction in prostate volume by 20–25% after 6 months of therapy. This statistically significant improvement was evident in both symptom scores and uroflows as compared to patients on placebo; the prostatic symptom score improved by a mean of 30%, while uroflow improved by 15–20% (1.5 mL s⁻¹). Moreover, this effect was maintained as long as the patient was on the drug, at least up to the end of a 6-year follow-up period. Additionally, it has been found that the finasteride improvement occurs within 6 months of therapy, probably by manifestation of decreased prostate size. However, after this 6-month period, there is no additional improvement observed, but improvement that has occurred is maintained at that level. Adverse events secondary to finasteride occur in less than 5% of patients and are mostly related to decreased libido, sexual dysfunction, and decreased ejaculatory volume, despite the fact that peripheral testosterone levels are normal in these patients. Gynecomastia has been noted in 0.4% of the patients.

More recently, it has been found that in addition to improvements in uroflow and symptom score, patients with large prostates (>40 cc) have a more significant improvement in symptom scores and uroflows compared with those with smaller prostates (<40 cc). Additionally, the hazard rate for BPH-related surgical intervention decreased by 40% and catheterization for urinary retention decreased by 57% in patients on finasteride therapy compared with those on placebo. The investigators in several of these studies felt that baseline prostate volume was a key predictor of treatment outcome. Furthermore, this has significant economic and public health implications because TURP is one of the most common surgical procedures in elderly men of this age group. However, important questions still remain. These include the fact that we may just be shifting the clock to a later date when, ultimately, even patients on finasteride will fail secondary to bladder decompensation. Cost is an additional issue, since only a small number of patients have benefited (1.5–5%) and it may not be justifiable to put 95–98.5% of the patients on treatment for this small benefit. In this regard, it is possible that using prostate volumes as an initial baseline parameter, one may select the patients that may benefit from finasteride therapy.

Finasteride therapy has been used in combination with α-blockers and the results revealed that there was no benefit to using the combination in reducing symptoms or improving uroflow measurements, especially in the average-sized prostate. This combination therapy was examined in a recent double-blind, placebo-controlled study comparing the α-blocker terazosin with finasteride. Significant improvement was demonstrated for the α-blocker, while finasteride produced little improvement overall and was not significantly more effective than placebo in treating moderately symptomatic BPH. However, a subanalysis of this study showed that while finasteride was poorly effective in patients with small prostate glands, a significant improvement was apparent in those with glands larger than 40 g.

With regard to PSA, finasteride partially suppresses the expression of PSA. In men on finasteride, the cumulative distribution of serum PSA levels at baseline is nearly identical to the distribution of twice the serum PSA level after 12 months of treatment.[5-7] In such circumstances, therefore, the upper PSA limit should be taken as 2 ng mL⁻¹ (instead of the normal 4 ng mL⁻¹), in which case a PSA level of 3 ng mL⁻¹ in a man on finasteride is just as elevated as a PSA of 6 ng mL⁻¹ in a man not on finasteride. Finasteride reduces serum PSA with the same kinetics in men with high (4–10 ng mL⁻¹) vs. low (<4 ng mL⁻¹) PSA levels.[8,9] However, finasteride also reduces serum PSA in men with known prostate cancer.[10,11] In some patients, ultimately diagnosed as having prostate cancer, the serum PSA did not increase in longitudinal follow-up.[6] Certainly, finasteride-induced suppression of the serum PSA does not appear to be a useful test for discriminating cancer from BPH. Further study is needed to determine whether finasteride will suppress the expected rise in PSA in men who develop prostate cancer while on therapy.[12-14]

The androgen regulation of finasteride in prostate cancer has been studied also at the molecular level. Use of leuprolide and flutamide in combination for 3 months does not abolish the expression of Type 2 of 5α-reductase enzyme. Orchiectomy suppresses but does not abolish the expression of Type 2 5α-reductase enzyme. In cancer cells, the Type 2 isoenzyme is present only in stromal cells. This suggests that if 5α-reductase inhibition has a role in suppressing prostatic cells, it may act by preventing DHT effects on epithelial luminal cells. This is being tested currently in the prostate cancer prevention trial, which is being conducted nationally in 200 centers within the USA. However, finasteride may not be the ideal choice for this trial since Type 1 isoenzyme-induced DHT from skin and liver may still influence prostatic epithelium in an endocrine fashion. There are currently agents in clinical trials that block both types of 5α-reductase enzyme; possibly these new agents will be more effective. Since 5α-reductase cannot be observed in prostatic cancer cells, the use of 5α-reductase inhibitors such as finasteride may not be helpful in treatment of established cancer.

1 Moore E, Bracken B, Bremner W et al. Proscar: five-year experience [published erratum appears in Eur Urol 1996; **29**(2): 234]. Eur Urol 1995; **28**(4): 304–9.
2 Tian G, Stuart JD, Moss ML et al. 17 beta-(N-tert-butylcarbamoyl)-4-aza-5 alpha-androstan-1-en-3-one is an active site-directed slow time-dependent inhibitor of human steroid 5 alpha-reductase 1. Biochemistry 1994; **33**(8): 2291–6.
3 Tian G. In vivo time-dependent inhibition of human steroid 5 alpha-reductase by finasteride. J Pharm Sci 1996; **85**(1): 106–11.
4 Thigpen AE, Silver RI, Guileyardo JM et al. Tissue distribution and ontogeny of steroid 5 alpha-reductase isozyme expression. J Clin Invest 1993; **92**(2): 903–10.
5 Roehrborn CG, Chinn HK, Fulgham PF et al. The role of transabdominal ultrasound in the preoperative evaluation of patients with benign prostatic hypertrophy. J Urol 1986; **135**: 1190–3.
6 Simonsen O, Moller-Madsen B, Dorfinger T et al. The significance of age on symptoms and urodynamic and cystoscopic findings in benign prostatic hypertrophy. Urol Res 1987; **15**: 355–8.

7 Donkervoort T, Zinner NR, Sterling AM *et al*. Megestrol acetate in treatment of benign prostatic hypertrophy. *Urology* 1975; **6**: 580–7.

8 Meyhoff HH, Ingemann L, Nordling J, Hald T. Accuracy in preoperative estimation of prostatic size. A comparative evaluation of rectal palpation, intravenous pyelography, urethral closure pressure, profile recording and cystourethroscopy. *Scand J Urol Nephrol* 1981; **15**: 45–51.

9 Mohr DN, Offord KP, Melton LJ. Isolated asymptomatic microhematuria; a cross-sectional analysis of test-positive and test-negative patients. *J Gen Intern Med* 1987; **2**: 318–24.

10 Mohr DN, Offord KP, Melton LJ. Isolated asymptomatic microhematuria; a cross-sectional analysis of test-positive and test-negative patients. *J Gen Intern Med* 1987; **2**: 318–24.

11 Messing EM, Young TB, Hunt VB. The significance of asymptomatic microhematuria in men 50 or more years old: findings of a home screening study using urinary dipsticks. *J Urol* 1987; **137**: 919–22.

12 Eri LM, Tveter KJ. Safety, side effects and patient acceptance of the luteinizing hormone-releasing hormone agonist leuprolide in treatment of benign prostatic hyperplasia. *J Urol* 1994; **152**(2 Pt1): 448–52.

13 Mebust WK, Holtgrewe HL, Cockett ATK *et al*. Transurethral prostatectomy: immediate and postoperative complications. A cooperative study of 13 participating institutions evaluating 3,885 patients. *J Urol* 1989; **141**: 243–7.

14 Holtgrewe HL, Valk WL. Factors influencing the mortality and morbidity of transurethral prostatectomy: a study of 2,105 cases. *J Urol* 1962; **87**: 450–9.

Role of Newer Agents and Combinations

14

T.C. Chai and W.D. Steers

INTRODUCTION

The medical treatment of lower urinary tract symptoms (LUTS) in men from bladder outlet obstruction due to benign prostatic hyperplasia (BPH) has evolved over the last decade. Decreased force, intermittent urinary stream, and straining to void are attributable to the static and dynamic components of BPH. The origins of irritative symptoms such as urinary urgency, frequency, and nocturia are not well delineated. More importantly, these irritative symptoms bother patients most, causing them to seek referral to urologists. The three most prevalent LUTS in men over the age of 50 years are nocturia, weak stream, and urinary frequency.[1] LUTS are multifactorial and may not relate entirely to BPH because they are equally present in elderly women.[2,3] Additionally, 15–30% of men complain of persistent irritative voiding symptoms, despite relief of outlet obstruction.[4,5] Therefore, future treatments for BPH will extend beyond reducing the size of the prostate or decreasing urethral resistance.

Since Caine et al.[6] first demonstrated α_1-adrenoreceptor-mediated contraction of prostatic smooth muscle, the usage and refinement of α_1-blocker therapy in BPH has rapidly evolved. The discovery of subtypes of α_1-receptors holds the promise of targeting prostate tissue-specific α_1-receptor(s), thereby reducing vascular or central nervous system side effects. However, the efficacy of α_1-blockade may not rest solely in reducing the smooth muscle tone in the prostate. The α_1-blockers reduce bladder outlet resistance through inhibition of both sympathetic and somatic outflow from the spinal cord.[7,8] Systemic and intrathecal α_1-blockade also abolish bladder hyperactivity of central origin.[9,10] Because norepinephrine released from descending pathways regulates bladder function,[11] α_1-receptors located in the sensory receiving areas of the dorsal horn of the spinal cord may modulate input from the bladder. It has been shown that terazosin can reduce voiding symptom scores independently of pretreatment peak flow rates, suggesting that the clinical effect of α_1-blockers may not lie solely in reducing outlet resistance at the prostate level.[12] Finally, it has been shown that doxazosin can induce apoptosis of the prostatic glandular epithelium and that the degree of apoptosis correlated strongly with degree of symptom relief, suggesting yet another pathway in the mechanism of action of α_1-blockers.[13]

Inhibition of 5α-reductase by finasteride reduces the prostatic size. This hormonal manipulation is another approach in the treatment of BPH Because of distinct modes of action for α_1-blockers and hormonal therapy, it is logical to investigate combination therapy for prostatism. However, future therapies will need adequately to treat the bladder and the nervous system, which can be altered by BPH.

The causes of irritative voiding symptoms in BPH are unclear. Given that the majority of patients with BPH today do not present with urinary retention, renal damage, urinary tract infection, or bladder stones, drugs that solely target irritative voiding can provide excellent relief from prostatism. To discover novel medical therapies for irritative LUTS, we need to understand the pathobiology of bladder outlet obstruction on the bladder smooth muscle, and its innervation. Animal models continue to provide insight into the myogenic and neurogenic events that occur as a consequence of bladder outlet obstruction. Obviously, the biology of prostatic growth also needs further investigations. Developments in these disciplines will advance the treatment and/or prevention of prostatism.

COMBINATION THERAPIES (α_1-BLOCKERS AND HORMONAL THERAPY)

The use of α_1-blockade combined with hormonal manipulation (5α-reductase inhibition) offers a theoretical benefit of reducing the dynamic as well as the static components of bladder outlet obstruction secondary to BPH. There may even be synergism in combination treatment. Lepor and colleagues[14] recently investigated combination therapy in a large double-blind, placebo-controlled study. Over 1000 men were treated over the course of 1 year in one of four treatment arms: terazosin+finasteride, terazosin+placebo, finasteride+placebo, placebo+placebo.

The study reveals no significant benefits from the combined use of terazosin+finasteride compared with terazosin+placebo. In fact finasteride+placebo has minimal salutary effects on peak urinary flow rates and AUA symptoms scores compared with placebo+placebo (Figure 14.1 and 14.2). Overall, terazosin+placebo is much more effective than finasteride+placebo. However, when the study subjects are stratified to those with <50 cm^3 and $\geq$ 50 cm^3 prostate volume, finasteride+placebo significantly increases the peak urinary flow rates in the $\geq$ 50 cm^3 group compared with the placebo+placebo group, although this increase is less than that accomplished by terazosin+placebo.[15] Finally,

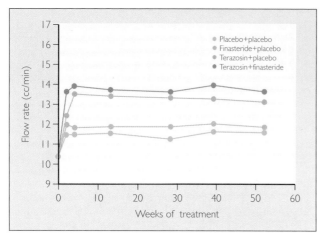

Figure 14.1 Effect of combination therapy on urinary flow rates

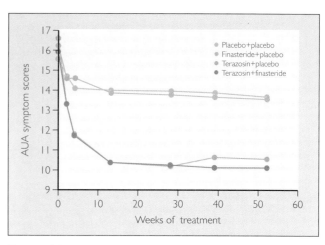

Figure 14.2 Effect of combination therapy on AUA symptom scores

the mean prostate-specific antigen (PSA) decrease is similar in both terazosin+finasteride and finasteride+placebo[16] treatment arms, reaffirming that terazosin does not affect PSA levels. These investigators conclude that combination therapy is not synergistic, and terazosin is significantly more efficacious than finasteride in treatment of symptomatic BPH. These findings are not surprising given the fact that (1) α_1-blockade works both "peripherally" (prostate) and "centrally" (spinal cord) and (2) BPH is primarily a stromal disease, and finasteride does not affect the stromal volume. As stated above, finasteride is clinically most effective in patients with large prostates. It has been shown that in a group of men with a mean prostate volume of 54 cm³, finasteride had a long-term beneficial effect, not only in reducing prostate volume, symptom scores, and increasing urinary flow rates, but also in decreasing the probability of requiring surgery.[17] Additionally, earlier symptom scores tended to weigh obstructive symptoms equally to or greater than irritative ones. These findings suggest targeting therapy by using specific variables such as prostate size and/or stromal/epithelial composition.

A clinical trial is underway to determine the effect of doxazosin+finasteride, doxazosin+placebo, finasteride+placebo, and placebo+placebo on men with LUTS. This long-term large multi-institutional study will also evaluate the natural progression of BPH and whether treatment alters the clinical course of BPH.

A combination trial of terazosin and flutamide, a testosterone receptor antagonist, vs. terazosin alone in the treatment of symptomatic BPH has been previously evaluated.[18] This study found no additional reduction in symptoms from the addition of flutamide compared with using terazosin alone. Even though flutamide alone does increase urinary flow rates in patients with BPH, its high incidence of side effects such as diarrhea, nipple tenderness, and gynecomastia probably precludes its routine use in treatment of BPH.[19]

NOVEL AND POTENTIAL NEW THERAPIES

PHYTOTHERAPEUTIC AGENTS

The treatment of voiding symptoms is often dictated by severity of patients' symptoms. Since urodynamic testing to diagnosis bladder outlet obstruction secondary to BPH is debatable in terms of cost effectiveness and prognostic capability, physicians continue to diagnose and treat patients empirically on severity of symptoms. Many patients seek alternative forms of treatment for their LUTS, be it from bladder outlet obstruction secondary to BPH or other causes. Patients use such compounds in the belief that natural products are safer and less costly than current medically accepted treatment regimens. Phytotherapeutic agents are plant extracts that have been used extensively in Europe and Asia for LUTS secondary to BPH. However, none is approved by the Food and Drug Administration for use in treatment of BPH in the USA. Scientific investigations of these agents have been mostly from Europe.

One of the more studied phytotherapeutic agents is a liposterolic extract of the palm plant *Serenoa repens* or *Sabal serrulata* (Permixon, Strogen, Curbicin, Prostavigol). This extract inhibits 5α-reductase, 3-ketosteroid reductase, receptor binding of androgens,[20,21] and smooth muscle contractions.[22] These findings suggest a possible use in treatment of BPH by reducing prostatic size as well as decreasing uninhibited bladder contractions. However, other studies have found contradictory results: namely, that Permixon in addition to six other plant extracts had no antiandrogen effects.[23] Permixon fails to decrease serum dihydrotestosterone, testosterone, follicle-stimulating hormone (FSH), or luteinizing hormone (LH) levels when given to male volunteers.[24,25] In clinical tests, some studies find that Permixon has no beneficial effect over placebo or α_1-blocker in reducing symptoms or increasing urinary flow rates.[26,27] Conversely, several double-blind studies show that *Serenoa repens* significantly decreased voiding symptoms, coupled with significantly increased urinary flow rates.[28-32] However, these patients were followed for less than 3 months, so the durability of the effect is unknown.

Another phytotherapeutic agent used for symptomatic treatment of BPH is *Pygeum africanum*, which is derived from the bark of the African plum. The mechanism of action is unknown, but it is believed that it does not act as a 5α-reductase inhibitor, α_1-blocker, or a potassium channel opener. Studies *in vitro* suggest that Tadenan (*Pygeum africanum* extract) works by inhibiting fibroblast hyperproliferation induced by basic fibroblast growth factors (bFGF).[33] Not only may this mechanism of action prevent prostatic hyperplasia, Tadenan also prevents detrusor contractile dysfunction induced by partial bladder obstruction.[34] A comprehensive review of published clinical experience with *Pygeum africanum* in 2262 patients has been published.[35]

A recent randomized, double-blind, placebo-controlled study of β-sitosterol (Harzol), which is a heterogeneous extract from plants containing phytosterols, shows that patients treated with β-sitosterol have significant improvement of both urinary flow rates and symptoms.[36] This is in contrast to another study showing that β-sitosterol has no benefit over placebo.[37] Other phytotherapeutic agents such as Cernilton (a pollen extract from several different plants), South African star grass (*Hypoxis rooperi*), and pumpkin seeds (*Cucurbita pepo*) have been used to treat BPH. Polyene antifungal macrolides such as candicidin and mepartricin have also been used. A double-blinded study of mepartricin shows improvement of pressure-flow data in treated patients.[38]

A recent review has highlighted many of the clinical studies published on phytotherapy and its use in BPH.[39] These agents must undergo both further basic research as well as more placebo-controlled clinical trials with longer follow-up. Additionally, because the manufacturing of these agents is not subject to quality control, the purity of the contents is not consistent. Most of these compounds are heterogeneous and the active ingredient is uncertain. Until more studies are conducted, it will be difficult to confirm the scientific validity of use of these agents in the treatment for LUTS secondary to BPH.

NERVE GROWTH FACTOR AND NEURALLY TARGETED THERAPY

In the final analysis, if urinary retention, infection, stones, or renal insufficiency are rare complications of BPH, treatment targeted at symptoms is an attractive first line of therapy. It stands to reason that irritative symptoms must somehow be mediated by nerves supplying the lower urinary tract. Indeed, partial bladder outlet obstruction in animals elicits urinary frequency which temporally correlates with changes in the neural pathways to the bladder.[40] These neural changes are orchestrated through increased nerve growth fact or (NGF) production by the smooth

muscle of obstructed bladders as a result of mechanical stretch.[41] The elevated NGF levels produce hypertrophy of parasympathetic motor and sensory neurons.[42-44] There is also a 40–60% increase in labeling of bladder afferents, especially in the vicinity of the sacral parasympathetic nucleus (motor area to bladder) as well as an increase in GAP-43, a protein marker for neuronal growth.[45] Therefore, one could postulate an increase in neural connections between sensory input and motor neurons. This formation of increased spinal connections in the micturition pathway secondary to bladder outlet obstruction is further confirmed electrophysiologically by demonstration of enhancement of a spinal micturition reflex in animals.[40] In man, an analogous spinal reflex manifested as a cooling reflex is detected as a positive ice-water test (see below). Finally, further to reaffirm that NGF plays a role in this neural plasticity or reorganization, NGF-immune animals with circulating anti-NGF antibodies fail to develop increased urinary frequency or neural changes after obstruction.[45]

Human studies reveal that obstructed bladders, but not normal or neurogenic bladders, have increased NGF content.[46] These observations suggest that a therapy that prevents sensory rearrangement could have therapeutic potential in the treatment of BPH. Agents that can decrease the production of NGF by the obstructed bladder, increase the degradation of NGF, and/or block the NGF receptor on sensory neurons in the bladder could all potentially alleviate the irritative voiding secondary to bladder outlet obstruction. NGF is also produced by the prostate and may even influence prostatic growth. In-vitro studies demonstrate that blockade of the trkA-NGF receptor on cultured prostate cells prevents proliferation.[47] Thus, NGF receptor antagonists may not only prevent sensory reorganization from the bladder, but also non-androgen mediated growth of the prostate.

Finally, results from ice-water cystometrograms (CMGs) on patients with bladder outlet obstruction further support the notion of sensory reorganization of the bladder. The ice-water CMG was initially described by Bors and Blinn.[48] Ice water infused into the bladder would either elicit a positive response (bladder contraction) or a negative response (no bladder contraction). Originally, this test was used to differentiate whether a neurogenic bladder was the result of an "upper motor neuron" or a "lower motor neuron" injury. In a normal individual, the ice-water test is negative. We have observed that the ice-water test is positive in 70% of patients with bladder outlet obstruction and no neurologic disease, whereas it is positive in 7% of patients without bladder outlet obstruction.[49] This finding again suggests that the sensory input in individuals with bladder outlet obstruction can be altered and that potential therapeutic intervention exists at this level.

CAPSAICIN AND TACHYKININS

It may not be possible to prevent or reverse sensory nerve reorganization secondary to BPH; however, the function of these sensory nerves can be diminished by selective toxins. As the bladder fills, a threshold pressure for micturition is reached. At this point, afferent signals are relayed to the spinal cord by thinly myelinated A-δ afferent fibers. From the spinal cord, the signal is relayed to a supraspinal center and a micturition reflex is initiated. In diseased states such as spinal cord injury or bladder outlet obstruction, the afferent signal to filling may be conveyed by a different subset of afferents, the unmyelinated C-afferents or capsaicin-sensitive afferents (CSA).[50] Many of the C-fibers are "silent" and require thresholds of stimulation to be activated. Disease states such as obstruction or inflammation may awaken these silent fibers. The CSA mediate a spinal micturition reflex with a shorter latency than the supraspinal micturition reflex. The predominance of the CSA as the major afferent pathway could explain the etiology of detrusor hyperreflexia in spinal cord injury and irritative voiding in bladder outlet obstruction.

CSA contain neuropeptides including tachykinins, such as substance P (SP) and neurokinin-A. Other peptides include calcitonin gene-related peptide (CGRP). Tachykinins mediate their effects through neurokinin receptors, NK-1, NK-2, and NK-3.[51] Capsaicin releases these neuropeptides from afferents, with subsequent bladder hyperactivity via spinal mechanisms (chemonocioceptive micturition reflex).[52-54] Chronic administration of capsaicin will deplete the CSA of their neuropeptides and thus "desensitize" a bladder in certain disease states such as the neurogenic bladder in spinal cord injury.[55-57] Resiniferatoxin, another compound with similar effects to capsaicin, has been studied in rats with bladder outlet obstruction.[58] Resiniferatoxin is more effective than capsaicin at desensitizing the CSA and may be of potential use in bladder hyperactivity.

Neurokinin receptor antagonists have been evaluated for their effects on micturition in normal and obstructed rats. NK-1 receptor in the spinal cord is involved in the micturition reflex induced by bladder filling in normal rats.[53,54,59] In rats with bladder outlet obstruction, an NK-1 receptor antagonist given intrathecally causes bladder areflexia,[59] again suggesting that the NK-1 receptor mediates the afferent signal to the micturition reflex. Interestingly, an NK-2 receptor antagonist, given either intra-arterially or intrathecally, prevents bladder hyperactivity induced by capsaicin in rats with bladder outlet obstruction. These observations suggest a potential use of neurokinin antagonists in patients with bladder hyperactivity secondary to BPH.

CALCIUM CHANNEL BLOCKERS
The contraction of bladder smooth muscle requires the presence of calcium ions from extracellular and intracellular stores.[60-63] Calcium is also involved in smooth muscle growth.[64-66] Because partial bladder outlet obstruction increases bladder weights in the experimental animal,[40,65] the role that calcium channel blockers play in the prevention of the bladder response to outlet obstruction has been studied.[67] Both verapamil and diltiazem blunt the bladder hypertrophic response to outlet obstruction. Additionally, calcium channel blockers reduce neuronal growth after obstruction by decreasing NGF production in the bladder. Unfortunately, these treated animals continue to manifest

urinary frequency. In contrast, the α_1-blocker, prazosin reduces the voiding frequencies of the obstructed animals. Clinically, it has been shown that the intravesical calcium channel blockers, terodiline and verapamil, reduced detrusor hyperactivity.[68,69]

These findings suggest a possibility of yet another combination therapy for BPH. Terazosin, an α_1-blocker, can be used to decrease voiding symptoms. However, α_1-blockers do not prevent the pathophysiologic myogenic and neurogenic sequelae of outlet obstruction. Calcium channel blockers do prevent or blunt some of these sequelae. Combining calcium channel blockers with an α_1-blocker may decrease outlet resistance as well as prevent associated pathology. It remains to be seen whether blunting obstructive changes in the bladder with calcium channel blockers will lead to hypocontractility or an increase in residual urine.

POTASSIUM CHANNEL OPENERS
For bladder smooth muscle to contract, depolarization of the smooth muscle membrane occurs by influx of calcium ions. Relaxation occurs when the membrane hyperpolarizes due to efflux of potassium ions out of the smooth muscle cells. An agent that "opens" the potassium channel would then hyperpolarize the smooth muscle and therefore make the muscle less excitable. This strategy has potential therapeutic advantage in treatment of idiopathic detrusor instability or that secondary to bladder outlet obstruction.

Potassium channel openers have a relaxant effect on experimental bladder.[70-72] However, most of the available potassium channel openers are not bladder selective and therefore have potential for adverse cardiovascular side effects such as hypotension. Clinically, utility of these agents in treatment of bladder instability secondary to BPH remains to be investigated.

PROSTATIC PEPTIDE GROWTH FACTORS
To discover other potential new areas in treatment of BPH, the biology of prostatic growth has been investigated. The prostate begins to form at the 10th gestational week as epithelial outgrowths or buds from the endodermal urogenital sinus and contacts the surrounding mesenchymal cells (stroma). The continued development of the prostatic glandular tissue depends on androgens, specifically dihydrotestosterone.[73] However, androgens have an indirect effect because androgen receptor positive mesenchymal cells directly mediate prostatic epithelial morphogenesis and proliferation.[74-79] This is evidenced by the fact that the extent of embryologic prostatic growth is determined by stromal content.[80] After birth, there is limited cessation of growth of the prostate followed by regrowth at puberty due to the surge in androgens. This growth continues until adulthood, at which time it stops.

McNeal studied the histopathology of BPH and made several important observations.[81] First, BPH arose in a small defined area periurethrally above the verumontanum, termed the transition zone. Secondly, he observed that BPH nodules originate through eccentric budding, suggesting localized stromal inductive effects. He suggested that the pathogenesis of BPH involves a "reawakening" of embryonic inductive interactions between mesenchyme and nascent glandular nodules. The mechanisms involved in this interaction may be due to humoral inducing agent(s) from the stroma that incite glandular proliferation.

There is ample evidence that stromal cells produce various peptide growth factors that regulate normal epithelial–mesenchymal interaction and growth.[78] One peptide growth factor produced by prostatic stromal cells implicated in pathogenesis of BPH is bFGF. Studies on int-2 transgenic mice support this theory.[82] The int-2 mice overexpress a peptide homologous to bFGF. The prostates from int-2 mice are 20 times larger than the prostates from wild-type mice. This increased prostatic size is mostly from epithelial hyperplasia. Interestingly, 5α-reductase inhibitors fail to cause cellular regression in this model.[83] The int-2 gene product is not normally expressed in adult tissues, but is detected in embryonic tissue during development,[82,84] supporting McNeal's theory that the events leading to BPH parallel embryonic prostatic development. The amount of mRNA for bFGF is also elevated in the human BPH specimens.[85,86]

Another peptide growth factor implicated in the pathogenesis of BPH is transforming growth factor $\beta2$ (TGF-$\beta2$). The mRNA for TGF$\beta2$ is elevated in human BPH tissue.[86,87]

Immunostaining for TGF$\beta1$, another member of the TGFβ family, reveals marked increased content in the stroma of BPH prostates.[88,89] It is hypothesized that TGFβ stimulates the growth and activity of stromal cells, which, in turn, increase production of other peptide growth factors, thereby causing epithelial growth. This explanation could explain the variability in hyperplasia of stromal and epithelial compartments seen in BPH.[90]

With the advancement of molecular biological techniques, new treatment strategies such as gene therapy in prevention or regression of BPH may be imaginable. We now have the capability to study the cellular mechanisms that control the transcription and translation of the genes encoding these growth factors involved in pathogenesis of BPH. By targeting these "control" points, we can potentially prevent or reverse the stromal–epithelial interactions leading to BPH. However, we need to gain further insight into fundamental stromal–epithelial interactions that occur in the development of BPH before we know which peptide growth factors to target.

TRANSURETHRAL INTRAPROSTATIC INJECTIONS OF ENZYMES

Because the fibromuscular stroma of the prostate contains abundant collagen and BPH is primarily a stromal disease,

Agent	Proposed mechanisms and/or effects
I. Phytotherapy	
A. *Serenoa repens/Sabal serrulata* (Permixon, Strogen, Curbicin, Prostavigol)	Antiandrogen activity (inhibition of 5α-reductase and/or inhibition of dihydrotestosterone binding to nuclear and cytosolic receptors)
B. *Pygeum africanum* (Tadenan)	Inhibition of fibroblast hyperproliferation induced by bFGF, prevents detrusor contractile dysfunction
C. β-Sitosterol (Harzol)	Unknown
D. Cernilton	Unknown
E. Mepartricin/candicidin (antifungals)	Effect mediated by cholesterol metabolism
II. NGF targeted therapy	
A. NGF immunity	Prevents both neuroplasticity and increased voiding frequency secondary to bladder outlet obstruction
B. NGF receptor (trk A) blockers	Prevents NGF's biologic actions
III. Capsaicin and tachykinins	
A. Capsaicin	Depletes afferent neuropeptides
B. Tachykinin receptor blockers	Blocks biologic effects of afferent neuropeptides
IV. Calcium channel blockers	
A. Diltiazem/verapamil	Blunts both bladder hypertrophy and neuroplasticity secondary to obstruction
B. Intravesical terodiline and verapamil	Decreases bladder hyperactivity
V. Potassium channel openers	Hyperpolarizes bladder smooth muscle, thereby decreasing smooth muscle activity
VI. Peptide growth factors	Regulates stromal/epithelial interactions in the prostate; manipulations of these factors may prevent or retard the development of BPH
VII. Enzymatic ablation	Collagenase and hyaluronidase to decrease prostatic size as well as urethral resistance

Table 14.1 Potential novel medical therapies for BPH

investigators have studied whether intraprostatic injections of collagenase and hyaluronidase can be used to treat BPH. Additionally, because of aging, collagen becomes less compliant owing to an increase in hydroxyproline residues. This rigidity of collagen in the prostatic stroma may play a part in bladder outlet obstruction secondary to BPH. Therefore, agents such as collagenase and hyaluronidase may decrease the size of the prostate and reduce urethral resistance. In the canine model, prostatic stromal atrophy occurred after enzymatic treatment with minimal morbidity.[91] This methodology may have merit in treatment of patients with BPH.

CONCLUDING REMARKS

Table 14.1 summarizes the potential new therapies for BPH. The medical treatment of BPH has advanced in the last 20 years with the advent of α_1-blockers and 5α-reductase inhibitors. Since then, no new medical breakthroughs have been discovered. Because a majority of patients do not present with severe morbidities secondary to BPH, such as renal failure, recurrent urinary tract infections, or refractory urinary retention, the primary treatment of BPH patients can be directed at relief of voiding symptoms. The fact that 15–30% of men have persistent voiding symptoms despite surgical relief of prostatic obstruction further exemplifies the need to better understand how voiding symptoms relate to BPH. In order to discover newer treatments, we need to understand basic changes in both the prostate and bladder that occur secondary to BPH. By identifying these biologic alterations, we can potentially arrive at efficacious therapies for BPH and even possibly prevent the development of BPH.

REFERENCES

1 Norman RW, Nickel JC, Fish D, Pickett SN. "Prostate-related symptoms" in Canadian men 50 years of age or older: prevalence and relationships among symtoms. Br J Urol 1994; 74: 542–50.
2 Lepor H, Machi G. Comparison of AUA symptom index in unselected males and females between fifty-five and seventy-nine years of age. Urology 1993; 42: 36–40.
3 Chai TC, Belville WD, McGuire EJ, Nyquist L. Specificity of AUA voiding symptom index: comparison of unselected and selected samples of both sexes. J Urol 1993; 150: 1/10–13.
4 Seaman EK, Jacobs BZ, Blaivas JG, Kaplan SA. Persistence or recurrence of symptoms after transurethral resection of the prostate: a urodynamic assessment. J Urol 1994; 152: 935–7.
5 Andersen JT. Detrusor hyperreflexia in benign obstruction: a cystometric study. J Urol 1994; 152: 523–34.
6 Caine M, Raz S, Zeigler M. Adrenergic and cholinergic receptors in the human prostate, prostatic capsule and bladder neck. Br J Urol 1975; 47: 193–202.
7 Danuser H, Thor KB. Inhibition of central sympathetic and somatic outflow to the lower urinary tract of the cat by the alpha 1 adrenergic receptor antagonist prazosin. J Urol 1995; 153: 1308–12.
8 Gajewski J, Downie JW, Awad SA. Experimental evidence for a central nervous system site in the effect of alpha-adrenergic blockers on the external urinary sphincter. J Urol 1984; 132: 403–9.
9 Yoshimura N, Sasa M, Yoshida O, Takaori S. Mediation of the micturition reflex by central norepinephrine form the locus coeruleus in the cat. J Urol 1990; 143: 840–3.
10 Dray A, Nunan L. Supraspinal and spinal mechanisms in morphine-induced inhibition of reflex urinary bladder contractions in the rat. Neuroscience 1987; 22: 281–7.
11 Sasa M, Yoshimura N. Locus coeruleus noradrenergic neurons as a micturition center. Microscopy Res Tech 1994; 29: 226–30.
12 Lepor H, Nieder A, Feser J et al. Effect of terazosin on prostatism in men with normal and abnormal peak urinary flow rates. Urology 1997; 49: 476–80.
13 Kyprianou N, Litvak JP, Borkowski A et al. Induction of prostate apoptosis by doxazosin in benign prostatic hyperplasia. J Urol 1998; 159: 1810–15.
14 Lepor H, Williford WO, Barry MJ et al. The efficacy of terazosin, finasteride, or both in benign prostatic hyperplasia. N Engl J Med 1996; 335: 533–9.
15 Lepor H et al. Does prostate volume (PV) predict response to terazosin and finasteride monotherapy and terazosin/finasteride

combination therapy? A subset analysis of the VA Cooperative BPH medical therapy study. J Urol 1996; 155(5): 574A (abstract 1052).
16 Williford WO, Lepor H, Dixon CM et al. Serum PSA levels after 52 weeks of therapy with finasteride, terazosin, combination, and placebo: results of the VA Cooperative Study #359. J Urol 1996; 155(5): 533A (abstract 890).
17 McConnell JD et al. (Finasteride Long-Term Efficacy and Safety Study Group). The effect of finasteride on the risk of acute urinary retention and the need for surgical treatment among men with benign prostatic hyperplasia. N Engl J Med 1998; 338: 557–63.
18 Lepor H, Machi G. The relative efficacy of terazosin versus terazosin and flutamide for the treatment of symptomatic BPH. Prostate 1992; 20: 89–95.
19 Narayan P, Trachtenberg J, Lepor H et al. A dose–response study of the effect of flutamide on benign prostatic hyperplasia: results of a multicenter study. Urology 1996; 47: 497–504.
20 Sultan C, Terraza A, Devillier C et al. Inhibition of androgen metabolism and binding by a liposterolic extract of "Serenoa repens b" in human foreskin fibroblasts. J Steroid Biochem Mol Bid 1984; 20: 515–19.
21 Weisser H, Tunn S, Behnke B, Krieg M. Effects of the Sabal serrulata extract IDS 89 and its subfractions on 5α-reductase activity in human benign prostatic hyperplasia. Prostate 1996; 28: 300–6.
22 Gutierrez M, de Boto G, Cantabrana B, Hidalgo A. Mechanisms involved in the spasmolytic effect of extracts from Sabal serrulata fruit on smooth muscle. Gen Pharmacol 1996; 27: 171–6.
23 Rhodes L, Primka RL, Berman C et al. Comparison of finasteride (Proscar), a 5α reductase inhibitor, and various commercial plant extracts in in vitro and in vivo 5α reductase inhibition. Prostate 1993; 22: 43–51 (1993).
24 Strauch G, Perles P, Vergult G et al. Comparison of finasteride (Proscar) and Serenoa repens (Permixon) in the inhibition of 5-alpha reductase in healthy male volunteers. Eur Urol 1994; 26: 247–52.
25 Casarosa C, Cosci di Coscio M, Fratt M. Lack of effects of a lyposterolic extract of Serenoa repens on plasma levels of testosterone, follicle-stimulating hormone, and luteinizing hormone. Clin Ther 1988; 10: 585–8.
26 Smith HR, Memon A, Smart CJ, Dewbury K. The value of Permixon in benign prostatic hypertrophy. Br J Urol 1986; 58: 36–40.
27 Grasso M, Montesano A, Buonaguidi A et al. Comparative effects of alfuzosin versus Serenoa repens in the treatment of symptomatic benign prostatic hyperplasia. Arch Esp Urol 1995; 48: 97–103.

28 Champault G, Patel JC, Bonnard AM. A double-blind trial of an extract of the plant *Serenoa repens* in benign prostatic hyperplasia. *Br J Pharmacol* 1984; **18**: 461–2.

29 Boccafoschi C, Annoscia S. Confronto fra estratto di serenoa repens e placebo mediate prova clinica controllata in pazienti con adenomatosi prostatica. *Urologia* 1983; **50**: 1257–68.

30 Emili E, Lo Cigno M, Petrone U. Risultati clinici su un nuovo farmaco nella terapia dell'ipertrofia della prostata (Permixon). *Urologia* 1983; **50**: 1042–8.

31 Tasca A, Barulla M, Cavazzana A et al. Trattamento della sintomatologia ostruttiva da adenoma prostatico conestratto di Serenoa Repens. *Minerva Urol Nefrol* 1985; **37**: 87–91.

32 Cukier P, Ducassou P, Le Guillou P et al. Permixon versus placebo: resultats d'une etude multicentrique. *C R Ther Pharmacol Clin* 1985; **4**: 15–21.

33 Paubert-Braquet M, Monboisse JC, Servent-Saez N et al. Inhibition of bFGF and EGF-induced proliferation of 3T3 fibroblasts by extract of *Pygeum africanum* (Tadenan). *Biomed Pharmacother* 1994; **48**(Suppl 1): 43–7.

34 Levin RM, Riffaud J-P, Bellamy F et al. Protective effect of Tadenan of bladder function secondary to partial outlet obstruction. *J Urol* 1996; **155**: 1466–70.

35 Andro M-C, Riffaud J-P. *Pygeum africanum* extract for the treatment of patients with benign prostatic hyperplasia: a review of 25 years of published experience. *Curr Ther Res* 1995; **56**: 796–817.

36 Berges RR, Windeler J, Trampisch HJ, Senge T. Randomised, placebo-controlled, double-blinded clinical trial of β-sitosterol in patients with benign prostatic hyperplasia. *Lancet* 1995; **345**: 1529–32.

37 Kadow C, Abrams PH. A double-blind trial of the effect of beta-sitosteryl glucoside (WA184) in the treatment of benign prostatic hyperplasia. *Eur Urol* 1986; **12**: 187–9.

38 Tosto A, Dattolo E, Serni S et al. A double-blind study of the effects of mepartricin in the treatment of obstruction due to benign prostatic hyperplasia. *Curr Ther Res* 1995; **56**: 1270–5.

39 Lowe FC, Ku JC. Phytotherapy in treatment of benign prostatic hyperplasia: a critical review. *Urology* 1996; **48**: 12–20.

40 Steers WD, de Groat WC. Effect of bladder outlet obstruction on micturition reflex pathways in the rat. *J Urol* 1988; **140**: 864–71.

41 Persson K, Sando JJ, Tuttle JB, Steers WD. Protein kinase C in cyclic stretch-induced nerve growth factor production by urinary tract smooth muscle cells. *Am J Physiol* 1995; **269**: C1018–24.

42 Steers WD, Ciambotti J, Erdman S, de Groat WC. Morphological plasticity in efferent pathways to the urinary bladder of the rat following urethral obstruction. *J Neurosci* 1990; **10**: 1943–51.

43 Steers WD, Ciambotti J, Etzel B, Erdman S, de Groat WC. Alterations in afferent pathways from the urinary bladder of the rat in response to partial urethral obstruction. *J Comp Neurol* 1991; **310**: 401–10.

44 Dupont MC, Persson K, Spitsbergen J, Tuttle JB, Steers WD. The neuronal response to bladder outlet obstruction, a role for NGF. *Adv Exp Med Biol* 1995; **385**: 41–54.

45 Steers WD, Creedon DJ, Tuttle JB. Immunity to nerve growth factor prevents afferent plasticity following urinary bladder hypertrophy. *J Urol* 1996; **155**: 379–85.

46 Steers WD, Kolbeck S, Creedon D, Tuttle JB. Nerve growth factor in the urinary bladder of the adult regulates neuronal form and function. *J Clin Invest* 1991; **88**: 1709–15.

47 Pflug BR, Dionne C, Kaplan DR, Lynch J, Djakiew D. Expression of a Trk high affinity nerve growth factor receptor in the human prostate. *Endocrinology* 1995; **136**: 262–8.

48 Bors EH, Blinn KA. Spinal reflex activity from the vesical mucosa in paraplegic patients. *Arch Neurol Psychiatry* 1957; **78**: 339–54.

49 Chai TC, Gray ML, Steers WD. Incidence of positive ice water test in bladder outlet obstructed patients: evidence for bladder neuroplasticity. *J Urol* 1998; **160**: 34–8.

50 Cheng CL, Ma CP, de Groat WC. Effects of capsaicin on micturition and associated reflexes in rats. *Am J Physiol* 1993; **265**: R132–8.

51 Maggi CA. The role of peptides in the regulation of the micturition reflex: an update. *Gen Pharmacol* 1991; **22**: 1–24.

52 Ishizuka O, Yasuhiko I, Mattiasson A, Andersson KE. Capsaicin-induced bladder hyperactivity in normal conscious rats. *J Urol* 1994; **152**: 525–30.

53 Lecci A, Giuliani S, Garret C, Maggi CA. Evidence for a role of tachykinins as sensory transmitters in the activation of micturition reflex. *Neuroscience* 1993; **54**: 827–37.

54 Lecci A, Giuliani S, Patacchini R, Maggi CA. Evidence against a peripheral role of tachykinins in the initiation of micturition reflex in rats. *J Pharmacol Exp Ther* 1993; **264**: 1327–32.

55 Fowler CJ, Jewkes D, McDonald WI et al. Intravesical capsaicin for neurogenic bladder dysfunction. *Lancet* 1992; **339**: 1239.

56 Fowler CJ, Beck RO, Gerrard S et al. Intravesical capsaicin for treatment of detrusor hyperreflexia. *J Neurol Neurosurg Psychiatry* 1994; **57**: 169–73.

57 Geirsson G, Fall M, Sullivan L. Clinical and urodynamic effects of intravesical capsaicin treatment in patients with chronic traumatic spinal detrusor hyperreflexia. *J Urol* 1995; **154**: 1825–9.

58 Ishizuka O, Mattiasson A, Andersson KE. Urodynamic effects of intravesical resiniferatoxin and capsaicin in conscious rats with and without outflow obstruction. *J Urol* 1995; **154**: 611–16.

59 Ishizuka O, Igawa Y, Lecci A et al. Role of intrathecal tachykinins for micturition in unanesthetized rats with and without bladder outlet obstruction. *Br J Pharmacol* 1994; **113**: 111–16.

60 Haugaard N, Levin SS, Buttyan R et al. Bladder function in experimental outlet obstruction: pharmacologic responses to alterations in innervation, energetics, calcium mobilization, and genetics. *Adv Exp Med Biol* 1995; **385**: 7–19.

61 Zderic SA, Duckett JW, Levin RM. Effect of partial outlet obstruction on the biphasic response to field stimulation at different concentrations of calcium. *Pharmacology* 1994; **49**: 167–72.

62 Saito M, Hypolite JA, Wein AJ, Levin RM. Effect of partial outflow obstruction on rat detrusor contractility and intracellular free calcium concentration. *Neurourol Urodyn* 1994; **13**: 297–305.

63 Zhao Y, Wein AJ, Levin RM. Role of calcium in mediating the biphasic contraction of the rabbit urinary bladder. *Gen Pharmacol* 1993; **24**: 727–31.

64 Kamm KE, Stull JT. The function of myosin and myosin light chain kinase phosphorylation in smooth muscle. *Annu Rev Pharmacol Toxicol* 1985; **25**: 593–620.

65 Malmqvist M, Arner A, Uvelium B. Contractile and cytoskeletal proteins in smooth muscle during hypertrophy and its reversal. *Am J Physiol* 1991; **260**: C1085–93.

66 Morgan JI, Curran T. Role of ion flux in the control of c-fos expression. *Nature Lond* 1986; **322**: 552–5.

67 Steers WD, Albo M, Tuttle JB. Calcium channel antagonists prevent urinary bladder growth and neuroplasticity following mechanical stress. *Am J Physiol* 1994; **266**: R20–6.

68 Ekstrom B, Andersson KE, Mattiasson A. Urodynamic effects of intravesical instillation of terodiline in healthy volunteers and in patients with detrusor hyperactivity. *J Urol* 1992; **148**: 1840–3.

69 Mattiasson A, Ekstrom B, Andersson KE. Effects of intravesical instillation of verapamil in patients with detrusor hyperactivity. *J Urol* 1989; **141**: 174–7.

70 Howe BB, Halterman TJ, Yochim CL et al. ZENECA ZD6169: a novel KATP channel opener with in vivo selective for urinary bladder. *J Pharmacol Exp Ther* 1995; **274**: 884–90.

71 Levin RM, Hayes L, Zhao Y, Wein AJ. Effect of pinacidil on spontaneous and evoked contractile activity. *Pharmacology* 1992; **45**: 1–8.

72 Andersson KE. Clinical pharmacology of potassium channel openers. *Pharmacol Toxicol* 1992; **70**: 244–54.

73 Imperato-McGinley J, Guerrero L, Gautier T *et al*. Steroid 5 alpha-reductase deficiency in man: an inherited form of male pseudohermaphrodism. *Science* 1974; **186**: 1213–15.

74 Cunha GR, Lung B. The possible influence of temporal factors in androgenic responsiveness of urogenital tisue recombinants from wild type and androgen insensitive (Tfm) mice. *J Exp Zool* 1978; **205**: 181–93.

75 Cunha GR, Young P, Reese B. Glandular epithelial induction by embryonic mesenchyme in adult bladder epitelium of BALB/c mice. *Invest Urol* 1980; **17**: 302–4.

76 Cunha GR, Fujii H, Neubauer BL *et al*. Epithelial–mesenchyme interactions in prostatic development. I. Morphologic observations of prostatic induction by urogenital sinus mesenchyme in epithelium of the adult rodent urinary bladder. *J Cell Biol* 1983; **96**: 1662–70.

77 Cooke PS, Young P, Cunha GR. Androgen receptor expression in developing male reproductive organs. *Endocrinology* 1991; **128**: 2867–73.

78 Cunha GR, Alarid ET, Turner T *et al*. Normal and abnormal development of the male urogenital tract: role of androgens, mesenchymal–epithelial interactions, and growth factors. *J Androl* 1992; **13**: 465–75.

79 Lasnitzki I, Mizuno T. Prostatic induction: interaction of epithelium and mesenchyme from normal wild type and androgen-insensitive mice with testicular feminization. *J Endocrinol* 1980; **85**: 423–8.

80 Chung LW, Cunha GR. Stromal–epithelial interactions. II. Regulation of prostatic growth by embryonic urogenital sinus mesenchyme. *Prostate* 1983; **4**: 503–11.

81 McNeal JE: Origin and evolution of benign prostatic enlargement. *Invest Urol* 1978; **15**: 340–5.

82 Muller WJ, Lee FS, Dickson C *et al*. The int-2 gene product acts as an epithelial growth factor in transgenic mice. *EMBO J* 1990; **9**: 907–13.

83 Tutrone RF Jr, Ball RA, Ornitz DM *et al*. Benign prostatic hyperplasia in a transgenic mouse: a new hormonally sensitive investigatory model. *J Urol* 1993; **149**: 633–9.

84 Jakobovitz A, Shackleford GM, Varmus HE *et al*. Two proto-oncogenes implicated in mammary carcinogenesis, int-1 and int-2, are independently regulated during mouse development. *Proc Natl Acad Sci USA* 1986; **83**: 7806–10.

85 Mydlo JH, Bulbul MA, Richon VM *et al*. Heparin-binding growth factor isolated from human prostatic extracts. *Prostate* 1988; **12**: 343–55.

86 Mori H, Maki M, Oishi K *et al*. Increased expression of genes for basic fibroblast growth factor and transforming growth factor type $\beta2$ in human benign prostatic hyperplasia. *Prostate* 1990; **16**: 71–80.

87 Story MT, Hopp KA, Meier DA *et al*. Influence of transforming growth factor beta 1 and other growth factors on basic fibroblastic growth factor levels and proliferation of cultured human prostate derived fibroblasts. *Prostate* 1993; **22**: 183–97.

88 Thompson TC, Truong LD, Timme TL *et al*. Transforming growth factor $\beta1$ as a biomarker for prostate cancer. *J Cell Biochem* 1992; **16H**: 54–61.

89 Truong LD, Kadmon D, McCune BK *et al*. Association of transforming growth factor-$\beta1$ with prostate cancer: a immunohistochemical study. *Hum Pathol* 1993; **24**: 4–9.

90 Steiner MS. Role of peptide growth factors in the prostate: A review. *Urology* 1993; **42**: 99–110.

91 Harmon WJ, Barrett DM, Qian J *et al*. Transurethral enzymatic ablation of the prostate: canine model. *Urology* 1996; **48**: 229–33.

COMMENTARY

In this chapter, Drs Chai and Steers have provided a comprehensive overview of the various new and combination therapies available for BPH and early LUTS.

There is evidence that α-blockers may act not only by reducing smooth muscle tone of the prostate and urethra but also by reducing outflow resistance mediated via autonomic and somatic outflow from the spinal cord. Recent studies also suggest a role for doxazosin in inducing apoptosis of prostatic epithelial cells, and further studies may be necessary to determine whether other α-blockers have similar actions. The use of 5α-reductase inhibition by finasteride reduces prostate size. This method of BPH treatment in combination with α-blockers has been tested recently. In over 1000 men treated in a four-arm trial, Lepor and the VA Cooperative Group of Investigators noted that the finasteride plus terazosin combination offered no advantage over terazosin alone. Additionally, the terazosin plus placebo group was superior to finasteride plus placebo arm. The mean prostate size in this study was under 30 cm³. In contrast to this data there is recent data that in a group of men with mean prostate volume of 54 cm³ finasteride not only had a long-term benefit of reducing prostatic volume, symptom scores, and improving urinary flow rates but also in decreasing the probability of needing surgery. These data suggest that targeting specific therapy using variables of prostate size and stromal–epithelial ratios may have relevance in optimizing therapy for BPH. Currently, a clinical trial is underway to determine whether long-term use of doxazosin and finasteride will alter the clinical course of BPH. The use of anti-androgens such as flutamide in BPH alone or in combination has also been tested. The side effects of currently available anti-androgens preclude their routine use in BPH.

Among other novel agents being tested for BPH are phytotherapeutic agents. The liposterol extract of palm plant *Serenoa repens* (saw palmetto) is commonly used as a health food by many patients. It is thought to have several effects including inhibition of 5α-reductase, androgen binding, and relaxation of smooth muscles. However, clinical trials have shown mixed results for saw palmetto's efficacy in reducing symptoms and improving uroflow. Other agents that are being used include *Pygeum africanum*, β-sitosterol, pollen extracts, and pumpkin seeds. However, controlled clinical trials are lacking.

Molecular approaches to LUTS treatment include, among others, neurally targeted therapy to decrease bladder stimulation. Possible targets include neural growth factors, sensory nerve inhibition by toxins such as capsaicin, and tachykinins such as substance P and neurokinin receptor antagonists.

Other innovative approaches are also possible based on blockage of smooth muscle contraction by calcium channel blockers, which have been extensively tested on humans in combination with α-blockers for treatment of hypertension and cardiac disease. These agents would not only inhibit prostatic smooth muscle but also abnormal bladder contractions, which are present in a significant number of patients with BPH, as pointed out by Cespedes and McGuire in Chapter 8, "Urodynamics in the Evaluation of Benign Prostatic Hyperplasia". Potassium channel openers are also another possibility for use in combination, although current agents have too many systemic side effects.

Finally, peptide growth factors are among agents being extensively investigated as important factors in the maintenance of prostate growth, as pointed out in Chapters 1 and 2. These agents may be involved in the autocrine loops of prostatic growth maintenance, which continues even after blockage of hormonal influences. Among these factors are bFGF and TGFβ2. The use of intraprostatic enzymes are also being investigated in this regard and this is another novel approach to management of BPH.

Phytotherapeutic Agents

P. Narayan and M. Patel

15

INTRODUCTION

Abundant literature has been published in the last 20–30 years claiming that the Western high-animal-fat diet is mainly responsible for the high incidence of chronic and degenerative diseases (such as prostate cancer and benign prostatic hyperplasia (BPH)) seen in Western Europe, USA, and Canada.[1-7] Epidemiological data have also suggested that an abundance of animal fat and beef in the diet appears to be associated with increased risk for BPH and prostate cancer, in comparison with a soy-rich, low-fat, low-animal-protein diets.[8] From these findings, increased attention has been focused on herbal treatment (phytotherapy) for the management of BPH. Even though medical management of BPH continues to be of primary interest, it would be of greater usefulness (and convenience to the patient) if a "natural" agent found in everyday foods with low side effects could be used in the treatment of BPH. This form of treatment has grown favorably in many countries, especially in Germany, where several millions of dollars are spent on herbal (plant extracts) agents.[9,10]

Additionally, since BPH has had a linear relationship with bladder outlet obstruction (BOO), new pharmaceutical agents have been developed over the past two decades in an attempt to reduce the urinary symptoms of clinically evident BPH. Men are not bothered by an enlarged prostate unless it produces urinary obstructive symptoms. This is of great importance, because the majority of men with BPH visit their urologists, not because of any life-threatening medical emergency, but because of bothersome urinary symptoms. Therefore, it is legitimate to find agents (even if they are herbal) that can reduce the obstructive symptoms, and some clinicians feel that a secondary gain in increased urinary peak flow rates and decreased residual urine is of minor importance. Therefore, the primary goal in the management of BPH with phytotherapy has been to find agents capable of reducing the bothersome symptoms and improving lifestyle.

The phytotherapeutic agents have not been tested in any rigorous clinical trials until recently. The reason for this is that it is difficult to do multicenter, placebo-controlled, randomized clinical trials using herbal medication. Firstly, it is very difficult to control the diet of people in the study; a certain favorite diet of a subject can change him from the placebo category to the treatment category or vice versa. Additionally, controlled trials are expensive and would require "diet control" in addition to testing agent

consumption for a certain period of time. Regardless of these drawbacks, further clinical studies need to be done using phytotherapeutic agents.

Two groups of agents have been used for phytotherapeutic management of BPH; these agents are lignans and isoflavonoids. These agents are of plant origin and have similar structures to those of steroids found in the human body, especially testosterone and estrogen (see Figure 15.1). The lignans developed from flavonoid precursors about 400 million years ago and the isoflavonoids developed from the same ancestry about 120 million years ago. However, the latter group is the more important group of phyto-agents. Isoflavonoids were first used in veterinary medicine as estrogen substitutes, but their utility in humans was not well studied until 1982. There is no clear-cut reason for introducing these agents for management of BPH, besides the fact that they are natural substances in everyday foods. Reportedly, however, there has been great patient satisfaction with these agents, as judged by their popular consumption despite inadequate data and high prices. One reason for this popularity is that phytotherapeutic agents can be purchased with ease (without a prescription), and they have no side effects.

THE AGENTS AND THEIR CONTENTS

Many authors have postulated that the high-animal-fat diet compared with a semi-vegetarian diet may alter hormone production, and alter cellular metabolism in BPH. Two groups of hormone-like diphenolic phyto-estrogens of dietary origin have been documented to reduce prostatic hyperplasia; these agents are lignans and isoflavonoids. The former is found in large amounts in linseed (flax seed), sesame seeds, cereals, grains, fruits, and vegetables; it contains a diglycoside named secoisolariciresinol. When ingested, this diglycoside is metabolized to two mammalian lignans, enterodiol and enterolactone, by the intestinal bacteria.[11] The main source of isoflavonoids in the human diet is from soya bean and other legumes such as clover, which contain two methylated compounds, named formononetin and biochanin A. These two compounds are converted to daidzein and genistein by intestinal bacteria, respectively. Daidzein can be further metabolized to an isoflavon compound, named equol. Interestingly enough, these isoflavonoids have been identified in beer and bourbon.[12,13]

Several compounds from these groups have been found to be abundant in plasma of men living in areas of low

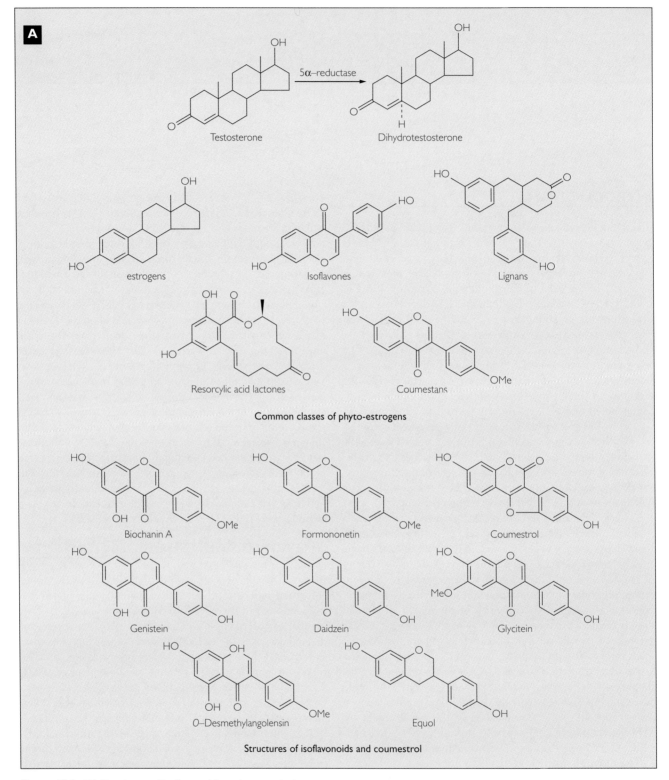

Figure 15.1 and associated structure labels:

A

5α–reductase

Testosterone → Dihydrotestosterone

estrogens

Isoflavones

Lignans

Resorcylic acid lactones

Coumestans

Common classes of phyto-estrogens

Biochanin A

Formononetin

Coumestrol

Genistein

Daidzein

Glycitein

O–Desmethylangolensin

Equol

Structures of isoflavonoids and coumestrol

Figure 15.1 (A) Structures of isoflavonoids and coumestrol

prostate cancer and BPH incidence. The precursors of these biologically active plant lignan and isoflavonoid glycosides are believed to be converted by intestinal bacteria to hormone-like compounds that possess weak estrogen activity.

Many plant lignan and isoflavonoid extracts have been used for the treatment of BPH, and several small clinical trials have shown that it works in improving urinary obstructive symptoms. The most frequently used products are the following:

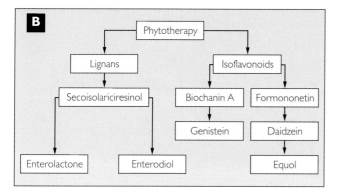

Figure 15.1 (B) Metabolism of isoflavonoids and lignans

(1) Saw palmetto berry – Fruits of the American Dwarf Palm (*Serenoa repens* or *Sabal serrulata*)
(2) bark of the African plum (*Pygeum africanum*)
(3) leaves of the trembling poplar (*Aspen* or *Populus tremula*)
(4) roots of the purple cone flower (*Echinacea purpurea*)
(5) pumpkin seeds (*Cucurbita pepo*)
(6) rye (*Secale cereale*)
(7) roots of the South African star grass (*Hypoxis rooperi*)
(8) roots of stinging nettle (*Urtica dioica*)
(9) unicorn root (*Aletrius farinosa*)
(10) pollen extract

There may be a common natural ingredient found in these products that is responsible for improving urinary symptoms. However, the exact ingredient that may be responsible for this effect is still unclear. Research in our labs shows that these plant extracts contain various amounts and proportions of free fatty alcohols, free fatty acids, and triterpenes and sterols (such as campesterol, lipoxin, lupenone, sitosterol, stigmasterol, tocopherol). Further investigation in the laboratory and clinical trials of specific ingredients is necessary to clarify their effects on BPH.

MECHANISM OF ACTION ON A MOLECULAR LEVEL

Many different mechanisms of action of plant extracts have been proposed, but very few have been proven by scientific methods. Two phyto-estrogenic isoflavones, daidzein and genistein, have been studied in great detail by many authors, and are the basis of our present knowledge of the physiology and mechanism of action of phytotherapeutic agents. Upon ingestion of daidzein and genistein plant extracts, the (highly polar) conjugated (natural) forms are hydrolyzed in the large intestine to the (non-polar) unconjugated forms via intestinal bacteria.[14] The extent of absorption of daidzein and genistein is dependent on the amount that is in the unconjugated form, because it is this form that is lipophilic enough to be readily absorbed across the intestinal cell membrane; therefore, the highly polar, conjugated form remains in the intestinal lumen and is eliminated with the stools.

The absorbed phyto-estrogenic isoflavonoids are then transported to the liver via the hepatic portal vein, where they are conjugated with glucuronic acid, and to a much lesser extent with sulfuric acid, by the liver.[14–17] (see Figure 15.2). Thus, in blood and urine, these compounds are found primarily conjugated to glucuronic acid. In plasma, the free and sulfated forms are biologically active, while the conjugated form is considered to be biologically inactive.[18]

The early molecular events involved in the initiation, promotion, and progression of BPH are testosterone dependent and may be influenced by endocrine changes induced by the estrogenic lignans and isoflavonoids.[19,20] Furthermore, it has been shown that these dietary compounds have the ability to stimulate sex hormone binding globulin synthesis in the liver, and also possess antiestrogenic properties, aromatase inhibitory properties, and 5α-reductase inhibitory properties.[21–24] Recent molecular studies have shown that soya and flax seed inhibit tumorigenesis in experimental animals, and genistein has been shown to inhibit tyrosine kinase, topoisomerase, and angiogenesis.[25–29] In addition to these properties, all lignans and isoflavonoids act as antioxidants, owing to their polyphenolic structure. Because of these known characteristics, lignans and isoflavonoids obtained through the diet influence (1) sex-hormone metabolism and biological activity, (2) intracellular and steroid metabolic enzymes, (3) protein synthesis (via inhibiting topoisomerase), (4) malignant cell proliferation, (5) calcium transport, (6) Na/K ATPase activity, (7) vascular smooth muscle cells, and (8) lipid oxidation and cell differentiation, making them candidates for a role as cancer-protective compounds.[6,7,11,30-33]

AGENTS USED IN THE TREATMENT OF BENIGN PROSTATIC HYPERPLASIA

There have been many theories postulated on how phytotherapeutic agents influence the prostate gland, but few have been proven scientifically.

SOY AND β-SITOSTEROL

Several histological studies have revealed that the prostate gland contains cholesterol, and its secretions contain cholesterol. It has been shown that plant extracts containing sitosterol (which is similar in structure to cholesterol) reduce prostatic cholesterol content, causing, in turn, a reduction in prostate size. Furthermore, it has been shown that prostatic hyperplastic tissue contains twice as much cholesterol as normal prostatic tissue. This finding has led to the theory that any agent that can lower the prostatic cholesterol levels would also be able to inhibit prostate growth; this would subsequently lead to a decrease in prostatic size with improvement in urinary obstructive symptoms. This unproven theory is the basis for which plant extracts containing sitosterol are used in the treatment of BPH. Structurally similar to cholesterol, sitosterols are poorly absorbed from the gastrointestinal tract even after unconjugation via hydrolysis. It is believed that sitosterol binds to cholesterol in the intestinal lumen and prevents its absorption, thereby

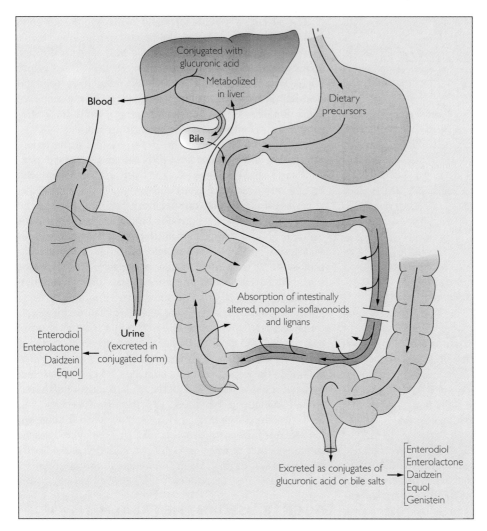

Figure 15.2 Physiology of phytotherapeutic agents

lowering plasma cholesterol levels. Lowering circulating cholesterol levels, in turn, will decrease the cholesterol content of the prostate, preventing enlargement of the gland. However, the downside of this is that approximately 10 g day^{-1} of sitosterol is needed to lower the plasma cholesterol by 10–20%, and the average daily diet consumed in the USA only provides 200 mg of sitosterol.[34]

In a 6-month, double-blind, placebo-controlled multicenter study, 200 patients with clinically evident BPH were randomized to receive either β-sitosterol (Harzol) 20 mg (t.i.d) or placebo.[35] The parameters measured were International Prostate Symptom Score (IPSS), urine flow, postvoid residual volume, prostate volume, and Boyarsky score. The latter being the primary endpoint, while the others were the secondary endpoints of the study. In the treated group, the modified Boyarsky score decreased by a mean value of 6.7 points in comparison with a 2.1-point decrease in the placebo group; this was statistically significant ($P < 0.01$). There was a decrease in IPSS by 7.4 points (14.9 to 7.5) in the β-sitosterol-treated group vs. a 2.3-point decrease (15.1 to 12.8) in the placebo group; this was statistically significant ($P<0.01$). The peak urinary flow rate increased from 9.9 mL s^{-1} to 15.2 mL s^{-1} ($\Delta=5.3$) in the treatment group,

and from 10.2 mL s^{-1} ($\Delta=1.2$) in the placebo group; this was also statistically significant ($P<0.01$). The postvoid residual volume (PVR) also showed a statistical difference between the two groups ($P<0.01$); treatment group decreased from 65.8 mL to 30.4 mL ($\Delta=35.4$), and the control group decreased from 64.8 mL to 54.3 mL ($\Delta=10.5$). Interestingly enough, there was no statistical difference in the prostatic volume between the two groups. The β-sitosterol treated group showed a 3.1 mL decrease in prostate volume compared with a 0.3 mL decrease in the control group ($P>0.01$); this shows that β-sitosterol does not have a substantial effect on the prostate volume. According to the authors, the significant improvement in symptoms and urinary flow parameters show the effectiveness of β-sitosterol in the treatment of benign prostatic hyperplasia. The authors state that there were no severe adverse events attributed to the β-sitosterol treatment; however, erectile dysfunction, loss of libido, constipation, and nausea were experienced in some patients taking β-sitosterol.

These excellent results were reproduced by Klippel and associates on behalf of the German BPH-Phyto study group.[36] This study was a 13-site multicenter, double-blind, placebo-controlled trial involving 177 patients with symptomatic BPH; these subjects were randomized to receive either β-sitosterol (phytosterol) 65 mg (b.i.d.) or placebo over a 6-month period. The primary endpoint of the study was the relative difference in the IPSS between the two groups, measured by the percent change from the initial values to the final office visit. In addition, the other parameters measured as secondary endpoints were the quality of life change, peak urinary flow rate, and PVR. After 6 months of treatment, there was a change in the IPSS from 16.0 to 7.8 ($\Delta=-8.2$) in the treated group, and 14.9 to 12.1 ($\Delta=-2.8$) in the placebo group. The change in the quality of life was a decrease of 1.9 (from 3.3 to 1.4) in the treatment group, and a decrease of 0.9 (from 3.1 to 2.2) in the control group. The peak urinary flow rate increased from 10.6 mL s^{-1} to 19.4 mL s^{-1} ($\Delta=8.8$) in the treated group, and from 11.3 mL s^{-1} to 15.7 mL s^{-1} ($\Delta=4.4$) in the placebo group. Finally, the PVR showed a decrease of 37.8 mL (from 63.4 mL to 25.6 mL) in the treatment group, and a decrease of 4.0 mL (from 63.1 mL to 59.1 mL) in the control group. All of these measured variables showed a statistically significant ($P<0.01$) improvement in the β-sitosterol treated group compared with the placebo group. The improvement in the primary endpoint (IPSS) with β-sitosterol and placebo was 51% and 19%, respectively. Of interest, the improvement in the assessed variables seen in the β-sitosterol group was more rapid during the first month of therapy than later. This is similar to those reported in other studies using α-blockers or finasteride for the treatment of BPH. Furthermore, finasteride showed an increase in the peak urinary flow rate of 4 mL s^{-1} after 12 months and the IPSS improved by 3.6 after 36 months of treatment.[37,38] These outcomes, calculated from baseline, are similar to the improvements seen in this German BPH-Phyto study. From the favorable results of this report, it appears that β-sitosterol is clinically proven to relieve BPH symptoms.

SAW PALMETTO BERRY (FRUITS OF THE AMERICAN DWARF PALM)

Saw palmetto berry is the most widely used plant extract for BPH. It is also commonly known as *Serenoa repens*, *Sabal serrulata*, or *Sabalis serrulata*. Historically, the saw palmetto berry is from the dwarf palm tree, a species from the Arenacea family, and was commonly used in the West Indies and the southeastern USA. It is extracted under supercritical conditions using carbon dioxide as the solvent. In the past, it has been used to treat numerous genitourinary problems, such as mucous membrane irritation.[39] It has also been shown to act as a nutritional tonic, and to increase testicular function.

As with all plant extracts, saw palmetto consists of a water-soluble extract and a pharmacologically active lipid-soluble extract. The latter consists of 85–95% fatty acids and sterols, mainly β-sitosterol, stigmasterol, cycloartenol, lupeol, lupenone, and methylcycloartenol.[39] Of these, β-sitosterol, similar in structure to cholesterol, is believed to be the most important; however, its influence on the prostate is still poorly understood.

Plant extracts have been postulated to have hormonal effects, such as the ability to inhibit 5α-reductase enzyme. *S. repens* plant extract is a complex mixture of various compounds. A number of pharmacodynamic effects have been demonstrated with the use of *S. repens*, suggesting multiple mechanisms of action including inhibition *in vitro* of 5α-reductase in human fibroblasts[40] and competitive inhibition of DHT binding to both cytoplasmic and nuclear androgen receptors in prostate cells.[40-44] It also is reported, through studies *in vitro*, to have anti-androgenic properties. Several other studies *in vitro*, using human metastatic prostate carcinoma cell lines, have shown that *S. repens* inhibits the 5α-reductase enzyme.[44,45] One of these studies showed that it caused a 50% reduction in the conversion of testosterone to DHT by inhibiting this enzyme. It has also been demonstrated *in vitro* that it has an anti-estrogenic effect. These findings are encouraging, but further studies involving the use of saw palmetto berries in relation to the PSA levels and prostate size need to be done. In order to claim that *S. repens* possesses 5α-reductase inhibitory properties, there should be an expected reduction in the PSA level and prostate gland size in subjects using this phytotherapeutic agent; the level of reduction should be comparable to that of finasteride – 50% decrease in PSA level and 29% reduction in gland size after 6 months of therapy.

In a histological study conducted by Weisser *et al*, it was shown that *S. repens* truly does have an impact on the prostate gland. Histology of BPH-affected prostate tissue from placebo-treated patients revealed marked edema with mucoid degeneration of the periglandular stroma, intraglandular congestion, and congestive periglandular prostatitis. However, in patients with BPH treated with *S. repens*, there was marked reduction in all these histological findings upon biopsy of the prostate gland.[46]

In a recent study conducted in France, the liposterolic extract of *S. repens* (Permixon) was used to examine cell proliferation *in vitro* of human prostate tissue obtained through biopsies.[47] Basic fibroblast growth factor (bFGF) and epidermal growth factor (EGF), both believed to be the etiologic agent for BPH, induced a 250% increase in human prostate cell proliferation, mainly evident in the glandular epithelium. The liposterolic extract inhibited the bFGF-induced prostatic cell proliferation when the extract was applied at a high concentration of 30 μ mL^{-1}; no effect was seen at lower concentrations. Even though there was no effect on basal proliferation, the authors felt that *S. repens* can be an effective agent for BPH management by inhibiting bFGF-induced prostatic cell proliferation.

It has been well documented that the infiltration of inflammatory cells (such as PMN) into the prostate gland is one of the etiologic factors involved in the development of BPH. It is believed that these PMN cells produce chemotactic mediators (such as leukotriene B4) via phospholipase A2 enzymatic action on arachidonic acid, contributing to the development of tissue hyperplasia. Phospholipase A2 in the cell membrane produces arachidonic acid, which is metabolized by lipoxygenase to produce leukotriene B4.

Paubert-Braquet and associates[48] described how *S. repens* influences the prostate by inhibiting the formation of the arachidonic acid derivatives, especially leukotriene B4, thereby reducing the inflammatory component of BPH. The authors showed that *S. repens* significantly inhibited the production of 5-lipoxygenase metabolites (such as 5-HETE, LTB4) at concentrations *in vitro* as low as 5 μ mL^{-1}. This same result was noted when 20 μ mL^{-1} of arachidonic acid was introduced into the culture of human PMN cells *in vitro*. Despite proving that *S. repens* does not inhibit the phospholipase A2 enzyme through the addition of f-MLP, the authors did not conclude the exact mechanism of the action of the extract.

In another study using *S. repens*, the effect of the liposterolic extract on castrated rats with hormonally induced prostate enlargement was examined.[49] The authors grouped the rats into three categories: (1) rats treated with *S. repens*; (2) castrated rats given estradiol and testosterone treatment; and (3) castrated rats given both hormone and *S. repens* treatment. After 3 months of continuous hormonal therapy with estrogen and testosterone, the prostates increased in size, reaching a maximum size by day 30; weights of the lateral prostate increased fourfold, the ventral region sevenfold, and the dorsal region 13-fold. However, the increase in size was inhibited in rats fed with *S. repens*; the dorsal lobe of the prostate was reduced first, followed later by the lateral and ventral regions. The latter lobe did not show any significant change (7.9% reduction) when compared with the untreated group ($P > 0.21$). This work has clearly established that *S. repens* does not equally reduce the size of all the lobes in the gland. But, more importantly, these findings demonstrated that *S. repens* administration in the diet inhibits the increase in hormonally induced prostate enlargement. However, it adds nothing about the *S. repens* effects on pathologically induced prostate enlargement.

In the first of three clinical studies, Braeckman[50] in 1994 evaluated 305 patients with symptomatic BPH after 3 months of 160 mg (b.i.d.) *S. repens* therapy. The IPSS decreased from 19.0 to 12.4 ($P < 0.0001$); peak urinary flow rate improved from 9.78 mL s^{-1} to 12.19 ml s^{-1} ($P < 0.0001$); and PVR decreased from 35.8 mL to 28.6 mL ($P < 0.0001$). Interestingly enough and contrary to the other *S. repens* studies, this trial showed a significant reduction in prostate volume, as measured by transrectal echography; there was a mean 9% decrease after 45 days, followed by a mean 10% decrease on day 90 ($P < 0.0001$). Furthermore, there was no noticeable change in the PSA level; 3.44 ng mL^{-1} at the beginning of the study to 3.28 ng mL^{-1} at day 90. The authors noted that the onset of action of *S. repens* occurred after 30–45 days of treatment. As for the side effects, most were abdominal symptoms (50%) – gastralgia, nausea, vomiting, constipation, and diarrhea. Several patients did experience chest pain, breathlessness, tachycardia, and dizziness.

In the second study done by Descotes *et al.*[51] in 1995, 271 patients participated in a 30-day single-blind placebo lead-in period, and only the responders (less than 30% improvement in peak urinary flow rate as characterized by

the authors) continued in the study. The 176 non-responders were then randomized to a double-blind treatment of *S. repens*, and they were followed for a 30-day period. The results showed a statistically significant difference in the peak urinary flow rate in the treated group (increased from 11.7 to 15.3 mL s^{-1}) in comparison with the placebo group (increased from 12.4 to 13.5 mL s^{-1}).[51] Regardless of these impressive results, the credibility of this study is hampered by following the study subjects for only a 1-month period, and also there was nearly a 15% drop-out rate with relatively few patients to begin with. In 1996, a large double-blind equivalence trial was conducted involving 1098 men with moderate BPH, who were randomized to receive either *S. repens* 160 mg (b.i.d.) or finasteride 5 mg (q.d.) for a 26-week period.[52] Of the 1098 men, only two-thirds of them responded to either form of treatment, with the authors noting that two-thirds responded in each treatment group. On the subjective sexual function questionnaire, the *S. repens*-treated group ($n=553$) had fewer complaints of decreased libido, abnormal ejaculation, and impotence than the finasteride-treated group ($n=545$). When comparing both groups after 26 weeks of treatment, there was a decrease in the IPSS from 15.7 to 9.9 (37% decrease) in the *S. repens* group in comparison with 15.7 to 9.5 (39% decrease) in the finasteride group; there was no significant difference between the two groups ($P=0.17$). The improvement in the quality of life showed a 38% increase in the *S. repens* group vs. 41% in the finasteride group ($P=0.14$). Furthermore, there was an equal percent change in the peak urinary flow rates in both groups, 25% (from 10.6 mL s^{-1} to 13.3 mL s^{-1}) in the *S. repens* group vs. 30% (from 10.8 mL s^{-1} to 14.0 mL s^{-1}) in the finasteride group ($P=0.035$). There was no statistical difference between the *S. repens* group and the finasteride group in all categories; note that all groups showed relatively equal amounts of change. This similarity ends when comparing the prostate volume and PSA levels between the two groups. The finasteride group showed an 18% reduction (from 44.0 mL to 36.7 mL) in prostate volume with a 41% decrease in the PSA value; in comparison, the *S. repens* group showed only a 6% reduction (from 43.0 mL to 41.5 mL) in size and no change in the PSA level. (Both are significant, $P < 0.001$.) These latter findings are of great importance because they show that *S. repens* clinically improves urinary obstructive symptoms perhaps in equal measure to finasteride, but with no change in the prostate volume size. This suggests that there must be another mechanism, separate from inhibition of 5α-reductase, by which *S. repens* works to reduce BPH symptoms. As a final thought, side effects seen in the *S. repens* group were hypertension (3.1%), decreased libido (2.2%, finasteride showed 3.0%), abdominal pain (1.8%), impotence (1.5%, finasteride showed 2.8%), and constipation (0.4%).

Pygeum Africanum (BARK OF THE AFRICAN PLUM)

There are numerous theories on how *P. africanum* (Tadenan) effects the prostate to relieve symptoms of BOO. One such theory is based on studies *in vitro* showing that *P. africanum* acts in a dose-dependent manner to inhibit the proliferation of rat prostatic stromal cells (fibroblasts) stimulated by growth factors, such as EGF, bFGF, and IGF-I. It has been shown that *P. africanum* extract inhibits both basal and stimulated growth at IC_{50} concentrations of 4.5 µg mL^{-1}, 7.7 µg mL^{-1}, and 12.6 µg mL^{-1} for EGF, IGF-I, and bFGF, respectively. It has been theorized that growth factors play an important role in the pathogenesis of BPH, and this growth factor influence can be inhibited by Tadenan. Yablonsky et al.[53] showed that *P. africanum* extract does inhibit growth factors responsible for the prostatic overgrowth seen in BPH, and believe that this may account for the clinical benefits observed in BPH patients taking *P. africanum* extract. To substantiate this, further studies both at the molecular and clinical level need to done.

One study on the use of *P. africanum* demonstrated that this agent in the diet protected the bladder against abnormal contractile forces in cases of partial BOO. This is of major significance since current research on BPH treatment is focusing on neurotransmitters that are involved in crosstalk between urethral pressure maintenance and bladder contraction. This study raised the possibility that plant extracts may have a direct action on the bladder muscle. In a study conducted by Malkowicz and associates using rabbits,[54] it was concluded that the bladder contractile mechanism can be elicited by three mechanisms: (1) field stimulation, where the release of acetylcholine neurotransmitter from the nerve endings causes activation of the muscarinic receptors, which in turn activate the actin/myosin contractile mechanism; (2) KCl stimulation, where the administration of KCl directly activates the actin/myosin contractile mechanism; and (3) bethanechol stimulation, where administration of bethanechol (similar to acetylcholine) acts on muscarinic receptors to activate the actin/myosin contractile mechanism. Fitzpatrick and Lynch[55] stated that an unpublished study was reconducted using rabbits fed with *P. africanum*. The results showed that the contractile responses to KCl, bethanechol, and field stimulation were significantly greater in these animals. It was felt that it possibly protected the status of the contractile apparatus and the level of muscarinic receptors by being a membrane stabilizer, but further studies would be required to confirm this.[56]

Levin and coworkers[57] conducted an animal experiment to determine whether *P. africanum* had any effects on the bladder during states of partial outlet obstruction. After 2 weeks of partial obstruction of the bladder, the *P. africanum* (100 mg kg^{-1} day^{-1}) pretreated rabbits (pretreated for 3 weeks) showed that Tadenan did not reduce the effect of partial outlet obstruction on the bladder mass. However, it did show that detrusor muscle strips from Tadenan-pretreated rabbits responded to all forms of stimulation, including field stimulation, bethanechol, and KCl. Moreover, the enzyme activities of citrate synthase (a marker for mitochondrial function) and calcium-ATPase (a marker for sarcoplasmic reticulum) were initially reduced following outlet obstruction in the *P. africanum*-treated

animals but returned to normal levels for the remainder of the experiment, whereas these enzyme levels were reduced in the non-treated rabbits. From these findings, the investigators conclude that Tadenan protected the bladder against contractile and metabolic abnormalities that are normally present during partial BOO.

In yet another study, using a similar rabbit model of partial BOO, Levin et al.[58] have identified three major cellular changes in the bladder wall that occur upon 2 weeks of obstruction. These changes progressively occur, beginning with denervation of the bladder, followed by mitochondrial dysfunction, and disturbances in calcium storage. According to the authors, they hypothesize that BOO results in bladder hypertrophy that induces ischemia due to increased cellular mass. This, in turn, leads to a release of intracellular calcium, leading to the activation of various enzymes and generation of numerous free radicals. These then attack the cell membrane of nerves, mitochondria, and sarcoplasmic reticulum, causing permanent damage. However, through the use of a rabbit model, the authors show that 3 weeks of pretreatment of rabbits with (100 mg kg^{-1} day^{-1}) *P. africanum* (Tadenan) significantly reduces the severity of both the contractile and metabolic dysfunctions seen in BOO. The contractile response of isolated strips of detrusor muscle to field stimulation in untreated rabbits showed a significant reduction in the contractile response to the stimuli. However, this same form of stimuli in the Tadenan-treated rabbits showed an initial decrease in contractile response, but then returned to control levels. There were significant reductions in the contractile responses to bethanechol, KCl, and ATP in the obstructed group without *P. africanum* pretreatment, whereas the responses to these three forms of stimulation in the obstructed group treated with Tadenan showed normal responses.[57,58] Secondly, the authors showed that pretreatment of the animals with *P. africanum* protected the bladder against the reduced mitochondrial and sarcoplasmic reticulum function. According to their findings, the authors feel that *P. africanum* protects the bladder from the development of both the contractile and metabolic dysfunctions that are induced by 2 weeks of partial BOO. This study shows promise, but further studies targeted towards identifying the mechanism of action of *P. africanum* should be done.

P. africanum has also been shown to inhibit fibroblast proliferation in a study *in vitro*.[59] This study showed that *P. africanum* inhibits the action of basic-fibroblast growth factor, and epidermal growth factor induced proliferation of 3T3 fibroblast cells. This finding is of great importance because it has been shown that there is an increase in basic-fibroblast growth factor in cases of BOO. It is believed that *P. africanum* may prevent the irreversible bladder changes seen in protracted obstructed cases by inhibiting basic-fibroblast growth factor. This theory needs to be explored in more detail.

In a study conducted in France, *P. africanum* was shown to express anti-estrogenic effects only at high doses, such as 150 mg day^{-1}.[60] In this simple study, 18 men with BPH were given 150 mg day^{-1} of *P. africanum* for 15–20 days. After this treatment period, there was a functional improvement in BPH symptoms. However, this improvement was only seen in patients with a prostate volume greater than 50 cc. They also noticed that the men with the large prostates initially benefited the most with *P. africanum* therapy, similar to the results seen in finasteride trials. These investigators, based on their previous work, conclude that *P. africanum* extract, owing to its anti-estrogenic effects, reduces the volume of true and large (>50 cc) prostatic hypertrophy. Interestingly enough, these authors also demonstrated that *P. africanum* extract possesses the ability to suppress hot flushes induced by noradrenaline and serotonin. Further studies are needed to examine this clinical effect in relation to BPH.

RYE POLLEN (*Secale Cereale*)

Rye pollen extract is derived from several plants originating from Sweden. There have been numerous reports of it being useful in the treatment of prostatodynia, prostatism, and prostatitis.[61,62] Once again, this extract contains an inactive water component and an active (acetone-based) lipid-soluble component, mainly consisting of β-sterols. However, the exact mechanism of action on the prostate gland is unknown.

Studies *in vitro* on rye have shown that it has the ability to inhibit arachidonic acid metabolism, thus preventing the formation of prostaglandin and leukotrienes.[63] According to the authors of this study, the fat-soluble fraction of the pollen was noted to have anti-congestive and anti-inflammatory properties. However, the results of this test, to some extent, are obscure, but it did suggest that inhibition of prostaglandin and leukotriene synthesis is the mode of action. Other studies *in vitro* have shown that pollen inhibits the proliferation of prostate carcinoma cell lines.[64]

In animal model experiments, pollen extract was shown to decrease the size of rat prostates,[65] and another report claimed that the extract caused smooth muscle relaxation in the urethra of pigs and mice, along with increased contraction of bladder wall musculature.[66]

In another experiment using rye pollen extract to examine prostate cell growth, the authors[64] demonstrated that the water-soluble fraction of rye selectively inhibits growth of some prostate cancer cells; a cyclic hydroxamic acid, DIBOA, has been isolated from this extract and mimics its cell growth-inhibitory properties.[67] Nine human-derived cancer and non-cancer continuous cell lines were employed to evaluate the relative *in vitro* activity of rye pollen extract (Cernitin). Responses of the cell lines to the extract were assessed by measuring growth and cell survival as determined by cell count. The results demonstrated that of the 9 continuous cell lines tested, only those derived from the human prostate were growth inhibited by the pollen extract, whereas the non-prostate derived cells showed variable degrees of cell growth. The authors suggested that the extract exerted a powerful mitogenic inhibition of the proliferation of fibroblasts and epithelial cells by effecting epidermal growth factor. Even though the data did not

show a significant statistical difference between the control and experimental groups, further tests need to be done to confirm these findings.

In England, a 6-month double-blind, placebo-controlled study involving 60 patients with urinary outlet obstruction due to BPH was conducted to evaluate the effect of a 6-month course of rye pollen extract; the Boyarsky symptom score was used, but each symptom was assessed individually.[61] Sixty-nine percent (21/31) of the patients (in the experimental group taking 4 capsules of Cernilton) subjectively showed improvement in their urinary obstructive symptoms compared with 30% (8/26) in the placebo group ($P<0.06$). All the symptoms improved in both groups with no statistical significance seen in the treatment group; the only factor that showed statistical significance in the treatment group in comparison with the placebo group was the "feeling of incomplete bladder emptying." Objectively, there was a significant decrease in the residual urine in the treated patients, and in the anteroposterior (A–P) diameter of the prostate on ultrasound. However, the differences in respect to peak flow rate and voided volume in the treated group in comparison with the placebo group were not statistically significant. It is concluded by the authors that rye pollen extract does have a beneficial effect in BPH and may have a place in the treatment of patients with mild or moderate symptoms of outflow obstruction. However, these results only show minor improvement.

In a study conducted in Poland consisting of 89 patients with BPH, the patients were randomized to receive 4 months of pollen extract (Cernilton) or placebo (Tadenan), after which they were analyzed using peak urinary flow rate, postvoid residual urine and prostate volume.[68] (Note that the author used Tadenan as the placebo, but Tadenan is the trade name for another marketed phytotherapeutic agent used for BPH, namely *P. africanum*. Thus, this study truly does not compare pollen extract with placebo, but with another phytotherapeutic agent.) Significant subjective improvement was found in 78% of the patients in the treatment group ($n=51$) compared with only 55% of the *P. africanum*-treated group ($n=38$). The obstructive and irritative symptoms responded best to the pollen extract therapy. In the Cernilton-treated patients, a significant improvement was seen via evidence of an increase in the peak urinary flow rate, a decrease in postvoid residual urine, and a decrease in prostate volume. Based on these findings, the author states that Cernilton is a more effective therapy for patients with BPH than *P. africanum*.

CONCLUSION

Plant extracts are widely used in Europe. In Germany, approximately 90% of all patients with BPH are treated with phytotherapeutic agents, and 50% of German urologists prefer plant-based agents to chemically derived agents.[69] The precise mode of action is not clear, but owing to their mixed chemical composition, these extracts may target their action at several different molecular levels rather than in a specific manner, as finasteride does.

REFERENCES

1 Dunn JE. Cancer epidemiology in populations of the United States, with emphasis on Hawaii and California, and Japan. *Cancer Res* 1975; **35**: 3240–5.

2 Trowell HC, Burkitt DP. *Western Diseases: Their Emergence and Prevention*. London: Edward Arnold 1981.

3 Reddy BS, Cohen LA (eds). Diet nutrition and cancer: a critical evaluation. *Macronutrients and Cancer*, Vol. VII. Boca Raton, FL: CRC Press 1986.

4 Reddy BS, Cohen LA (eds). Diet nutrition and cancer: a critical evaluation. *Micronutrients Nonnutritive Dietary Factors, and Cancer*, Vol. VII. Boca Raton, FL: CRC Press 1986.

5 Rose DP, Boyar AP, Wynder EL. International comparison of mortality rates for cancer of the breast, ovary, prostate, and colon, and per capita food consumption. *Cancer* 1986; **58**: 2363–71.

6 Adlercreutz H. Western diet and Western diseases: some hormonal and biochemical mechanisms and associations. *Scan J Clin Lab Invest* 1990; **50** (Suppl 201): 3–23.

7 Griffiths K, Adlercreutz H, Boyle P et al. *Nutrition and Cancer*. Oxford: ISIS Medical Media 1996.

8 Le Marchand L, Kolonel LN, Wilkens LR et al. Animal fat consumption and prostate cancer – a prospective study in Hawaii. *Epidemiology* 1994; **5**: 276–82.

9 Dreikorn K, Richter R, Schoenhoefer, Konservative PS, Nicht-Hormonell Behaundlung der Benignen Prostatahyperplasie. *Urologe A* 1990; **29**: 8–16.

10 Dreikorn K, Shoenhoefer Ps. Stellenwert von Phytotherapeutika bei der Behandlung der benignen Prostatahyperplasie (BPH). *Urologe A* 1995; **34**: 119–29.

11 Setchell KDR, Adlercreutz H. Mammalian lignans and phyto-estrogens. Recent studies on their formation, metabolism and biological role in health and disease. In: Rowland IR (ed) *Role of the Gut Flora in Toxicity and Cancer*. London: Academic Press: 1988; 315–45.

12 Rosenblum ER, Campbell IM, Van Thiel DH, Gavaler JS. Isolation and identification of phytoestrogens from beer. *Alcohol Clin Exp Res* 1992; **16**: 843–5.

13 Van Thiel DH, Galvao-Teles A, Monteiro E et al. The phytoestrogens present in de-ethanolised bourbon are biologically active: A preliminary study in postmenopausal women. *Alcohol Clin Exp Res* 1991; **15**: 822–3.

14 Setchell KD, Borriello SP, Hulme P et al. Nonsteroidal estrogens of dietary origin: possible roles in hormone-dependent disease. *Am J Clin Nutr* 1984; **40**(3): 569–78.

15 Axelson M, Setchell KD. Conjugation of lignans in human urine. *FEBS-Lett* 1980; **122**(1): 49–53.

16 Setchell KD, Lawson AM, Conway E et al. The definitive identification of the lignans trans 2, 3-bis (3-hydroxybenzyl)-gamma-butyrolactone and 2, 3-bis (3-hydroxybenzyl) butane 1, 4-diol in human and animal urine. *Biochem J* 1981; **197**(2): 447–58.

17 Setchell KD, Lawson AM, Borriello SP et al. Lignan formation in man–microbial involvement and possible roles in relation to cancer. *Lancet* 1981; **4** 2 (8236): 4–7.

18 Adlercreutz H, Markkanen H, Watanabe S. Plasma concentrations of phyto-oestrogens in Japanese men. *Lancet* 1993; **342**: 1209–10.

19 Griffiths K, Davies P, Eaton CL et al. Endocrine factors in the initiation, diagnosis and treatment of prostatic cancer. In: Voigt KD, Knabbe C (eds) *Endocrine Dependent Tumors*. New York: Raven Press 1991; 83–130.

20 Griffiths K, Akaza H, Eaton CL et al. Regulation of prostatic growth. In: Cockett ATK, Khoury S, Aso U et al. (eds) *The 2nd International Consultation on Benign Prostatic Hyperplasia (BPH), Paris, France, 1993 June 27–30*. Jersey: Scientific Communication 49–75.

21 Waters AP, Knowler JT. Effect of a lignan (HPMF) on RNA synthesis in the rat uterus. *J Reprod Fertil* 1982; **66**: 379–81.

22 Adlercreutz H, Bannwart C, Wahala K et al. Inhibition of human aromatase by mammalian lignans and isoflavonoid phytoestrogens. *J Steroid Biochem Mol Bio* 1993; **44**: 147–53.

23 Evans BAJ, Griffiths K, Morton MS. Inhibition of 5α-reductase and 17β-hydroxysteroid dehydrogenase in genital skin fibroblasts by dietary lignans and isoflavonoids. *J Endocrinol* 1995; **147**: 295–302.

24 Adlercreutz H, Hockerstedt K, Bannwart C et al. Effect of dietary components, including lignans and phytoestrogens on enterohepatic circulation and liver metabolism of estrogens and on sex hormone binding globulin (SHBG). *J Steroid Biochem* 1987; **27**: 1135–44.

25 Hawrylewicz WJ, Huang HH, Blair WH. Dietary soybean isolate and methionine supplementation affect mammary tumor progression in rats. *J Nutr* 1991; **121**: 1693–8.

26 Serraino M, Thompson LU. The effect of flaxseed supplementation on the initiation and promotional stages of mammary tumorigenisis. *Nutr Cancer* 1992; **17**: 153–9.

27 Akiyama T, Ishida J, Nakagawa S et al. Genistein, a specific inhibitor of tyrosine-specific protein kinases. *J Biol Chem* 1987; **262**: 5592–5.

28 McCabe MJ Jr, Orrenius S. Genistein induces apoptosis in immature human thymocytes by inhibiting topoisomerase – II. *Biochem Biophys Res Commun* 1993; **194**: 944–50.

29 Fotsis T, Pepper M, Adlercreutz H et al. Genistein, a dietary-derived inhibitor of in vitro angiogenesis. *Proc Natl Acad Sci USA* 1993; **90**: 2690–4.

30 Messina M, Messina V, Setchell K. *The Simple Soybean and Your Health*. Garden City Park, NY: Avery 1994.

31 Messina MJ, Persky V, Setchell KDR, Barnes S. Soy intake and cancer risk – a review of the in vitro and in vivo data. *Nutr Cancer* 1994; **21**: 113–31.

32 Adlercreutx CHT, Goldin BR, Gorbach SL et al. Soybean phytoestrogen intake and cancer risk. *J Nutr* 1995; **125**: 757S–70S.

33 Adlercreutz H. Phytoestrogens: epidemilogy and a possible role in cancer protection. *Environ Health Perspect* 1995; **103**: 103–12.

34 Dreikorn JL, Rambeaud JJ, Deschaseaux P, Faure G. Placebo-controlled evaluation of the efficacy and tolerability of Permixon® in benign prostatic hyperplasia. In: Ackerman R, Schroeder FH (eds) *New Developments in Biosciences 5, Prostatic Hyperplasia*. New York: Walter de Gruyter 1989; 109–31.

35 Berges RR, Windeler J, Trampisch HJ, Senge I. Randomized placebo-controlled, double-blind clinical trial of beta-sitosterol in patients with benign prostatic hyperplasia. *Lancet* 1995; **345**: 1529–32.

36 Klippel KF, Hiltl DM et al. A multicentric, placebo-controlled double-blind clinical trial of beta-sitosterol (phytosterol) for the treatment of benign prostatic hyperplasia. *Br J Urol* 1997; **80**: 427–32.

37 Lepor H, Stoner E. Long-term results of medical therapies for benign prostatic hyperplasia. *Current Opin Urol* 1995; **5**: 18–24.

38 The MK-906 (Finasteride) Study Group. One-year experience in the treatment of benign prostatic hyperplasia with finasteride. *J Androl* 1991; **12**: 372–5.

39 Murray M, Pizzorno J. *Encyclopedia of Natural Medicine*. Seattle, John Bastyr University 1994.

40 Sultan C, Terraga A, Devillrer C et al. Inhibition of androgen metabolism and binding by a liposterolic extract of "Serenoa repens B" in human foreskin fibroblasts. *J Steroid Biochem* 1984; **20**: 515–19.

41 Briliey M, Carilla E, Fauran F. Permixon, a new treatment for benign prostatic hyperplasia, acts directly at the cytosolic androgen receptor in rat prostate. *Br J Pharmacol* 1983; **79**: 327P.

42 Briley M, Carilla E, Roger A. Inhibitory effect of Permixon on testosterone 5 alpha reductase activity of the rat ventral prostate. *Br J Pharmacol* 1984; **83**: 401P.

43 Carilla E, Briley M, Fauran F, Sultan C, Duvilliers C. Binding of Permixon, a new treatment for prostatic benign hyperplasia, to the cytosolic androgen receptor in the rat prostate. *J Steroid Biochem* 1984; **20**: 521–3.

44 Di Silverio F, D'Eramo G, Lubrano C et al. Evidence that *Serenoa repens* extract displays an antiestrogenic activity in prostatic tissue of benign prostatic hypertrophy patients. *Eur Urol* 1992; **21**: 309–314.

45 Delos S, Iehle C, Martin PM et al. Inhibition of the activity of "basic" 5-alpha reductase (type 7) detected in DU-145 cells and expressed in insect cells. *J Steroid Biochem* 1994; **48**: 347–52.

46 Weisser H, Behnke B, Helpap-B et al. Enzyme activities in tissue of human benign prostatic hyperplasia after three months' treatment with the *Sabal serrulata* extract IDS 89 (Strogen) or placebo. *Eur Urol* 1997; **31**(1): 97–101.

47 Paubert-Braquet M, Cousse H, Raynand JP et al. Effect of the lipidosterolic extract of *Serenoa repens* (Permixon) and its major components on basic fibroblast growth factor-induced proliferation of cultures of human prostatic biopsies. *Eur Urol* 1998; **33**(3): 340–7.

48 Paubert-Braquet M, Mencia-Herta JM et al. Effect of the lipidic lipidosterolic extract of *Serenoa repens* (Permixon) on the ionophore A23187-stimulated production of leukotriene B4 (LTB4) from human polymorphonuclear neutrophils. *Prostaglandins. Leukot Essent Fatty Acids* 1997; **57**(3): 299–304.

49 Paubert-Braquet M, Richardson FO et al. Effect of *Serenoa repens* extract (Permixon) on estrodiol/testosterone-induced experimental prostate enlargement in the rat. *Pharmacol Res* 1996; **34** (3–4): 171–9.

50 Braeckman J. The extract of *Serenoa repens* in the treatment of benign prostatic hyperplasia: A multicenter open study. *Curr Ther Res* 1994; **55** 7: 776–8.

51 Descotes JL, Rambeaud JJ, Deschaseaux P, Faure G. Placebo-controlled evaluation of the efficacy and tolerability of Permixon® in benign prostatic hyperplasia after exclusion of placebo responders. *Clin Drug Invest* 1995; **9**: 291–7.

52 Carraro JC, Raynaurd JP, Koch G et al. Comparison of phytotherapy (Permixon) with finasteride in the treatment of benign prostatic hyperplasia: a randomized international study of 1,098 patients. *Prostate* 1996; **29**: 231–40.

53 Yablonsky F, Nicolas V et al. Antiproliferative effect of *Pygeum africanum* extract on rat prostatic fibroblasts. *J Urol* 1997; **157**: 2381–7.

54 Malkowicz SB, Wein AJ, Whitmore K et al. Acute biochemical and functional alterations in the partially obstructed rabbit urinary bladder. *J Urol* 1986; **136**: 1324–9.

55 Fitzpatrick JM, Lynch TH. Phytotherapeutic agents in the management of symptomatic benign prostatic hyperplasia. *Urol Clin North Am* 1996; **22**: 407–12.

56 Kirby R, McConnell JD et al. *Textbook of Benign Prostatic Hyperplasia*. London: ISIS Med Media, 1996; 334.

57 Levin RM, Riffand JP, Bellamy F et al. Effects of Tadenan pretreatment on bladder physiology and biochemistry following partial outlet obstruction. *J Urol* 1996; **156**: 2084–8.

58 Levin RM, Levin SS et al. Cellular and molecular aspects of bladder hypertrophy. *Eur Urol* 1997; **32** (Suppl 1): 15–21.

59 Paubert-Braquet M, Monboisse JC, Servent-Saez N et al. Inhibition of bFGF and EGF-induced proliferation of 3T3 fibroblasts by extract of *Pygeum africanum* (Tadenan®). *Biomed Pharmacother* 1994; **48** (Suppl 1): 435–75.

60 Mathe G, Hallard M et al. A *Pygeum africanum* extract with so-called phyto-estrogenic action markedly reduces the volume of true and large prostatic hypertrophy. *Biomed Pharmacother* 1995; **49**: 341–3.

61 Buck AC, Cox R, Rees RW et al. Treatment of outflow tract obstruction due to BPH with the pollen extract Cernilton: A double-blind, placebo-controlled study. *Br J Urol* 1990; **66**: 398–404.

62 Rugendorff EW, Weidner W et al. Results of treatment with pollen extract (Cernilton) in chronic prostatitis and prostatodynia. *Br J Urol* 1993; **71**: 433–8.

63 Loschen G, Ebeling L. Inhibition of the arachidonic acid metabolism by an extract from rye pollen. In: IVahlensieck W, Rutischauser G (eds) *Benign Prostatic Disease*. Stuttgart: Georg Theieme 1992; 65–72.

64 Habib FK, Ross M, Buck AC, Ebeling L, Lewenstein A. In vitro evaluation of the pollen extract, Cernitin T-60, in the regulation of prostate cell growth. *Br J Urol* 1990; **66**: 393–7.

65 Ito R, Ishii M et al. (1986) Cernitin pollen extract (Cernilton): anti-prostatic action cernitin pollen extract (Cernilton). *Pharmacometrics* 1986; **31**: 1–11.

66 Kimura M, Kimura I, Nakase K et al. Micturition activity of pollen extract: contract effects on bladder and inhibitory effects on urethral smooth muscle of mouse and pig. *Planta Med* 1986; **2**: 148–51.

67 Roberts KP, Iyer RA et al. Cyclic hydroxamic acid inhibitors of prostate cancer cell growth: selectivity and structure activity relationships. *Prostate* 1998; **34**(2): 92–9.

68 Dutkiewicz S. Usefulness of Cernilton in the treatment of benign prostatic hyperplasia. *Int Urol Nephrol* 1996; **28**(1): 48–53.

69 Krzeski T, Kazon M, Borkowski A et al. Combined extracts of *Urtica dioica* and *Pygeum africanum* in the treatment of benign prostatic hyperplasia: double-blind comparison of two doses. *Clin Ther* 1993; **15**: 1011–20.

COMMENTARY

Phytotherapeutic agents are a popular treatment for diseases such as BPH for several reasons. These agents are natural agents found in everyday foods with low side effects. Secondly, there are data that a high-fat diet and animal protein in excess can cause several diseases, including heart disease and diseases of aging. Finally, the increasing recognition that BPH is a non-life-threatening disease that affects quality of life, and that pharmaceutical agents may have benefit in reducing symptoms has led to the impetus to find new agents that may have similar benefits with fewer side effects. Two groups of agents that are being used for phyotherapeutic management of BPH are lignans and isoflavonoids. These agents are of plant origin and of similar structure to steroids found in the human body. The main source of lignans are sesame seeds, cereals, fruits, and vegetables. The main source of isoflavonoids in the human diet is from soybean and other legumes. Among the active ingredients that may result from these agents after dietary conversion include daidzein and genistein. Among the plant lignan and isoflavonoid extracts that have been used for BPH are saw palmetto, *Pygeum africanum* (the bark of the African plum), leaves of the trembling poplar (aspen or *Populus tremula*), and a host of others as detailed in this chapter.

Many different mechanisms of action of these plant extracts have been proposed but very few have been proven by scientific methods. Two phyto-estrogenic isoflavonoids, daidzein and genistein have been studied in great detail by many authors and are the basis of our present knowledge of the physiology and mechanism of action of most phytotherapeutic agents. Testosterone required for BPH growth and maintenance may be influenced by estrogenic influences of lignans and isoflavonoids. Additionally, these dietary compounds also have the ability to stimulate sex hormone binding globulins, inhibit aromatase, and possibly inhibit 5α-reductase. Recent molecular studies have also shown that soya and flax seed inhibit tumorigenesis in experimental animals and humans, and genistein has been shown to inhibit tyrosine kinase activity, topoisomerase and angiogenesis. In addition to these properties, lignans and isoflavonoids also act as anti-oxidants owing to their polyphenolic structure. One postulated theory of how phytotherapeutic agents can influence the prostate gland is by lowering of cholesterol levels. Since the prostate is induced by steroid hormones, it is thought that this may have some benefit. In a clinical placebo-controlled double-blind study of patients treated with β-sitosterol (soy-based isoflavonoid) or placebo, there was a clinically significant decrease in American Urological Association (AUA) PSS symptom scores by 7.4 points in the β-sitosterol-treated group vs. a 2.3-point decrease in the placebo group. However, the prostatic volume did not change in the treated group.

In the USA, saw palmetto berry has become popular as a treatment for BPH over the past several years. The active ingredient in saw palmetto is a lipid-soluble extract of fatty acids and sterols but the exact ingredient that may have activity against BPH is still unknown. Studies *in vitro* have shown that the saw palmetto berry inhibits 5α-reductase enzyme. In clinical trials, saw palmetto has been shown to cause a statistically significant decrease in the IPSS score and improve uroflow in comparison with placebo. There have been mixed results about saw palmetto's influence on prostate volume and PSA levels; some studies have shown a reduction in prostatic volume without altering the PSA level, but others have not.

P. africanum is another agent that has been used. This agent may act in a dose-dependent manner to inhibit the proliferation of prostatic stromal cells stimulated by various growth factors. These studies have been mostly performed in preclinical trials. However, a 6-month clinical trial in England and another study in Poland have shown *P. africanum* to be clinically effective in reducing BPH-associated symptoms. Another agent being tested is rye pollen, which has been shown to inhibit arachidonic acid metabolism. In conclusion, it may be stated that plant extracts are becoming increasingly important in the management of many diseases including BPH. Presently, it appears that they have some benefit in decreasing BPH symptoms in limited controlled clinical trials. Their precise mode of action is unclear and owing to their mixed composition these agents may target their action at several different molecular levels, which are difficult to quantify based on existing data.

Section IV

LASER TREATMENT

Section IV Overview

LASER TREATMENT
P. Narayan

Laser prostatectomy has evolved from an investigative procedure to an accepted method of treatment for benign prostatic hyperplasia (BPH). With experience, the initial overenthuslasm that accompanies all new technologies has given way to a realistic understanding of benefits and limitations. Laser technology has also spurred the use of several minimally invasive techniques for BPH. All of these developments should ultimately serve to bring down the cost of therapy while improving or at least maintaining acceptable efficacy. The advent of interstitial laser technology and the holmium:YAG laser (which can be used for both stone disease and BPH) may also herald the initial attempts towards cost containment and consolidation within this industry.

What is not controversial at this point is that laser prostatectomy can produce results that are 70–80% comparable with that of traditional transurethral resection of the prostate (TURP). Laser prostatectomy also remains the least morbid among minimally invasive therapies and, indeed, sets the standards for such procedures in terms of hospitalization cost, anesthetic requirement, and complications such as bleeding, fluid absorption, retrograde ejaculation, impotence, and incontinence. In recent randomized trials comparing lasers with standard TURP, the immediate and long-term (12 month) complication rates were 5% and 10% for lasers vs. 30% and 35% for standard TURP.[1,2] There

is also a shorter learning curve for urologists in training, and therefore complications related to laser techniques are low. This is a major issue in TURP, where training and technique is critical for optimal outcome. Another advantage to laser is its ability to be used in patients on anticoagulation without the need for stopping or changing medications.

What is more controversial, however, is the type of laser energy that is ideal, the fiber that is optimal, and the technique that is universally applicable. Indeed, it may turn out that no single fiber or technique is universally applicable. Among various surgeons and in different countries, the unique aspects of technology available, training obtained, and insurance laws may dictate the type of laser and technique that is viable for use. The disadvantages of laser therapy include the fact that capital costs are high, the technology is still evolving, and postoperative retention and irritative symptoms remain issues.

In conclusion, it may be stated that laser therapy for BPH will remain a viable option. It is clear from the review of many clinical trials in several countries that patients have benefited from laser therapy and continue to have long-term positive outcomes. With continued evolution of techniques and technology, we should see a consolidation within the industry resulting in availability of laser technology that is cost effective and efficacious.

1 Cowles RS III, Kabalin JN, Childs S et al. A prospective randomized comparison of transurethral resection to visual laser ablation of the prostate for the treatment of benign prostatic hyperplasia. Urology 1995; 6: 155–60.

2 Anson K, Nawrocki J, Buckley J et al. A multicenter randomized, prospective study of endocropic laser ablation versus transurethral resection of the prostate. Urology 1995; 46: 305–10.

Principles of Laser Therapy

W.H. Nau Jr, D.F. Milam, R.J. Roselli, and J.A. Smith

16

INTRODUCTION

Laser prostatectomy has evolved from an investigative technology to an accepted urologic procedure. As with any new technique, the early period was characterized by optimism and hyperbole. With experience, practitioners came to understand both its indications and limitations. Controversy surrounding the method largely dissipated following publication of several articles demonstrating meaningful postoperative results.[1-6] Manuscripts published to this point show AUA symptom score reductions at 3 and 6 months comparable with transurethral resection of the prostate (TURP), and peak urinary flow rate increases of approximately two-thirds of that produced by TURP. Although early works only reported a small number of patients, initial results have been confirmed by larger current series.[7,8] Laser prostatectomy now remains among the least morbid operative procedures for benign obstructive prostatism, and indeed sets the standard for minimally invasive procedures in terms of hospitalization, blood loss, bladder neck contracture, and rate of occurrence of retrograde ejaculation. It is important to note that each of the many laser prostatectomy methods is not equally appropriate for all patients. Therefore, the purpose of this chapter is to guide the practitioner in selecting the appropriate treatment method through knowledge of the underlying principles of laser thermal therapy.

LASER GENERATORS AND TISSUE EFFECTS

LASER is an acronym for light amplification by stimulated emission of radiation. Within a laser, extremely high-intensity light from a flashlamp bombards a resonator cavity with photons with a wide range of wavelengths. Photons from the flashlamp excite electrons in the resonator cavity to higher energy states. Less than 5% of incident photons are absorbed within the resonator cavity by the active medium, however. Most photons pumped into the system by the flashlamp are wasted in the form of heat. Medical lasers require elaborate cooling devices incorporating either a radiator similar to that seen in automobiles or a continuous source of cooling water.

Photons that are absorbed cause electrons to jump to higher, "excited state" orbitals. Inherent instability of excited state orbitals causes many of the electrons to decay to the ground state within nanoseconds. The decay process emits a photon with a wavelength dependent upon the energy difference between the excited and ground states of the atom. This process is termed spontaneous emission of radiation. Table 16.1 illustrates the relationship between wavelength and photon energy. Since the emitted photon results from a specific orbital decay of the lasing medium, it possesses the specific quanta of energy necessary to interact with other excited atoms. Should the emitted photon encounter another atom in an excited state, the photon will stimulate electron orbital decay, and photon emission. This emitted photon will have the same wavelength, phase angle, and travel in the same direction as the incident photon. This process, termed stimulated emission of radiation, is the operating principle of lasers.

Photon energy	E	=	$E_y - E_x$
	E	=	hf
where h		=	Planck's constant
		=	6.625×10^{-34} J s^{-1}
f		=	frequency of photon (Hz)
Photon wavelength	λ	=	c/f
		=	3.00×10^{8} m s^{-1} f^{-1}
		=	3.00×10^{17} nm s^{-1} f^{-1}

Table 16.1 Relationship between laser wavelength and photon energy

Within a laser cavity, photons travel through the resonator until other excited state atoms are encountered (Figure 16.1). These interactions lead to further emission of identical wavelength photons. This binomial expansion causes the energy "gain" of the resonator cavity. Laser photons exit the resonator cavity as a collimated and coherent "laser" beam. Most urologists associate the wavelength of a particular laser with the active medium through which it is generated. For that reason, we discuss different wavelengths by laser type.

NEODYMIUM:YTTRIUM–ALUMINUM–GARNET LASER (1064 nm)

Since its introduction into clinical practice in 1979, the neodymium:yttrium–aluminum–garnet (Nd:YAG) laser has been, and remains the most frequently used laser in urologic surgery. The active medium consists of neodymium atoms embedded in an yttrium–aluminum–garnet rod. The

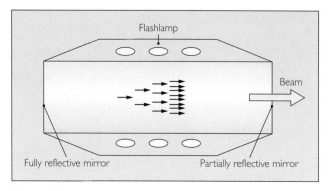

Figure 16.1 Design of a conventional laser, illustrating energy gain through spontaneous emission of radiation

Nd:YAG laser emits invisible, infrared light at a wavelength of 1064 nm. Light at this wavelength is poorly absorbed by water and body pigments compared with other medical laser wavelengths. Owing to poor absorption, 1064 nm light penetrates relatively deeply into tissue. Tissue coagulation extending more than 1 cm is not uncommon during laser prostatectomy.

In a fluid environment, the poor optical absorption results in thermal coagulation of surface and subsurface tissue. However, the tissue retains its structural integrity. After non-contact Nd:YAG laser treatment, prostatic hemostasis is total. The coagulated tissue acquires a white, cadaveric appearance. Other than this change in tissue appearance, little else is noticeable. After coagulation, the tissue sloughs over a period of several weeks. Complete healing may take up to 3 months.

The Nd:YAG laser may also be used for tissue vaporization and desiccation. Vaporization techniques involve higher energy density exposure for longer periods of time. Surface carbonization results in a marked increase in superficial laser light absorption and further increases the energy density by limiting the depth of penetration (Figure 16.2). Tissue

vaporization may facilitate early catheter removal following laser prostatectomy, and will be discussed in more detail later in this chapter.

KTP LASER (532 nm)

A "KTP" laser produces 532 nm wavelength green light by using a potassium titanyl phosphate crystal to double the frequency of an Nd:YAG laser. KTP light can be transmitted by the same standard optical fiber used for Nd:YAG laser treatment.

The 532-nm wavelength provides an intermediate level of vaporization and coagulation. Tissue coagulation with this laser reaches only half the depth produced by 1064-nm Nd:YAG laser light. Reducing the depth of penetration can produce important consequences, however. Higher energy per unit tissue volume can produce increased vaporization and desiccation. Many urologists have used this effect to incise the bladder neck and prostate. Combined techniques for treatment of BPH, using coagulating energy followed by vaporization of prostate tissue with a KTP laser, have been described.

HOLMIUM:YTTRIUM–ALUMINUM–GARNET LASER (2100 nm)

The holmium:yttrium–aluminum–garnet (Ho:YAG) laser emits light in the mid-infrared region of the electromagnetic spectrum (2100 nm). Unlike the continuous wave lasers described above, energy emission from a holmium laser occurs in a series of rapid pulses over a few milliseconds (Q-switched laser). A different flexible optical fiber is required from that used for 1064 nm or 532 nm laser light. Ho:YAG laser light is strongly absorbed by water and produces tissue cutting by explosive vaporization of tissue water. Since vaporization is the predominant tissue effect, the hemostatic properties of this laser are less than a continuous wave Nd:YAG laser. However, it may still be used to coagulate soft tissues. The primary application of the Ho:YAG laser has been for fragmentation of urinary tract stones. Ho:YAG lasers have been used for laser prostatectomy, but are used less commonly for that purpose than Nd:YAG or diode lasers.[9,10]

DIODE LASERS

A diode laser is one of two principal semiconductor photon sources. The other photon source, the light-emitting diode (LED) is commonly used in instrument displays, optical storage, and communications devices. A LED emits light of relatively wide bandwidth. The laser diode, on the other hand, emits narrow bandwidth, nearly monochromatic, light. Diode lasers are used to read information from audio and computer compact disks.

A typical diode laser is constructed from a cleaved semiconducting material sandwiched between a voltage potential. Two polished parallel surfaces act as mirrors to increase laser gain. Laser light exits the side of the semiconductor (Figure 16.3). Structural differences between diode and conventional lasers produce important differences in the type of laser light produced, and help to

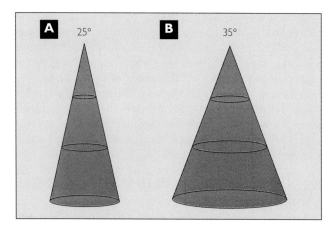

Figure 16.2 Relationship between power density and spot size: (A) distance 1 cm; energy 40 W; exposure area 0.154 cm^2; power density 259 W cm^{-2}; (B) distance 1 cm; energy 40 W; exposure area 0.312 cm^2; power density 128 W cm^{-2}

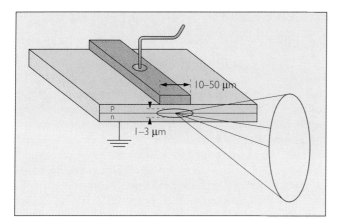

Figure 16.3 Semiconducting diode laser design. An electrical potential placed across the p and n terminals energizes the laser. Beam output is elliptical

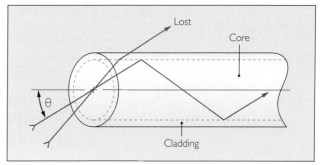

Figure 16.4 Propagation of light through an optical fiber. The lower refractive index of the cladding material assures transmission through the fiber by total internal reflection

explain the potential advantages of diode laser sources for medical therapy.

Semiconductor laser gain is high compared with conventional laser sources. That property allows diode lasers to be considerably more efficient than conventional medical lasers. Conventional medical lasers convert less than 5% of electrical input into laser light. Inefficiency is the reason many medical lasers require 50-A 220-V energy sources, cooling water, radiators, and noisy fans. Diode lasers have high gain, which allows for more efficient generation of the photon stream. Currently available medical diode laser sources are small, portable boxes powered by 110 V wall current. Special connections are not required, permitting the laser to be hand-carried from the operating room to the clinic setting.

Laser light emitted from a diode is not as tightly collimated as that from a conventional source. Conventional sources generate a narrow Gaussian beam profile producing a small spot size. As illustrated in Figure 16.3, laser diodes produce an elliptical beam profile. Fortunately, native spot size is not particularly important to urologists, since laser light is usually carried through an optical fiber before contacting tissue.

DESIGN AND FABRICATION OF OPTICAL FIBERS

Laser prostatectomy waveguides are manufactured from fused silica glass. The high purity of the material minimizes optical absorption and scattering. Propagation of light through the core fiber occurs by a series of total internal reflections from one side wall to the opposite wall. The fiber core is covered by a layer of lower refractive index glass or plastic, termed cladding. When light obliquely traverses the core fiber, energy loss is prevented by reflection from the cladding interface back into the core (Figure 16.4).

Fiber-optic waveguide systems are extraordinarily efficient in most applications. Actual loss of energy within the

length of the fiber utilized in medical applications is less than 1%. However, as much as 25% of the incident energy may be lost in coupling of the laser to the fiber. Energy may also be lost when the beam is redirected laterally into prostatic tissue. These facts reinforce the importance of calibrating the fiber before treatment; otherwise, unexpected undertreatment may result.

TISSUE EFFECTS

Laser thermal therapy involves deposition of laser light into tissue. The effects of laser radiation on tissue may be classified as photothermal, photochemical, or photomechanical in nature. For the purposes of this chapter, only photothermal interactions, or tissue heating, will be considered. Tissue heating occurs from the optical distribution of deposited laser energy, as well as diffusion of the resulting heat into surrounding tissue.

The distribution of light will depend on the amount of light that is reflected from the tissue surface, and the amount scattered before being absorbed. Photons of laser light experience three possible interactions during passage through tissue. Initially, photons pass through tissue in the original incident direction. This is termed through transmission. Interaction with cellular structures within tissues causes photons to be scattered away from the direction of the incident light. Scattering causes the beam to form a plume, and is highly wavelength dependent. Absorption of laser light in tissue depends upon the amount and type of absorbers present. The main absorbing materials in tissues are water and the tissue pigments hemoglobin and melanin. Absorption by tissue pigments is strongly wavelength dependent. Once a photon is absorbed by tissue, its energy is liberated as heat. Thermocoagulation will occur if enough laser energy is used to achieve tissue temperatures of 60–70°C for more than a few seconds.

Many factors affect tissue temperature distribution, the most important of which are laser parameters and tissue optical properties. Laser parameters include wavelength, power, spot size, beam profile, and scanning velocity. The optical parameters of importance are surface reflection and the tissue absorption and scattering coefficients.

Tissue optical characteristics define the effect of a specific laser delivery system. Three parameters are most important for laser prostatectomy. These are energy loss due to urethral reflection, and the prostatic light absorption and scattering coefficients. Loss due to urethral reflection represents less than 5% of incident energy, and is therefore considered negligible in many clinical applications. Light distribution in tissue for a given wavelength source can be estimated by the Lambert–Beer's law:

$$I_x = I_0 \, e^{-\varepsilon x} \qquad (1)$$

where I_0 is the intensity of the incident beam, I_x is the intensity of the beam at a tissue depth of x cm, and ε is the total tissue attenuation coefficient (absorption + scattering). The Lambert–Beer's law, however, does not differentiate between the effects of true absorption (μ_a) and scattering (μ_s) of light, and underestimates the fluence rate in tissue.

A more universally applicable model is the solution to the radiative transfer equation[12-15]

$$\frac{1}{c}\frac{\partial}{\partial t}\,\phi\,(r,\,t) - D\nabla^2\,\phi\,(r,t) + \mu_a\,\phi\,(r,\,t) = S(r,\,t) \qquad (2)$$

where c is speed of light in tissue, t is time, ϕ is the photon fluence rate at position r, and S is the photon source term. D is the optical coefficient expressed in terms of the optical absorption coefficient (μ_a), scattering coefficient (μ_s), and the anisotropy coefficient (g, mean cosine of the scattering angle), as $\{3[\mu_a + (1 - g)\mu_s]\}^{-1}$.

Once the distribution of light in tissues is known, the production of heat due to absorption of photons (Q in J cm^{-3}) can be determined by:

$$Q_L = \mu_a\phi \qquad (3)$$

Temperature distributions in tissue can then be calculated through the solution of the Pennes bioheat equation:[16]

$$\rho c_t\,\frac{\partial T}{\partial t} = k\,\nabla^2\,T + Q_L + Q_M - wc_b\,(T - T_a) \qquad (4)$$

where ρ is the density of tissue, c_t is the specific heat of tissue, T is temperature, t is time, k is the thermal conductivity, Q_L is the optical power deposition in tissue, calculated by equation (3), and Q_M is the metabolic heat generation. Note that thermal energy carried away by convective blood flow is included in the last term in equation (4), where w is the blood mass perfusion, c_b is the specific heat of blood, and T_a is arterial blood temperature. Although it is still unclear whether convective heat loss due to blood perfusion has a significant role in temperature distributions during laser prostatectomy, recent studies using canine models have shown that prostatic blood perfusion more than doubles from 0.19 mL min^{-1} g^{-1} to 0.41 mL min^{-1} g^{-1} during laser irradiation.[17A]

As tissue is heated, proteins become denatured, resulting in cell damage. Henriques proposed a model for predicting tissue damage based on first-order Arrhenius rate theory.[17B] This tissue damage integral (Ω) is defined by:

$$\Omega = \left(\frac{kT}{h}\right)\int_0^t \exp\left(\frac{-\Delta G}{RT}\right)\,dt \qquad (5)$$

where k is the Boltzmann constant, T is temperature (K), h is Planck's constant, R is the universal gas constant, t is the exposure time, and ΔG is the free energy difference between the normal and denatured states of molecules. A value of $\Omega = 1$ defines the threshold for irreversible tissue damage.

Continued development and application of mathematical models such as these can help lead to optimal treatment strategies for laser thermal therapy of BPH. Several studies have demonstrated the wavelength dependency of the absorption coefficient in a typical biological tissue.[18,19] This is the principal mechanism causing differing tissue effects with different wavelength lasers. Rapid superficial vaporization seen with the CO_2 laser is a consequence of the tissue absorption coefficient being greater than 1000 times that of the Nd:YAG laser operating at 1064 nm.

APPLICATION OF THEORY TO SIDEFIRING LASER THERAPY

Surface carbonization markedly affects the tissue absorption coefficient. Carbon black is a near perfect absorber of all visible and infrared wavelengths. During Nd:YAG laser prostatectomy, surface char can alter the treatment session, producing a superficial effect similar that of the CO_2 laser. This has been theorized to be the causative mechanism for 40 W exposure proving clinically superior to 60 W exposure in one coagulation prostatectomy series.[1] Surface charring should be avoided if coagulation of deep tissue is the goal. This can be accomplished by slight probe movement during static exposure or increasing probe movement during scanning exposure.

Laser parameters affect tissue treatment. These include wavelength, power, spot size, beam profile, and scanning velocity. The importance of wavelength is largely determined by tissue absorption and scattering coefficients, as discussed earlier. While near-infrared light from the Nd:YAG (1064 nm) laser provides good results, other sources in the 800–1000 nm range may also be used. High power (25–50 W) diode lasers are competitive alternatives to the continuous wave Nd:YAG laser source. While diode lasers may achieve results comparable with the volume of prostatic coagulation achieved using the Nd:YAG laser, exposure at these wavelengths would not be expected to achieve superior clinical or experimental results. All "poorly absorbed" near-infrared lasers produce similar coagulation zones. Other commonly available medical laser sources (CO_2, holmium, alexandrite, KTP, and argon) are too strongly absorbed by tissue pigment or water to be useful for sidefiring non-contact coagulation prostatectomy. More highly absorbed sources can be used for vaporization prostatectomy or incision, however.

Laser power is an important determinant of the extent of tissue injury. Coagulation prostatectomy requires tissue temperatures of 60–70°C for about 3 s to affect reliable protein denaturation. The extent of surface heating at a given power is also a function of spot size. Indeed, power density (power/spot size) coupled with the prostatic optical absorption coefficient are the critical determinants of surface tissue heating. The sidefire laser beam profile is often considered analogous to spot size. Christiaan van Swol et al. have demonstrated variations in visible laser beam profile between different sidefiring devices (Table 16.2).[20] These data are useful for determination of optimal exposure techniques. For maximum treatment depth, narrow beam profile devices require probe movement, while those producing widely divergent beams may be used for static treatment.

Initial laser prostatectomy studies using the Urolase device were performed with a static exposure technique using a divergent laser fiber (low power density).[1-4] This technique treated a large volume of tissue, minimized surface charring, and facilitated laser scattering. Static treatment is clearly not appropriate for other fibers with a narrow divergence angle and higher power density.

Several devices with narrow divergence angles have less than a 3 mm spot size under usual cystoscopic conditions. Laser light scattering of 1064 nm throughout prostate tissue is not sufficient to insure thorough coverage of an entire prostate without probe movement. Analytic and finite element mathematical models are being developed to help predict optimum tissue exposure. Roselli et al. predicted the volume of coagulated tissue assumed to occur when tissue temperature rose above 70°C to be 36–109% greater with a laser scanning rate of 1 mm s^{-1} than with an identically powered laser source where the beam is stationary for 60 s (RJ Roselli et al., personal communication). Intuitively, the optimal scanning rate would be as slow as possible without causing tissue charring. In addition to a slow scan rate, thorough treatment may be facilitated by an initial static dwell period. During probe movement, tissue ahead of the probe is heated owing to forward scatter of the laser light. Tissue treated at the beginning of a laser pass is not exposed to energy from prior forward scatter. Undertreatment of the initial region may occur unless the fiber is held static for 2–3 s before initiating movement. Intuitively, one should dwell for as long a period as possible without creating tissue carbonization.

CONSIDERATION OF TREATMENT TECHNIQUE

The first decision point in laser prostatectomy is whether to attempt tissue coagulation or tissue vaporization. Coagulation is a rapid, low-energy process. While only 300 J g^{-1} are technically required to coagulate prostatic tissue, the techniques used to assure adequate coverage of the prostatic urethra require the use of at least 1000 J g^{-1} Tissue removal occurs by delayed urethral passage of sloughed acellular prostatic debris. Acute urinary retention due to debris does not occur. Tissue loss following coagulation prostatectomy is slow. Most tissue is lost within 6 weeks. However, cystoscopy as long as 3 months after laser prostatectomy may show residual shaggy, gray necrotic tissue.[21] It is essential to minimize tissue carbonization during coagulation treatment, as the presence of substantial carbon prevents penetration of laser light deep into tissue. Carbonization can be avoided by moving the fiber (scanning beam) to broaden tissue exposure and reduce power density in a given area.

The second decision point in selecting an appropriate laser prostatectomy technique is determination of whether

Device name	Manufacturer	Exit angle (degrees)	Divergence (degrees in air)	
			parallel	perpendicular
Urolase	Bard (Covington, GA)	95	25	60
Ultraline	Circon-ACMI (Stamford, CT)	75	21	30
ADD	LaserSonics (Milpitas, CA) Laserscope (San Jose, CA)	70	14	42
SideFire	Myriadlase (Forest Hill, TX)	105	15	15
TULIP	Intrasonix (Burlington, MA)	90	25	25
Prolase II	Endocare (Cytocare) (Aliso Viejo, CA)	35	20	not measured

Table 16.2 Demonstrates the differing properties of the exit beam from individual fibers. The first two fibers listed produce widely divergent beams while the remaining fibers have narrower divergence angles

Source: Modified from Christiaan FP, van Swol RM, Verdaasdonk JM, Boon TA. Physical evaluation of laser prostatectomy devices. In: Watson GM, Steiner RW, Johnson DE, (eds) Lasers in Urology, Proc. SPIE 1994; 2129: 25–33

antegrade ejaculation is a priority. Retrograde ejaculation can often be prevented by minimizing bladder neck treatment. That technique is discussed later. Other important factors that play a role in selecting one technique over another are prostate size and geometry. These will also be discussed in detail.

REFLECTIVE SIDEFIRING DEVICES

Reflective systems utilize a gold-plated stainless steel reflector to deflect the laser beam laterally. Other materials have been tried. However, gold, being one of the least reactive elements, experiences little surface decay during treatment. The Urolase (Bard Corporation, Marietta, GA) device does not preserve the beam diameter, but produces beam divergence of 60° along the perpendicular axis and 25° parallel to the fiber. Reflective systems absorb more energy than refractive systems. Consequently, heat dissipation and device heating are a design concern. Contact of the hot fiber with surrounding tissue may cause reflector degradation and loss. Current systems, while having sufficient longevity for non-contact coagulation treatment, do not tolerate energy-intensive treatment sessions (100,000+ J) required for vaporization prostatectomy.

REFRACTIVE SIDEFIRING DEVICES

Glass-capped refractive sidefiring devices having a narrow divergence angle, and can be used either for coagulation or high-energy vaporization. For coagulation, the Nd:YAG laser is set to produce 40 W output. Higher wattage produces more carbonization and has been shown not to increase coagulation depth.[22] The probe is positioned 1–5 mm away from the tissue surface. We begin treatment at the bladder neck. The probe should initially remain in place for about 3 s. This initial "dwell" period produces a coagulation defect at the initial probe location similar to that produced later during the pass. Tissue treated in locations other than the initial zone is preheated by lateral scatter of laser light before the fiber actually reaches that location. Preheating due to lateral photon scatter causes deeper coagulation. Tissue located immediately below the starting location does not benefit from preheating. Our work indicates that the depth of coagulation at the initial site may be only half that of later treated regions, although the surface effects are the same.[23] This explains the importance of the initial dwell period. Why could this problem not be solved by repeated treatment? Coagulation of prostatic tissue results in changes in the absorption and scattering coefficients that govern light penetration in such a way as to limit the depth of coagulation that can be produced by further treatment. Clearly, the best chance for deep coagulation is afforded by a properly conducted first pass. Dwell periods longer than 3 s can produce extensive carbonization and are counterproductive.

After the initial dwell period, the probe is pulled or rotated slowly along the urethral surface. A tissue surface velocity of about 1 mm^{-1} appears to produce maximum coagulation depth and minimum carbonization. Use of a methodical treatment regimen assures tissue coverage, reduces carbonization, and permits deep tissue heating. Treatment continues until the entire prostatic urethral surface becomes cadaveric white in appearance. When a particular area is adequately treated once, we move to an untreated region. Repeated treatment of the same area after the tissue has been allowed to cool does not appear to extend the depth of coagulation. Adequate treatment requires over 1000 J g^{-1} of prostatic tissue. These general guidelines can be applied to different techniques of prostatic exposure including longitudinal and radial scanning, and rocking exposure.

LONGITUDINAL SCANNING

The original scanning exposure technique involved longitudinal treatment from the bladder neck to the verumontanum. This method was employed by the TULIP investigational protocol (IntraSonix Corporation, Burlington, MA). Probe movement began after an initial 3-s dwell period at the bladder neck and proceeded at 1 mm s^{-1}. After a pass was complete, the probe was rotated 30° and a new scan was begun. These treatment parameters are remarkably similar to current longitudinal scanning methods. We would expect to achieve similar results with optically guided fibers moved in the same way.

A longitudinal scanning treatment begins at the bladder neck if retrograde ejaculation is not an issue. Bladder neck treatment will produce retrograde ejaculation in 5–15% of individuals. The chance of retrograde ejaculation can be reduced to almost 0% if longitudinal scans begin 1 cm distal to the bladder neck (Figure 16.5). We sense that beginning the treatment distal to the bladder neck compromises treatment only minimally. However, no data have been published to support that belief. For most patients, the pass begins proximal to the bladder neck after an initial 3-s dwell period. The probe is pulled at 1 mm s^{-1} until the verumontanum is reached. As with TURP, treatment may continue slightly past the verumontanum if the patient has a substantial amount of apical tissue. One must be aware of the exit angle of the laser beam when treating apical tissue. Optical fibers that forward direct the laser beam provide a margin of safety that reduces the chance of sphincter zone coagulation. Fibers that direct the beam back toward the surgeon should be used with great care near the prostatic apex.

After the first pass the probe is rotated slightly so that the second pass coagulates tissue immediately adjacent to the first pass. This process is repeated until the entire prostatic fossa has been coagulated and appears a cadaveric gray-white color. Using the longitudinal technique, tissue coagulated by a prior pass has cooled sufficiently by the time of the next pass that heating from the second pass does not deepen the coagulation defect produced by the prior pass. Similarly, repeat treatment of white coagulated urethral tissue does not deepen the depth of coagulation. Non-contact coagulation laser prostatectomy using the longitudinal scanning technique produces reliable results that are comparable to other techniques described.

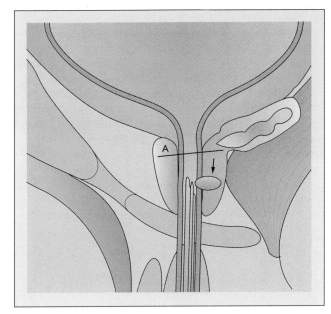

Figure 16.5 Non-contact laser prostatectomy using the longitudinal scanning technique. Beginning the pass 1 cm distal to the bladder neck (A) markedly decreases the incidence of retrograde ejaculation. Arrow indicates areas of lesion

Source: Adapted from Milam DF, Smith JA. *Laser Prostatectomy in Profiles in Urology.* Surgical Communications 1993

RADIAL SCANNING

Like the longitudinal method, a radial scanning session begins at the bladder neck. Probe movement begins after an initial dwell period of 3 s. The fiber is slowly rotated over the 360° urethral circumference at a surface speed of 1 mm s^{-1} (Figure 16.6). It is easy to rotate the fiber too rapidly using this method. Movement of the probe at an aiming beam surface velocity of only 2 mm s^{-1} will markedly decrease coagulation depth. After the first 360° treatment is complete, we withdraw the fiber 5 mm distally and perform

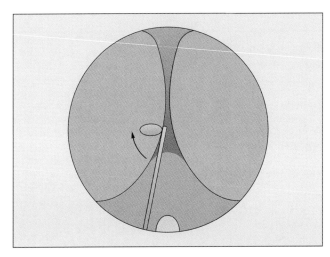

Figure 16.6 Radial scanning non-contact laser prostatectomy

another treatment. Circumferential exposures are done at 5-mm increments until the verumontanum is reached. At that point the entire prostatic urethra should appear coagulated and no further treatment is necessary. It has been suggested that, by limiting treatment of the prostatic floor near the verumontanum, the possibility of ejaculatory duct obstruction may be minimized (A Shanberg, personal communication). Radial scanning is a methodical technique for minimizing wasted treatment energy and time. Good clinical results are achieved with this method. Another method, using a rocking exposure pattern, has a theoretic advantage that may translate into deeper coagulation.

ROCKING EXPOSURE

A theoretic advantage of the rocking technique is the accumulation of heat in subsurface tissue. For protein denaturation to occur, tissues must be exposed to temperatures greater than 56°C for over 3 s.[24] Convective heat loss due to either prostatic blood flow or urethral irrigation fluid will decrease prostatic temperature in the treated zone. Coagulation volume is maximized by exposing a packet of prostatic tissue for as long as possible while minimizing carbonization. The rocking technique does just that.

As with radial scanning, a rocking treatment is begun at the bladder neck. The Nd:YAG laser is set at 40 W energy, and a narrow divergence angle fiber is used. After a 3-s dwell period, the fiber is rotated using the radial technique so that the aiming beam scans over tissue at a 1 mm s^{-1} surface velocity. Once 30° of urethral circumference has been traversed, however, the rotation is reversed to re-treat the same 30° region. We rock back and forth over a treatment area four to six times before moving on to another 30° region. Approximately 12 segments are treated separately in each 360° urethral circumference. The probe is withdrawn 5 mm with each traverse of the urethral circumference until the verumontanum is reached and treatment is complete. This strategy allows heat to accumulate during treatment within a finite 30° tissue segment. Increased subsurface temperature causes deeper coagulation due to conductive heat transport. Rocking exposure is a more time- and energy-intensive method, however. We use almost 2000 J g^{-1} of prostate tissue with this method.

INTERSTITIAL LASER THERMOTHERAPY

Interstitial laser thermotherapy devices are now available in the USA. The technique initially involved the transurethral placement of bare optical fibers into the prostate under cystoscopic guidance. This method did not achieve complete success. Prostatic heating was unsatisfactory owing to incomplete exposure of the entire prostate to laser light. Current fibers utilize diffuser tips at least 2 cm long, which attempt to distribute the laser energy evenly throughout the prostate. Numerous transurethral punctures are required. However, the entire prostate can be treated within 1 h. Interstitial laser thermotherapy has been used extensively in Germany and is discussed in detail later in this book.[25]

CONTACT VAPORIZATION PROSTATECTOMY

Contact vaporization prostatectomy differs considerably from the coagulation procedures described previously. Tissue ablation occurs in real time, creating an open prostatic fossa similar to TURP. During vaporization prostatectomy, the structural components of tissue are carbonized and the water component is vaporized. Equipment capable of withstanding large amounts of energy must be used.

Contact vaporization prostatectomy is performed using either a durable glass-capped fiber or the Contact Laser system. When using the Contact Laser™ system (Surgical Laser Technologies, Oaks, PA), a 7-mm-diameter round contact probe (MTRL 10) is threaded on to a 600 μm optical fiber.[26] A black absorbent coating deposited on to the contact probe surface during manufacture absorbs approximately 30% of the laser energy, causing intense heating. Contact between the hot probe and tissue produces tissue vaporization and desiccation. Passage of laser energy through the probe into tissue further enhances vaporization and facilitates hemostasis due to subsurface vascular coagulation. Contact Laser systems utilize a conventional fiber-optic waveguide surrounded by a cooling channel made of plastic material.

Durable, internally reflecting, glass-capped optical fibers may also be used for vaporization prostatectomy. Fournier and Narayan performed an extensive investigation using the Ultraline II (Haraeus LaserSonics, Milpitas, CA) fiber.[22] The authors compared lesions created in tissue contact at 60–100 W with lesions created with the probe 1 and 2 mm away from the tissue surface. Their results argue strongly that vaporization prostatectomy with a sidefiring fiber should be performed in contact with tissue.

Only the most durable of sidefiring fibers can be used for this very energy-intensive technique. Fournier and Narayan noted initial fiber pitting at 30,000 J and complete probe failure at 150,000 J.[22] As with the Contact Laser system, vaporization prostatectomy using a sidefiring fiber involves treatment times similar to TURP.

Vaporization prostatectomy has been performed after non-contact coagulation prostatectomy. The goal of that method is typically not to vaporize the entire prostate, but to open a channel that facilitates early catheter removal. One option is to use a dual wavelength Nd:YAG/KTP laser. After coagulating the prostate with Nd:YAG light, the same fiber can be used to vaporize briefly or incise the bladder neck and prostatic tissue with KTP energy. Catheter removal as early as the first postoperative day can be accomplished with this method. Although vaporization may play a role in some practices as an adjunct to coagulation prostatectomy, we would not expect the eventual clinical result to be influenced by the addition of tissue vaporization, since a similar volume of tissue is eventually removed.

CONCLUSIONS

Laser prostatectomy has become an accepted technique for treatment of bladder outlet obstruction due to benign prostatic hyperplasia (BPH). Several studies have shown laser prostatectomy to be an effective treatment for BPH. Questions remain regarding the relative effectiveness of individual methods. Factors such as prostatic size and geometry, laser equipment, and physician experience must be considered when selecting the appropriate treatment method for an individual patient. Thorough knowledge of laser principles and tissue interaction can serve as a guide for the practicing urologist.

Laser prostatectomy is competing with other alternative technologies for treatment of obstructive prostatism. Laser prostatectomy has an objective record of producing symptomatic and urodynamic results similar to electrosurgical resection, while substantially reducing patient morbidity. Elimination of bleeding complications and dilutional hyponatremia along with a marked reduction in the incidence of bladder neck contracture and retrograde ejaculation assures that laser prostatectomy will continue to play an important role in BPH treatment.

REFERENCES

1 Kabalin JN. Laser prostatectomy performed with a right angle firing neodymium: YAG laser fiber at 40 watts power setting. *J Urol* 1993; **150**: 95–9.

2 Norris JP, Norris DM, Lee RD, Reubenstein MA. Visual laser ablation of the prostate: clinical experience in 108 patients. *J Urol* 1993; **150**: 1612–14.

3 Kabalin JN, Gill HS, Leach GE *et al*. Visual laser assisted prostatectomy (VLAP) using Urolase right angle fiber: preliminary results with 60 watts protocol, Abstract #4, American Urological Association Meeting 1993.

4 Dixon C, Machi G, Theune C, Lepor H. A prospective, double-blind, randomized study comparing laser ablation of the prostate and transurethral prostatectomy for the treatment of BPH. *J Urol* 1994; **151**: 229A.

5 McCullough DL, Roth RA, Babayan RK *et al*. Transurethral ultrasound-guided laser-induced prostatectomy: National Human Cooperative Study results. *J Urol* 1993; **150**: 1607–11.

6 Costello AJ, Bowsher WG, Bolton DM *et al*. Laser ablation of the prostate in patients with benign prostatic hypertrophy. *Br J Urol* 1992; **69**(6): 603–8.

7 Krautschick AW, Weber HM, Benkin N *et al*. VLAP – single center experience with more than 110 patients. *J Urol* 1995; **153**: 416A.

8 Kabalin JN, Gill HS, Bite G, Wolfe V. Comparative study of laser versus electrocautery prostatic resection: 18-month followup with complex urodynamic assessment. *J Urol* 1995; **153**: 94–8.

9 Gilling PJ, Cass CB, Cresswell MD, Fraundorfer MR. Holmium laser resection of the prostate: preliminary results of a new method for the treatment of benign prostatic hyperplasia. *Urology* 1996; **147**: 48–51.

10 Johnson DE, Cromeens DM, Price RE. Transurethral incision of the prostate using the holmium: YAG laser. *Lasers Surg Med* 1992; **12**(4): 364–9.

12 Wilson B, Adam GA. Monte Carlo model for the absorption and flux distributions of light in tissue. *Med Phys* 1983; **10**(6): 824–30.

13 Arridge S, Cope M, Delpy D. The theoretical basis for the determination of optical pathlengths in tissue: temporal and frequency analysis. *Phys Med Biol* 1992; **37**(7): 1531–60.

14 Jacques S, Prahl S. Modeling optical and thermal distributions in tissue during laser irradiation. *Lasers Surg Med* 1987; **6**: 494–503.

15 Patterson M, Chance B, Wilson B. Time resolved reflectance and transmittance for non-invasive measurement of tissue optical properties. *Applied Optics* 1994; **28**(12): 2331–6.

16 Roemer R, Cetas C. Applications of bioheat transfer simulations in hyperthermia. *Cancer Research* 1984; Suppl 4788s–98s.

17A Nau WH, Roselli RJ, Milam DF. Quantitative measurement of blood flow in the prostate during laser irradiation using radiolabeled microspheres. In *Modeling Photocoagulation of the Prostate During Exposure to Laser Radiation*, Doctoral Dissertation in Biomedical Engineering, Vanderbilt University, Nashville, TN, 1996, pp. 80–99.

17B Henriques FC, Moritz, AR. Studies of thermal injury. V. The predictability and the significance of thermally induced rate processes leading to irreversible epidermal injury. *Arch. Pathol.*, 1947; **43**: 489–502.

18 Anvari B, Rastegar S, Motamedi M. Modeling on intraluminal heating of biological tissue: implications for treatment of benign prostatic hyperplasia. *IEEE Trans Biomed* Eng 1994 **41**(9): 854–64.

19 Orihuela E, Motamedi M, Cammack T, Torres J. Comparison of thermocoagulation effects of low power, slow heating versus high power, rapid heating Nd:YAG laser regimens in a canine prostate model. *J Urol* 1995; **153**(1): 196–200.

20 Christiaan FP, van Swol RM, Verdaasdonk JM, Boon TA. Physical evaluation of laser prostatectomy devices. In: Watson GM, Steiner RW, Johnson DE (eds) *Lasers in Urology, Proc SPIE* 1994; **2129**: 25–33.

21 Marks LS. Serial endoscopy following visual laser ablation of prostate (VLAP). *Urology* 1993; **42**: 66–71.

22 Fournier GR Jr, Narayan P. Factors affecting size and configuration of neodymium: YAG (Nd:YAG) laser lesions in the prostate. *Lasers Surg Med* 1994; **14**(4): 314–22.

23 Nau WH, Roselli RJ, Milam DF. Finite element modeling of heat transfer in the prostate. In: *Lasers in Urology*, GM Watson, RW Steiner, DE Johnson (eds), Proceedings of SPIE, 1994; **2129**, 34–41.

24 Jacques S, Prajl SA. Modeling optical and thermal distributions in tissue during laser irradiation. *Lasers Surg Med* 1987; **6**(6): 494–503.

25 Muschter R. Laser induced interstitial thermotherapy of benign prostatic hyperplasia and prostate cancer. In: Brown SG, Escourrou J, Frank F *et al.* (eds) *Medical Applications of Lasers II. SPIE Proc.* 1994; **2327**: 287–92.

26 Gomella LG, Lotfi MA, Rivas DA, Chancellor MB. Contact laser vaporization techniques for benign prostatic hyperplasia. *J. Endourol* 1995; **9**: 117–23.

COMMENTARY

In this chapter, Drs Nau *et al.* have discussed the various factors governing the use of lasers in BPH and provided a rational basis for choosing a particular type of fiber and technique, based on the individual patient's need and expectations.

Laser prostatectomy has evolved from an investigative technology to an accepted urologic procedure. With experience, practitioners now understand both its indications and its limitations. Many of the initial controversies surrounding use of laser for BPH have now dissipated because data on efficacy and side effects on a variety of laser techniques have been published. The summary of these studies (Tables 17.2 and 17.3, and 18.1 and 18.2 Chapter 18) reveal that laser techniques reduce symptoms by 64–68% at 6–12 months after surgery, while improving uroflow by 97–140%. This is about 70–100% of the efficacy achieved by TURP. Over 2000 patients have been reported in clinical trials and possibly several thousands of others have been treated over the last 5 years.

Among the factors influencing the success of therapy are the wavelength of the beam, medium of transmission, and the type of fiber as well as fiber tip used to deposit the energy on tissue. The tissue effects of laser are based on photothermal, photochemical, or photomechanical reaction. Only photothermal interactions are important for BPH therapy. Many factors affect tissue temperature distribution. Most important of these are wavelength, power, spot size, beam profile, and scanning velocity. Mathematical models are also being developed to optimize treatment strategies. The knowledge of these factors is important in preforming optimal therapy. For example, it is known that surface carbonization affects tissue absorption; therefore, surface char can alter treatment, producing a superficial

effect. This can be avoided by increasing probe movement during exposure. This is the rationale for doing a 30° degree side-to-side movement in several techniques of laser prostatectomy. Wavelength is important because this determines absorption and scattering coefficients. Nd:YAG is a good wavelength for the prostate, since it is not absorbed in the water medium through which the procedure is done. However, it is absorbed by hemoglobin and tissue, which is helpful in prostatic treatment. Similarly, higher power is important for causing vaporization, as is rapid deposition of energy by using narrow divergence angles. The type of fiber that allows close contact without melting, such as quartz, is also important in being able to cause vaporization. Among treatment techniques, the first issue is whether coagulation is the end goal or whether vaporization is the end goal. The second decision is whether antegrade ejaculation is a priority. Finally, cost of the fiber and side effects are issues that merit consideration.

Important questions still remain regarding the relative effectiveness of individual methods and their advantages. Factors such as prostate size, geometry, and physician experience as well as laser equipment must be considered when selecting an appropriate treatment method for an individual patient. Knowledge of laser principles and tissue interactions can only serve as a guide to the practicing urologist. However, it is clear that laser prostatectomy now remains among the least morbid operative procedures for BPH and indeed sets the standard for minimally invasive procedures in terms of decreased hospitalization, blood loss, bladder-neck contracture, impotence, and incontinence. The continuing evolution of techniques and fibers will ultimately decide the role of lasers in the management of BPH.

Laser Therapy: Rationale, Technique, and Results of Vaporization

17

B.S. Stein and P. Narayan

Laser energy is a type of electromagnetic radiation that requires no medium for its transmission. Several types of laser energy are available for treating human tissue. These include CO_2 Nd:YAG, KTP, argon, diode, holmium, excimer, and pulsed dye. Depending on the wavelength, the properties of the laser energy are variable. For example Nd:YAG with a wavelength of 1064 nm is close to the infrared portion of the electromagnetic spectrum and therefore is unabsorbed in water and hemoglobin (Figures 17.1 and 17.2). Nd:YAG can, therefore, be used in a fluid medium. CO_2, for example, is absorbed by water and so cannot be used in a fluid medium, which makes it difficult for use in prostatic therapy. Since Nd:YAG energy can be delivered through quartz fibers, it can be used for endoscopic ablation. Other laser wavelengths that are delivered through quartz include KTP (wavelength 532 nm), holmium (wavelength 2100 nm), and diode laser (832 nm).

LASER EFFECTS ON TISSUE

The key features regulating laser effects on tissue is power density (Figure 17.3). The power of a laser source is expressed in watts. The product of power, in watts, multiplied by time, in seconds, is expressed as the unit of energy, joules. Power density (PD) is the area of target tissue to which power is delivered and is given by the formula $PD = (power/area) = (watts/\pi r^2)$. PD expresses the strength

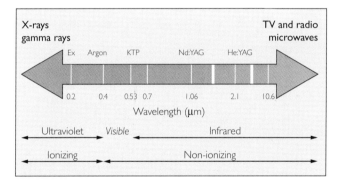

Figure 17.1 Electromagnetic spectrum. Ex=Excimer

Source: Modified from Childs SJ. Basic laser physics. In: Childs SJ (ed) Laser-Assisted Transurethral Resection of the Prostate (TURP). Baltimore: Williams & Wilkins 1993

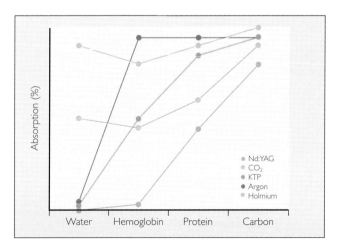

Figure 17.2 Percentage absorption of various lasers in different body tissue components

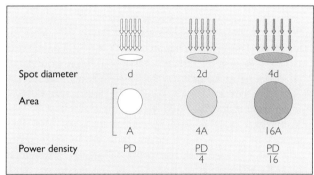

Figure 17.3 Relation between spot size, area, and power density

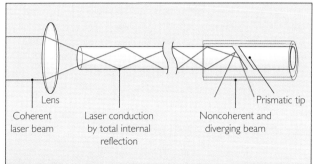

Figure 17.4 Phenomenon of internal reflection and beam divergence. Mechanism of laser beam transmission through fibers

231

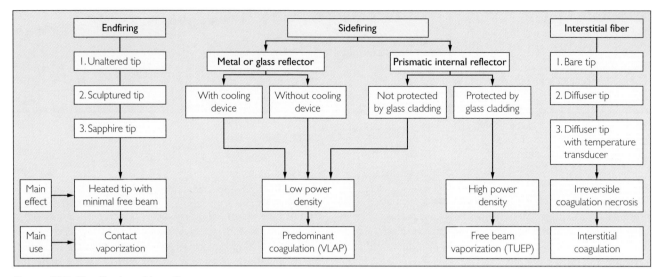

Figure 17.5 Classification of laser fibers

of the laser at a spot and is directly proportional to the power of the laser source and inversely related to the area. If a spot size increases twofold, then PD will drop fourfold and vice versa. This also means that the beam divergence and the distance of the beam from the tissue will influence the amount of energy delivered. The implications of these factors on laser effects are discussed further in Chapter 16, "Principles of Laser Therapy".

LASER DELIVERY SYSTEMS

The laser energy travels in a fiber by means of total internal reflection (Figure 17.4). The most commonly used fiber for laser energy transmission has an inner core of silicon dioxide (quartz) and an outer coat of Teflon cladding. A variety of fiber types have been described for delivering laser energy to prostate tissue (Figure 17.5). The initial attempts at using bare quartz fiber led to the development of the transurethral laser-induced prostatectomy (TULIP). This consisted of a transurethral ultrasound transducer, incorporating a sidefiring YAG laser probe. This was surrounded by a balloon inflated to a pressure of 2 atmospheres with sterile water. Although efficacious, the complexity and the high price of the system gave way to the sidefiring quartz fiber, allowing visual laser ablation of the prostate (VLAP). This 600-µm fiber can easily be introduced through an ordinary cystoscope.

Currently four fiber systems are available for use in the prostate. These include: endfiring fibers, either bare tipped or modified for contact, sidefiring fibers, and interstitial fiber.

MECHANISMS OF LASER-INDUCED PROSTATIC DESTRUCTION

There are both technical as well as tissue factors that influence laser effects on tissue (Figure 17.6). The effects of laser energy on tissue include reflection, scattering,

transmission (penetration) through tissue, and absorption (resulting in heat). Among the primary objectives in using a specific type of laser energy and fiber are to reduce reflection and scattering outside tissue, increase absorption inside tissue, and to cause adequate penetration of the

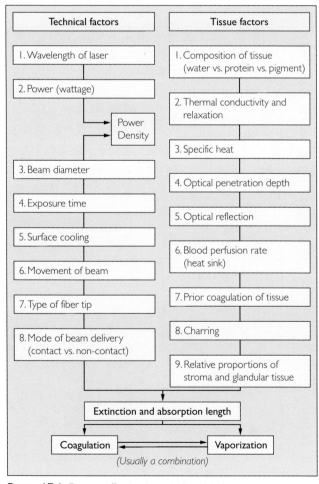

Figure 17.6 Factors affecting laser-induced lesions

adenoma but prevent laser effects on extraprostatic tissue. These factors have been discussed in recent reviews and are also discussed in Chapter 16.[1]

COAGULATION vs. EVAPORATION

Coagulation is the process of causing molecular breakdown of organic compounds (proteins) by raising their temperatures (Table 17.1). Sander and Beisland[2] and Shanberg and associates[3] were some of the earliest investigators to use coagulation laser techniques for human prostate. Subsequently, Kandel and associates[4] performed canine experiments. The initial technique of VLAP was first reported by Johnson and colleagues,[5] then followed by Costello *et al.*[6] and Kabalin.[7,8] The use of coagulation alone in BPH makes the procedure imprecise, and it can be especially hazardous when working close to the external sphincter. During vaporization, there is a change in the physical state of tissue water into steam (approximately 2500 J g^{-1} is required to change the temperature from 37 to 100°C). The kinetic energy of escaping vapor causes mini explosions within tissue, further adding to mechanical rupture of membranes. The rate of ablation is determined by the rate of deposition of laser energy into the tissue. It is not the total duration of the energy application but rather the intensity of the application that determines vaporization. The initial rate at which the energy penetrates is determined by the laser wavelength. What one attempts to do is raise the amount of energy deposited per unit volume of tissue to bring cells to vaporization temperature quickly. If the cells are brought only to coagulation temperature, they then become half as penetrable to laser energy, and this will halt the forward progress of ablation and will increase backscatter and surrounding coagulation. This implies that increasing the duration of the laser application at lower power density will only result in a greater depth of coagulation and possible periprostatic injury rather than creation of a channel defect.

Molecular effect	Temperature range (°C)
Boiling of tissue with carbonization and vaporization	over 100
Irreversible coagulation	60–100
Beginning of coagulation	50–60
Desiccation and reduction in enzyme activity	45–50
Heating and tissue retraction	30–45

Table 17.1 Approximate temperatures of coagulation and evaporation

TISSUE EXPERIMENTS

Studies *in vitro* conducted in our laboratory on liver and human prostate tissue demonstrated that, at any given power setting, the proximity of the beam to the tissue is the single most important determinant of lesion size and configuration.[9] Contact not only causes a substantial increase in laser-induced lesion size and volume compared with a non-contact mode of energy delivery but also substantial tissue evaporation. Craters up to 2 cm deep can be created in the prostate with 3600 J of energy delivered to a single spot. Part of this effect is due to an accelerated evaporation that occurs when energy is concentrated on tissue, causing superheated gas bubbles to form. The gas bubbles, which are trapped in tissue for a while, enhance evaporation because they allow the beam to be more effective without the intervening presence of fluid causing loss of heat or reflection of beam. This powerful evaporative effect is characterized by a vigorous outpouring of gas and charred material from the lesion. We have termed this the "accelerated evaporation phenomenon" (AEP). It is important to recognize the occurrence of AEP, since it can be used to enhance evaporation rapidly in prostates that have large volumes; on the other hand, AEP should not be allowed to occur near the apex or at the prostate capsule (toward the end of the procedure), to prevent injury to periprostatic tissues. The depth of the evaporation cavity, however, can be readily controlled by altering the time of laser irradiation such that cavities <1 cm in depth can be reliably created by not irradiating a single spot for longer than 30 s.

Dragging the fiber tip in contact with the target during laser irradiation maximizes the amount of tissue destroyed by both evaporation and coagulation. The area of evaporation is also enhanced by a 30° side-to-side rocking movement as dragging is performed. Increasing the laser beam power from 60 to 100 W causes a greater proportion of the tissue to be evaporated rather than coagulated without substantially increasing the overall drag lesion volume.

ADVANTAGES OF VAPORIZATION OVER COAGULATION

The types of fiber used for laser energy delivery have an impact on how energy is deposited and end results on tissue. If energy is deposited in large quantity with close contact (Nd:YAG energy, quartz fibers, contact, narrow beam, sidefiring), there will be evaporation of tissue secondary to steaming, and explosion of cells and tissue will be removed as smoke, resulting in a cavity. If energy is deposited in smaller quantity in smaller amounts (wide beam, non-contact, gold-tipped fibers), then coagulation will occur with slow reabsorption and sloughing. It is important to note that coagulation will occur even in tissues where evaporation is occurring because at a deeper plane less energy is deposited – enough for coagulation but not evaporation. With the evaporation technique, therefore, one can get an immediate open fossa as well as a deeper coagulation. The question then arises, why bother with coagulation at all as a technique? The major advantages of coagulation technique is that it does work – though unpredictably – in many patients, requires less time, is less wearing on fibers – thus is cost effective – and is better tolerated by patients under intravenous sedation or prostate block. Therefore, when cost-effective considerations are paramount, the coagulation technique is quite acceptable. The disadvantages of the vaporization technique include longer duration of therapy, requirement of more anesthesia and fiber wear-out, often necessitating the use of two fibers, which increases costs. The newer technique of interstitial laser thermal therapy (ILTT) tries to combine the best of both by using coagulation technique but only inside the adenoma. By sparing the urethral lumen, the hope is that the most unacceptable complication of VLAP, i.e. prolonged retention, can be reduced and yet provide patients symptomatic relief. In our preliminary experience with 25 patients, as well as the experience of others, this appears to be holding true. VLAP and ILTT are discussed further in Chapters 18 and 20, respectively. The impact of holium (Ho:YAG) using bare fibers is discussed in the section overview.

VAPORIZATION TECHNIQUES AND RESULTS

The technique of vaporization, which requires high power density and short pulse duration, is best undertaken with refractive quartz fibers that can be placed close or in contact with tissue (Figure 17.7). We developed this technique after extensive animal and tissue experimentation.[9,10] Power settings of 80–100 W are employed. During treatment of the median lobe, it is important to restrict treatment of the bladder neck to the area between the 5 and 7 o'clock position. This preserves antegrade ejaculation in 70% of patients. To treat the rest of the prostate, the fiber is slowly dragged through the lateral lobe to the verumontanum being careful not to treat beyond this area. The drag rate should be slow enough to ensure adequate vaporization as determined visually. We have found a drag rate of 1 cm per 20 s to be acceptable. Simultaneously with dragging, a 30° side-to-side rocking movement is performed. This avoids extensive charring, ensures even evaporation, and increases

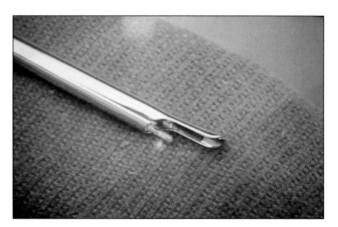

Figure 17.7 Ultraline quartz laser fiber

the area under treatment so that, in many cases, the initial four troughs are all that are necessary to accomplish adequate vaporization. After creating four troughs, at 2, 4, 8, and 10 o'clock areas, any remaining untreated tissue is lased until the entire prostate has been treated. Owing to charring and tissue color change, attempts at retreatment to areas already vaporized does not result in deeper penetration. Approximately 1500–2000 J of energy are delivered per gram of tissue, in this technique. A catheter will be required postoperatively for only 1–3 days.

The results of the vaporization technique in 61 patients were first published by us in 1994. Subsequently, an updated series of 168 patients was reported in 1996. The initial set of 61 patients had American Urological Association (AUA) symptom scores of greater than 8, uroflow of less than 15, and patients in retention were also treated. An Ultraline fiber with power settings of 60–80 W was used, and a total of 32,000–225,000 J were delivered to various sized prostates. The catheter was removed on day 2 in 43 patients and on days 3 to 7 in the remaining 18 patients. Only 5 patients required recatheterization. Two of the 61 patients required transurethral resection of the prostate

Authors	Fiber	Number of patients	Baseline PFR (mL s⁻¹)	% improvement in PFR		Baseline IPSS	% change in IPSS
				6 months	1 yr		
Narayan et al.	Ultraline	61	9.3	42	166.5	27.5	76
de la Rosette et al.	Ultraline	43	7.8	85.9	107.7	21.2	67.5
Gottfried et al.	Ultraline	232	7.5	156	164	26	77
Leidich et al.	Ultraline	90	–	152	–	–	72
Narayan et al.	Ultraline	100	8.7	101	–	23.8	68
Pinto et al.	Ultraline	21	7.4	a	–	23.3	a
Narayan et al.	Ultraline	168	8.2	120.7	121.9	20.6	65
Krautschick et al.	Ultraline	112	6.9	–	–	32	–
Corrica et al.	Ultraline	143	12.6	47.7	–	17.6	51.1
Mean	–	970	8.55	100.8	140	24.0	68.09

a100% of patients had >50% improvement

Table 17.2 Results of transurethral evaporation using side firing fibres in contact with tissue

(TURP) for residual adenoma and were considered failures. All 12 patients in retention voided well. There were complications in only 4.9% of patients, and most were due to infection. Results are given in Table 17.2. In a recent update, we assessed the safety and efficacy of transurethral electrovaporization of the prostate (TUEP) on a total of 168 patients. Peak flow rate, AUA Symptom Index and postvoid residual were assessed at baseline, and at 3, 6, and 12 months of follow-up. We found a statistically significant decrease in mean AUA Symptom Index from 20.6 at baseline to 7.2 at 12 months (mean difference 10, 122% increase, $P<0.0001$). The most frequent complications were irritative voiding symptoms in 22.6% of patients and urinary tract infections in 4.8%. There were no additional major complications. From these results, we confirmed that TUEP was safe and effective for treatment of BPH at 12 months of follow-up (Figures 17.8–17.10). We also compared results between various prostate sizes and determined that large-sized prostates and patients in retention were equally well treated by this technique, provided an adequate amount of energy was delivered.[11] The updated results of vaporization reported by Narayan and associates are similar to those of Drs Stein and associates, as well as others (Table 17.3).

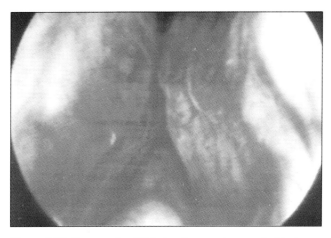

Figure 17.8 Preoperative BPH view from cystoscope just below bladder neck

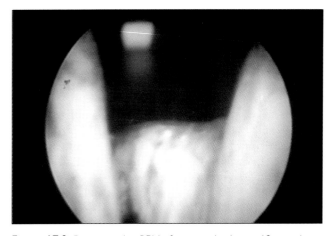

Figure 17.9 Postoperative BPH after vaporization at 12 months, after follow-up

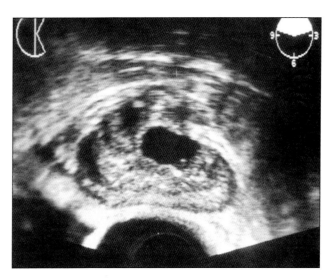

Figure 17.10 Postoperative TUR defect 6 months after vaporization

COMPARISON OF VARIOUS LASER THERAPIES WITH TRANSURETHRAL RESECTION OF THE PROSTATE

Almost every technique of laser prostatectomy fares better than TURP in safety. Additionally, laser prostatectomies require shorter hospitalization and often can be performed as an out-patient procedure under local anesthesia and intravenous sedation.[12,13]

Bleeding is the main complication of TURP, resulting in problems such as clot retention, and transfusions with associated complications.[14] The incidence of hemorrhage needing blood transfusion is 3.9%, and it increases by twofold (>7%) if the resected tissue is more than 45 cm³ or resection time is greater than 90 min.[14] Such hemorrhagic complications are unheard of in all forms of laser prostatectomy and more than one series has established its safety even in patients on anticoagulant therapy.[11,15] In over 20 studies to date, <0.1% of patients have experienced bleeding after laser prostatectomy.[16]

Fluid absorption during TURP results in a 2% incidence of transurethral resection (TUR) syndrome either due to dilutional hyponatremia, glycine-induced ammonia intoxication, or direct toxic effect of glycine.[14] As with bleeding, fluid absorption increases with larger glands and longer resection times. This has never been a problem with any laser technique, and our studies have clearly demonstrated that TUEP can be safely used in glands larger than 80 cm³ in volume.[11,15] The main reason for lack of complications is the zone of coagulation that always accompanies any laser procedure, including vaporization. This results in "real time" sealing-off of venous sinuses, preventing fluid absorption. In our initial 40 patients who had intraoperative continuous monitoring of body weight using the in-bed urological scale (Model 2900, scale Tronix, Wheaton, IL), there was no significant change in weight after the procedure (mean 0.8 lb; range 0.0–2.5 lb).[17]

Incidence of impotence following TURP is 4–13%.[14] Etiology is thought to be due to diffusion of electrical

Authors	Fiber	Number of patients	Baseline PFR (mL s^{-1})	% improvement in PFR		Baseline IPSS	% change in IPSS
				6 months	1 yr		
Leach et al.	Urolase	28	8.1	60.5	–	21	55.2
Kabalin	Urolase	190	6.7	144.8	176	20.4	54.9
Norris et al.	Urolase	108	7.5	60	–	22.3	58.7
Anson and Watson	Urolase	23	9.7	116.5	106.2	19.3	48.2
de la Rosette	Urolase	47	7.8	85.9	–	21.1	61.6
Leach et al.	Urolase	117	7.4	93.2	116.2	21.0	59
Buckley et al.	Urolase	77	9.9	76.8	–	19.0	68.4
Costello and Crowe	Urolase	35	8.7	80.5	139	19.9	55.8
Anson and Watson	Myriadlase	23	9.5	67	62.1	20.5	60
Kabalin et al.	Urolase	62	7.7	105.2	–	20.9	52.6
Shanberg et al.	Urolase/ADP	25	5.7	136.8	–	26.5	70.6
	Prolase	25	6.5	123.1	–	25.6	79.7
Krautschick et al.	Ultraline	39	7.3	164.4[a]	–	32	84.4[a]
Gill et al.	Prolase II	50	10.5	58.1[a]	–	18.9	94.8[a]
Anson et al.	Lateralase	12	11	18.2	–	23	60.9
Dixon et al.	Urolase	20	9.2	53.3	–	16.5	27.9
Orihiela et al.	Urolase	15	5	166	21.6	27.3	82.4
Orihiela et al.	Urolase	14	4.5	228.9	196	26.1	85.6
Kabalin et al.	Urolase	13	–	141	154	–	78
Bolton et al.	ND	7	9.2	68.5[b]	–	21.2	67[b]
Costello et al.	Myriadlase	33	8.5	79.3[a]	–	21.5	55.8[a]
Mean	–	1035	8.03	97.71	125.3	22.14	64.8

[a] 3-month data
[b] Boyarski score: (1) VLAP; (2) extensive VLAP; (3) 15 W for 180 s; (4) 50 W for 60 s

Table 17.3 Results of non-contact visual laser ablation

current into the cavernosal nerves, which travel quite close to the prostatic apex, or interference with penile arterial flow, which occasionally depends partly on prostatic vascularity. Overall incidence of impotence following all forms of laser prostatectomy is rare. Norris and colleagues[18] reported that, of 108 patients who underwent VLAP, 56 were sexually active prior to procedure (intercourse more than once per month) and 37 patients were sexually active postoperatively at 3–6 months. Dixon and associates[19] compared TURP with VLAP and found that 2/21 patients in VLAP group developed impotence at 3 months. Leach and associates reported loss of potency in 5/117 (4.3%) men following VLAP.[20]

Retrograde ejaculation, which occurs in up to 90% of patients undergoing TURP, is less common following various laser prostatectomies that allow relative preservation of bladder neck integrity. Norris et al.[18] found retrograde ejaculation in only 3/37 patients and Kabalin observed it in <10% of patients following VLAP.[7,8] Only 3% of patients develop retrograde ejaculation 3 months following TULIP.[21] Following TUEP, if the patient wishes to retain antegrade ejaculation, the technique is modified to preserve bladder neck.[11,15] Following interstitial laser prostatectomy, up to 93% of the patients have retained antegrade ejaculation.[16]

The incidence of urethral stricture after TURP is 3.1% and, if bladder neck contractures are included, it approaches 5%.[14] Etiology is thought to be large size of resectoscope and use of coagulating (low intensity) current,

which penetrates deeper into tissue compared with cutting currents. Since laser procedures do not use electrical current and cystoscopes are smaller in size, the incidence of stricture and bladder neck contracture are lower following laser procedures. However, strictures of urethra have been reported following laser prostatectomy.[16,17] Three instances of bladder neck contractures have been reported by Leach and two by Dixon and Lepor following VLAP.[22–24] It has also been noted to be a significant feature of VLAP European trials (see Chapter 18, Sakr & Watson). Longer follow-up is necessary to determine the actual incidence of these complications.

The incidence of UTI following TURP is 15.5% (median) and epididymitis is 1.2%.[14] UTIs have been reported to be between 1 and 20% following laser prostatectomy and epididymitis occurs in 5–7% of patients. We and others have noted that, with postoperative antibiotic prophylaxis, the incidence of UTI is less than 1%.[11,15] Similar need for long-term antibiotics following laser prostatectomy has been noted by others.[25]

Most series of laser prostatectomy have noted a high incidence of postoperative urinary retention following most laser techniques lasting from a few days to several weeks.[26,27] The incidence varies between 20 and 32% and is higher than the 6.5% incidence following TURP.[14] To overcome this problem, some investigators have resorted to use of stents in postoperative phase following VLAP.[28] However, prolonged postoperative retention following the TUEP technique of laser prostatectomy is 5%, which is comparable with TURP.[11,14,15,17] The need for reoperations following VLAP is 9%, while it is 2% every year with TURP and 0–4% in the first year after TUEP.[11,12,14,15]

A complication unique to most laser prostatectomies is the high incidence of irritative voiding symptoms during the initial few weeks postoperatively. This problem occurs owing to coagulated necrotic tissue that has not yet sloughed, as well as raw and unepithelialized mucosa. This is less common (30%) after TUEP.

Incidence of urinary incontinence is rare following all forms of laser prostatectomy.

FINANCIAL IMPLICATIONS

Due to the high initial expenses for the laser delivery system (approximately $50,000–$80,000) compared with the TURP electrocautery ($8400), there has been a concern about the cost effectiveness of laser prostatectomy. In addition to this cost, there is a recurring, high maintenance cost, namely laser fibers that sell in the range of $225–$850.[12] Although the laser delivery system is expensive, it is only a one-time expenditure, and it can be used for various other procedures besides BPH. Furthermore, in 1996, nearly 50% of the medical centers in the USA were found to have already purchased a laser delivery system for the urologic department. Additionally, VLAP has been found by several authors to be less expensive than other forms of treatment, specifically electrocautery. Fugate and associates reported that VLAP was $2000 less expensive than TURP.[29] This gap in expenditure is only going to widen as technology advances, resulting in fibers that are more durable, efficient, and reusable (with detachable tips). The competition among manufacturers to produce these fibers will also result in lower overhead costs.

From a patient's perspective, the main advantage of using laser prostatectomy is that it can be performed as an out-patient procedure, requiring no postoperative irrigation or pathology report expenses. Postoperatively, there are no costs related to TURP syndrome and clot retention, which would necessitate hospitalization and blood transfusions. The lower incidence of other complications from laser should also result in less cost overall.

CONCLUSIONS

The role of laser prostatectomy in the management of BPH is still evolving. The main limiting factor for common utilization of this technique is the cost of fiber and availability of several equally safe and efficacious techniques such as TUEP. However, in today's world of cost-effective therapy, especially in the USA, the TUEP technique is giving way to ILTT, because of the ILTT's inherent ease and reasonable efficacy.

REFERENCES

1 Narayan P. Laser evaporation. In: *Smith's Textbook of Endourology*, Vol. 2. 1996; 1054–77.

2 Sander S, Beisland HO *et al*. Laser in the treatment of localized prostatic cancer. *J Urol* 1984; **132**: 280–1.

3 Shanberg AM, Tansey LA *et al*. The use of neodymium YAG laser in prostatectomy *J Urol* 1985; **133**: 331 (Abstract).

4 Kandel L, Harrison L *et al*. Transurethral laser prostatectomy: creation of a technique for using the neodymium:yttrium aluminum garnet (YAG) laser in the canine model. *J Urol* 1986; **135**: 110 (Abstract).

5 Johnson D, Levinson AK *et al*. Transurethral laser prostatectomy using a right angle delivery system. *SPIE Proc* 1991; **1421**: 36–8.

6 Costello A, Bowsher W *et al*. Laser ablation of the prostate in patients with benign prostatic hypertrophy. *Br J Urol* 1992; **69**(6): 603–8.

7 Kabalin J. Laser prostatectomy performed with a right angle firing neodymium:YAG laser fiber at 40 watts power setting. *J Urol* 1993; **150**(1): 95–9.

8 Kabalin J, Gill H. Urolase laser prostatectomy in patients on warfarin anticoagulation: a safe treatment alternative for bladder outlet obstruction. *Urology* 1993; **42**(6): 738–40.

9 Fournier GJ, Narayan P. Factors affecting size and configuration of neodymium:YAG (Nd:YAG) laser lesions in the prostate. *Lasers Surg Med* 1994; **14**(4): 314–22.

10 Breza A, Aboseif S *et al*. Transurethral Nd: YAG laser prostatectomy with a laterally firing fiber: Local effects on tissue associated with erectile dysfunction. *Laser Surg Med* 1995; **17**(4): 364–9.

11 Narayan P, Tewari A *et al*. Impact of prostate size on the outcome of transurethral laser evaporation of the prostate for benign prostatic hyperplasia. *Urology* 1995; **45**(5): 776–82.

12 Dixon C. Lasers for the treatment of benign prostatic hyperplasia. *Urol Clin North Am* 1995; **22**(2): 413–22.

13 Mebust W. Editorial comment. *J Urol* 1995; **153**: 98.

14 Mebust W, Holtgrewe H *et al*. Transurethral prostatectomy: immediate and postoperative complications. A cooperative study of 13 participating institutions evaluating 3,885 patients. *J Urol* 1989; **141**: 243–7.

15 Narayan P, Tewari A *et al*. Impact of prostate size and techniques of laser prostatectomy (evaporation vs coagulation) on the outcome of therapy for benign prostatic hyperplasia. *J Urol* 1995; **153**: 231A.

16 Muschter R, Perlmutter A *et al*. Interstitial laser coagulation of benign prostatic hyperplasia: three years experience. In: Marberger M (ed) *Application of Newer Forms of Therapeutic Energy in Urology: SIU Report*. Oxford: Isis Medical Media 1995; 179–87.

17 Narayan P, Fournier G *et al*. Transurethral evaporation of prostate (TUEP) with Nd:YAG laser using a contact free beam technique: results in 61 patients with benign prostatic hyperplasia. *Urology* 1994; **43**(6): 813–20.

18 Norris J, Norris D *et al*. Visual laser ablation of the prostate: clinical experience in 108 patients. *J Urol* 1993; **150**(5 Part 2): 1612–14.

19 Dixon C, Machi G *et al*. A prospective double-blind, randomized study comparing laser ablation of the prostate and transurethral prostatectomy for the treatment of BPH. *J Urol* 1993; **149**: 6 (Abstract).

20 Dixon C, Machi G *et al*. A prospective double-blind, randomized study comparing the safety, efficacy and cost of laser ablation of the prostate and transurethral prostatectomy for the treatment of BPH. *J Urol* 1994; **151**: 229A.

21 McCullough D, Roth R *et al*. Transurethral ultrasound-guided laser-induced prostatectomy: National Human Cooperative Study results. *J Urol* 1993; **150**(5 Part 2): 1607–11.

22 Leach G, Dmochowski R *et al*. Visual laser assisted prostatectomy (VLAP) using Urolase right angle fiber: Multicenter 60 Watts protocol. *J Urol* 1994; **151**(Suppl): 230A.

23 Leach G, Sirls L *et al*. Outpatient visual laser-assisted prostatectomy under local anesthesia. *Urology* 1994; **43**(2): 149–53.

24 Dixon C, Lepor H. Laser ablation of the prostate. *Semin Urol* 1992; **10**(4): 273–7.

25 Perlmutter A, Muschter R *et al*. A comparison of the free beam side fire irradiation effects of 805 to 1000 nm in the canine prostate. *J Urol* 1995; **153**(4): 414A.

26 Gottfried H, Frohnberg D *et al*. Transurethral laser ablation of prostate (TULAP) – experience of a European multicenter study using Ultraline® fiber. *J Urol* 1995; **153**(4): 230A.

27 Schulze H, Martin W *et al*. Transurethral ultrasound-guided laser-induced prostatectomy: clinical outcome and data analysis. *Urology* 1995; **45**(2): 241–7.

28 Petas A, Talja M *et al*. Bioresorbable PGA-Urospiral preventing urinary retention in VLAP. *J Urol* 1995; **153**(4): 534A.

29 Fugate D, Sirls LT *et al*. Detailed cost analysis of high power visual laser assisted prostatectomy vs. transurethral prostatectomy. *J Urol* 1995; **153**: 362 (Abstract).

COMMENTARY

Several types of laser energy are available for treating human tissue. These include CO_2, Nd:YAG, KTP, argon, diode, holmium, excimer, and pulsed dye. The key feature regulating laser effects on tissue is power density. Power density expresses the strength of the laser at a spot, is directly proportional to the power of the laser source, and is inversely related to the area. This also means that the beam divergence and the distance of the beam from the tissue will influence the amount of energy delivered. The most commonly used fiber for laser energy transmission has an inner core of silicone dioxide (quartz).

A variety of fiber types have been described for delivering energy to prostate tissue. Initial attempts at using bare quartz fiber led to the development of the TULIP system. This subsequently gave way to the less costly alternative of using sidefiring quartz fibers to cause coagulation. The mechanisms of laser-induced prostatic destruction involve both technical as well as tissue factors (Figure 17.6). Among the primary objectives in using a specific type of energy and fiber are attempts to reduce reflection and scattering outside tissue, increase absorption inside tissue, and to cause adequate penetration of the adenoma by the laser energy, without causing laser effects on extraprostatic tissue.

Coagulation is a process of causing molecular breakdown of organic compounds by raising their temperatures. After coagulation, there is gradual absorption of tissue that is necrosed. One side effect is a variable period of postoperative urinary retention in 20% of the patients. The major advantages of the coagulation technique are that it requires less time, is less wearing on fibers, and therefore cost effective. It is also better tolerated by patients under intravenous sedation or prostate block.

During vaporization there is a change in the physical state of tissue water into steam. Tissue is removed as smoke and steam, leading to immediate cavitation and a TUR-like effect. In initial studies conducted by the Editor and his associates, it was found that at any given power setting the proximity of the beam to the tissue is the single most important determinant of lesion size and configuration. Holding the beam in close contact with tissue also causes an accelerated evaporation phenomenon. The advantages of the vaporization technique are that an immediate TUR-like cavity can be created and coagulation also occurs underneath the area of vaporization. This combination of effects results in not only the traditional advantages of laser prostatectomy such as lack of bleeding, fluid absorption, and decreased hospitalization but also captures some of the traditional advantages of TURP, such as immediate ability to void with minimal catheterization time and decreased postoperative irritative side effects. The disadvantages of the vaporization technique include a longer duration of therapy, requirement of deeper anesthesia, and fiber wear-out, often necessitating the use two fibers, which increases cost.

In a series of 168 patients followed over 12 months, the Editor and his associates demonstrated that the evaporation technique results in symptom improvements in 65–76%, and uroflow improvements of 121–166%. The complications were low with irritative voiding symptoms in 22.6% of patients lasting from a few days to 3 weeks, and urinary tract infections in 4.8% of patients. Additionally, small as well as large prostates can be treated with this technique as well as patients in retention. The procedure failed in only 3% of patients, owing to residual adenoma that was not satisfactorily treated at initial operation. Similar results have been noted by others (Table 17.2).

Almost every technique of laser proctectomy fares better than TURP in safety. Additionally, laser prostatectomies require shorter hospitalization and currently are performed as an out-patient procedure.

In conclusion, the role of laser prostatectomy in the management of BPH is still evolving. The main limiting factor for common utilization of the vaporization technique is the cost of the fiber and the current availability of equally safe and efficacious techniques such as interstitial laser, modified VLAP, and newer minimally invasive techniques. It remains to be seen which of these techniques will ultimately be the most common one used for BPH therapy.

Visual Laser Ablation of the Prostate

G. Sakr and G. Watson

18

INTRODUCTION

The terms used in laser prostatectomy have been imprecise. Words such as "ablation" have crept in to use and this should be abandoned. A more correct term would be coagulation. Visual laser ablation of the prostate (VLAP), endoscopic laser ablation of the prostate (ELAP), and sidefire laser prostatectomy all denote coagulative laser prostatectomy.

There are basically two ways in which a laser can have an effect on prostatic tissue: vaporization and coagulation. Vaporization can be achieved by using a high power density that raises the tissue temperature to several hundred degrees. Another way of vaporizing tissue is by using a wavelength that is more powerfully absorbed by the prostate or by using a tip that increases the absorption (such as carbon coating after contact with tissue or coating the tip with an infrared absorber). Coagulation occurs at tissue temperatures of 70–90° C. It is usually achieved using a laser beam with wide scattering and deep penetration, such as the neodymium:yttrium–aluminum garnet (Nd:YAG) laser. The total energy delivered and the time during which this energy is applied are important determinants of the photothermal tissue effect.

Equally important is the power density of a laser beam, which is defined as the amount of power per unit area. If the power density is high, such as with a narrow beam, tissue vaporization occurs, whereas with a wide beam, the power is distributed over a larger surface area and coagulation occurs. The laser beam is delivered under cystoscopic control via either a sidefiring or a forward-firing fiber. The beam can also be delivered via a balloon within the prostatic urethra, as with the TULIP system. When the prostate is coagulated, proteins are denatured and the gland becomes whitish and shrinks. The tissue swells for a transitory period, causing urinary retention. The necrotic tissue is then sloughed and passes urethrally or is absorbed.

Laser vaporization techniques will be discussed in separate chapters. This chapter will therefore focus on laser coagulation of the prostate.

SIDEFIRE LASER COAGULATION OF THE PROSTATE: DOSIMETRY

The first laser prostatectomy was a sidefire procedure performed in 1992 by Costello et al.[1] The dosimetry formula was developed from a small number of procedures performed in dogs.[2] The Nd:YAG laser energy was delivered through a sidefiring fiber (Lateralase), which reflected the beam at 90°. Energy was applied at 60 W for 60 s in four separate quadrants (Figure 18.1) and resulted in large volume coagulative necrosis of the canine prostate. Based on this, the dosimetry formula was extrapolated to man. But the prostate of the dog is different from the human gland: the shape is different and the epithelial tissue is predominant.[3]

Since then modifications have involved three areas: the delivery fibers, the dosimetry formula, and the number of spots lased.

Improvements in the sidefiring fibers involved increasing the durability of the fiber. The tips of the new fibers do not melt after a certain amount of laser energy delivery. A variety of sidefiring fibers are available. Figure 18.2 shows the Urolase sidefiring fiber.

Anson et al.[4] provided a comparative optical analysis of some fibers. They demonstrated that there is considerable variation in the angles of exit from the launch fiber and that the spot sizes vary markedly (Figures 18.3 and 18.4). Therefore, the choice of fiber is important in determining the tissue effect. Moreover, when used to deliver Nd:YAG energy, all these fibers have the ability to vaporize tissue if used close enough so that the spot size decreases and the power density increases. Figure 18.5 shows the angulation and conical distribution of an Nd:YAG laser beam produced by the Urolase dish reflector tip.

Changes in the dosimetry formula involved changing the ratio between power setting and time of delivery. The ideal ratio to achieve maximal tissue coagulation is still being debated. After a certain amount of energy delivery at one spot, superficial tissue carbonization occurs and delivery of further energy would result in tissue vaporization because of superficial absorption. This would prevent deeper penetration of the laser beam, and less prostatic tissue would be coagulated. An array of formulae appeared in the literature, some advocating 40 W for 60 s, others 40 W for 90 s or 60 W for 60 s.

The initial four-spots technique was modified as experience was gained. More applications were added to ensure blanching of the lateral lobes.[5] Other investigators advocated the use of two sets of four quadrants. Kabalin[6], using the Urolase™ fiber to deliver Nd:YAG laser energy, used the four-quadrants application in 1993 (see Figure 18.1),

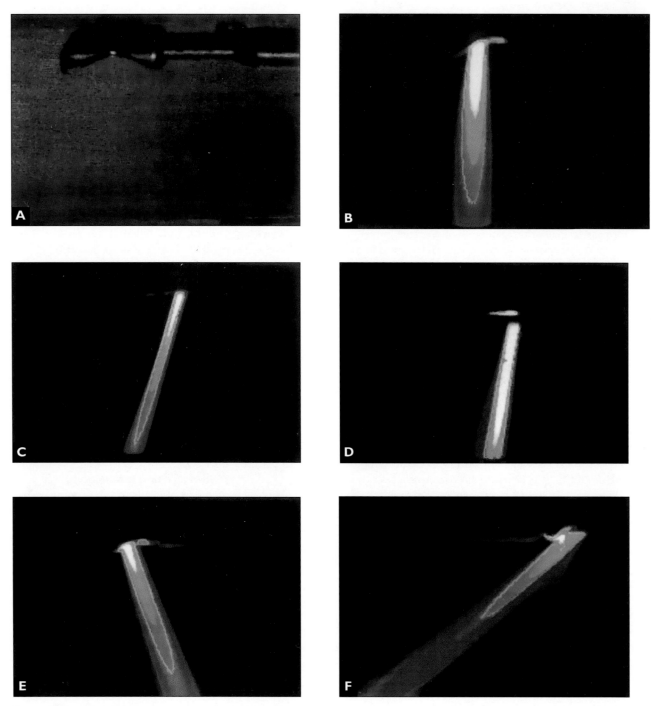

Figure 18.1 Lateral fluorescence intensity profiles for each device; (A) device in cuvette; (B) Urolase; (C) angle delivery device; (D) Ultraline; (E) Myriadlase; (F) Prolase. Scale 1×1.3 cm

Source: Anson K *et al. Br J Urol* 1995; **75**(3): 328–34, with permission of Blackwell Science Ltd.

while later he changed the technique to a multiple-fixed-spots application, as shown in Figure 18.5.[7,22] We changed our technique to a continuous set of spot applications. The beam is delivered at a certain spot until complete blanching of the tissue occurs, then the laser beam is moved to an adjacent non-blanched area and so on, until blanching of the whole gland is completed. We adopted this as part of our hybrid technique, and this resulted in more tissue

destruction. The hybrid technique will be described in detail later in the chapter. A continuous firing is needed for a certain time to achieve coagulation. If, for example, 60 s are needed to achieve coagulation of a certain amount of tissue, the same amount of coagulation will not be achieved if the energy is applied in two sets of 30 s each. Interrupting the laser beam will allow the tissue to cool and the deeper tissue will not be heated enough to coagulate.

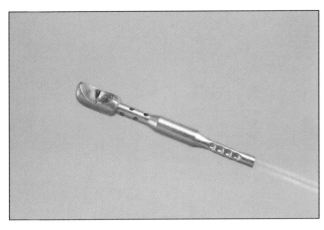

Figure 18.2 The Urolase device

RESULTS AND ADVANTAGES OF LASER PROSTATECTOMY

RESULTS

Laser prostatectomy provides an efficacious treatment for symptomatic bladder outlet obstruction due to benign prostatic hyperplasia. Early studies documented the short-term efficacy and safety of laser prostatectomy.

Costello *et al.*[1] in his pioneering study used the Lateralase fiber to deliver Nd:YAG laser energy at 60 W power for 60 s in four quadrants. He treated 17 patients, with a resultant decrease in the Madsen–Iversen symptom score from 15 preoperatively to 4 at 6 weeks, and an increase in flow rate from 5 to 9 mL s⁻¹ at 6 weeks. Norris *et al.* treated 108 patients with the four-quadrants technique and the 60 W for 60 s protocol. Additional applications were given, if necessary, to ensure complete blanching of the lateral lobes. With a follow-up of 3–6 months, flow rates increased from

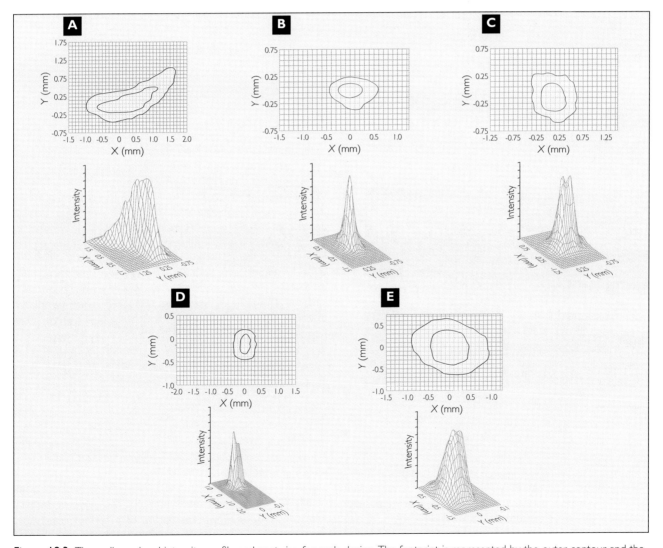

Figure 18.3 Three-dimensional intensity profile and spot size for each device. The footprint is represented by the outer contour and the half-maximum intensity by the inner contour: (A) Urolase; (B) angle delivery device; (C) Ultraline; (D) Myriadlase; (E) Prolase

Source: Anson K et al. Br J Urol 1995; **75**(3): 328–34, with permission

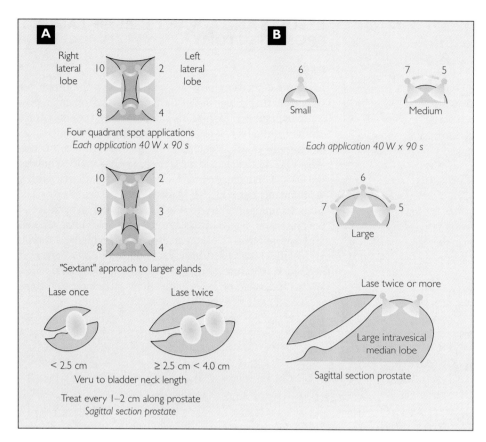

Figure 18.4 (A) Basic four-quadrant and expanded operative approaches to laser coagulation of prostatic lateral lobes with multiple fixed spot applications; (B) operative approach to laser coagulation of median lobe with multiple fixed spot applications. Veru, verumontanum

Source: Kabalin JN *et al. J Urol* 1996; **155**(1): 181–5, with permission

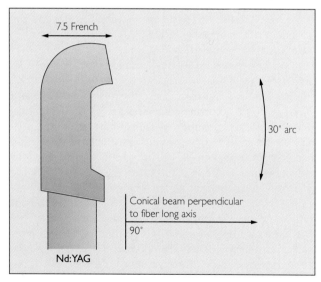

Figure 18.5 Angulation and conical distribution of Nd:YAG laser beam produced by Urolase dish reflector tip

7.6 to 12 mL s^{-1} and American Urological Association (AUA) symptom scores decreased from 22.3 to 9.2 postoperatively.[5] In 1994 Costello *et al.*[8] provided 3-month follow-up data on 33 patients. AUA symptom scores decreased from 21.5 to 9.5, and maximal flow rates increased from 8.5 to 15.2 mLs^{-1} postoperatively. Kabalin *et al.*[9] had a decrease in AUA symptom score from 21 to 10 at 3 months and 9.8

at 6 months. Peak flow rates increased from 7 to 13 and 12 mL s^{-1} at 3 and 6 months, respectively.

Anson *et al.*[10] reported their experience with 16 patients. AUA symptom scores fell from 20 preoperatively to 9.5 at 12 weeks and 7.2 at 26 weeks. Maximal flow rates increased from 10.2 mL s^{-1} to 23 mL s^{-1} at 12 weeks and 22.3 mL s^{-1} at 26 weeks. But the transrectal ultrasound volume of the prostate and the PSA did not change significantly.[10] Kabalin *et al.*[7] treated 227 patients, the last 156 patients being treated by the more aggressive method described previously (Figure 18.5). Peak flow rates increased from 7.3 mL s^{-1} preoperatively to 15.2 mL s^{-1} at 3 months, 17 mL s^{-1} at 1 year, 18.3 mL s^{-1} at 2 years and 18.5 mL s^{-1} at 3 years. AUA-6 symptom scores fell from 20.3 preoperatively to 10 at 3 months, 8 at 1 year, 8.6 at 2 years, and 5.7 at 3 years.

LASER COAGULATIVE PROSTATECTOMY vs. TRANSURETHRAL RESECTION OF THE PROSTATE

Several comparative studies on laser prostatectomy and transurethral resection of the prostate (TURP) have been done. A multicenter randomized prospective study was done in the UK, comparing laser prostatectomy with TURP.[11] Anson *et al.* used the Urolase fiber to deliver 60 W of Nd:YAG laser energy for 60 s in four quadrants. Two sets of four quadrants were given for longer prostates, and the median lobe was treated if significantly enlarged. AUA symptom scores decreased from 18.2 to 6.4 and 5.1 at 3 months and 1 year, respectively, in the TURP group, whereas the symptom score decreased from 18.1 to 8.7 and 7.7 at 3 months and 1 year, respectively, in the laser group. Maximal flow rates increased from 10 mL s^{-1} to 21.3 mL s^{-1} and 21.8 mL s^{-1} at 3 months and 1 year, respectively, in the TURP group. In the laser group, flow rates increased from 9.5 mL s^{-1} to 15.9 mL s^{-1} and 15.4 mL s^{-1} at 3 months and 1 year, respectively. Group comparison favoured TURP in maximum flow rates and symptom scores, but both groups showed significant improvements in all efficacy parameters. They concluded that laser prostatectomy is a useful alternative to TURP. In their comparative study, Dixon et al.[12] had a decrease in AUA symptom score from 16.5 preoperatively to 11.9 at 6 months in the laser group vs. a decrease from 20.3 preoperatively to 7.6 at 6 months in the TURP group. Peak flow rates increased from 9.2 mL s^{-1} preoperatively to 14.1 mL s^{-1} at 6 months in the laser group compared with an increase from 8.5 mL s^{-1} preoperatively to 14.9 mL s^{-1} at 6 months in the TURP group. Greater symptomatic improvement was found in the TURP group, but the improvement in peak flow rates was not statistically different.

LASER PROSTATECTOMY RESULTS WITH URODYNAMIC ASSESSMENT

Proof that laser prostatectomy is capable of relieving bladder outlet obstruction due to benign prostatic hyperplasia has been presented in several studies. James et al.[13] had 79 patients treated by free beam coagulation (72 patients) or by SLT contact vaporization. Patients treated by free beam coagulation had increases in flow rates from 6.5 mL s^{-1} preoperatively to 10.6 mL s^{-1} at 3 months, with a concomitant decrease in voiding pressure from 74 cmH$_2$O preoperatively to 54.2 cmH$_2$O at 3 months. AUA symptom scores decreased from 21.4 to 9.4 at the 3-month follow-up. Similarly, patients treated by SLT laser contact vaporization experienced increases in flow rates from 5.4 mL s^{-1} preoperatively to 13.9 mL s^{-1} with a concomitant decrease in voiding pressure from 82.8 cmH$_2$O to 51.1 cmH$_2$O at the 3-month follow-up. AUA symptom scores decreased from 20.4 preoperatively to 4.1 at 3 months. Te Slaa et al.[14] reported the results obtained with 79 patients treated with the Nd:YAG laser free beam. The International Prostate Symptom Scores (IPSS) decreased from 21.3 to 5.3 at 6 months and maximal flow rates increased from 7.9 to 17.8 mL s^{-1} at the 6-month follow-up. Eighty per cent of the patients were obstructed preoperatively by pressure-flow studies according to the Abrams–Griffiths nomogram, compared with 5% at the 6-month follow-up. Kabalin et al.[15] randomized 25 patients to undergo either TURP or laser prostatectomy with the Urolase™ right-angle fiber. Patients were assessed at 1 year. In the laser group, peak flow rates increased from 8.2 to 21.6 mL s^{-1} and maximal detrusor pressure decreased from 91.3 to 54.6 cmH$_2$O. AUA symptom scores decreased from 20.9 to 4.3. In the TURP group, peak flow rates increased from 8.3 mL s^{-1} to 21.6 mL s^{-1}, maximal detrusor pressure decreased from 92.7 to 58.7 cmH$_2$O, and AUA symptom scores decreased from

18.8 to 6.3. They concluded that laser prostatectomy is equivalent to TURP in bringing about similar disobstruction in patients suffering from bladder outlet obstruction due to benign prostatic hyperplasia.

ADVANTAGES OF LASER PROSTATECTOMY

The results of the pilot studies and of the multicenter trials attest to the efficacy of laser prostatectomy being close to that of transurethral resection in the short term. But why should laser prostatectomy be chosen over conventional resection? Laser prostatectomy carries the advantages of being virtually bloodless; there is no risk of the transurethral resection (TUR) syndrome; the procedure can be performed as a day case; operative time is relatively short; there is less chance of retrograde ejaculation and finally the procedure is less stressful to the patient in the immediate perioperative period.

Coagulation of the prostate by Nd:YAG laser energy is a hemostatic action rather than a blood-letting one. The lack of bleeding has been documented in several studies.[6,11,12] Anson et al.[11] reported a decrease in the hemoglobin level from a mean of 14.4 to a mean of 12.7 following TURP, compared with a decrease from a mean of 14.4 to 14.3 following laser prostatectomy. He reported a 16.7% transfusion rate in the TURP group, compared with no transfusions in the laser group. Costello et al.[16] have treated a cohort of 22 patients on full anticoagulation therapy using the Urolase sidefire without any bleeding ensuing. Isolated case histories of bleeding have been described in verbal communications (these rare events are best treated by resection of the prostate down to capsule or by retropubic prostatectomy in the case of a very large prostate).

Blood vessels are not opened and there is therefore no risk of intravasation of irrigant, which might otherwise cause the TUR syndrome. There is no reported case of a TUR syndrome occurring after laser prostatectomy. Cummings et al.[18] demonstrated the lack of fluid absorption during laser prostatectomy by adding ethanol to the irrigation fluid and measuring the expired air ethanol levels. Only four patients were studied, but the expired ethanol levels were zero throughout the procedures. The serum sodium following laser prostatectomy does not fall significantly, in contrast to the mean serum sodium following TURP.[1,7,11]

The average operating time to perform a four-quadrant laser prostatectomy is less than 30 min. However with the more aggressive laser prostatectomy protocols, and especially with the hybrid technique, the operating time can be the same as a full TURP.

The percentage of patients who were sexually active prior to the procedure and who subsequently developed retrograde ejaculation is lower with laser prostatectomy than with TURP. Anson et al.[11] reported a 33% retrograde ejaculation, Kabalin et al.[7] a 27% rate (using the higher energy protocol), and Norris et al.[5] reported a rate of 3 out of 37. Kabalin observed that some patients had prograde ejaculation postoperatively but subsequently lost it, presumably as the prostatic tissue was sloughed or resorbed.

DISADVANTAGES OF LASER PROSTATECTOMY

The early complications of laser prostatectomy include the complications of instrumentation and the complications of leaving necrotic tissue behind in a patient who is obstructed, resulting in a temporary increase in their obstruction. Kabalin reported urethral strictures in 1.8%, bladder neck contracture in 4.4%, low-grade bacterial prostatitis in 2.6%, and a 5.3% conversion to TURP. Bladder neck contracture was noted particularly in patients with smaller glands (i.e. the group where a laser coagulation without incision is conceptually inappropriate). The low-grade bacterial prostatitis cases all responded to a prolonged course of antibiotics. Narayan et al.[19] reported a longer catheterization time and greater reoperation rate in patients having transurethral laser coagulation than in patients having laser vaporization of the prostate. He reported urinary tract infection in 1 of 32 patients and a 15.6% reoperation rate. Anson et al.[11] reported 28 positive urine cultures in 76 patients having laser coagulation of the prostate out of which two had epididymoorchitis and five needed retreatment within the first year. One patient had a secondary bleed after 24 days, after being placed on warfarin anticoagulation for a DVT. Forty-one percent of patients had moderate perineal discomfort or dysuria at 4 weeks, compared with 15% after TURP.

The incidence of longer-term complications following sidefire coagulation of the prostate is low. Urethral strictures occur in as many 16% of TURPs.[20,21] After laser prostatectomy, the incidence is 0 and 1.8% in the series of Anson and Kabalin, respectively. One would expect to produce a lower incidence of strictures after laser than TURP because smaller-caliber cystoscopes are used and because there is no risk of electrical leakage being transmitted down the instrument. The incidence of bladder neck contracture is equivalent to that after TURP. Case selection is important here. All small prostates should be treated by incision through the bladder neck and prostate capsule.

The absence of tissue for histology is of concern to some urologists. One might counter this by pointing out that TURP can also miss cancers. After all TURP is just a resection of the transitional zone without taking the peripheral zone. With the use of prostate-specific antigen (PSA), rectal examination, and transrectal ultrasound, the chance of missing cancer of the prostate is thought to be small. Therefore, one might argue that exclusion of prostate cancer should be made prior to treatment and that, once prostate cancer is excluded, any therapeutic modality can be chosen on its merits.

This still leaves us with concerns about the duration of irritative symptoms after sidefire laser coagulation, the requirement for catheter drainage after the procedure, and the amount of residual tissue. The irritative symptoms are almost certainly due to the fact that the patients are voiding urine in a state of partial obstruction over necrotic prostatic tissue. This tends to produce fissures in the prostate and a prostatitis temporarily in many; in addition, it predisposes the individual to infection. Early disobstruction by combining a laser transurethral incision of the prostate (TUIP) is

one way of bringing about earlier disobstruction. It is also probably helpful to have the patient on urinary drainage for at least 7 days without attempting to void. Whenever there is a bulk coagulation of the prostate, therefore, one should probably accept a prolonged period of catheterization as necessary. It is balanced by the fact that the patient can go home with the catheter on the same day as the surgery if necessary. Inevitably, the longer catheterization time will result in a high rate of bacteriuria, and this should be covered with antibiotics at least at the time of catheter removal. Finally, there is no doubt that laser sidefire coagulation prostatectomy removes less tissue than TURP. The long-term data of Kabalin and Costello suggest that, after 5 years, patients are still voiding well after the Urolase™ procedure.

We have recently reviewed the results of patients in Eastbourne treated as part of the British multicenter trial comparing Urolase™ with TURP.[11] Sixteen patients were treated by laser and 16 by TURP. Of the 16 TURP patients, only 1 patient has had a second procedure and he had cancer of the prostate. Of the 16 laser patients six have been reoperated on using TURP or TUIP. It is only when the poor-outcome patients have been weeded out that we are left with a group of patients who compare very favorably with TURP in both symptom score and flow rate. If we were to look at the long-term data of patients from centers with itinerant populations (i.e. all major cities), then we might miss a very significant failure rate. The 6 laser-treated patients who required conversion to conventional surgery failed in 3 cases because of bladder neck stenosis, and in 3 cases because of residual adenoma. The deficiencies in the protocol used in the British study have been addressed by the hybrid approach of incorporating a TUIP into the standard laser treatment and thereby avoiding bladder neck stenosis. The problem of residual prostatic tissue is addressed at least in part by treating the prostate with more energy and lower powers. Kabalin's latest technique[7] using the Urolase fiber at 40 W for 90 s at multiple points is probably as good as any technique.

HOW TO PERFORM A PURE SIDEFIRE COAGULATIVE PROSTATECTOMY

PATIENT SELECTION

The ideal patient for this treatment has a prostate size of greater than 30 cm^3 and less than 70 cm^3. If the prostate is smaller than 30 cm^3 then there is a high risk that bladder neck dyssynergia is an element of the obstruction. In our opinion, coagulation is not likely to resolve this problem. Incision is required. If the prostate is larger than 70 cm^3, sidefire coagulation is unlikely to extend deeply enough into the tissues and retreatment may be required. Also deployment of the sidefire probe is difficult because of the tight space between the prostatic lobes. The ideal indications are the patient who wants the maximum chance of retaining prograde ejaculation and the patient who is at most risk from bleeding – as for example a patient on anticoagulants.

PREOPERATIVE COUNSELLING

Patients should be warned that they will require a catheter for 7 days and occasionally longer. They should be warned that an improvement in symptoms is delayed and that the flow will not start to improve for at least 6 weeks. They should be warned that the risk of losing ejaculation is still present, even though it is reduced. Bleeding still occurs albeit rarely. There is a risk of urinary tract infection, and this should be looked for in the early postoperative weeks.

Prostate cancer should be excluded prior to surgery by performing at least a PSA and rectal examination. If biopsies are to be taken at the time of the procedure, then we recommend taking them transperineally rather than inoculating the prostate with fecal organisms at the time of causing coagulative necrosis.

PREOPERATIVE CHECKS OF INSTRUMENTATION

Choose a Nd:YAG or semiconductor diode laser with which you are familiar. The sidefire device should be known to you. The protocol for one fiber is not necessarily applicable to another, although in practice the devices are used in identical ways. If the sidefire device has been used before, be sure that it still transmits the laser beam effectively. One can check the transmission using power levels of 2 W from the laser and directing the resultant beam on a power meter in air. Proprietary devices are available for checking sidefire devices in water at high power.

PERFORMING THE PROCEDURE

The procedure is performed under laser-safe conditions. The patient is prepared as for a cystoscopy with general anesthesia, spinal anesthesia or, rarely, local anesthesia. If using local anesthesia, a suprapubic catheter is recommended so that the patient and surgeon are not inconvenienced by distention of the bladder. A cystoscopy is performed and particular attention paid to the configuration of the prostate and the bladder neck region. The ideal prostate has a trilobar obstruction. If the bladder neck is circular, it should be left intact during lasering. A 23.5 Ch cystoscope with working bridge is used to deliver the sidefire device. Start at the bladder neck side of the prostate and work systematically towards the apex always starting with the easily accessible areas of the prostate and then continuing to the less easily accessible. This is because some shrinking of the lobes will occur during the procedure, and access can become easier. Deep penetration of heat into the depths of the prostate is the aim of the technique, and it will only occur if the laser is delivered continuously and to an area that does not become charred. Having chosen the area to start lasering, empty the bladder so that lasering can continue for as long as possible. Keep the sidefire device as far away as possible from the area to be lasered so that maximum use is made of the beam divergence. Using 40 W for 90 s, deliver the laser energy without interruption. If it is necessary to stop the delivery of the energy, the build-up of heat deep in the tissues ceases. Unless one can recom-

mence within seconds, the laser energy should be delivered for a further 90 s. If charring occurs, the heat does not penetrate deeply and one should move to an adjoining area for the rest of the 90 s in the hope that the deep heat build-up will be maintained. If the space between the prostate lobes is too little and charring tends to occur, one can slowly rotate the device backwards and forwards to adjust for the smaller spot size. As the procedure progresses, the prostate tends to shrink somewhat making further laser delivery easier. Move to an adjacent spot and, having emptied the bladder, restart the process. In a prostate of 40 cm³ one might expect to deliver six spots at any transverse section of the prostate and repeat these six spots at 1 cm steps until 0.5 cm from the vermontanum. In addition, a middle lobe should be treated with at least two spots, although the bladder neck should be left intact. The operator might prefer a continuous delivery of the laser energy, moving from a spot to adjoining virgin tissue only once the tissue has achieved total blanching. It is important, however, that the new area is contiguous. This promotes deep heat build-up. Again, start where there is most space in the prostate and creep towards the areas where space is limited. One can laser the prostate to within 5 mm of the verumontanum. The blanching of the tissue should extend into the apical tissue but not the sphincter active area. The procedure is complete only when the entire prostatic urethra is intensely white from apex to bladder neck, but not including the bladder neck.

We recommend inserting a urethral catheter for 7 days.

THE HYBRID PROCEDURE

The pure sidefire procedure is associated with minimal perioperative trauma and, in particular, little or no bleeding. On the negative side, however, there is a failure rate due to bladder neck obstruction and insufficient prostatic removal. Narayan et al.[19] have argued for using a sidefire device with a high power density in order to vaporize a cavity in the prostate. The hybrid procedure is a combination of sidefire coagulation of the prostate with contact incision through the prostate from verumontanum to trigone. The incisions are made with a contact tip of the SLT system (SLT Corporation, Oak, PA) or using a carbonized ball tip. The incisions are made from verumontanum to trigone right through the capsule and bladder neck. We favor performing the incisions first in order to open up the prostatic fossa as much as possible. This then creates more space for deploying the sidefire device. Others perform the incisions after sidefiring, on the basis that any charring from the incisions interferes with deep penetration of the laser beam. The counter to this argument is that the charred areas are avoided when delivering the sidefire laser energy. The hybrid technique thus combines an immediate disobstruction from the incisions with a delayed debulking from the sidefire coagulation.

We have found that a triple incision through the prostate is superior to a single incision. We start at the 6 o'clock position, incising through to fat. We then make incisions at 10 and 2 o'clock down to capsule. The contact fiber is replaced with a sidefiring device and used at 40 W to effect complete blanching of the intervening prostatic tissue. A catheter is then placed urethrally for a week.

Our first experience with the hybrid technique dates back to 1991. For the incisions, we used a KTP laser (Laserscope, San Jose, CA) using a ball tip with a diameter of 2.5 mm at 532 nm and 30 W. For subsequent coagulation, we used a bare fiber (forward firing) and a power of 60 W. Our results are shown in Table 18.1.

	Preop.	3 months	6 months	12 months
AUA score	23	7	6	3
Q_{Max} (mL s^{-1})	7.4	15.7	20	16

Table 18.1 Results using hybrid laser technique

We have used the hybrid approach using the SLT (Oak, PA) chisel tip for incisions and the sidefire attachment for standard sidefire coagulation. We are currently exploring the use of a semiconductor diode laser for hybrid treatment. We have used the Diomed laser (Diomed Company, Cambridge, UK) which is a 60 W maximum output gallium arsenide laser. The device is portable and plugs into a standard household electrical socket. Using a triradiate incision with a 3-mm ball tip, we then irradiate at 35–40 W with a sidefiring device. Our results using this combination are shown in Table 18.2.

	Preop.	3 months	6 months
AUA score	21.1	7.2	2.8
Q_{Max} (mL s^{-1})	8.1	18.8	24.6

Table 18.2 Results using hybrid laser technique: Diomed laser

It has long been our contention that, using the PSA and the transrectal ultrasonography (TRUS) volume, we can look at the degree of debulking that we achieve using any modality. In Table 18.3, we summarize all the data of our series.

The hybrid laser patients have a reduction of PSA that is greater than with other laser techniques, and they have a reduction in TRUS volume close to that of the sidefire group. Perhaps the incisional element of the hybrid treatment expands the outer capsule, while the coagulation debulks.

CONCLUSIONS

Laser prostatectomy has developed, evolved, and diverged. It is still a technique where the clinician should continue to evaluate all his patients. There are patients in whom laser prostatectomy is preferred over standard TURP; any patient in whom there is an increased risk of bleeding is best treated by laser. This includes patients on anticoagulants or with clotting disorders, patients with incompatibility to blood transfusion, and patients who are very frail. Another relative indication for laser surgery is the patient with an enlarged obstructing prostate who wishes to maximize his chance of maintaining prograde ejaculation. A pure sidefire prostatectomy is the treatment of choice.

There are relative contraindications to laser prostatectomy. The patient in retention who wishes to lose his catheter at the first opportunity would be better treated by TURP. (Combination of laser with temporary stenting is a development that might make laser prostatectomy effective for this group.) The patient with chronic retention may have a failing detrusor and may be best treated by TURP with its greater debulk of the prostate. A patient in whom the increased risk of urinary tract infection may be more serious, as in the patient with valve disease who might get subacute bacterial endocarditis, is also possibly better treated by TURP, unless meticulous attention is paid to urine bacteriology over the ensuing 2 months.

Pure sidefire laser prostatectomy does not make sense for small prostates of up to 25 cm^3, and in our opinion it is better used in combination with contact laser incisions as part of the hybrid technique. We only use the pure sidefire laser technique when treating patients with full anticoagulation or patients who want to maximize the chance of maintaining prograde ejaculation.

	TRUS volume			PSA		
	Preop.	Postop.	% drop	Preop.	Post-op.	% drop
TURP	47.3	26.9	43.1	5.6	2.2	60.7
Contact laser (SLT)	43.3	42.8	1.1	7.5	6.0	20.0
Sidefire (Urolase)	35.0	29.0	17.1	6.5	5.9	9.2
Hybrid	37.2	31.5	15.3	4.0	2.2	45.0

Table 18.3 The reduction in TRUS volume and PSA following TURP and different laser treatments

REFERENCES

1 Costello AJ, Bowsher WG, Bolton DM *et al*. Laser ablation of the prostate in patients with benign prostatic hypertrophy. *Br J Urol* 1992; **69**: 603–8.
2 Johnson DE, Levinson AK, Greskovish FJ. Transurethral laser prostatectomy using a right-angled laser delivery system. *SPIE Proc* 1991; **1421**: 36–41.
3 Helty R, Mettfeld T, Gottfried HW *et al*. The critical role of the epithelium–stroma ratio in the laser treatment of BPH. *J Urol* 1995; **153**(Suppl): 231A.
4 Anson K, Buonaccorsi G, Eddowes M *et al*. A comparative analysis of laser sidefiring devices – a guide to treatment. *Br J Urol* 1995; **75**: 328–34.
5 Norris JP, Norris DM, Lee RD, Rubenstein MA. Visual laser ablation of the prostate: clinical experience in 108 patients. *J Urol* 1993; **150**: 1612–14.
6 Kabalin JN. Laser prostatectomy performed with a right-angled firing Nd:YAG laser fiber at 40 watts power setting. *J Urol* 1993; **150**: 95–9.
7 Kabalin JN, Bite G, Doll S. Neodymium:YAG laser coagulation prostatectomy: 3 years of experience with 227 patients. *J Urol* 1996; **155**: 181–5.
8 Costello AJ, Shaffer BS, Crowe MR. Second generation delivery systems for laser prostatic ablations. *Urology* 1994; **43**: 262–6.
9 Kabalin JN, Harcheran SG, Leech GE *et al*. Visual laser assisted prostatectomy (VLAP) using Urolase right angle fiber. Preliminary results with 60 watts protocol. *J Urol* 1993; **150**: 214A.
10 Anson K, Seenivasagam K, Watson GM. Letter to the editor "Visual laser ablation of the prostate." *Urology* 1994; **43**: 276.
11 Anson K, Nawocki J, Buckley J *et al*. A multicentre randomised prospective study of endoscopic laser ablation versus transurethral resection of the prostate. *Urology* 1995; **43**: 305–10.
12 Dixon C, Machi G, Theune C *et al*. A prospective double-blind randomised study comparing the safety, efficacy and cost of laser ablation of the prostate and transurethral resection prostatectomy for treatment of BPH. *J Urol* 1994; **151**: 229A.
13 James MJ, Harris DR, Ceccherini A *et al*. A urodynamic study of laser ablation of the prostate and a comparison of techniques. *Br J Urol* 1995; **76**: 179–83.
14 Te Slaa E, De Wildt M, Rosier D *et al*. Urodynamic assessment in the laser treatment of benign prostatic enlargement. *Br J Urol* 1995; **76**: 604–10.
15 Kabalin J, Harcheran SG, Bite G, Wolfe V. Comparative study of laser versus electrocautery prostatic resection: 18 months follow-up with complex urodynamic assessment. *J Urol* 1995; **153**: 94–8.
16 Costello A, Crowe HR. A single institution experience of reflecting laser fiber over 4 years. *J Urol* 1994; **152**: 229A.
17 Leach G, Sirls E, Ganabathi K *et al*. outpatient visual laser-assisted prostatectomy under local anesthesia. *Urology* 1993; **43**: 149–53.
18 Cummings J, Parra RO, Bouiller JA *et al*. Evaluation of fluid absorption during laser prostatectomy by breath ethanol techniques. *J Urol* 1995; **154**: 2080–2.
19 Narayan P, Teweri A, Aboseif S, Evans C. A randomised study comparing visual laser ablation and transurethral evaporation of prostate in the management of benign prostatic hyperplasia. *J Urol* 1995; **154**: 2083–8.
20 Cowles RS, Kabalin JN, Childs S *et al*. A prospective randomised comparison of transurethral resection to visual laser ablation of the prostate for the treatment of benign prostatic hyperplasia. *Urology* 1995; **46**: 155–8.
21 Meyhoff HH, Nordling J. Long term results of transurethral and transvesical prostatectomy: a randomised study. *Scand J Urol* 1986; **20**: 27.
22 Kabalin JN, Gill HS, Bite G. Laser prostatectomy with a right angle neodymium:YAG laser fiber at 60 watts power setting. *J Urol* 1995; **153**: 1502–5.

COMMENTARY

In this chapter Drs Watson and Sakr, who have been pioneers in coagulation laser prostatectomy, present the rationale and results of this technique. There are basically two techniques in which lasers can be used on the prostate (i.e. vaporization or coagulation). Each technique requires a specific type of fiber tip (quartz or sapphire vs. gold), energy delivery system (example: narrow vs. wide beam) and surgical technique (example; contact vs. non-contact) to achieve optimum results. The coagulation technique involves slow heating with resulting coagulation and subsequent necrosis with reabsorption or sloughing of tissue. The technique also causes thrombosis of blood vessels, resulting in essentially a bloodless surgical technique.

Initially, coagulation techniques were based on studies in canine models, which revealed that low-density laser energy delivered using widely divergent beam techniques in non-contact mode could effectively slough a majority of the prostate within 6 weeks, resulting in a widely open prostatic frosa. Initial trials were then undertaken in humans by Costello in Australia, Kabalin and others in the USA, and Watson and associates in Europe. However, it soon became apparent that treatment parameters as extrapolated from canine studies were not totally applicable to human prostatic tissue, which differed significantly in its composition and sensitivity to laser energy from canine tissue. Additionally, the initial laser fibers lacked durability and the ability to withstand heat in close contact with tissue. A combination of these drawbacks resulted in mixed results of BPH therapy due to incomplete and uneven prostatic destruction.

In this chapter, Drs Watson and Sakr reiterate their dissatisfaction with the initial methodology and techniques used for VLAP. These drawbacks resulted in the initial four-quadrant technique being changed to a continuous spot technique in which the entire prostate is coagulated. Currently, they have further evolved to using a hybrid technique in which TUIP is performed using an SLT fiber and, subsequently, a continuous spot coagulation (modified VLAP) technique is used to complete the prostatectomy procedure. In the Editors opinion this technique has excellent scientific rationale especially in small and medium sized prostates (under 40 cc). In the USA also, Kabalin and others (Table 18.4) increased laser power (wattage) and

	AUA Score pre	AUA Score 6 months	AUA Score 12 months	Uroflow pre	Uroflow 6 months	Uroflow 12 months
Stein, Zabbo[1] Laser	19.4	11.4	13.9	7.2	10.7	8.1
TURP	20.5	6.0	6.2	7.1	16.2	14.6
Kabalin[2] Laser	20.9	4.6	4.3	8.5	20.5	21.6
TURP	18.8	5.7	6.3	9.0	22.9	21.6
UK Study[3] Laser	18.1	–	7.7	9.5	–	15.4
TURP	18.2	–	5.1	10.0	–	21.3
Dixon[4] Laser	16.5	11.9	–	9.2	14.1	–
TURP	20.3	7.6	–	8.5	14.9	–

Table 18.4 Urolase™ results

duration of treatment to increase tissue destruction by VLAP. These modifications have resulted in the VLAP coagulation technique's providing improved AUA symptom scores as well as improvement in uroflow and other urodynamic parameters.

Randomized trials of VLAP to TURP have revealed that both techniques result in improved AUA symptom scores and uroflow. While initial results among the four quadrant techniques revealed less benefit from laser, other trials using more energy revealed symptom improvements that were comparable (see Table 18.4).

However, all trials have shown that the most common complications of VLAP were related to prolonged catheterization, irritative symptoms, and significant reoperation rates. In the original study conducted by Bard[1-5] 11% in the VLAP group had a reoperation at 6 months and 30% had prolonged retention. The need for reoperation was even greater in patients with acute retention and VLAP appears to be a poor choice for this group of patients. In a study comparing the evaporation technique with that of the coagulation method, the Editor and his associates also noted a 15% incidence of immediate reoperation using the coagulation technique.[6] In a study comparing TURP with laser coagulation using Urolase™, Watson noted a 5% vs. 30% reoperation rate for TURP vs. laser.[2,6]

In summary, laser coagulation prostatectomy is still an evolving technique in many countries. In the USA, it has been abandoned by most urologists in favor of either an evaporation technique or, more recently, an interstitial technique.

1 Stein BS, Zabbo A. Personal experience.
2 Kabalin JN, Gill HS, Bite G et al. Comparative study of laser versus electrocautery prostatic resection:18-month followup with complex urodynamic assessment. J Urol 1995; 153: 94–8.
3 Anson K, Seenivasagam K, Watson GM. Letter to the editor "Visual laser ablation of the prostate." Urology 1994; 43: 276.
4 Dixon C, Machi G, Theune C, Olejniczak G, Lepor H. A prospective double-blind randomized study comparing the safety, efficacy and cost of laser ablation of the prostate and transurethral resection prostatectomy for treatment of BPH. J Urol 1994; 151: 229A.

5 Cowles RS III, Kabalin JN, Childs S et al. A prospective randomized comparison of transurethral resection to visual laser ablation of the prostate for the treatment of benign prostatic hyperplasia. Urology 1995; 46: 155–60.
6 Narayan P, Tewari A, Abosief S, Evans C. A randomized study comparing visual laser ablation and transurethral evaporation of prostate in the management of benign prostatic hyperplasia. J Urol 1995; 154: 2083–8.

Contact and Interstitial Laser Treatment Methods

19

T.A. McNicholas and J. Hines

INTRODUCTION

Currently, the most popular methods of laser treatment of lower urinary tract symptoms (LUTS) secondary to bladder outlet obstruction (BOO) use a miniature reflector or prism at the end of a "sidefiring" fiber. This is visual laser ablation of the prostate or VLAP. The laser beam strikes the prostatic adenoma almost perpendicularly, which appears to increase the coagulating effect, and the beam-deflecting mechanism allows reasonably easy access for the beam to all relevant parts of the prostatic adenoma.

To achieve a primarily coagulating effect, the neodymium:yttrium–aluminum–garnet (Nd:YAG) laser is fired at a power of between 40 and 90 W (usually 60 W) for 40–120 s (usually 60 s) and repeated in quadrants circumferentially, i.e. at 2, 4, 8, and 10 o'clock. Further "shots" can be fired according to the anatomy and size of the gland, particularly at the bladder neck or any middle lobe.

Alternatively, the complete tissue surface may be "painted" by moving the beam steadily over the whole surface of the adenoma. A combination of "painting" and focal 60–120-s "shots" may also be used. The aim is to create extensive tissue changes within the adenoma. Usually, a mixture of superficial vaporization and tissue disruption results (because of the production of steam) with underlying deeper coagulative necrosis.

There are four main problems with VLAP:

(1) lack of control over the distribution of energy;
(2) an immediate post-treatment phase of considerable obstruction;
(3) a variable period of post-treatment discomfort and irritable bladder symptoms;
(4) the unpredictability of the eventual result.

The VLAP procedure is only "visual" up to the point that the laser is fired at the surface of the prostatic adenoma. Once laser light has entered the tissue, the distribution of energy and its effects are largely invisible. In practice, the procedure is relatively unpredictable. This may result in apical tissue being relatively spared by the cautious operator in order to avoid sphincteric injury, and this can lead to a degree of residual obstruction at this point.

Investigation of the process of VLAP in dogs and man suggests that, after laser irradiation, significant tissue edema develops.[1,2] This contributes to the immediate postoperative

obstructive phase, during which bladder emptying may be difficult without a catheter. Subsequently (overlapping with the obstructive phase) ulcerated areas develop in the ischemic laser-treated sites.[3,4] This adds to the dysuria that may last for 1–4 weeks or more. The ulcerated tissue sloughs and is passed as small amounts of gelatinous material, usually without difficulty. In theory, a series of confluent cavities develop leading to improved voiding by 6–12 weeks. Complete healing may take considerably longer.[5,6]

The delayed voiding and dysuria experienced following endoscopic VLAP treatment has encouraged exploration of methods that either preserve the urethral lining (interstitial laser coagulation, ILC) or remove some tissue immediately so that postoperative voiding is more successful (contact tip laser methods using contact tips [CT]).

CONTACT LASER METHOD

The direct application of laser-heated probes (CT) was intended to achieve enough immediate tissue removal to allow unobstructed postoperative voiding. Synthetic sapphire tips fixed to the fiber end absorb energy and become very hot. This allows cutting with an otherwise "coagulating" wavelength for incision of bladder neck muscle (BNI) (Figure 19.1) or prostate. The original tips were 1.5 mm in diameter. Reasonable results have been reported by Watson *et al.*[7] with average peak flow rates (Q_{max}) rising from 9 to 18 mL s^{-1} and (American Urological Association, AUA) symptom scores falling from 18 to 5 in 30 men, though they reported great difficulty in creating the intended "TUR-like cavity" in prostates over 40 g. As a result, even larger diameter CTs (4–5 mm) have been used, at higher powers (55 W rather than 35 W), through modified resectoscopes[8] to try to achieve an immediate cavity. Most recently 10-mm diameter tips (MTRL-10) and right-angle "sidefiring" tips (VaporMax) (Figures 19.2 and 19.3) have been introduced. As with other laser methods, hemorrhage has not been a problem but the relative inefficiency of laser vaporization is such that the treatment of moderately sized or large prostates is time consuming.

CONTACT LASER: METHOD

Patients can be treated under general or regional anesthesia or under intravenous sedation with or without urethral anesthetic gel or local periprostatic block. Following traditional endoscopy of the lower urinary tract, the CT fiber

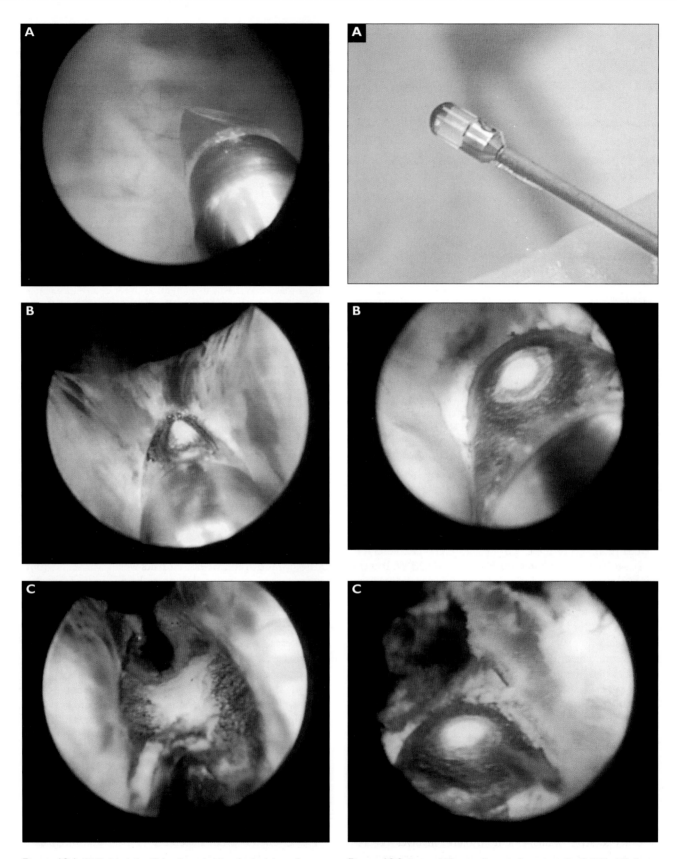

Figure 19.1 SLT chisel tip. This allows cutting for incision of bladder neck muscle (BNI) or prostate: (A) SLT chisel tip in bladder; (B) SLT chisel tip at bladder neck prior to incision; (C) SLT chisel tip after first cut at bladder neck

Figure 19.2 Large (10-mm diameter) contact tip (MTRL-10) for use on prostate: (A) MTRL-10 fixed to laser fiber; (B) MTRL-10 prior to prostatic vaporization; (C) MTRL-10 during prostatic vaporization

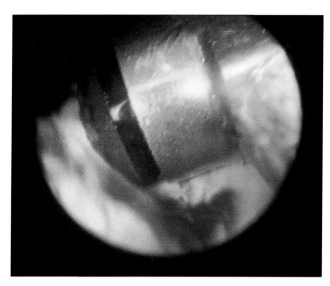

Figure 19.3 Endoscopic view of right-angle "sidefiring" contact tip (SLT VaporMax)

system is introduced through the endoscope. Since the CT itself is large, it is usually necessary to load the endoscope with the fiber and then screw on the CT once the fibre protrudes through the cystoscope sheath distal end. The endoscope is then passed down the urethra with the CT device *in situ*. Recently, purpose-built endoscopes that accommodate these devices more easily have been demonstrated by major endoscope manufacturers and may allow withdrawal of the CT and fiber to facilitate changes of the CT model if required (e.g. to change from the large coagulating MTRL-10 to a cutting CT "chisel tip" for BNI).

The CT is placed just above the level of the verumontanum marking the upper edge of the distal sphincter, and the laser is fired at a power of approximately 20 W. It is better to dwell at the starting point for a few seconds to allow temperatures at the zone of CT and tissue contact to rise to the point of vaporization. Once small bubbles start to form, the operator "pushes" the tip against the prostatic adenoma so as to slowly create a furrow of vaporized and coagulated tissue extending upward to the bladder neck. It is important to follow the natural curve of the prostatic capsule in a similar manner to the resection of chips during transurethral resection of the prostate (TURP), so as to avoid undermining the bladder neck and trigone. Repeated passes are made from distal to proximal, aiming to smooth out the ridges that are created between the furrows. Finally, a bladder neck incision can be made (with the chisel tip) if desired, this is more likely to lead to retrograde ejaculation. Fibres can be used approximately three times and sapphire tips up to six times each. However, effects can become less predictable with a greater number of uses.

Postoperative management usually involves a 24-h period of urethral catheter drainage and a short period of broad-spectrum antibiotic cover. There is usually some minor hematuria and mild discomfort. We advise men to refrain from sexual activity for 2 weeks and from vigorous physical activity for 4 weeks, i.e. slightly shorter periods than following TURP.

CONTACT LASER: RESULTS

The quality of data on CT methods has been poor so far, but has been markedly strengthened by preliminary data from the Oxford laser prostate trial.[9] This double-blind, randomized, controlled trial (RCT) of contact tip methods (72 men) vs. TURP (76 men) remains the only study published so far that was designed with the statistical power to detect a difference between the two arms in the symptomatic response to either treatment. This was taken to be a reduction of 5 points on the AUA question symptom score (AUA7SS),[10] which they felt would be evident to patients as a moderate improvement.[11]

The study showed no statistically significant difference between the two arms in terms of AUA7SS response or flow rates at 3-month follow-up. Other parameters (blood loss, hospital stay, and length of catheterization) favored the CT laser arm. Interestingly, three men were found to have prostatic adenocarcinoma and one lymphoma on pathological examination of the TURP chips. No details of the significance of these findings were given, and no such pathology has been found in the CT laser group (so far).

Catheters were removed at a median of 1 night after laser and 2 nights after TURP. Seventeen (28%) men in the CT laser arm failed to void after removal of the catheter compared with 8 (12%) in the TURP arm. This appears to support the contention that CT methods may allow earlier voiding than purely coagulative laser techniques, but a significant proportion of men managed in this way by CT will still have a delay before voiding freely. Of 10 men carefully selected for "day-case prostatectomy" by CT laser,[12] 9 were discharged the same day catheter free, 2 developed clot retention within 48 h, and 2 failed to void and needed catheterization for 2 weeks. Patients were later sent a questionaire and 8 reported they were happy to be treated as day cases. This experience suggests day-case CT laser prostatectomy is feasible but not problem free.

Twelve-month follow-up data are now available[13] on 127 of 152 men recruited by the close of the study. There was still no statistically significant difference with regard to absolute change in symptom scores, but significantly more men achieved a large change in AUA7SS (8 points or more, likely to be perceived by the patient as a marked improvement) after TURP than after CT. The reoperation rate was 6.6% in the TURP group (three urethral strictures and two bladder neck stenoses) compared with 18.4% for CT laser, including four (5.5%) perioperative conversions to TURP due to "cystoscope trauma" and six (8.3%) who later underwent TURP because of poor symptomatic response.

An economic evaluation of the Oxford CT laser prostate trial[14] suggests TURP will remain more cost effective than CT laser methods until the cost of laser consumables is reduced to 20% of the (then) list price or there is a more aggressive approach to postoperative management, e.g. reducing in-patient stay to 1 night and community nurses removing catheters at home. CT laser costs US$200 more than a TURP, mainly owing to the cost of theater consumables (even though fibers were used three times and sapphire tips up to six times each). These devices are expensive and, if damaged, the use of a second device will negate any hospital cost saving. Community costs could also be higher, and this needs to be considered.

The well-designed Oxford study will presumably provide outcome data over the longer term. For now, we can conclude that CT laser prostatectomy appears an effective option in the short term and overcomes three of the four problems complicating VLAP. It may be 5 years before we know the overall failure or retreatment rates, which will define the cost effectiveness of this laser technique.

INTERSTITIAL LASER TECHNIQUES

Inserting a small, relatively atraumatic fiber into the prostatic tissue transurethrally, transrectally, or percutaneously under ultrasound guidance and heating it up directly (ILC) reduces energy losses by reflection into the irrigant so that low power Nd:YAG or 830–950 nm diode laser light (2–20 W) can cause high temperatures, characteristic ultrasound appearances (with some devices), and localized coagulative necrosis, while preserving the prostatic urethral lumen.[15-17] Intraprostatic necrotic tissue is separated from the urinary stream and is resorbed by the normal processes of tissue repair. It is hoped, but by no means yet proven, that this will reduce the postoperative dysuria that a significant proportion of men complain of following endoscopic laser coagulation or vaporization of the prostatic urethral lining. This raises the question of just what causes the discomfort and why it does not affect all treated men. Also, since there is no generally agreed system for quantifying post-laser symptoms, it is difficult to compare the aftereffects of one method with those of another in any meaningful way.

METHODS AND RESULTS

The laser fiber conducting the light energy can be introduced into the prostate transurethrally, transrectally, or percutaneously through the perineal skin. In practice, the transurethral approach is most attractive as it is most familiar to urologists and the procedure can be combined with a transurethral endoscopic review of the lower urinary tract, allowing a detailed assessment of prostatic urethral anatomy. Patients have been treated under general or regional anesthesia or under intravenous sedation with or without urethral anesthetic gel or local periprostatic block. Following endoscopy, the fiber system is introduced through the prostatic urethral lining into the prostatic adenoma. The position of the puncture is determined visually and the depth of fiber penetration can be controlled under ultrasound guidance or by counting depth markers on the shaft of the fiber device. A series of punctures are made sequentially along the length of the prostate on each side, and the laser fired for a duration according to the protocol being followed. The number and position of punctures will depend on the size and shape of the prostate. One puncture

and heating cycle per 5–8 g of measured prostate is currently recommended. Tissue heating to approximately 100°C produces small bubbles of gas and a degree of tissue disruption, which can be visualized on transurethral ultrasonography, allowing a degree of real-time control of the process. There is little to see ultrasonically if temperatures are controlled below this level. As with VLAP, the best results are to be expected if the lesions are produced so as to overlap and blend into each other.

Postoperative management usually involves a period of urethral, suprapubic catheter drainage or clean intermittent self-catheterization (CISC) and a short period of broad-spectrum antibiotic cover. There is usually some minor hematuria and mild discomfort. We advise men to refrain from sexual activity for 2 weeks and from vigorous physical activity for 4 weeks.

There are three systems by which laser energy can be introduced into prostatic tissue for ILC.

(1) A simple bare fiber is cheap and easily repairable but may not resist high intraprostatic temperatures, leading to breakage of the silica glass fiber itself within the prostate. The fiber and tissue heating effects are readily visible by transrectal ultrasonography (TRUS).[16]

(2) A more complex fiber with a distal "diffusor tip" attached is shown in Figure 19.4. This acts to diffuse the emitted laser light over a relatively large surface area and prevents excessive heating and tissue charring on the tip surface. It is not clear whether the presence of tissue carbonization or charring is detrimental to the process of ILC or not. Most ILC device design assumes carbonization is to be avoided, but the theoretical advantages of more complex fiber systems have certainly not been proven.[18] Amin *et al.* investigated ILC *in vivo* in a study comparing Nd:YAG wavelengths (1064 nm, 1320 nm) and 805 nm diode using bare fibers implanted in rat liver with and without "pre-charring". Using the more strongly absorbed

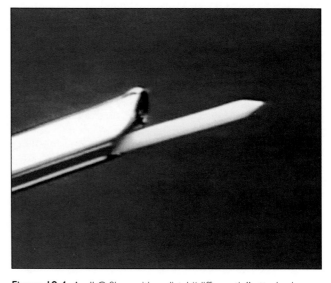

Figure 19.4 An ILC fiber with a distal "diffusor tip" attached (Indigo model)

wavelengths (805 and 1320 nm) and pre-charring, the fiber tip gave more extensive thermal damage than 1064-nm light and a fiber without charring.[19] This is contrary to the commonly accepted view that the optimal combination was 1064 nm light with careful temperature control to avoid charring. Carbonization may or may not be helpful but does certainly lead to high focal temperatures at or near the device, which may damage it unless it is adequately protected. There is also a mechanical weak point at the junction of the fiber and diffusor tip that may be prone to failure. As yet, no real-time ultrasound-visible tissue heating changes have been described, presumably because temperatures are maintained below 100°C.

In 1994 Muschter *et al.* described in an abstract the results of several diffusor tip interstitial fibers in 172 men treated by the transperineal or the transurethral approach. Average AUA symptom scores fell from 25.1 to 5.7 and mean peak flow rates rose from 5.8 to 16.2 mL s^{-1} at 6 months. Over 350 men have been treated by the Munich group since 1991, though by a series of different protocols and fibers, making comparison difficult. Of 221 men with 12-month follow-up, AUA symptom scores fell from 25.4 to 6.1, peak flow rates increased from 7.7 to 17.8 mL s^{-1}, and TRUS-measured prostatic volume decreased by 40%.[20]

Muschter and Hofstetter[21] also described the results of several different diffusor tip fibers (Sharplan, Dornier, and various prototypes) in 239 men treated by the transperineal ($n=75$) or the transurethral interstitial approach. Twelve-month follow-up data were reported on 127 men. AUA symptom scores fell from 25 to 6, peak flow rates rose from 8 to 18 mL s^{-1} at 12 months. Irritative symptoms were noted in 12.6%, 4% developed urethral strictures, and 7% retrograde ejaculation. No previously potent man developed impotence.[21]

Orovan *et al.*[22] reported 16 men treated transurethrally with the Dornier fiber at a power of 7 W for 10 min for each lateral lobe and for 5 min for the median lobe. Average AUA7SS fell from 16.3 to 5.8, and flow rates increased from 8.8 to 11.9 mL s^{-1} at 3 months. Side effects were minimal and it was stated, without further details, that there were "less irritative symptoms than seen with other laser procedures and shorter periods of catheterization."

Arai *et al.*[23] reported less dramatic changes in 61 men treated by Dornier fiber transurethral ILC (during which three fibers broke). AUA7SS scores fell from 18.9 to 7.7 (59%) and flow rates increased from 6.7 to 10.0 (49%) mL s^{-1} at 3 months. There was no reported erectile dysfunction. Indeed 53% claimed an improved sex life! All were catheterized for 2–3 days, after which 25 (41%) developed acute retention or a significant increase in postvoid residual (PVR) urine and were managed by CISC or indwelling catheter for a mean of 12 days (2–28). This was thought to be "unacceptable," though irritative voiding symptoms such as urgency and pain were not significant.

Preliminary (promotional) data reported for the Indigo diffusor tip fiber and 830-nm diode laser (Indigo, Palo Alto, CA) was in line with ILC results outside the German experience. Multicenter RCTs comparing the

Indigo diffusor tip fiber and 830-nm diode laser to TURP are under way. One small study has been reported of 25 men treated with this laser and fiber system.[24] Results included mean symptom score improvement from 20.6 to 9.4 at 1 month and 6.9 at 3 months. Peak flow rate (Q_{max}) increased from 9.1 to 14.1 and then to 20.3 mL s^{-1}. The system senses temperatures at the fiber tip and adjusts power output with the intention of maintaining a temperature of 100°C throughout the treatment cycle. Temperatures reached and power levels required varied according to the site of puncture, with apically placed lesions requiring less energy to achieve and maintain target temperature. Presumably the heat-losing mechanisms are less effective at the prostatic apex. Since this report, the laser source and system has been "enhanced," so we await new data from studies of the new system before we can really define the effectiveness of the Indigo method of ILC.

(3) A recent compromise between these two basic fiber types is a bare fiber within a cannula through which saline flows to protect the cannula and the fiber from these high temperatures (Figure 19.5). Canine[25] and clinical studies[26] show characteristic ultrasound-visible changes during prostatic heating.

In our study of 31 men with symptomatic BOO (mean prostatic volume 40 cm^3, range 24–72) treated with transurethral saline-cooled interstitial laser fiber coagulation, preoperative AUA7SS of 22 (18–29) fell to 6.3 (0–25) and peak flow rates increased from 9.3 (4–14) to 14.6 mL s^{-1} (7–32) at 3 months. They were treated with a mean total energy of 11,400 J (5560–17,600 J) at powers of 5–10 W over a mean laser exposure time of 22 min (6.5–45 min). Patients were taught CISC without difficulty for postoperative bladder drainage and were discharged on the first postoperative day. They were reviewed 1 week

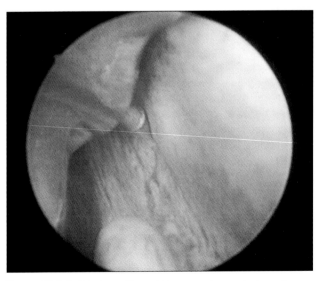

Figure 19.5 ILC by bare fiber within a metal cannula through which saline flows to protect the cannula and the fiber from high temperatures. Cannula shown puncturing left lateral lobe of prostate

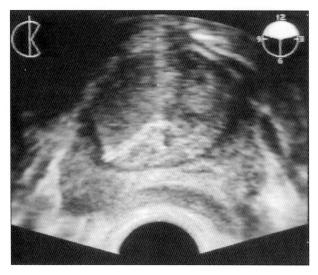

Figure 19.6 TRUS scan during treatment, showing the saline-cooled ILC cannula and fiber *in situ* before heating

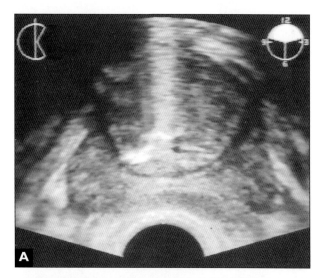

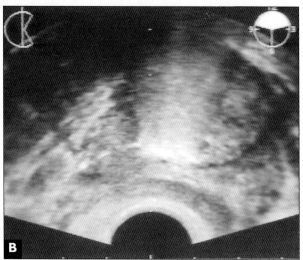

Figure 19.7 TRUS during treatment showing the ILC thermal changes within the prostate during heating: (A) changes seen as heating begins; (B) thermal (white) changes spread out as heating progresses

post-treatment, with an average of 3.7 days (0–7) of CISC being required. However, not all men benefited greatly, with four failing to respond and another four responding only moderately. Of those with a good response, the average symptom score change was 17 (8–28), with an average Q_{max} change of 6.6 mL s^{-1} (2–17).

Most of the patients tolerated the treatment very well. Only one patient developed significant dysuria in the immediate postoperative period and required TURP. Most of the patients noticed improvement in their symptoms as well as in their flow rate on the fourth week post-treatment. Complications were otherwise minor. There were no effects on ejaculation in these studies.

TRUS during treatment showed the cannula *in situ* and the thermal changes within the adenoma as heating occurred (Figures 19.6 and 19.7). TRUS on the fourth week post-treatment showed a zone of mixed hyper- and hypodense echoes corresponding to the site of coagulation. By the sixth week, cystic changes appeared in the center of the treated zone surrounded by rim of hyperdense tissue. By the third month post-treatment, these characteristic changes become very distinct (Figure 19.8) with the cystic changes becoming larger in size and often extending along the complete length of the adenoma.

CONCLUSIONS

Currently, it would appear that there are so many different variations on a theme of "laser prostatectomy" that no one method is clearly best, though a trend towards higher power, higher power density (PD), vaporizing methods can be discerned. It could be said that variability in methods and results is to be expected, since we do not know the answers to the basic questions of which wavelength to use; whether to use it for a short time at high power or at a low power for a longer duration; whether to aim for vaporization or coagulation; and whether there is a "right" amount of energy for any particular prostate. We do not even know how much tissue we have to destroy to guarantee a good, long-term result (it is probably less than we thought). Certainly, VLAP laser techniques have been shown to overcome obstruction in trials incorporating pressure-flow studies, despite relatively modest tissue removal compared with TURP,[27,28] and it is highly likely that CT methods will be as effective in view of the good early flow rate and symptomatic response seen.

The sidefiring beam deflectors (e.g. VLAP and the more vaporizing transurethral laser evaporation of the prostate) are best known and simplest to use, but this may disguise a lesser degree of accuracy and control once the energy has hit the prostate. VLAP gives delayed results compared with CT methods, but data on vaporizing methods are now available[29] that suggest less postoperative obstruction than VLAP

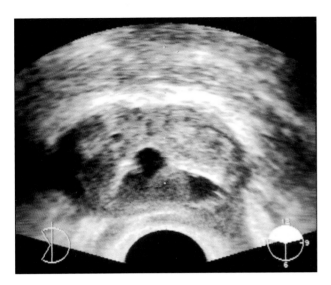

Figure 19.8 TRUS at 11 months post-ILC treatment by saline-cooled ILC cannula and fiber showing characteristic cystic changes within the prostate

and comparable periods of post-treatment catheterization to CT. Similarly, the development of transurethral electrovaporization of the prostate (TUEVP)[30] will be a challenging competitor for CT. The case for contact tip methods has been greatly strengthened by the Oxford study but more studies are needed.

Interstitial methods may well have a role in older, sicker men with larger prostates. Interstitial methods remain promising but unfulfilled due to the lack of good prospective, randomized studies, and partly because the technique is still in evolution – which is true of all methods of laser prostatectomy. Fundamentally, it is still not clear whether preserving the prostatic urethral mucosa is worth the degree of temporary extra obstruction following interstitial heating. Otherwise, the method has minimal morbidity and can be applied to both moderately sized and large prostates in all age groups.

Whatever method we choose, we need to determine the longevity of the initial response to laser treatment and the incidence of retreatment over many years. Only when we have these data will we be able to define the role of different forms of laser prostatectomy.

REFERENCES

1 Bosch J, Groen J, Schroder F. Treatment of benign prostatic hyperplasia by transurethral ultrasound-guided laser induced prostatectomy (TULIP): effects on urodynamic parameters and symptoms. *Urology* 1994; **44**(4): 507–11.

2 Costello A, Shaffer B, Crowe H. Second generation delivery systems for laser prostatic ablation. *Urology* 1994; **43**: 262–6.

3 Marks L. Serial endoscopy following visual laser ablation of prostate. *Urology* 1993; **42**(1): 66–71.

4 Norris J, Norris D, Lee R, Rubenstein M. Visual laser ablation of the prostate: clinical experience in 108 patients. *J Urol* 1993; **150**: 1612–14.

5 Anson K, Watson G, Shah T, Barnes D. Laser prostatectomy: our initial experience of a technique in evolution. *J Endourol* 1993; **7**(4): 333–6.

6 Costello A, Bolton D, Ellis D, Crowe H. Histopathological changes in human prostatic adenoma following neodymium:YAG laser ablation therapy. *J Urol* 1994; **152**: 1526–9.

7 Watson G, Anson K, Janetschek G *et al.* An in depth evaluation of contact laser vaporisation of the prostate. *J Urol* 1994; **151**(5): 231A.

8 Bartsch G, Janetschek G, Watson G, Anson K. The development of an endoscope and of contact probes for transurethral laser surgery of the prostate. *J Urol* 1994; **151**(5): 333A.

9 Keoghane S, Cranston D, Lawrence K *et al.* The Oxford laser prostate trial: a double blind, randomised, controlled trial of contact vaporisation against transurethral resection: preliminary results. *Br J Urol* 1996; **77**: 382–5.

10 Barry M, Fowler F, O'Leary M *et al.* The American Urological Association symptom index for benign prostatic hyperplasia. *J Urol* 1992; **148**: 1549–57.

11 Barry M, Williford W, Chang Y *et al.* Benign prostatic hyperplasia specific health status measures in clinical research: how much change in the American Urological Association symptom index and the benign prostatic hyperplasia impact index is perceptible to patients? *J Urol* 1995; **154**: 1770–4.

12 Keoghane S, Millar J, Cranston D. Is day case prostatectomy feasible? *Br J Urol* 1995; **76**(5): 600–3.

13 Keoghane S, Lawrence K, Doll H, Cranston D. The Oxford laser prostatectomy trial: one year data from a randomised, controlled trial. *Br J Urol* 1996; **77**(Suppl 1): 8.

14 Keoghane S, Lawrence K, Gray A *et al.* The Oxford laser prostate trial: economic issues surrounding contact laser prostatectomy. *Br J Urol* 1996; **77**: 386–90.

15 McNicholas T, Steger A, Charig C, Bown S. Interstitial YAG laser coagulation of the prostate. *Lasers Med Sci* 1988; **3** (Abstracts issue): abstract 446.

16 McNicholas T, Steger A, Bown S. Interstitial laser coagulation of the prostate: an experimental study. *Br J Urol* 1993; **71**: 439–44.

17 Muschter R, Hofstetter A, Anson K, Perlmutter A, Vaughan D. Nd:YAG and diode lasers for interstitial laser coagulation of benign prostatic hyperplasia: experimental and clinical evaluation. *J Urol* 1995; **153**(Suppl): 229A.

18 Nolsoe C, Torp-Pedersen S, Holm H *et al.* Ultrasonically guided interstitial Nd-YAG laser diffuser tip hyperthermia: an in vitro study. *Scand J Urol Nephrol* 1991; (Suppl 137): 119–24.

19 Amin Z, Buonaccorsi G, Mills T *et al.* Interstitial laser photocoagulation. *Lasers Med Sci* 1993; **8**(2): 113–20.

20 Muschter R, Zellner M, Hessel S, Hofstetter A. Lasers and benign prostatic hyperplasia – Experimental and clinical results to compare different application systems. *J Urol* 1994; **230A**: 151. *J Urol* 1994; **151**(Suppl): 230A.

21 Muschter R, Hofstetter A. Interstitial laser therapy outcomes in benign prostatic hyperplasia. *J Endourol* 1995; **9**(2): 129–35.

22 Orovan W, Whelan J. Neodymium YAG laser treatment of BPH using interstitial thermometry: a transurethral approach. *J Urol* 1994; **151**: 230A.

23 Arai Y, Ishitoya H, Okubo K, Suzuki Y. Transurethral interstitial laser coagulation for BPH: treatment outcome and quality of life. *Br J Urol* 1996; **78**(1): 93–8.

24 de la Rosette J, Muschter R, Lopez M, Gillatt D. Interstitial laser coagulation in the treatment of benign prostatic hyperplasia using a diode-laser system with temperature feedback. *Br J Urol* 1997; **80**(3): 433–8.

25 Hoopes J, Williams J, Harris R *et al.* Interstitial laser coagulation

(ILC) of the canine prostate with ultrasound and thermal monitoring. *J Urol* 1994; **151**(5): 334A.

26 McNicholas T, Alsudani M. Interstitial laser coagulation therapy for benign prostatic hyperplasia. In: Anderson E, Rox R (eds) *Lasers in Surgery: Advanced Characterisation, Therapeutics and Systems VI,* Vol. 2671. Bellingham, WA: SPIE: International Society for Optical Engineering 1996; 300–8.

27 James M, Hariss D, Ceccherino A *et al*. A urodynamic study of laser ablation of the prostate and a comparison of techniques. *Br J Urol* 1995; **76**: 179–83.

28 De Wildt M, Testa E, Rosier P *et al*. Urodynamic results of laser

treatment in patients with benign prostatic hyperplasia. Can outlet obstruction be relieved? *J Urol* 1995; **154**: 174–80.

29 Narayan P, Tewari A, Schalow E *et al*. Transurethral evaporation of the prostate for treatment of benign prostatic hyperplasia: results in 168 patients with up to 12 months of follow-up. *J Urol* 1997; **157**(4): 1309–12.

30 Patel A, Fuchs G, Gutierrez-Aceves J, Ryan T. Prostate heating patterns comparing electrosurgical transurethral resection and vaporization: a prospective randomized study. *J Urol* 1997; **157**(1): 169–72.

COMMENTARY

In this chapter, Drs McNicholas and Hines, who are pioneers of laser therapy of the prostate, have discussed in detail the evolution and current status of laser prostatectomy. As analyzed by them very succinctly, the four problems with VLAP are (1) lack of control of distribution of energy; (2) a variable post-treatment period of obstruction and (3) irritability; and (4) most importantly, the unpredictability of the eventual result.

The contact laser technique used by their team and others appears to be efficient and a reasonable alternative to VLAP. However, even in the contact laser technique, there was an 18.4% reoperation rate, which was comparable to the 16% rate noted by us and others after aggressive VLAP.[1,2] A significant point raised by Dr McNicholas is the lack of economic feasibility of the contact laser technique until cost of fibers is reduced by 20%. One hope that the urologist had was that the fiber cost would decrease with competition and volume of use, yet this has not occurred in the USA, and it seems to be the case in the UK as well. The Ho:YAG laser which uses a bare tip may solve this problem, since the fiber tip is broken off when degraded and the fiber is reused. There are, however, minimal published results of BPH therapy with this technique.[3,4] Dr McNicholas also discusses the ILC technique in which he is an expert. The ILC technique initially started with insertion of a bare tip, but successive modifications included a diffuser tip and, most recently, the Indigo laser system which has had both a diffuser tip and a temperature sensor to adjust the laser power to maintain a temperature of 85°C. (Indigo Laser, Johnson & Johnson, Cincinnati, OH, USA) Indigo ILC is further discussed in Chapter 20 "Interstitial Laser Thermal Therapy for Benign Prostatic Hyperplasia."

The European experience with a variety of ILC fibers and techniques has revealed that the ILC technique is simple to use, user friendly, and is associated with moderate improvements in AUA score and uroflow. However, acute retention needing CISC for about 12 days occurs in about 41% of patients. This, however, is not necessarily a major problem in our experience. We find most patients are willing to use CISC for 1–2 weeks, provided they can have guaranteed relief of symptoms with no side effects. We, therefore, routinely advise all our patients to learn CISC after laser ILT procedures, even though only about 20% require it.

A novel technique of ILC that is being used by Dr McNicholas is with saline-cooled bare fibers to prevent fiber deterioration and yet save costs, since bare fibers are less expensive. Preliminary results, however, suggest that this technique was only moderately successful, perhaps because the cooling of the fiber may have prevented adequate prostatic destruction.

In summary, a variety of contact and interstitial laser techniques are currently evolving. It remains to be seen which of these techniques will eventually survive in the marketplace based upon efficacy, side effects, and costs.

1 Narayan P. Laser evaporation. In: *Smith's Textbook of Endourology,* Vol. 2. 1996; 1054–77.

2 Dixon C, Machi G *et al*. A prospective double-blind, randomized

study comparing laser ablation of the prostate and transurethral prostatectomy for the treatment of BPH. *J Urol* 1993; **149**: 6 (Abstract).

Interstitial Laser Thermal Therapy for Benign Prostatic Hyperplasia

20

M.M. Issa, N.P. Symbas, and M.S. Steiner

INTRODUCTION

Interstitial laser thermal therapy (ILTT) is a new minimally invasive thermal treatment for symptomatic benign prostatic hyperplasia (BPH). The treatment achieves intraprostatic thermal tissue ablation ($>60°C$), often in the range of $80–90°C$, and attempts to preserve the prostatic urethra. The relatively lower therapeutic temperatures of ILTT, urethral preservation, and lack of tissue evaporation/resection make this treatment different from conventional transurethral free beam laser prostatectomy despite its "laser" name. Therefore, ILTT seems to fit better as a minimally invasive thermal therapy along the same lines as microwave, radiofrequency (RF), and high-intensity focused ultrasound (HIFU) therapies.

NOMENCLATURE

Various nomenclatures are used in the literature to describe the same procedure. These include interstitial laser thermal therapy (ILTT), interstitial thermal therapy (ITT), interstitial laser therapy (ILT), interstitial laser coagulation (ILC), laser-induced thermal therapy (LITT), and laser delivered interstitial therapy (LDIT).

PATIENT SELECTION

Any patient with clinical BPH, as judged by the standard subjective parameters such as symptom and bother scores, and by standard objective parameters such as prostate size, peak flow rate, postvoid residual (PVR) urine volume, and pressure-flow studies, may be considered as a suitable candidate for ILTT. Every attempt should be made by urologists to ensure that the patients' voiding symptoms are not due to other pathologies such as prostate cancer, urethral stricture, primary bladder neck dysfunction/contracture, urinary infection, detrusor muscle dysfunction from neurogenic conditions, interfering medications (α-agonists and anticholinergics), interstitial cystitis, prostatitis, bladder stones, or bladder cancer. Such concomitant conditions may prove responsible for subsequent suboptimal outcomes. Prostate size is not a deciding criteria, although limited experience/results are available regarding ILTT for the treatment of relatively small (<15 cm³) and large (>100 cm³) prostates. Median lobe BPH can also be treated. Patients with chronic urinary retention secondary to BPH can be considered for ILTT. Furthermore, ILTT may have a potential in the treatment of chronic non-bacterial prostatitis and prostatodynia syndromes. However, current data are limited.

In our opinion, ILTT is best positioned for BPH patients who fail, are unable to tolerate, or are unwilling to take medical therapy, and who are not candidates for transurethral resection of the prostate (TURP). Non-suitability for TURP may be due to patients' personal preference, which is often influenced by their unwillingness to accept retrograde ejaculation, impotence, spinal/general anesthesia, hospitalization, and the potential for significant blood loss/transfusion. On the other hand, it may be due to medical reasons, such as the presence of significant comorbidity, which put them at high surgical risk.

TISSUE EFFECT AND DOSIMETRY

The therapeutic effect of ILTT results from the irreversible coagulative necrosis achieved inside the prostate. This thermal tissue ablation has been studied radiologically and histologically by a number of investigators.[1-7] Based on the results of these studies, the amount of thermal ablation, i.e. depth of coagulation or size the lesion, seems dependent on various factors: (1) wavelength of the laser energy; (2) wattage power during treatment session; (3) duration of treatment; (4) number of treatments; (5) tissue vascularity; and (6) ratio of fibromuscular to glandular elements.

In general, treatment parameters are established for the various interstitial laser systems so as to establish spherically/elliptically shaped thermal ablation lesions measuring approximately 1–2 cm in diameter. The size and contour of these lesions seem anatomically and therapeutically appropriate for the prostate, as they are maintained at a safe distance from the prostatic capsule, urothelium, and bladder neck. During this process, it is important to heat the prostate slowly, in order to avoid tissue overheating and carbonization (charring), which takes place when the temperature reaches $>100°C$. Such tissue carbonization forms an insulating layer, which limits further tissue coagulation. Newer systems are now capable of tissue temperature monitoring, feedback control, and automated adjustment of energy delivery to overcome this problem and optimize the heating process.

URETHRAL PRESERVATION DURING INTERSTITIAL LASER THERMAL THERAPY

Preservation of the integrity of the prostatic urothelium is important for any minimally invasive BPH therapy, including ILTT. It minimizes postoperative urothelial inflammation, edema, and subsequent tissue sloughing, which results in a significant decrease in the postoperative catheterization, irritative voiding symptoms, hematuria, and retrograde ejaculation. This aspect of the treatment has been shown to depend on the operative technique and operator experience.[7-9] Furthermore, since the prostatic urothelium is relatively more sensitive to pain, its preservation allows for the procedure to be performed under local anesthesia.

INSTRUMENTATION

There are a number of systems currently in use worldwide. Each system consists of a laser generator and a flexible optical fiber with the ability to deliver laser energy into the prostate using standard cystoscopic equipment. The generator laser energies vary in wavelengths depending on the system generator, and include diode lasers (800–1000 nm), neodymium:yttrium–aluminum–garnet (Nd:YAG) (1064 nm), and holmium:yttrium–aluminum–garnet (Ho:YAG) (2120 nm). Similar variability exists between different laser optical fibers regarding their distal tip designs and the configuration of their laser emission. In general, they all emit lasers in a radical or conical fashion inside the prostatic tissue so as to produce the final therapeutic effect of coagulative necrosis.

Currently, the most widely used system in the USA is the Indigo LaserOptic system (Indigo Medical, Johnson & Johnson, Cincinnati, OH, USA). In Europe, it is the Dornier ITT System (Dornier, Germering, Germany and Kennesaw, GA, USA). Other systems are emerging, such as Ho:YAG Pulse Laser System BLM-800 (Baasel, Starberg, Germany). However, current literature and experience are limited.[10] Niedergethmann *et al.*[10] have recently shown the Indigo diode laser and the Dornier Nd:YAG systems to have similar ablative capacity. While the two systems seem similar with regard to the their laser tissue penetration and final thermal effect on the prostate, they are significantly different with regard to features and cost. Overall, the Indigo system has a number of advantages over the Dornier system in providing a more compact, more energy efficient, less noisy, and less expensive generator, and by its automated energy delivery through a feedback temperature monitoring system.

LASER GENERATORS

INDIGO LASER GENERATOR (MODEL 830E)

This portable generator (Figure 20.1) measures $40 \times 34 \times 16$ cm and weighs 12.7 kg. It is a diode laser generator, which utilizes a diode pump source and gallium–aluminum–arsenide as a lasing medium to generate a 830-nm wave-

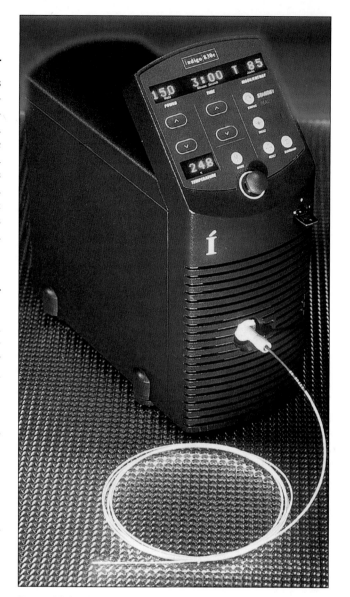

Figure 20.1 The Indigo diode laser generator

length laser with a power range of 2–20 W. The energy is transported from the lasing medium to the laser fiber through semiconductor integrated circuits with relatively low energy loss. The generator has a fully automated energy delivery program, which continously adjusts the power wattage to achieve an efficient and smooth rise in the intraprostatic temperature to 85°C. The generator receives feedback from an optical sensor at the tip of the laser fiber, which monitors intraprostatic temperatures during treatment. It uses the principle of reflectance ("black body radiation") which calculates tissue temperature changes according to the changes in the emitted light signal amplitude as the tissue temperature changes during treatment. The generator has a built-in safety feature that recognizes breakage of the laser fiber immediately, shuts off the laser energy delivery within few seconds, and warns the operator to that effect on its digital display panel.

DORNIER LASER GENERATOR

This generator (Figure 20.2) measures $108 \times 61 \times 42$ cm and weighs 100 kg. It is a conventional laser generator, which utilizes a kryptic arc pump source and Nd:YAG crystal as a lasing medium to generate 1064-nm wavelength laser energy with a power range of 2–100 W. The energy is transported from the lasing medium to the laser fiber through tubes with relatively high energy loss.

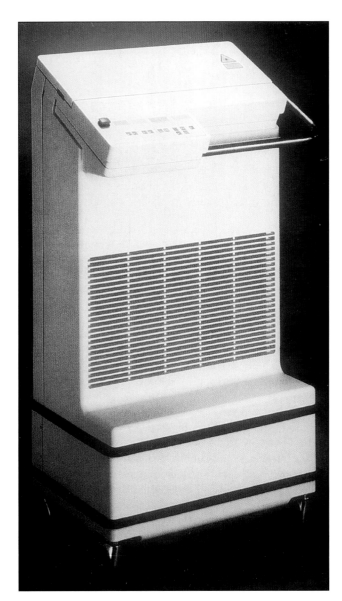

Figure 20.2 The Dornier Nd:YAG laser generator

LASER FIBERS

THE INDIGO DIFFUSER-TIP LASER FIBER

This is a 3-m long optical fiber (Figure 20.3) made of silica–silica with an outer diameter of 1.8 mm (5.4 French). It is relatively flexible with a radius stress tolerance of >8

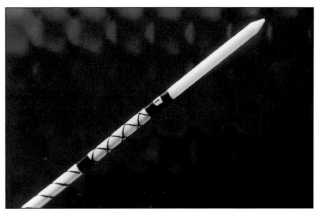

Figure 20.3 The Indigo diffuser-tip laser fiber

cm. Its distal end is designed to emit laser energy in a radial (360° angle) fashion along a 1-cm segment located near the tip. The distal tip of the fiber is beveled into a sharp point to allow its insertion, penetration, and advancement into the prostate.

THE DORNIER ITT LIGHT GUIDE LASER FIBER (MODEL TF-360)

This is a 3.5-m-long optical fiber (Figure 20.4) made of silica–silica with an outer diameter of 1.9 mm (5.7 French). At the distal end of the fiber is a 2-cm quartz glass cap, designed to emit laser energy in a radial (360° angle) fashion. The tip of the cap is similarly beveled into a sharp point to allow its insertion, penetration, and advancement into the prostate. The fiber requires a specially designed adaptor to be connected to the generator.

SURGICAL TECHNIQUE

The patient is placed in the dorsolithotomy position and a standard 21-French cystoscope is used to insert the laser fiber transurethrally into the prostatic adenoma (Figure 20.5). Laser energy is then delivered according to the treatment parameters set by the specific laser system in use. Using the Nd:YAG system, a 10-min irradiation time at 5–7 W power produces maximum coagulation volume without the risk of carbonization. It is possible to induce a more rapid heating using higher laser power. However, this increases the risk of carbonization unless the wattage power is adjusted to maintain a tissue temperature of <100°C. Using the Indigo diode laser system, the process of energy delivery is automated through the feedback tissue-temperature-monitoring system described earlier. The intraprostatic temperature reaches the target therapeutic temperature of 85°C within 1 min and is maintained at that level for the remainder of the 3-min treatment session (Figure 20.6). The length of procedure is dependent on the number of treatment sites (lesions) and the time needed to treat each site. The former is determined by the size and contour of the prostate, and the latter by the capability of the individual laser system.

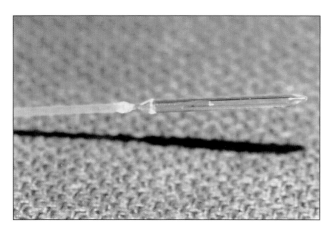

Figure 20.4 The Dornier ITT light guide laser fiber

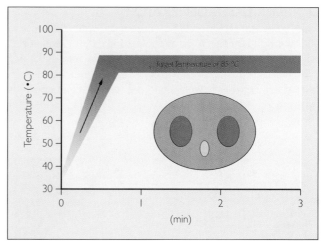

Figure 20.6 A graph of the intraprostatic temperature during the 3-min ILTT treatment session. The delivery of the laser energy into the tissue is automated by the aid of the generator feedback temperature monitoring system. An intraprostatic temperature in the region of 85°C is reached within the first minute and is maintained for the remainder of the treatment session (>2 min)

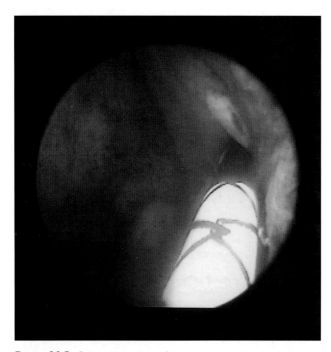

Figure 20.5 Cystoscopic view of the prostate at the level of the verumontanum, showing the laser fiber placed inside the lateral lobe of the prostate

The amount of tissue ablation per prostate volume required for the desired therapeutic effect varies and continues to be a topic of discussion. Many investigators, including ourselves, are in favor of treating the prostate with lower number of lesions and ensuring precise fiber placement to minimize overlaps. On the other hand, other investigators advocate a more aggressive approach, such as a minimum of one lesion per 5–7 cm^3 of prostate tissue.[6] The differences in these treatment recommendations can be explained by the differences between the laser systems and surgical techniques. The main concern about overtreatment with too many lesions is the potential to trade-off the minimally invasive morbidity profile of the procedure for additional objective improvement, i.e. higher peak flow rates, yet without further improvement in symptoms. Using

the new automated Indigo LaserOptic system, the lower number of treatment sites seems to result in similar efficacy. This suggests that the large number of fiber insertions by other laser systems may result in overlapping of lesions rather an increase in tissue ablation. We currently treat prostates measuring under 40 cm^3 in sonographic volume at one plane, i.e. one lesion per lobe. Larger prostates require two or more treatment planes. It is possible that these recommendation may change in the future as more research data become available.

The exact positioning of the laser fiber tip within the prostate plays an important role regarding thermal injury of the adjacent prostatic urothelium. Using the conventional technique, the laser fiber tends to be placed close to the urethra (Figures 20.7A and 20.8A), which in turn leads to significant edema, inflammation, and subsequent tissue sloughing. Consequently, there is an increased likelihood of prolonged postoperative Foley catheterization, exacerbation of irritative voiding symptoms, and the potential for retrograde ejaculation. Recently, we reported a new modified technique of intraprostatic laser fiber insertion to minimize urethral thermal injury.[9] Using this technique, the laser fiber is placed deeper inside the prostate at a safe distance from the urothelium (Figures 20.7B and 20.8B). More consistent urethral preservation is achieved with this technique, resulting in significantly fewer postoperative complications. This new technique is only possible with the Indigo laser fiber, owing to the inherent physical properties (torque capability) of its fused silica material. The Dornier laser fiber is not suitable for this technique, because of its inability to bend at its quartz glass distal tip.

Other important technical points include the proper positioning of the laser fiber for satisfactory treatment of the apical BPH tissue. This is achieved by inserting the laser fiber more distally and laterally into the apical shoulder of

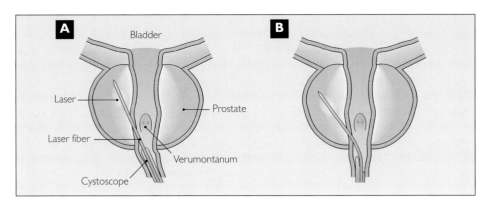

Figure 20.7 An illustration showing the anatomical relationship of the interstitial laser fiber using two different techniques. The fiber is seen in close proximity to the midline (urethra) using the conventional technique (A), and at a safe distance from the midline (urethra) using the modified technique (B)

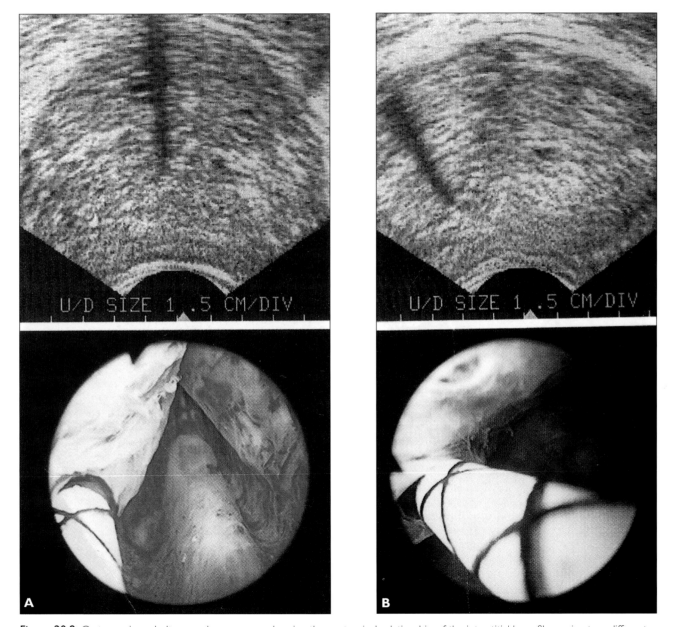

Figure 20.8 Cystoscopic and ultrasound appearance showing the anatomical relationship of the interstitial laser fiber using two different techniques. The fiber is seen in close proximity to the midline (urethra) using the conventional technique (A), and at a safe distance from the midline (urethra) using the modified technique (B)

the lateral lobe (Figure 20.9). Extra care should be exercised to refrain from pushing the fiber tip under the trigone and from penetrating into the bladder when treating smaller prostates with relatively short prostatic urethra. The operator must also avoid excessive trauma to the urothelium during the insertion of the fiber. This occurs when the fiber's sharp distal tip is allowed to scratch the urothelium repeatedly during insertion attempts.

Additional trauma such as iatrogenic lifting of a urothelial mucosal flap may result when the fiber is inserted at a more parallel, rather than perpendicular, angle into the prostatic lobe. The latter can be avoided by using our modified insertion technique,[9] or by using a modified cystoscope with a separate working channel, which ends at the level of the telescope for optimal stabilization of the fiber tip during insertion (R Muschter, personal communication).[11]

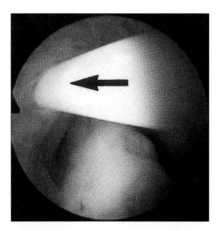

Figure 20.9 A cystoscopic view of the prostate at the level of the verumontanum, illustrating the insertion of the laser fiber into the lateral aspect of the apical shoulder of the prostatic lobe. The arrow demonstrates the lateral direction of the laser fiber toward the inner region of the prostate

ANESTHESIA REQUIREMENT

There continues to be a wide diversity in the anesthesia requirement for ILTT among various urologists and institutions. This is explained by the variability in urologists' preference, patients' pain threshold, and rules and traditions of different medical institutions. The spectrum includes pure local anesthesia with and without sedation, regional prostatic block, and spinal and general anesthesia. Indeed, it is reasonable to perform the first few procedures under spinal or general anesthesia to facilitate the initial learning process and ensure "one less thing to be concerned about." With more experience, most patients (>95%) can undergo ILTT under local anesthesia or regional prostatic

block without the need for sedation, spinal or general anesthesia. We routinely use the perineal approach for prostate block. Recent anatomical and clinical studies suggest that this approach produces the most effective anesthetic block.[12] A study of intraoperative pain using various visual analog pain scales in a series of 42 patients undergoing Indigo ILTT, confirmed highly satisfactory pain control in >95% of patients.[13] For the perineal prostatic block to be successful, a familiarity/experience with the technique, as well as a clear understanding of the anatomical neural innervation of the prostate are required.

RESULTS

Several studies have shown ILTT to be an efficacious treatment for symptomatic BPH, as judged by the improvement in patients' subjective and objective parameters.[1,7,13-21] The widest experience to date comes from Muschter and co-workers in Munich, Germany, who have been instrumental in researching and refining this technology. A recent review of the world literature on ILTT,[20] included a total of 785 patients (14 series, 1994–96) with a follow-up of 2–12 months. Overall improvement in the American Urological Association symptom score averaged 70% (22.8–6.8; $n=875$) with improvement in individual series ranging between 32% (19.9–13.5; $n=25$) and 92% (31.0–2.3; $n=48$). Similar improvements were noted in the peak flow rates with an average of 98% (8.1–16.0 cm³ s⁻¹; $n=875$) for all the series combined and a range of 35.2% (6.7–10.0 cm³ s⁻¹; $n=16$) to 203% (8.2–24.9 cm³ s⁻¹; $n=42$) for individual series. The variation in results between individual series can be explained by the fact that ILTT is a new procedure and the technology is evolving. Therefore, ongoing modifications in the systems/instrumentations and surgical techniques, as well as increasing experience, may continue to influence the results. Improvement in other objective parameters such as PVR urine volume, prostate volume, and detrusor pressures has also been reported.[1,8,14,16,20,21] The reported decrease in the prostate volume following ILTT ranges between 8.3% (57.0–52.3 cm³)[15] and 41.6% (47.1–27.5 cm³).[20] Finally, the current durability data are limited owing to the fact that the technology is new. The re-treatment rate ranges from 0 to 15.4% at 12 months follow-up.

ADVERSE EVENTS/MORBIDITY PROFILE

Urinary tract infection is the most common adverse event seen following ILTT, reported in 27–35% of patients during the early postoperative period.[8,16,17] This high incidence is attributed to the inconsistent use of antibiotics and to the prolonged duration of the bladder catheters in the initial postoperative period. With the use of prophylactic antibiotics, the incidence decreased to 16.5%.[22] In our institution, urinary infection is prevented by the use of prophylactic fluoroquinolone antibiotics, which is continued for 5 days through the postoperative period.[9] Irritative voiding symptoms with tissue sloughing is seen in only 11–12% of patients which is significantly less than with the conventional free beam laser prostatectomy.[8,7,16,17]

Significant postoperative bleeding is rare (<2%) and so is the need for blood transfusion (0.4%).[8,16] Transient stress urinary incontinence has been reported in a single patient (0.4%) in one series of 239 patients.[8] The combined rate of urethral strictures and bladder neck contractures is <5% at 1 year follow-up. Postoperative erectile sexual dysfunction has not been reported. The incidence of retrograde ejaculation ranges between 3% and 11.9%.[6,7,16,22]

It is to be emphasized that ongoing improvements in this technology as well as increasing experience will continue to impact positively on the morbidity profile of ILTT. For example, the 10–14 days requirement of bladder catheterization has been decreased significantly following recent modifications in the surgical technique. In particular, the protection of the prostatic urothelium from thermal injury seems to play an integral role. In our institution, we compared the results of a new technique (six patients) with the standard conventional technique (six patients) of intraprostatic laser fiber insertion.[9] In this preliminary comparison, the duration of Foley catheterization decreased from an average of 13.3 days (range 9–30) to 0.5 days (range 0–2). Gross hematuria similarly decreased from an average of 16.5 days (range 6–20) to 4.25 days (range 0.5–10). Using a questionnaire, the patients reported improvement of the voiding symptoms, beginning at an average of 4.25 days (range 3–5) after ILTT using the new technique compared with 16.5 days (range 6–20) using the conventional technique.[9]

CONCLUSION

Interstitial laser thermal therapy is an exciting new minimally invasive treatment for symptomatic BPH. Favorable treatment outcome and morbidity profile are dependent on instrumentation, surgical technique, and operator experience. Continued refinement in the technology is expected to impact positively on the results as ILTT moves toward optimizing tissue thermal ablation while preserving the prostatic urothelium. Cost saving is expected with ILTT when compared with standard TURP and conventional laser prostatectomy, owing to the omission of hospital and anesthesia fees. Long-term cost feasibility awaits future durability results.

ACKNOWLEDGMENT

The authors would like to thank Lois Elayne Miller, Katrina Anastasia, and Anthony Labadia for their contribution to the minimally invasive BPH therapy program at The Atlanta Veterans Affairs Medical Center, Atlanta, GA. The authors also would like to thank Douglas C. Durham, Denis Roy, and Peter Grattan at the Department of Medical Media, Atlanta Veterans Affairs Medical Center, Atlanta, GA, for preparing the illustrations.

REFERENCES

1 McNicholas TA, Steger AC, Bown SG. Interstitial laser coagulation of the prostate: an experimental study. Br J Urol 1993; 71: 439–44.

2 Johnson DE, Cromeens DM, Price RE. Interstitial laser prostatectomy. Lasers Surg Med 1994; 14: 299–305.

3 Pow-Sang M, Orihuela E, Motamedi M, Pow-Sang JE, Cowan DF, Dyer R, Warren MM. Thermocoagulation effect of diode laser in the human prostate: acute and chronic study. Urology 1995; 45(5): 790–4.

4 Mueller-Lisse UG, Heuck AF, Schneede P, Muschter R, Scheidler J, Hofstetter AG, Reiser MF. Postoperative MRI in patients undergoing interstitial laser coagulation thermotherapy of benign prostatic hyperplasia. J Comput Assist Tomogr 1996; 20(2): 273–8.

5 Mueller-Lisse UG, Heuck AF, Thoma M, Muschter R, Schneede P, Weninger E, Faber S, Hofstetter A, Reiser MF. Predictability of the size of laser-induced lesions in T1-weighted MR images obtained during interstitial laser-induced thermotherapy of benign prostatic hyperplasia. J Magn Reson Imaging 1998; 8: 31–9.

6 Arai Y, Ishitoya S, Okubo K, Suzuki Y. Transurethral interstitial laser coagulation for benign prostatic hyperplasia: treatment outcomes and quality of life. Br J Urol 1996; 77: 93–8.

7 Muschter R. Interstitial laser therapy. Curr Opinion Urol 1996; 6: 33–8.

8 Muschter R, Hofstetter A. Interstitial laser therapy outcomes in benign prostatic hyperplasia. J Endourol 1995; 9(2): 129–35.

9 Issa MM, Townsend M, Jiminez VK, Miller LE, Anastasia K. A new technique of intra prostatic fiber placement to minimize thermal injury to prostatic urothelium during Indigo interstitial thermal therapy. Urology 1998; 51: 105–10.

10 Niedergethmann M, Henkle TO, Kohrmann KU. The ablative capacity for the standardized comparison of interstitial laser systems. J Urol 1998; 159(5): 247.

11 Sroka R, Muschter R. Interstitial holmium:YAG laser application. A new procedure for prostatic tissue ablation. J Urol 1997; 157(4): 153.

12 Issa MM, Ritenour C, Grenberger M, Hollabaugh R, Steiner M. The prostate anesthetic block for outpatient prostate surgery. World J Urol 1998; 16: 378–83.

13 De La Rossette JJMCH, Muschter R, Lopez MA. Interstitial laser coagulation in the treatment of BPH using a tissue adaptive laser system. J Endourol 1996; 10(Suppl 1): 93.

14 Horninger W, Janetschek G, Pointner J, Wartson G, Bartsch G. Are TULIP, interstitial laser and contact laser superior to TURP? J Urol 1995; 153: 413.

15 McNicholas T, Alsudani M. Interstitial laser coagulation therapy for benign prostatic hyperplasia. SPIE Proc 1996; 2671: 300–8.

16 Muschter R, Hofstetter A. Technique and results of interstitial laser coagulation. World J Urol 1995; 13: 109–14.

17 Muschter R, De La Rossette JMCH, Whinfield H, Pellerin J, Maderbacher S, Gillatt D. Initial human clinical experience with diode laser interstitial treatment of benign prostatic hyperplasia. Urology 1996; 48: 223–8.

18 Muschter R, Perlmutter AP. The optimization of laser prostatectomy. Part II: other laser techniques. Urology 1994; 44: 856–61.

19 Te Slaa E, de La Rosette JMCH. Lasers in the treatment of benign prostatic obstruction: past, present, and future. Eur Urol 1996; 30: 1–10.

20 Muschter R. Interstitial laser therapy of benign prostatic hyperplasia. In: Graham SD Jr, Glenn JF (eds) *Glenn's Urological Surgery*, 5th edn. Philadelphia: Lippincott-Raven 1999.
21 Roggan A, Handke A, Miller K, Moller G. Laser induced interstitial thermotherapy of benign prostatic hyperplasia – basic investigations and first clinical results. *Min In Medizin* 1994; **5**: 55–63.
22 Muschter R, Sroka R, Perlmutter AP, Schneede P, Hofstetter A. High power interstitial laser coagulation of benign prostatic hyperplasia. *J Endourol* 1996; **10**(Suppl 1): 197.

COMMENTARY

Among the minimally invasive surgical treatments for BPH, microwave thermotherapy, lasers, and transurethral needle ablation (TUNA) are among the most widely used currently. Sonablation and stents are less common, although useful in select situations. TUIP, as pointed out in Chapter 28 ("Transurethral Incision of the Prostate") by Drs Sall and Bruskewitz, still has a small but significant incidence of retrograde ejaculation and bleeding. TUIP, however, is a highly cost-effective procedure, especially because of the lack of need for specialized expensive instrumentation.

ILTT using the Indigo laser system has become a popular therapy in the USA recently because of the simplicity of the procedure and because it is reimbursed by Medicare. As described by Dr Issa and associates in this chapter, the procedure can be performed in about 20 min using existing cystoscopic equipment familiar to all urologists. The Indigo device with which the editor is very familiar utilizes a technique of irreversible coagulation necrosis by achieving an 85°C core temperature within adenomatous tissue. Necrotic coagulated tissue is subsequently reabsorbed in the body, allowing increased prostatic urethral compliance and possibly a decrease in prostatic volume over time. The temperature-monitoring systems allow slow heating, avoiding charring and mini-explosions in tissue, and the interstitial placement of the fiber allows preservation of the urethral lining, thereby reducing the incidence of postoperative irritative voiding symptoms and edema. The preservation of the urethral lining also procedure to be performed under local anesthesia in select patients who can tolerate a rigid cystoscope and some mild pain. As discussed herein the histologic lesions are elliptical and conform to the shape of the prostate, allowing satisfactory therapy of the enlarged area. The insertion technique is simple and avoids potential damage to the capsule and nerves, although in our experience the technique does require some skill, which can be acquired over 5–10 cases. The automated temperature-monitoring system not only allows ease of therapy but also prevents inadvertent injury to the bladder by shutting the system down when the bladder neck is penetrated by deep insertion of the fiber, which can occur in short prostatic lengths.

Additional advantages of the ILTT system include elimination of the need for pretreatment procedures such as transrectal ultrasound (required for TUNA) and direct visualization of the prostate and treatment areas during therapy. One disadvantage we have noted is a requirement for prolonged postoperative catheterization, which may be required for 1–2 weeks in 20% of patients. However, as reported herein and based on our own limited results, in approximately 25 patients, the procedure appears to be effective in relieving symptoms, improving uroflow, with a low incidence of complications. The incidence of retrograde ejaculation, bleeding, or impotence is very rare, although pink urine for several days is common. The procedure can be performed under IV sedation in some patients and certainly in an ambulatory setting (day surgery) in all patients.

The cost of the instrumentation is in the range of $50,000 in the USA and the disposable fibers cost approximately $600 each. The device does require laser precautions, and specialized protective eyewear, which are expensive.

This compares with TUNA capital instrumentation costs in the range of approximately $30,000 and disposable costs of $700/catheter. The TUNA device also requires a special rod–lens system, which costs about $2000. While the rod–lens system may be included in the initial generator cost, subsequent replacement lenses may be required occasionally due to damage or deterioration over time.

The microwave devices discussed in Chapter 22 ("Transurethral Thermotherapy") are currently the most expensive among minimally invasive therapies, and require cost sharing among urologists/hospitals owing to heavy capital equipment costs of between $150,000 and over $500,000 at present. The advantages and disadvantages of microwave devices are further discussed in Chapter 22.

Section V

OTHER MINIMALLY INVASIVE TREATMENTS

Section V Overview

OTHER MINIMALLY INVASIVE TREATMENTS
P. Narayan

Various forms of minimally invasive therapy have recently emerged, the majority of which are in the field of thermotherapy. These therapies utilize various energies such as radiofrequency, microwave, laser, and high-intensity ultrasound, all of which cause tissue coagulative necrosis inside the prostate. Irrespective of the type of energy employed, the final objective is to heat the prostate to a desired temperature. In general, thermotherapy with temperatures in the range of 45–55°C causes limited tissue ablation, often with insufficient success. On the other hand, thermotherapies with temperature ranges between 60 and 100°C or higher result in significant tissue ablation and successful outcomes.

Transurethral needle ablation (TUNA) using radio-frequency energy is one such type of thermotherapy. Radio-frequency is a unique form of energy, which can be applied through tissue contact. Total heat dissipation is limited and is determined by the amount of tissue contact and duration of therapy. This allows a precise, customized and targeted tissue ablation. The TUNA system consists of an energy generator, and an endoscopic instrument for delivering energy into the prostate. Energy delivery is performed using an automated software program. The machine also has a urethral cooling system to prevent urethral heat injury. Prevention of urethral injury is a key feature in avoiding prolonged postoperative edema and retention. The mechanism of TUNA efficacy is believed to be tissue coagulative necrosis, which results in scarring, softening, and a decrease in volume of the prostate. Histologic lesions also show that there is destruction of α-adrenergic receptors following the TUNA procedure. The TUNA needles and technique of insertion maximize treatment of the adenomatous portion of the prostate, while preventing periprostatic structural damage. The procedure can be performed under combined topical and regional anesthesia in over 50% of patients in the Editor's experience, and in a higher percentage in others'

experience. The average symptom improvement in a combined analysis of over 500 patients reveals that there is an improvement of 58% in 1 year, 60% in 2 years, and 66% in 3 years. The improvement in peak flow rate is also in the range of 60–80%, although there is some variability in these results. The side effects of the procedure continue to be urinary retention in 30–41% of patients, but the retention in most instances is transient, lasting less than a week. Bleeding is rare, and the TUNA procedure can be performed in patients on coumadin and aspirin. As with any new technology, further refinements in instrumentation and technique continue to occur with the TUNA procedure. The problems that remain include the need for a preoperative ultrasonography, which increases costs, the requirement for a special endoscopic device, and duration of treatment, which currently is 30–40 min. However, the efficacy of the technology has been established and the capital costs are lower than those for lasers. The procedure may also have better durability and long-terms results due to the higher volume of tissue treated compared with interstitial laser.

Transurethral microwave thermal therapy or TUMT is also a technique of heat destruction of the prostate, based upon microwave heat energy. Microwaves are transverse electromagnetic waves with frequencies in the range of 30–300 Hz. These travel in a given medium and within the prostatic tissues cause drift, free charge, and polarization of atoms. The initial devices of microwave used the transrectal approach, but subsequently the transurethral approach, which is now called thermotherapy, was utilized to achieve intraprostatic temperatures in excess of 45°C without having to go through heating the rectum. There are several devices in existence now, and some of the more common ones are the Prostatron and the Targis systems. Even the Prostatron device has undergone an evolution from a 2.0 software to a 2.5 software, the latter having the ability to use higher levels of power and higher levels of heating. The

TUMT procedure involves placement of the microwave antenna in the urethra, monitoring by ultrasonography in the rectum, and urethral cooling, which is automated based on temperature elevations set at a certain threshold above body temperature. Treatments using microwave therapy, especially using the 2.0 system, can be performed in most patients under local anesthesia, although the time taken is close to 1 h. Owing to poor results with the 2.0 system, the 2.5 system was developed and, although this achieves higher intraprostatic temperatures, it requires more anesthesia. While the Prostatron system appears to be satisfactory in relieving symptoms and improving uroflow in 1-year trials, 4-year follow-up trials reveal that more than 50% of patients require an additional treatment in the form of TURP or another invasive procedure. In fairness to the microwave therapy results, it must be stated that most other systems, such as the interstitial laser and TUNA, do not have 5-year follow-up results. In trials where TUMT was compared with TURP, initial results at 1–2 years appear to be similar in both treatments as far as symptom reduction is concerned, but uroflow improvement is higher in the TURP group. Also, urodynamic studies of patients undergoing thermotherapy have revealed that only 15% of patients in the thermotherapy group are considered to have no obstruction at 6 months, while 40% of patients in the TURP group are considered to have no obstruction. A side effect of the thermotherapy appears to be urinary retention, which occurs in as many as 70–80% of patients and lasts up to 2 weeks. Other complications include hematuria, urinary tract infections, and sexual dysfunction in a small percentage of patients.

High-intensity focused ultrasonography (HIFU) is a method of causing heat-induced prostatic destruction using ultrasonic energy. Normally in biological tissue, mechanical ultrasonic energy is converted to heat. By increasing the intensity of the ultrasonic energy and focusing it on a specific area, temperatures between 80 and 200°C can be achieved. This level of temperature will produce irreversible coagulation necrosis and, by focusing the ultrasonic beam, intervening tissues are not injured. The instrumentation consists essentially of a piezoceramic transducer, which changes in thickness in response to electric current. This change causes acoustic waves with a frequency of 0.5 mHz, which are then focused on target tissues. For a variety of safety and technical reasons, transrectally applied HIFU appears optimal to target the prostatic adenoma. Transrectal devices incorporate both imaging and treatment systems on a single or a separate probe and are available with varying focal lengths to accommodate different prostate sizes. Phased-array transducers with varying focal lengths have also recently become available. The preliminary conclusions on HIFU by investigators who have been pioneers in the work related to its clinical application is that HIFU is an attractive minimally invasive therapy for both BPH and carcinoma of the prostate. The procedure can be performed under IV sedation in some patients. The HIFU probe is targeted at the prostate using a transrectal approach and creates lesions of 2–10 mm in a circumferential manner. To date, only 250 patients have been treated worldwide in Phase II trials. There is a 47% improvement in uroflow and a 53% decrease in symptom scores at 1 year following therapy. However, pressure-flow studies have shown only a moderate improvement in objective parameters using the Abrams–Griffiths nomogram. Therefore, in its present form, the technique may be applicable only in patients with moderate but not severely obstructed prostates. Side effects include urinary retention, resolved currently by placement of a suprapubic catheter for 6 days. Other injuries such as rectal complications are rare at less than 2%. The experience with HIFU in the USA is quite limited. One of the disadvantages of the technique is the requirement of capital expense of equipment, which is significant.

Urethral stents offer a safe and effective treatment for urethral obstruction due to a variety of causes. Stents may be used as temporary or permanent devices. For stents to work properly, they have to be biochemically compatible, chemically inert, memory shaped, have adequate tensile strength, and low internal to external diameter. Current stents are both hollow and solid with side channels. The original side effects of encrustation and obstruction have been somewhat resolved by using new techniques of woven mesh. Migration has also decreased with use of anchoring devices at the bladder and sphincter ends. The European experience which has been more extensive than that in the USA has utilized stents in a variety of indications, yet mostly in patients who are at poor risk for surgery. Biodegradable stents are especially attractive for temporizing patients recovering from other procedures and may indeed be useful even as a permanent technique for relieving obstruction when they could be exchanged or replaced every 6 months. In the USA the only stent that has been approved for use is the urolume wall stent, which is made of a super alloy of steel in mesh form with an inner diameter of 24 French, and which is inserted using a special cytoscopic-guided device. In a multicenter study of 126 patients in which the Editor participated, 2-year data reveal a significant decrease in symptom scores, which has been maintained in the 35 patients available for follow-up for up to 5 years. Complications included encrustation, migration, poor deployment, and severe irritative symptoms necessitating removal of the stent in up to 31% of the patients at 5 years. In summary, urethral stents can be utilized in select patient populations to keep the urethra open. Current downsides of available stents appear to be the irritative symptoms and the operative procedure necessary to remove them from patients when indicated.

Radiofrequency Thermal Therapy for Benign Prostatic Hyperplasia by Transurethral Needle Ablation of the Prostate

21

M.M. Issa and J.E. Oesterling

INTRODUCTION

The increasing demand for less invasive and more economical surgical therapies alternative to the conventional transurethral resection of the prostate (TURP) have influenced the direction of research in the field of benign prostatic hyperplasia (BPH). In an effort to meet these demands, a new concept of thermal therapy for BPH was introduced. With thermal therapy, various forms of energy are utilized to heat the prostate to temperatures above 45°C (usually above 60°C), resulting in improvement in the BPH symptoms. However, the exact mechanisms responsible for this remain undetermined and not fully understood. One form of such minimally invasive thermal therapy that has gained increasing popularity during the past few years is transurethral needle ablation (TUNA). This therapy utilizes radiofrequency (RF) energy for thermal ablation. It is the aim of this chapter to discuss all aspects of this new technology and to present the latest clinical results.

RADIOFREQUENCY

PHYSICAL PROPERTIES

RF has a number of unique physical properties that distinguish it from other forms of energy used for thermal ablation. To start with, RF can be applied into tissue only through direct contact and, once in the tissue, it causes thermal ablation through inductive heating of water molecules and by friction. The magnitude of tissue ablation is of limited distance dissipation and is determined by the amount of tissue contact, the amount of wattage energy, and the duration of therapy. Such physical properties give RF energy the following unique advantages:

(1) Targeted tissue ablation: thermal ablation occurs only in the region directly in contact with the metal transmitting the RF signal.
(2) Precise tissue ablation: thermal tissue ablation is exact and accurately localized, therefore adjacent tissue and organs are protected from thermal injury.
(3) Customized tissue ablation: the size and extent of thermal tissue ablation can be altered by changing the treatment settings appropriate to individual situations.

MEDICAL AND SURGICAL APPLICATIONS

Although the application of radiofrequency tissue ablation (RFTA) is new to urology, it has previously been used in other medical specialties. It offers precise tissue ablation in conditions affecting vital organs such as the heart and central nervous system, where accurate ablation of the abnormal tissue is mandatory, while excess ablation is undesirable and dangerous. In cardiology, RFTA is used for ablation of aberrant pathways in Wolff–Parkinson–White syndrome[1] and in neurosurgery for precise stereotactic ablation of abnormal neural tissue.[2]

In urology, the same principle of RFTA is applied to treat BPH with the TUNA procedure.

RADIOFREQUENCY IN BENIGN PROSTATIC HYPERPLASIA

During the TUNA procedure, thermal ablation of the BPH tissue is achieved by delivering low-wave RF (465 kHz) energy transurethrally into the prostate through needles. The amount of thermal ablation and the subsequent therapeutic effects are determined by the rate of increase, the range, and the duration of the temperatures achieved inside the prostatic adenoma during the procedure. During the TUNA procedure an intraprostatic target temperature of 60–90°C is achieved for a period of 1–2 min. In contrast to other forms of surgical therapies, the prostatic urethra is preserved during the TUNA procedure. Furthermore, adjacent structures such as the prostatic capsule, urinary sphincter, and rectum remain completely protected from the thermal effect. Such properties render the procedure minimally invasive and minimally morbid.

Preservation of the Prostatic Urethra

The concept of prostatic urethral preservation is new and a subject of much discussion. The advantages of urethral preservation are twofold:

(1) it allows the TUNA procedure to be performed under local Xylocaine anesthesia without the need for spinal and general anesthesia by protecting the pain-sensitive region of prostatic urothelium;
(2) it minimizes postoperative morbidity of irritative voiding symptoms, hematuria, and urinary retention.

The main question is whether urethral preservation compromises treatment efficacy. Using TURP as the gold standard suggests that the anatomical debulking, which includes urethral resection, is the hallmark for its highly efficacious results. Disputing this theory are the increasing reports on newer therapies such as the TUNA, showing significant efficacy despite urethral preservation. Such findings suggest that urethral resection is not an integral part for treatment success, which makes the concept of urethral preservation when achieved without compromising treatment efficacy very advantageous.

Protection of Adjacent Tissues

The precise nature of RFTA prevents heat dissipation and injury to adjacent structures, namely the prostatic capsule, neurovascular bundles, rectum, and urinary sphincter. Intraoperative temperatures in these regions are maintained within normal limits, thus preserving urinary and fecal continence as well as erectile function.

The minimization of energy wastage allows the entire RF energy to be utilized for heat generation inside the prostatic adenoma. Consequently, lower wattage energy can achieve higher temperatures (approaching 100°C) within a relatively shorter time (within 5 min) without the need for interruptions and cooling.

DOSIMETRY

Much of the dosimetry research on RFTA was performed in the early 1990s by Goldwasser and colleagues in Israel and Schulman and colleagues in Belgium. They used animal tissue model *ex vivo* (turkey breast)[3] and canine prostatic tissue model *in vivo*[4] to quantitate and qualitate the amount of RFTA and its effect on adjacent tissues (rectum, urethra, and bladder base). Following this, they experimented with human prostatic tissue *ex vivo* and *in vivo* to establish the optimal RF setting and technique.[3,5,6]

LESION SIZE AND PARAMETERS

The extent of RFTA, as judged by the size of the lesion created by the RF signal, depends on three factors: (1) the length of the needles; (2) the wattage energy of the RF; (3) the duration of treatment session.

A maximum lesion size (in excess of 10 mm) is achieved with 7–10 mm needle length at 6–9 W energy for 3–5 min treatment duration. Thermal mapping using an infrared thermal imaging system confirmed temperatures of 40–50°C at the periphery of the lesion, which increased progressively towards the center of the lesion to approach 80–100°C. Shorter needle length and shorter treatment duration decreased the amount of tissue ablation. Interestingly, higher wattage energy adversely affected the size of the tissue ablated. This is explained by the fact that higher wattage energy heats tissues to temperatures >100°C, which causes water evaporation and tissue charring. This tissue charring produces an insulating and non-conductive barrier, which limits further thermal tissue ablation.

HISTOPATHOLOGY

Macroscopically

Lesions were evident in the transition zone of the prostate gland treated with TUNA. The gross appearance of the lesions corresponded to the region of the needles and varied depending on the recovery time of the specimen, i.e. the duration *in vivo* after the procedure. After 3 hours, the lesions appeared minimally hemorrhagic with diffuse edges. At 1 week, the changes were more pronounced. At 2 weeks, the lesions appeared dark brown in color and were well demarcated (Figure 21.1). The appearances at 4 weeks were similar to those at 2 weeks. The appearance of the TUNA lesions in the human prostate *in vivo*, as seen in Figure 21.1, is markedly different from the human prostate

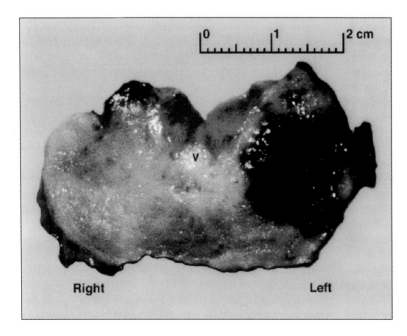

Figure 21.1 Transverse section of a human prostate at the veru montanum (v) plane demonstrating the gross appearance of a TUNA lesion. The thermal ablation lesion is seen within the left lobe 2 weeks *in vivo* following the TUNA procedure as compared with the right untreated lobe (control). The well-demarcated thermal ablation lesion (1.3-cm diameter) appears congested and severely hemorrhagic

Source: With permission from *Infections in Urology*, Liggot Publishing Co, A division of SCP/Liggot Communications Inc., 1998

in vitro model in Figure 21.2. In the latter, the lesion appears pale and has a firmer texture. The development of cavitations and cystic changes in the prostate have been inconsistent.[6,8]

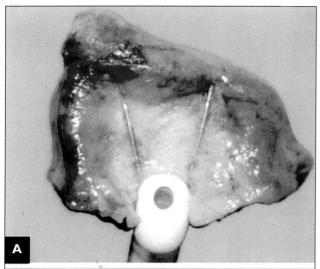

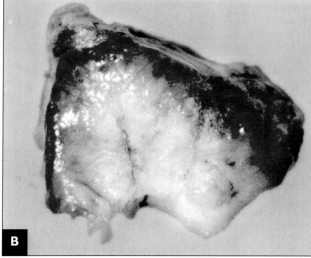

Figure 21.2 Transverse section of a prostatic lobe (*in vitro*) showing the pale gross appearance of the TUNA lesion: (A) with the needles *in situ*; (B) without the needles

Source: With permission from *Infections in Urology*, Liggot Publishing Co, A division of SCP/Liggot Communications Inc., 1998

Microscopically

Lesions showed extensive early inflammation with edema followed by coagulative and hemorrhagic necrosis of both glandular and stromal components. The necrosis was extensive and extended for 1–3 mm beyond the macroscopic margin.

Immunohistochemically

Absence of staining for prostate-specific antigen (PSA), smooth muscle actin, stroma, vascular component, neural tissue, α-adrenergic receptors as well as nitrinergic receptors was prominently evident in the RF ablated BPH tissue. The NOS receptors were most vulnerable to damage

following the TUNA treatment, as evidenced by the complete lack of their immunohistochemical staining within the initial hours. On the other hand, the damage to α-adrenergic receptors was more evident and pronounced 1–2 weeks later.

Ultrastructural studies

Thermal damage was evident in the glandular and stromal component of BPH within hours following the TUNA procedures and included epithelial and endothelial damage as well as smooth muscle degeneration.

THE TUNA PROCEDURE

The TUNA procedure is performed with the patient in the lithotomy position using 2% local Xylocaine anesthesia per urethra. The local anesthesia is supplemented with intravenous sedation when necessary. The appropriate length of the needles to be deployed and the number of the planes to be treated are calculated based on the sonographic transverse diameter measurement of the prostate and the cystoscopic prostatic urethral length, respectively. The length of the needle deployed (L) in millimeters is calculated using the formula $L = 1/2TD - 6$ (TD is the transverse diameter of the prostate on ultrasound in millimeters). This ensures that the tips of the needles stay within the prostate approximately 6 mm from the prostatic capsule. The shields are deployed out for 5–6 mm to cover the base of the needles adjacent to the TUNA catheter. The number of treatment planes is calculated based on the length of the prostatic urethra. One treatment plane is delivered for a prostatic urethral length <3 cm, two planes for 3–4 cm, and an additional plane for every additional centimeter of prostatic urethra. These planes are equidistant from each other in each lobe. The TUNA catheter is inserted transurethrally into the prostatic urethra and its tip positioned at the desired treatment plane. The needles and shields are then deployed and advanced into the prostatic lobe to their appropriate lengths. A 5-min treatment is delivered, during which the amount of energy is continuously adjusted manually by the operator to achieve a steady temperature rise of 3°C min^{-1} at the peripheral rim of the ablation region in the prostate as measured by the thermosensor located at the tip of the shields. The shield temperature is increased from a body temperature of 37°C to 40°C at 1 min, 43°C at 2 min, 46°C at 3 min, 49°C at 4 min, and 52°C at 5 min. This ensures at least 2 min of thermal therapy (>45°C) at the peripheral rim of the ablation region in the prostate, which translates into core temperatures approaching 100°C at the center of the ablation region in the prostate (Figure 21.5). With the new TUNA generators, the delivery of thermal therapy is an entirely automated process, which follows pre-set target temperatures as illustrated in Figure 21.5.

ANESTHESIA REQUIREMENT DURING TUNA

There continues to be a wide variation in the anesthesia requirement for TUNA between various urologists and

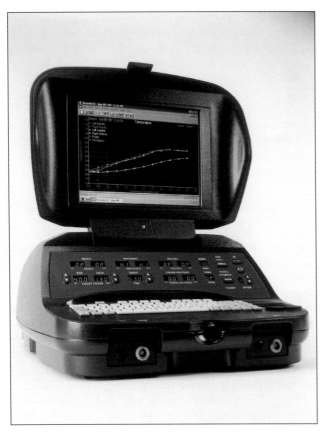

Figure 21.3 The TUNA generator

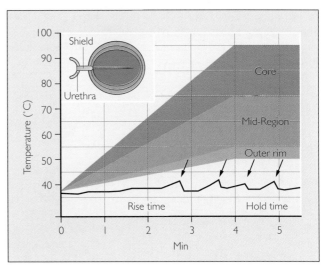

Figure 21.5 A graph of the temperatures inside the ablation lesion during the TUNA procedure. The delivery of RF energy for thermal ablation of the prostate is automated by the generator's computer to follow the preprogrammed target "outer rim" temperature (50–55°C) and "core" temperature (75–95°C). Note the tendency of the urethral temperature to rise during treatment and the cooling effect of fluid irrigation as demonstrated by the arrows

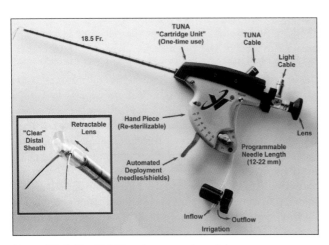

Figure 21.4 The TUNA catheter consists of three components (red labels), the TUNA cartridge, the TUNA fibroptic lens, and the TUNA handpiece

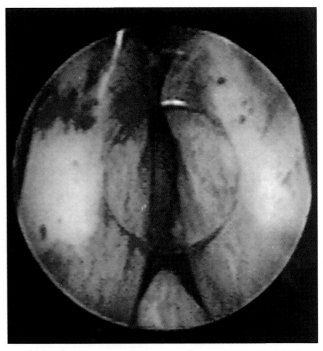

Figure 21.6 A view of the prostatic urethra at the level of the veru montanum with the lens in the normal forward position. The transparent "see-through" design of the distal sheath allows for a wide field of vision

institutions. This can be explained by the variability in urologists' preference, patients' pain threshold, and in rules and traditions of various medical institutions. Indeed, it is reasonable for the urologist to request spinal or general anesthesia for the first few TUNA cases. This ensures patient's comfort during the initial learning process. With more experience, most of the patients (>95%) can undergo the TUNA treatment under combined topical and regional anesthesia without the need for conscious sedation, spinal or general anesthesia. In our institution, we favor the transperineal prostatic block with intraurethral instillation of lidocaine gel as the primary method without supplemental sedation or narcotics. This omits the need for conscious sedation monitoring, which makes it possible to perform the procedure in the outpatient clinic without the need for elaborate and extensive set-up. Furthermore, it significantly reduces the global cost of the TUNA procedure by omitting operating room and anesthesia charges.

CLINICAL RESULTS

The first series of 12 TUNA procedures in the USA were performed in 1994.[9] The procedure then underwent extensive evaluation through various clinical trials to determine safety, efficacy and durability. A major clinical trial undertaken in the USA to compare TUNA with TURP in a randomized controlled way showed favorable outcome.[16] Based on the results of this study, the FDA approved TUNA in the USA in October 1996. The procedure was also approved globally in North and South America, Europe, Africa, Asia and Australia. In general, improvement is seen fairly early (within 1–2 weeks), and it is usually complete within 6 weeks following TUNA treatment. Occasionally, there is an impressive and complete resolution of the irritative voiding symptoms in the first few days. Conversely, a few patients experience delayed and slow recovery extending to 3 months. Possible explanation for this includes: very small prostates, poor patient selection, suboptimal surgical technique leading to urothelial thermal injury, thermal ablation bladder necks, and treatment of enlarged median lobes. These are purely observations, mostly anecdotal on our part, and have not been studied specifically.

SUBJECTIVE IMPROVEMENT

Significant subjective improvement in the symptoms score has been reported in various series (Table 21.1). The overall average improvement is 58% at 1 year (546 patients in 10 series), 60% at 2 years and 66% at 3 years. Exclusion of the series with the lowest and highest improvement (to minimize bias) did not impact the results. These results are statistically significant when compared with baseline and surpassed the expected placebo range of 30%. With regard to the bother score and quality of life score, improvements were similar and parallel to the improvement in symptom score. In the US randomized trial comparing TUNA with TURP, the improvements in all subjective parameters were similar with both procedures.[16]

OBJECTIVE IMPROVEMENT

Uroflowmetry

The improvement in the peak flow rate (Q_{max}) reported in the majority of the worldwide literature fall in the range of 60–80% (Table 21.1). There are, however, two series showing significantly higher improvement at 121% and 280%.[23,25] Conversely, there are other series with notably lower improvement, 30%[22] and 33%[21] compared with the expected >50%.[9,16–20,23–25] None the less, the latter two series reported significant improvement in the symptom score, 66%[22] and 54%,[21] respectively. A summary of the worldwide literature shows an overall average improvement in peak flow rate (Q_{max}) to be 77% at 1 year (546 patients in 10 series), 82% at 2 years, and 92% at 3 years. As with the results of symptom score, these peak flow rate results are statistically significant when compared with baseline and surpass the expected placebo range of 30%.

Postvoid Residual Urine

The decrease in the postvoid residual (PVR) urine volume ranged between 13% and 80%.[16,18,19,24] The interpretation and clinical value of PVR has traditionally been overrated. Its current utility has been surpassed by the various other parameters. Therefore, less emphasis is currently placed on PVR, and many series have stopped reporting on this parameter.[20,22,23,25]

Prostate Size

There is no convincing evidence that prostate size is significantly reduced following TUNA.[8,17,21,25] A statistically significant decrease in the ultrasound size of the prostate has been reported; however, one must interpret this finding cautiously and question its clinical significance.[9] This result may simply reflect the low sensitivity and reliability of our current technique of transrectal prostate ultrasound in accurately measuring small changes in prostatic volume. Intraoperator variability is common and has to be taken into consideration so as not to overestimate volume changes measured by ultrasound.

Endoscopic Appearance of the Prostatic Urethra

In general, there are no significant changes in the cystoscopic appearance of the prostate. Mild alterations in the urothelial color (pallor) and contour (retraction) may be seen immediately following the treatment. These changes are probably a result of the pressure exerted by the tip of the TUNA catheter onto the prostate during the treatment. On follow-up of 1 month and longer, the prostate appears the same as before treatment. Rarely, more significant urothelial retraction and formation of "urothelial divots" and "urothelial tunnels" are seen (Figure 21.8). It is tempting to declare this as the mechanism of TUNA action; however, this appearance is exceptional rather than the rule.

Pressure Flow Studies

At least five independent studies address detrusor pressures before and after TUNA (Table 21.2). The two largest series

Study Group	No. of patients	Months of follow-up	Symptom score			Peak flow rate		
			Baseline	Post-TUNA	% change	Baseline	Post-TUNA	% Change
US/Pilot Study (Issa)[9]	12	6	25.6	9.8	−61	7.8	13.5	+73
US/Multicenter Study (Roehrborn et al.)[17]	130	12	23.7	11.9*	−50	7.8	14.6*	+68
US/Multicenter Randomized Study (Bruskewitz et al.)[16]	65	12	24.7	11.1*	−55	8.7	15.0	+72
Brussels, Belgium (Schulman et al.)[18]	36	12	21.6	7.8*	−64	9.9	16.8*	+69
	25	24	21.6	8.5*	−61	9.9	15.5*	+57
	17	36	21.6	7.6*	−65	9.9	16.2*	+64
Harlow, UK (Virdi et al.)[19]	71	12	22.3	10.0	−55	7.0	13.8	+97
	71	24	22.3	9.4	−58	7.0	14.8	+111
	71	36	22.3	7.4	−67	7.0	14.2	+103
Milan, Italy (Campo et al.)[20]	72	12	20.8	6.2*	−70	8.2	15.9*	+93
	42	18	20.8	6.7*	−67	8.2	14.1*	+71
European Multi center (Ramon et al.)[21]	68	12	22.0	7.5*	−66	8.7	11.6*	+33
Sheffield, UK (Chapple et al.)[22]	58	12	22.0	10.0*	−54	8.8	11.5*	+30
Ioannina, Greece (Giennakopoulos et al.)[23]	50	12	22.4	9.1*	−59	7.6	16.8*	+121
Johannesburg, SA (Steele et al.)[24]	41	12	22.4	7.0*	−68	6.6	10.2*	+54
	38	24	22.4	9.5*	−57	6.6	11.0*	+66
Australia (Steele et al.)[25]	20	12	19.0	8.2*	−56	3.0	11.4*	+280
Summary (World Literature)	546	12	22.2	9.1*	−58	7.8	13.8*	+77
	176†	24	21.8	8.5*	−60	7.6	13.9*	+82
	88	36	22.1	7.4*	−66	7.5	14.5*	+92

* P<0.01–0.0001.
† Includes one series with 18-month follow-up

Table 21.1 Worldwide results of TUNA of the prostate

Study Group	No. of patients	Months of follow-up	Maximum detrusor pressure (cmH$_2$O			
			Baseline	Post-TUNA	% Change	P-value
US Pilot Study (Issa)[9]	12	6	91.8	70.9	−22.7	0.094
	(12)*	(6)*	(74.5)*	(56.3)*	(−24.4)*	0.046
Milan, Italy (Campo et al.)[20]	108	3	85.3	53.2	−37.6	<0.01
	86	6	85.3	61.3	−28.1	<0.01
	72	12	85.3	63.7	−25.3	<0.01
	42	24	85.3	67.8	−20.5	<0.01
Johannesburg, SA (Steele et al.)[24]	41	1	92.4	77.0	−16.6	<0.05
	39	3	92.4	68.5	−25.8	<0.05
	34	6	92.4	54.8	−40.6	<0.05
	29	12	92.4	72.9	−21.1	<0.05
	12	24	92.4	58.9	−36.2	<0.05
Sheffield, UK (Chapple et al.)[22]	39	3	97.0	79.0	−18.5	>0.05
	39	12	97.0	84.0	−13.4	>0.05
Australia (Millard et al.)[25]	20	6	70.7	59.9	−15.8	0.90

* indicated detrusor open pressure

Table 21.2 Detrusor pressures following transurethral needle ablation (TUNA) of the prostate

regarding the mechanism responsible for therapeutic improvement following TUNA.

POTENTIAL VARIABILITY IN RESULTS

The rapid pace of research and development in the field of RF thermal therapy is responsible for potential variability in results. Prolonged clinical trials using single protocols are becoming less favorable in the assessment of a new technology. The pursuit to improve results forces early implementation of better instrumentation, computer software and technique during ongoing trials. Such enthusiasm tends to accelerate the process of development; however, it also casts a shadow of uncertainty. Therefore, both patients and urologists need to temper their enthusiasm until convincing results become available. At the same time, there should be an equal resistance not to overlook arbitrarily a good technology, based on attitude rather than facts.

In general, it is a good policy to review various reports and exclude the ones with "the best" and "the worst" results to minimize the likelihood of bias. Also, it is important to be

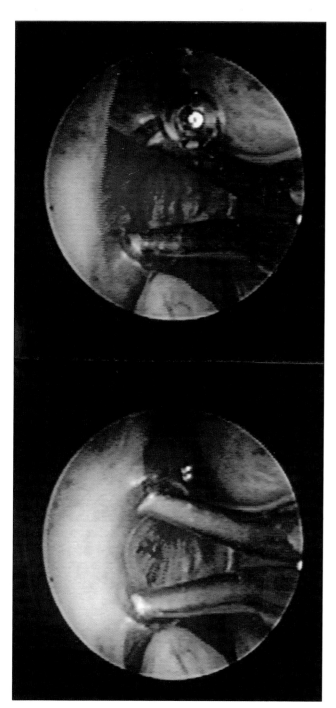

Figure 21.7 Intraoperative views of the needles and shields through the TUNA catheter during deployment into the right lateral lobe of the prostate (top view) and at the end of deployment, i.e. invisible inside the lateral lobe (bottom view). In both views, the lens is in the retractable position, showing the two metal housings for the needles and shields within the transparent body of the distal sheath

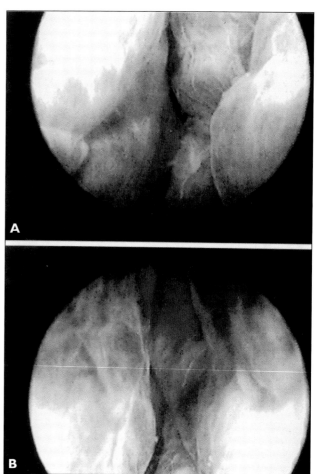

Figure 21.8 Cystoscopic appearance of the prostate 6 months after the TUNA procedure. The prostatic urothelium is markedly retracted at the site of the TUNA treatment in the distal region (apex) of the left prostatic lobe (A). These changes are more prominent in the proximal region of the left prostatic lobe giving the appearance of "tunneling" (B)

indicate that maximum detrusor pressure decreases significantly after TUNA.[20,24] The remaining three studies,[9,22,25] one of which had equivocal results,[9] suggest that obstruction persists despite the improvement in other subjective as well as objective parameters. This raises important questions

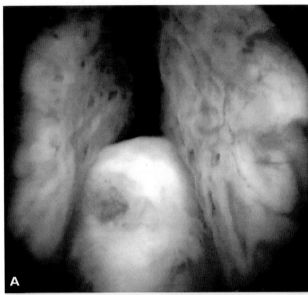

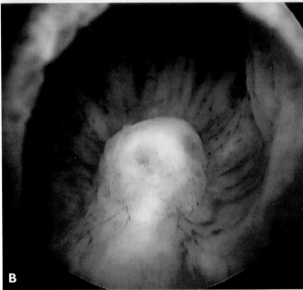

Figure 21.9 Cystoscopic appearance of the prostate 3 months after the TUNA procedure during the "static" phase (A) and during the "dynamic" voiding phase (B)

aware of the various changes in instrumentation and technique during clinical trials and how they impact the final outcome. For example, the TUNA system has undergone improvement in the optics, generators and technique during the course of its clinical trials over a period of 3 years (1994–1997). Using the original system, the endoscopic visualization was suboptimal, which led to difficulties in proper placement of the needle inside the prostate. Also, the original manual generator was a challenge to operate, which often resulted in suboptimal thermal lesions. Consequent variability in the results is expected and is simply a reflection of the various improvements discussed. Changes usually have a positive impact on outcome, since they tend to be specifically designed to correct problems.

ADVERSE EVENTS

To date, no mortality has been reported with the TUNA procedure. Morbidity is relatively insignificant and include the following.

Urinary Retention

The rate of postoperative urinary retention ranges from 13.3% to 41.6.[9,16–18,23,24] The retention is transient (12–48 h) in the majority of patients. During the initial learning phase, urinary retention is usually in the 40% range; however, this rate improves with more experience.

Hematuria

A mild degree of transient macroscopic hematuria is noted in most patients for a period of up to 24 h. Patients with significant coagulopathy may experience more pronounced hematuria and should be counseled about this preoperatively. It is recommended that such coagulopathy be corrected before the procedure. Anti-platelet agents such as aspirin and non-steroidal anti-inflammatory medications usually post no major problems; however, patients are advised to discontinue these for 7–10 days before TUNA if possible.

Irritative Voiding Symptoms

Dysuria and increased urinary frequency without urinary infection may develop in approximately 40% of patients during the initial postoperative period. These are mild and transient in nature, usually lasting 1–7 days and rarely more than 2–4 weeks.

Urinary Infection and Epididymitis

Postoperative urinary infection and epididymitis occur rarely (0–3.1%).[8,9,16,17,20,24] The risk of postoperative infection can be minimized by ensuring urine sterility preoperatively and by the use of antibiotics. In our experience, fluoroquinolone antibiotics (500 mg of ciprofloxacin twice a day) given preoperatively and continued for 5 days postoperatively has been effective in preventing urinary infection and epididymitis. Urinary manipulation of an infection-susceptible organ such as the prostate in a setting of tissue necrosis requires full antibiotic coverage.

Urethral Strictures

Urethral strictures occur in 0–1.5% of patients and are related to instrumentation of the urethra.[8,9,11,16,17,20,24] The relatively small diameter of the TUNA catheter and the short duration of the treatment put the patient at lower risk for development of urethral stricture than after standard TURP. In the US randomized clinical trial, the rate of urethral strictures was significantly lower following TUNA (1.5%) than TURP (7.3%).

Retrograde Ejaculation

No objective evidence currently exists in the literature that retrograde ejaculation occurs following TUNA. However, a marginal decrease in the amount of ejaculatory fluid has been suggested in limited cases (without objective proof).[8,9,17] In one series, 13% of TUNA patients noticed some change.[17] It is possible that more aggressive TUNA therapy to the region of the bladder neck is responsible for this.

Erectile Dysfunction

The incidence of erectile dysfunction is negligible (0–<2%) following the TUNA procedure in the majority of the world literature.[6,8,9,11,17–20,24,25] In one series of 38 sexually active patients, Ramon and colleagues[21] reported a surprising improvement in "sexual function" in 42% of patients after the TUNA procedure. Also, a puzzling 16% deterioration and 21% both deterioration and improvement in sexual function were reported in the same series. To date this report remains unique, unexplainable and inconsistent with the majority of the worldwide literature.

TUNA IN PATIENTS WITH URINARY RETENTION

Few reports currently exist regarding the efficacy of TUNA in the treatment of urinary retention secondary to BPH.[25–27] Millard et al. reported an 85% (17/20) initial success rate, which later became 75% (15/20), when two patients underwent TURP for persistent voiding symptoms.[25] Similarly, Zlotta and associates reported a 79% (30/38) success rate in patients with urinary retention.[27]

MECHANISM OF ACTION OF TUNA

The insignificant changes in prostate size and the disproportional improvement in subjective parameters compared with objective parameters raise important questions regarding the mechanism of TUNA action. Anatomical debulking is not significant, and improvements in the peak flow rates and maximum detrusor pressures are less pronounced than after anatomical debulking procedures such as TURP. Yet the improvement in the voiding symptoms matches those of TURP. Therefore, one must question the traditional thinking of anatomical debulking in BPH treatment and whether it is essential for the success of the treatment. This issue is a topic of much debate and requires closer analysis of BPH symptoms.

The American Urological Association Symptom Score explores seven symptoms, both obstructive and irritative. Although it is difficult to categorize the various symptoms into obstructive and irritative, approximately three are obstructive (weak stream, hesitancy, and intermittency) and three are irritative (frequency, urgency, and nocturia). The remaining symptom (feeling of incomplete bladder emptying) falls in-between the two categories. Since an anatomical debulking procedure aims to unobstruct the prostatic urethra, it is likely to improve the obstructive voiding symptoms. By design, this approach does not aim to address the irritative voiding symptoms specifically. None the less, in the majority of patients (approximately 70–80%) improvement in the irritative voiding symptoms follows. Traditional thinking indicates that irritative symptoms are a result of obstruction and that they should, therefore,

improve once the obstruction is treated. This theory is supported by the results of anatomical debulking procedures. However, this thinking may be challenged in the following scenarios:

(1) patients who continued to experience voiding symptoms following TURP, laser prostatectomy, intraprostatic stents, yet their prostatic urethras appear non-obstructing on cystoscopy;
(2) patients who have significant and bothersome voiding symptoms, yet their prostates appear small and non-obstructing on cystoscopy;
(3) patients who are responding satisfactorily to treatments with α-adrenergic blockers without decrease in the size of their prostate;
(4) patients who are treated successfully with thermal therapies without a significant decrease in the size of their prostate. Instead, the prostatic urethra seems to open widely, suggesting that there is an alteration in the physiological function of the prostate (Figure 21.9);
(5) patients with cystoscopically obstructing prostate who are asymptomatic.

Further analysis shows that the amount of bother experienced by patients is influenced more by their irritative rather than obstructive symptoms. Indeed, patients are distressed by their inability to do basic daily activities such as driving, watching a movie or game without interruption (frequency); inability to sleep through the night (nocturia); the embarrassment of rushing to the bathroom (urgency); and the occasional urge incontinence. All of these are related to the irritative aspect of BPH. On the other hand, less bother is generally felt by patients as they watch their intermittent weak stream or take an extra minute to complete voiding once they reach the bathroom.

For many years, urologists have designed procedures to treat BPH, a condition of obstructive and irritative symptoms, that aim specifically to treat obstruction even though the irritative symptoms cause the majority of bother. The advent of thermal therapies has brought a new understanding of BPH symptoms. They prove that patients can be treated successfully in a minimally invasive way without necessarily resulting in TURP-like flow rates and detrusor pressures.

There is increasing evidence that the mechanism of action responsible for the therapeutic effect of TUNA is explained by intraprostatic neuromodulation, which alters the physiological function of voiding (dynamic component of BPH). Thermal neural ablation, including "surgical" α-receptor blockade has been demonstrated by various researchers.[28–30]

COST

The TUNA procedure is performed as an outpatient clinic procedure under pure local/regional anesthetic (prostatic block) without the need for general, spinal anesthesia or intravenous sedation. These criteria have been reported to dictate the true cost effectiveness of the procedure.[8,31] Utilization of the operating room, anesthesia team, recovery room and conscious sedation monitoring significantly increase the cost as well as challenge the concept of "minimally invasive therapy". A significant cost saving, in the range of 40–70%, is seen with the TUNA procedure when compared with other surgical treatments such as TURP.[8,31]

THE FUTURE

As with any new technology, further refinement in instrumentation and technique is expected in the future. As with all thermal therapies, combined research and development efforts will further improve efficacy and durability. Furthermore, additional widespread experience is expected to enhance patient selection for prediction and optimization of the results.

CONCLUSIONS

The currently available treatment options for symptomatic BPH show a profound gap between medical and surgical therapies. The simplicity and the convenience of medical therapies at one end have limited efficacy and are well distant from the highly invasive surgical therapies at the other end. The arrival of minimally invasive thermal therapies such as the TUNA has filled the gap between the two extremes of treatment options.

Transurethral needle ablation is an exciting new minimally invasive treatment for symptomatic BPH. The procedure is tolerated well by patients under regional prostatic block in a clinic setting without the need for hospitalization. The treatment has a particular role in elderly patients with high surgical risk. Furthermore, the lack of significant risks, specifically those of urinary incontinence and sexual dysfunction, makes this treatment more attractive than TURP for many patients.

ACKNOWLEDGEMENT

The authors would like to thank Ms Lois Elayne Miller, RN, Ms Katrina Anastasia, PA, and Mr Anthony Labadia, PA, for their contribution to the minimally invasive BPH therapy program at The Atlanta Veterans affairs Medical Center, Atlanta, GA. The authors also would like to thank Mr Douglas C. Durham, Mr Denis Roy, and Mr Peter Grattan at the Department of Medical Media, Atlanta Veterans affairs Medical Center, Atlanta, GA, for preparing the illustrations.

REFERENCES

1 Calkins H, Langberg J, Sousa J et al. Radiofrequency catheter ablation of accessory atrioventricular connections in 250 patients. Abbreviated therapeutic approach to Wolff–Parkinson–White syndrome. Circulation 1992; 85: 1337–46.

2 Organ LW. Electrophysiologic principles of radiofrequency lesion making. International Symposium on Radiofrequency Lesion Making Procedures, Chicago, Illinois, 1976. Appl Neurophysiol 1976; 39: 69–76.

3 Rasor JS, Zlotta AR, Edwards SD, Schulman CC. Transurethral needle ablation (TUNA): thermal gradient mapping and comparison of lesion size in a tissue model and in patients with benign prostatic hyperplasia. Eur Urol 1993; 24: 411–14.

4 Goldwasser B, Ramon J, Engleberg S et al. Transurethral needle ablation (TUNA) of the prostate using low-level radiofrequency energy: an animal experimental study. Eur Urol 1993; 24: 400–5.

5 Ramon J, Goldwasser B, Shenfeld O et al. Needle ablation using radiofrequency current as a treatment for benign prostatic hyperplasia: experimental results in ex vivo human prostate. Eur Urol 1993; 24: 406–410.

6 Schulman CC, Zlotta AR, Rasor JS et al. Transurethral needle ablation (TUNA): safety, feasibility, and tolerance of a new office procedure for treatment of benign prostatic hyperplasia. Eur Urol 1993; 24: 415–23.

7 Issa MM, Kabalin JN. Transurethral needle ablation of the prostate: report of initial United States clinical trial. J Urol 1995; 153(4): 535A (abstract 1226).

8 Issa MM, Oesterling JE. Transurethral needle ablation of the prostate (TUNA™): an overview of radiofrequency thermal therapy for the treatment of benign prostatic hyperplasia. Curr Opin Urol 1996; 6: 20–7.

9 Issa MM. Transurethral needle ablation of the prostate: report of initial United States clinical trial. J Urol 1996; 156: 413–19.

10 Heaton JPW. Radiofrequency thermal ablation of the prostate: the TUNA* technique. Techniques Urol 1995; 1(1): 3–10.

11 Schulman CC, Zlotta, AR. Transurethral needle ablation of the prostate for treatment of benign prostatic hyperplasia: early clinical experience. Urology 1994; 45: 28–33.

12 Campo B, Bergamaschi F, Ordesi G et al. TUNA in BPH patients: urodynamic assessment at 18th month followup. J Urol 1996; 155(5): 403A (abstract 371).

13 Lynch TH, Eardley I, Frick J et al. Transurethral needle ablation for the treatment of symptomatic benign prostatic hyperplasia. J Urol 1996; 155(5): 709A (abstract 1591).

14 Rosario DJ, Woo HH, Byrne L et al. 12 month follow-up of the safety and efficacy of TransUrethral Needle Ablation (TUNA™). J Urol 1996; 155(5): 705A (abstract 1575).

15 Oesterling JE, Issa MM, Roehrborn CG et al. A single blind, prospective randomized clinical trial comparing transurethral needle ablation (TUNA™) to transurethral resection of the prostate (TURP) for the treatment of benign prostatic hyperplasia (BPH). J Urol 1996; 15(5): 403A (abstract 372).

16 Bruskewitz R, Issa MM, Roehrhorn CG et al. A prospective, randomized 1-year clinical trial comparing transurethral needle ablation (TUNA) to transurethral resection of the prostate for the treatment of symptomatic benign prostatic hyperplasia. J Urol 1998; 159: 1588–94.

17 Roehrhorn CG, Issa MM, Bruskewitz R et al. Transurethral needle ablation (TUNA) for benign prostatic hyperplasia: 12-month results of a prospective, multicenter US study. Urology 1998; 51: 415–21.

18 Schulman CC, Zlotta AR. Transurethral needle ablation (TUNA) of the prostate: clinical experience with 3 years follow-up in patients with benign prostatic hyperplasia (BPH). Eur Urol 1998; 33 (Suppl 1): 586.

19 Virdi JS, Pandit A, Rajagopalan S. Transurethral needle ablation of the prostate (TUNA). Eur Urol 1998; 33 (Suppl 1): 9.

20 Campo B, Bergamaschi F, Corrada P, Ordesi G. Transurethral needle ablation (TUNA) of the prostate: a clinical and urodynamic evaluation. Urology 1997; 49: 847–50.

21 Ramon J, Lynch TH, Early I *et al*. Transurethral needle ablation of the prostate for the treatment of benign prostatic hyperplasia: a collaborate multicenter study. *Br J Urol* 1997; **80**(1): 128–35.

22 Chapple CR, Rosario KJ, Hastie KJ *et al*. The long term follow-up of patients undergoing TUNA. *Eur Urol* 1996; **30**(2): 983.

23 Giennakopoulos X, Grammeniatis E, Gartzios A *et al*. Transurethral needle ablation (TUNA) of the prostate: preliminary results using the new generation TUNA III catheter on patients with symptomatic BPH controlled by a series of 50 patients using TUNA II device. *Eur Urol* 1996; **30**(2): 986.

24 Steele GS, Sleep DJ. Transurethral needle ablation of the prostate: a urodynamic based study with two year follow-up. *J Urol* 1997; **158**(5): 1834–8.

25 Millard RJ, Harewood LM, Tamaddon K. A study of the efficacy and safety of transurethral needle ablation (TUNA) for benign prostatic hyperplasia. *Neurol Urodynamic* 1996; **15**: 916–29.

26 Harewood LM, Laurence KC, O'Connell HE, Pope AJ. Transurethral needle ablation of the prostate (TUNA): clinical results and ultrasound, endoscopic, and histologic findings in pilot study of patients in urinary retention. *J Endourol* 1995; **9**: 407–12.

27 Zlotta AR, Peny MO, Matos C, Schulman CC. Transurethral needle ablation of the prostate: clinical experience in patients in urinary retention. *Brit J Urol* 1996; **77**: 391–7.

28 Issa MM, Wojno KJ, Pilat MJ *et al*. Histopathologic and biochemical study of the prostate following transurethral needle ablation (TUNA); insight to the mechanism of improvement in BPH symptoms. *J Endourol* 1996; **10**: 109.

29 Schulman CC, Zlotta AR. Possible mechanism of action of transurethral needle ablation of the prostate on benign prostatic hyperplasia: a neurohistochemical study. *J Urol* 1997; **157**: 894–9.

30 Peranchino M, Bozzo W, Puppo P *et al*. Does transurethral thermotherapy induce a long-term alpha blockade? An immunohistochemical study. *Eur Urol* 1993; **23**: 299–301.

31 Naslund MJ. A cost comparison of TUNA vs. TURP. *J Urol* 1997; **157**(4): 155.

COMMENTARY

Various forms of minimally invasive therapy have recently emerged, the majority of which are in the field of thermotherapy. These therapies utilize various energies such as RF, microwave, laser, and high-intensity ultrasound to achieve tissue coagulative necrosis inside the prostate. Irrespective of the type of energy employed, the final objective is to heat the prostate to a desired temperature of over 45°C. In general, thermotherapy with temperatures in the range of 45–55°C causes limited tissue ablation, often with insufficient success. Thermotherapies, on the other hand, with temperature ranges between 60 and 95°C result in significant tissue ablation and successful outcomes. Transurethral needle ablation is one such type of therapy, which utilizes RF energy. RF energy is a unique form of energy, which can only be applied through proper tissue contact. Once all of the energy gets into tissue, it is transformed into thermoenergy through inductive heating of water molecules as well as friction. The extent of heat dissipation is limited and is determined by the amount of tissue contact, wattage power, and duration of therapy. This allows the following advantages: targeted tissue ablation, precise ablation, and customized ablation. While the TUNA therapy has been used in the past for treatment of other conditions, its maximal experience has been in the field of BPH. The TUNA system consists of an energy generator and endoscopic instrumentation to deliver energy into the prostate. The energy delivery is performed in an automated fashion, using a computer-designed software program with a "rise time" of 4 min which allows gradual gradation of temperature from room temperature to between 75 and 95°C at the core of ablation. A "hold time" of 1.5 min allows the target temperature to be maintained sufficiently long to achieve the desired therapeutic ablation. The machine has automated safety features and also allows for urethral cooling, which is thought to be one of the key features in avoiding postoperative edema and prolonged retention. The mechanism of TUNA efficacy is believed to be tissue coagulative necrosis, which results in scarring, softening, and a decrease in volume of the prostate. However, histopathologic lesions also show that there are α-andrenergic and nitrinergic receptors that are thermally damaged following the TUNA procedure. This may be a significant mechanism by which this technique produces relief of symptoms.

The TUNA needles and the technique of insertion are designed to maximize treatment of the adenomatous portion, while the safety features of the ultrasound measurement prior to the therapy prevents damage of periprostatic structures. The anesthesia requirement during TUNA is variable and depends on the urologist's, as well as the patient's, preference. The procedure can be done under combined topical and regional anesthesia or some may prefer spinal or general anesthesia. In the Editor's experience, the TUNA procedure can be done in over 50% of patients using a combination of local and prostatic block anesthesia. This reduces operative costs by limiting operating room and anesthesia charges, while allowing treatment in a friendly, ambulatory setting.

With regard to the TUNA results, the average symptom improvement is 58% in 1 year, 60% in 2 years, and 66% in 3 years (see Table 21.1). The results shown in Table 21.1 are statistically significant compared with baseline, and surpass placebo results of 30%. Additionally, the bother and quality-of-life scores also improve in a comparison of TUNA with TURP. The improvement in peak flow rate is also in the range of 60–80%, although there is some variability in these results, depending on the series. However, the overall improvement in peak flow rate when comparing 546 patients in 10 series is 77% at 1 year, 82% at 2 years, and 93% at 3 years. There are currently no convincing data that prostate size is significantly reduced following TUNA. Several studies have addressed the results of pressure flow after transurethral needle ablation. These studies have found that the reduction in DMP during voiding is equivocal after TUNA.

The Editor's experience with the TUNA technique, which was recently published, is as follows: we treated large prostates with an average size of 48 cm^3 (range 20–185 cm^3). The IPSS decreased from a mean of 20.9 at baseline to 16.1 at 3 months and 9.9 at 1 year. The peak flow rate improved from a baseline of 8.3 to 14.9 at 1 year and the quality-of-life from baseline at 4.8 to 1.03 at 12 months. In two patients the procedure failed: one had reported a bladder neck incision at 3 months and the other a transuretheral resection. Foley catheters were left in place in all patients for an average of 4.85 days. Owing to the larger prostate size and the four-quadrant technique that we used, the duration of treatment was 79 min on average.

The side effects of the procedure have been urinary retention, which ranges from 13 to 41%. However, in most series the retention is transient and lasts only 1–2 days. The irritative symptoms following TUNA procedures were also less than after laser procedures and lasted for a shorter duration in the range of 1–2 weeks. Bleeding was rare. The Editor has performed the TUNA procedure in patients who are on Coumadin and aspirin without having to stop the therapy for any period of time. Most important, the incidence of erectile dysfunction, impotence, and incontinence is very rare following the TUNA procedure.

As with any new technology, further refinement in instrumentation and technique continues to occur with the TUNA procedure. Currently the problems that remain include the need for a preoperative ultrasound, which increases costs, and the requirement for a special endoscopic TUNA device instead of standard cystostophic equipment, the lack of visualization of the entry points of the needle during needle placement and, finally, the time required for treatment, which is 30–40 min. However, the efficacy of the technology has been established; it has lower capital costs than laser, does not require laser precautions, and may in fact have better durability and long-term results because of the higher volume of tissue treated compared with interstitial laser.

Transurethral Thermotherapy

P. Narayan and A. Tewari

22

INTRODUCTION

Although transurethral resection of the prostate (TURP) is considered the gold standard for surgical treatment of benign prostatic hyperplasia (BPH), there is a small but significant incidence of impotence, incontinence, bleeding, fluid overload, and retrograde ejaculation associated with this procedure. In most instances, patients undergoing TURP also stay overnight, adding to its costs. Because of the higher morbidity and costs associated with TURP, newer modalities such as transurethral needle ablation (TUNA), thermotherapy, lasers, the VaporTrode, and stents have been developed.

Thermotherapy recently received Food and Drug Administration approval and is appealing to many urologists primarily because of its ease of use, minimal morbidity, and impressive safety profile compared with TURP. The object of microwave hyperthermia has been to produce heat-induced tissue damage in neoplasms that cannot augment their blood supply in response to heat-induced stress. Microwave hyperthermia for BPH can be performed by the transurethral route or the transrectal route, but transurethral thermotherapy is more effective than the transrectal form. Regardless of this, in both techniques, the tissues closest to the microwave probe (prostatic urethra and rectal mucosa) are cooled to prevent tissue damage while the microwave heat is maximized to the area of the transition zone. The object is to achieve a temperature greater than 45°C at the transition zone. Results from several studies using transurethral thermotherapy indicate that 62% of patients have improvement in symptom scores and 74% have improvement in urinary flow.

SCIENTIFIC FOUNDATION

Most minimally invasive therapies use heat to destroy tissue. Heat destruction can be achieved by high-frequency current, radiofrequency (RF) current, laser beams, microwaves, or ultrasonic heating. When treating prostatic and most other tissues, the lesions created depend on the intensity of heat delivered, the rapidity with which it is deposited in tissues, and the surface area in which it is deposited. In general, low-level heat applied to large volumes of tissue causes coagulation, while high-intensity heat deposited rapidly in small volumes of tissue will cause vaporization. Table 17.1 in

Chapter 17 shows tissue changes that occur when heat is applied at various temperatures.

Minimally invasive procedures that cause vaporization achieve temperatures over several hundred degrees at the tissue. Minimally invasive procedures that cause coagulation reach temperatures between 45 and 100°C. The closer the temperatures are to 100°C, the higher the degree of coagulation and better the tissue ablation.

Thermotherapy was designed to apply microwave energy deep within the lateral prostatic lobes, while simultaneously cooling the urethral mucosa. Many thermotherapy devices have been developed for treatment of BPH. Most experience is available with the Prostatron device (see Figures 22.1–22.3), which has been used with three software programs with different features, as will be discussed later. Version 2.0 is the most widely used software, and the results achieved for symptomatic improvement and changes in urinary performance were encouraging. Since clinical outcome could possibly be enhanced with higher intraprostatic temperatures, resulting in enhanced thermal ablation and, thus, cavity formation, modifications to the operating software have been made. Early reports (discussed later in this chapter) on this high-energy software version (Prostasoft 2.5) show a good subjective response and excellent improvement in the objective parameters.

MECHANISM OF ACTION

Microwaves are transverse electromagnetic waves with frequencies in the 30–300 Hz range. These electromagnetic waves travel in a given medium and are reflected or scattered by media with differences in impedance.

Microwaves heat by transferring energy to cause the displacement or drift of free charge, polarization of atoms and molecules, and orientational polarization of existing dipoles. This kinetic energy raises the temperature of tissues. The amount of energy absorbed by the prostate is dependent on its size and shape, composition (i.e. glandular vs. stroma), vascularity, frequency, intensity of the microwaves, and the size and shape of the applicator. As the frequency and size of the microwave increases, the depth of tissue penetration decreases.

The first devices heated the prostate from 42 to 44°C using a transrectal probe. The International Consensus Conference on BPH in 1991 defined hyperthemia as no higher than 44°C. Owing to the disappointing results, a transurethral catheter was developed that offers more predictable and direct energy to the prostate. Results with this route improved, but up to 10 sessions lasting 30–60 min each were needed. Also, temperatures were still not high enough to achieve cellular toxicity and demonstrable histologic changes within the prostate.

With the development of catheters that could simultaneously cool the urethral mucosa, higher intraprostatic temperatures could be reached. With higher temperatures, usually one treatment lasting 60 min was all that was needed to achieve objective and subjective improvement. This newer technology was called thermotherapy, and intraprostatic temperatures in excess of 45°C were achieved.

A popular microwave device used today is the Prostatron. The Prostatron catheter employs a combination of radiative microwave heating and superficial urethral cooling. The Prostatron's components include a power oscillator, urethral cooling system, temperature-monitoring system, and a control console. The position of the urethral catheter is checked with ultrasound imaging. A probe placed in the rectum is used to measure rectal wall temperatures. The microwave energy levels and cooling system are both controlled by a software program responding to present temperatures in the urethra and rectum. The cooling fluid that circulates in the treatment catheter maintains the temperature of the urethra within a normal range, usually lower than 44.5°C. This prevents pain, necrosis, and bleeding of the urethra while the prostatic tissue deeper within the gland reaches temperatures as high as 70°C.

Simultaneous urethral cooling allows this procedure to be performed under local anesthesia. The entire procedure lasts approximately 1 h. Because of disappointing results with the 2.0, software that provides a maximum power of 70 W was developed. Rectal threshold temperatures are set at 43.5°C. It is believed the rectal wall is protected by its excellent blood supply, which dissipates heat. During transurethral microwave thermotherapy (TUMT) extraprostatic temperatures in the first 0.8 cm outward from the applicator have been found to drop at a rate of 6 to 7°C per centimeter. At distances of 0.8–1.2 cm, temperatures decrease at 3–5°C per centimeter. Periprostatic and rectal wall temperatures were found not to exceed 39.5°C.

The mechanism by which thermotherapy improves symptomatology is not entirely understood. Thermotherapy has been shown to produce coagulation necrosis of the prostate at distances of up to 17 mm from the urethra, with preservation of the urethral surface and periprostatic structures. In a study by de Wildt and associates,[1] high-energy thermoablation effects of TUMT caused an average prostatic volume reduction of 10.5 mL (=3.5 mL) at 52 weeks. Additionally, at 3 months, a cavity similar to one that develops following TURP was observed in 43% of patients. The presence of a cavity was positively correlated with improvement in urinary performance and relief of bladder outlet obstruction.

Another possible mechanism responsible for improvement in symptomatology is the destruction of the sympathetic nerve fibers. Perachino[23] performed TUMT in 10 patients prior to prostatectomy and demonstrated damage and disappearance of neural tissue.

In another study of 157 patients with BPH who were treated with TUMT; they performed histological studies on enucleated prostates after TUMT. Their study revealed degenerative changes of the nerve fibers upon immunohistochemical staining. Furthermore, in another study using rabbit prostates, examination *in vitro* revealed that the isometric contraction force of the prostatic tissue, measured after exposure to various temperatures (ranging from 37°C to 50°C), did not change with increased temperature until reaching 46°C. At 48°C and higher, the nerve-mediated contractions became completely depressed; however, the phenylephrine and KCl-induced contraction were only partially suppressed. After reaching a temperature of 50°C, no contractions were induced by any type of stimuli. From these findings, the investigators conclude that good symptomatic improvement after TUMT results from both neural and muscular damage to the prostate. Furthermore, magnetic resonance imaging (MRI) findings on men who have undergone TUMT show that the prostate undergoes a hemorrhagic necrosis (with apoptosis), which is eventually absorbed within 12 weeks, resulting in a widened prostatic urethra.[3]

TRANSURETHRAL MICROWAVE THERMOTHERAPY CLINICAL STUDIES

In a study conducted in Europe, 32 patients with BPH were enrolled to evaluate the clinical outcome of TUMT (Prostcare device at 915 MHz) treatment, and they were followed postoperatively for 12 months.[4] The Madsen symptom score decreased from a baseline value of 13.5 points to 2.9 after 12 months of having the microwave treatment; this was a statistically significant difference ($P<0.001$). The peak urinary flow rate also improved from 10.0 mL s^{-1} before treatment to 17.1 mL s^{-1} after treatment, showing a significant difference ($P<0.001$). The authors stated that in this study, 78% of the patients were satisfied with their microwave therapy.

Similar results were obtained in another US trial, where 78 men with symptomatic BPH were treated with microwave (Prostatron 2.0) and followed-up for 3 months.[5] There was a decrease in the AUA symptom score from 19.6 at baseline to 11.2 at the 3-month postoperative period ($P<0.0001$). The peak urinary flow rate improved from a baseline value of 8.5 mL s^{-1} to 12.8 mL s^{-1} at 3 months, resulting in a 50.5% improvement ($P<0.0001$). Mean postvoid residual volume decreased from 56.8 mL to 22.0 mL ($P<0.0001$). These results are somewhat misleading because the investigators did not use a sham-controlled study.

In a study conducted by de Wildt, 74 patients showed a 58% improvement in peak urinary flow rate and the Madsen symptom scores from baseline at 1-year follow-up; there was a 33% improvement in peak flow rate, and the mean symptom scores improved by 60% (Tables 22.1 and 22.2).[1,6] Patients with bigger prostate glands (>40 g) and patients

Study	Device used	No of patients enrolled	Duration of study	Baseline symptom score	Symptom score (% improvement)					
					at ≤2 months	at 3 months	at 6 months	at 1 year	at 2 years	at ≥4 years
Blute et al. 1993	Prostatron 2.0	150	12 months	13.7	–	–	4.1 (70.1)	5.4 (61)	–	–
Eliasson et al. 1998	Prostcare	32	12 months	13.5	–	5.5 (59)	3.8 (72)	2.9 (79)	–	–
Stravodimos et al. 1998	Prostatron 2.0	78	3 months	19.6	–	11.2 (43)	–	–	–	–
Glass et al. 1998	Leo Microthermer	67	48 months	10.18	–	–	7.3 (28.3)	–	6.45 (37)	–
Walden et al. 1998	Prostasoft 2.0	38	6 months	12.1	–	–	2.6 (78.5)	–	–	–
Hallin et al. 1998	Prostatron 2.0	187	4 years	12.2	–	–	–	5.9 (51.6)	7.1 (42)	7.7 (37)
Keijzers et al. 1998	Prostasoft 2.0	231	5 years	12.1	–	–	–	4.0 (67)	4.0 (67)	7.6 (37)[a]
Tubaro et al. 1993	Prostatron	144	12 months	11.73	8.39 (28.5)	4.9 (58)	4.4 (62.4)	4.2 (64)	–	–
Blute et al. 1992	Prostatron	60	3 months	13.9	6.2 (55.4)[b]	4.8 (65.5)	–	–	–	–
Van Cauwelaert et al. 1993	Prostatron	150	12 months	11.3	2.2 (80.5)	2.1 (81.4)[c]	–	Not reported	–	–
Lancaster et al. 1997	UroWave	93	12 months	22.66	–	–	–	11.94 (47.3)	–	–
Baba et al. 1996	Prostatron	135	2 years	18.2	–	11.7 (35.7)	10.6 (42)	10.6 (42)	10.1 (44.5)	–
Eliasson et al. 1995	Prostcare	172	12 months	12.7	–	7.0 (45)	6.9 (46)	6.6 (48)	–	–
de Wildt et al. 1996	Prostatron 2.5	85	12 months	13.9	–	6.7 (52)	5.7 (59)	5.8 (58.3)	–	–
de Wildt and D'Ancona et al. 1996	Prostasoft 2.0	305	3 years	12.9	–	–	–	5.6 (56.6)	6.1 (53)	8.1 (37.2)[d]
de la Rosette et al. 1996	Prostasoft 2.5	116	12 months	13.6	9.4 (31)	6.0 (56)	5.5 (59.6)	4.9 (69)	–	–
Ramsey et al. 1997	Targis Urologix	154	12 months	20.1	12.0 (40.3)	8.8 (56.2)	8.5 (57.7)	8.8 (56.2)	–	–

[a]at 5 years; [b]at 6 weeks; [c]at 4 months; [d]at 3 years

Table 22.1 Summary of symptom score results from different TUMT studies

Study	Device used	No of patients enrolled	Duration of study	Baseline Q_{max} (mL s^{-1})	Peak urinary flow rates (Q_{max}) (% improvement)					
					at ≤2 months	at 3 months	at 6 months	at 1 year	at 2 years	at ≥4 years
Blute et al. 1993	Prostatron 2.0	150	12 months	8.5	–	–	11.0 (29.4)	11.3 (33)	–	–
Eliasson et al. 1998	Prostcare	32	12 months	10.0	–	15.3 (53)	14.2 (42)	17.1 (71)	–	–
Stravodimos et al. 1998	Prostatron 2.0	78	3 months	8.5	–	12.8 (51)	–	–	–	–
Glass et al. 1998	Leo Microthermer	67	48 months	7.92	–	–	11.6 (32)	11.4 (31)	11.55 (31.4)	–
Walden et al. 1998	Prostasoft 2.0	38	6 months	8.4	–	–	11.7 (39)	–	–	–
Hallin et al. 1998	Prostatron 2.0	187	4 years	10.1	–	–	–	10.5 (−4)	–	8.2 (19)
Keijzers et al. 1998	Prostasoft 2.0	231	5 years	9.4	–	–	–	12.8 (36)	12.3 (31)	11.3 (20)[a]
Tubaro et al. 1993	Prostatron	144	12 months	8.97	–	12.6 (43)	13.1 (46)	13.3 (48)	–	–
Blute et al. 1992	Prostatron	60	3 months	8.9	11.6 (30.37)[b]	13.1 (47)	–	–	–	–
Van Cauwelaert et al. 1993	Prostatron	150	12 months	9.2	14.4 (56.5%)	14.9[c] (62)	–	Not reported	–	–
Lancaster et al. 1997	UroWAVE	93	12 months	8.23	–	–	–	11.33 (37.7)	–	–
Baba et al. 1996	Prostatron	135	2 years	8.3	–	10.2 (23)	10.3 (24.1)	11.2 (35)	11.8 (42.2)	–
Eliasson et al. 1995	Prostcare	172	12 months	9.8	–	10.3 (5.1)	10.7 (9.2)	10.9 (11.2)	–	–
de Wildt et al. 1996	Prostatron 2.5	85	12 months	9.4	–	15.8 (68.1)	14.4 (53.2)	14.9 (58.5)	–	–
de Wildt and D'Ancona et al. 1996	Prostasoft 2.0	305	3 years	9.1	–	–	–	11.4 (25.3)	11.2 (23.1)	11.9 (31)[d]
de la Rosette et al. 1996	Prostasoft 2.5	116	12 months	9.6	9.8 (2.1%)	15.2 (58.3)	14.1 (47)	14.5 (51)	–	–
Ramsey et al. 1997	Targis Urologix	154	12 months	9.3	11.9 (28%)	13.6 (46.2)	13.8 (48.4)	13.4 (44.1)	–	–

[a] at 5 years; [b] at 6 weeks; [c] at 4 months; [d] at 3 years

Table 22.2 Summary of peak urinary flow rate results from different TUMT studies

with more severe bladder outlet obstruction appeared to be the best responders.

The long-term results of Prostatron have not always been encouraging. In a recent study, Hallin and Berlin[7] reported the results of Prostatron TUMT treatment in 187 patients with a 4-year follow-up. Men who were not satisfied with the result of treatment were offered additional treatment, which reduced the number of patients during the follow-up period, resulting in only 56 patients after 4 years. In the 4-year follow-up period of these 56 men, the peak urinary flow rate decreased significantly from 10.1 mL s^{-1} at baseline to 8.2 mL s^{-1} after 48 months ($P=0.0141$). Furthermore, the total Madsen symptom score decreased significantly from 12.2 at baseline to 5.9 points at 12 months after the surgical procedure ($P<0.001$), but then increased to 7.7 points 48 months after treatment ($P<0.001$, but $P=0.0054$ when 12 months is compared with 48 months). According to the authors, they stated that this increase in total symptom score from 12 months to 48 months was mostly due to an increase in obstructive score (3.1 to 4.7, $P=0.001$), rather than irritative score (from 2.8 to 3.0, $P<0.001$). However, the number of satisfied patients noted at the 1-year follow-up period (62%) was significantly reduced after 4 years; only 23% of the TUMT-treated patients felt satisfied with their results after 4 years. Two-thirds of the initially treated patients had received supplementary BPH treatment. By using the Kaplan–Meier analysis, the authors estimated that the mean time for need of a supplemental BPH treatment was 45 months after having the TUMT procedure. Finally, the investigators concluded that patients with a preoperative peak urinary flow rate greater than 10 mL s^{-1} and an irritative score less than 5 were the best candidates for the TUMT procedure. Prostate volume or energy delivered to the prostate did not influence the results.

Similar 5-year results are noted by other authors who examined the long-term results of TUMT.[8] In the study by Keijzers *et al.*[8] 231 patients with BPH and lower urinary tract symptoms were treated with lower energy transurethral microwave thermotherapy (Prostasoft 2.0) and followed for 5 years. The Madsen symptom score decreased from 12.1 at baseline to 4.0 at 24 months, and then it increased to 7.6 at 5 years. The Madsen symptom score showed minimal fluctuation between the 12- and 24-month period. Furthermore, the peak urinary flow rate increased by approximately 3 mL s^{-1} from baseline at the 1-year follow-up period, and this improvement was consistently maintained for the next 4 years. Regardless of this, overall, 57% of the patients received additional treatment within 5 years of follow-up with 41% receiving invasive re-treatment and 17% receiving only pharmacologic therapy. Furthermore, the incidence of side effects from the TUMT was not trivial. Thirteen percent of the patients complained of erectile dysfunction, while 8% reported retrograde ejaculation, 8% had recurrent urinary tract infections, and only one patient had urethral stricture. Prostate volume did not modify the outcome. In conclusion, the investigators stated that patients older than 65 years of age with a preoperative Madsen symptom score

of less than 15, a postvoid residual volume of 100 mL or less, and a baseline peak urinary flow rate of greater than 10 mL s^{-1} are the better responders to low-energy TUMT procedure. Furthermore, the authors noticed that the risk of re-treatment occurred within the first 1–2 years after TUMT surgical treatment. In addition, the investigators concluded that patients younger than 65 years of age with high symptom scores, low peak flow rates, and high residual urine volumes have worse results after TUMT and, therefore, should be considered for invasive treatment.[8]

From these aforementioned clinical trials, it is evident that TUMT has an excellent effect on certain patients, while in others there is only a marginal effect. Therefore, it is important to determine the clinical factors of patients who are best suited for TUMT, and to define those variables that can predict a poor outcome. In a study conducted by Walden and associates,[9] they identified clinically predictive variables useful in selecting patients suitable for TUMT. In their study, 38 men with symptomatic BPH were enrolled and treated with TUMT. There was a significant improvement in the Madsen symptom score from 12.1 points at baseline to 2.6 points, 6 months after treatment. Moreover, the peak urinary flow rate increased from 8.4 mL s^{-1} to 11.7 mL s^{-1}, and the postvoid residual volume decreased from 97 mL to 66 mL. The investigators also noticed that TUMT significantly reduced bladder outlet obstruction, but the improvement in obstruction and peak flow rate was significantly less than that observed in TURP. Nonetheless, the investigators concluded that urodynamic evidence of obstruction was best correlated with improvements after TUMT.

Similar results were obtained by Glass and associates[10] in the UK. They conducted a long-term follow-up study of 4 years to examine the therapeutic value of TUMT in patients with symptomatic BPH. In this study, 67 patients were enrolled, and had undergone TUMT treatment. There was a significant improvement in the peak urinary flow rates from 7.9 mL s^{-1} at baseline to an increase of 11.6 mL s^{-1}, 3 months after TUMT; and this figure remained relatively stable after 48 months, at which the peak flow rate was 11.5 mL s^{-1} ($P<0.001$ at both time points). Furthermore, the Boyarsky symptom score significantly improved from a baseline value of 10.2 to 6.2 at the conclusion of the 4-year study ($P<0.02$). According to the authors, 58% of the patients who have undergone TUMT 4 years earlier were satisfied with their treatment, and of these satisfied patients, 55% had a greater than 50% reduction in their symptom scores. However, 31% of the patients had undergone another treatment for their BPH pathology. According to the authors, this 31% re-treatment rate at 4 years was greater than the re-treatment rate of 2% per year seen in TURP treatment.

The data from two TUMT studies have been separated and subgrouped into categories of responders and non-responders. The results are listed in Table 22.3. In one study, there was a 56% (77/139) response rate to microwave therapy; whereas the more recent study showed a 47% (136/292) success rate.

Study	Device used	Total No. of patients enrolled		Symptom score (% improvement)		Peak flow rate, Q_{max} (% improvement)	
				Baseline	After TUMT	Baseline (mL s^{-1})	After TUMT
de Wildt et al. 1995	Prostatron	292	136 Responders	13.7	3.2 (76.6)	8.8	16.0 (82)
			156 Non-responders	13.9	9.6 (31)	8.3	7.9 (−5)
Berg et al. 1993	Prostatron	139	77 Responders	12.9	3.74 (71)	9.14	17.46 (91)
			62 Non-responders	12.3	10.33 (16)	8.15	9.3 (14)

Table 22.3 TUMT data of responders vs. non-responders

THERMOTHERAPY VERSUS TRANSURETHRAL RESECTION

Published reports have shown thermotherapy to be a good alternative to TURP in the short term. However, in long-term follow-up more than 30% of patients require alternative surgical interventions. In a European study, D'Ancona and associates[11,12] compared the outcome of TURP and high-energy microwave thermotherapy in patients with BPH. Fifty-two men aged 54–89 years (average age 69) with BPH were randomized (thermotherapy-to-transurethral resection ratio 3:2) into the trial (Table 22.4).

Follow-up visits were scheduled at 3, 6, 12 and 24 months after treatment. Urodynamic investigation with pressure-flow study analysis was performed at baseline and 26 weeks after treatment. Ultrasound of the prostate was repeated at 12 and 52 weeks. All thermotherapy treatments were performed on an outpatient basis using the Prostatron device, and treatment duration was 60 min with increasing thermal dose up to 70 W. Before treatment, a 100-mg diclofenac suppository was administered and 2 mg midazolam was injected intramuscularly. During treatment, no additional anesthesia was given but, if necessary, intravenous sedation was administered when patients experienced major discomfort, which was mostly expressed as an intense urge to void that sometimes was combined with an urge to defecate. All patients were given a urethral catheter with a leg bag immediately after treatment.

TURP was performed using standard techniques. Statistical analysis was done with Wilcoxon's test for paired samples and the Mann–Whitney 2-sample U-test for independent samples (non-parametric). No statistically significant difference was found between the pretreatment measures and scores of the two groups. At baseline, 52 patients entered the study, of which 31 underwent thermotherapy and 21 underwent TURP. At 1 year of follow-up, 44 patients were available for analysis. Mean operative time was 51 min (range 35–70) with a mean resected weight of 32 g (range 8–100). At 12 months, 2 patients failed in the TUMT group and 2 in the TURP group. At 12 months the mean Madsen symptom score improved by 84% for the transurethral resection group and by 68% for the

thermotherapy group. Mean maximum flow rate improved significantly from 9.3 mL s^{-1} at baseline to 17.1 mL s^{-1} at 12 months in the TUMT group, while the TURP group showed an improvement from 9.3 mL s^{-1} at baseline to 19.3 mL s^{-1}. For the thermotherapy group, a prolonged need for catheterization was noted compared with the transurethral resection group (mean 12.7 vs. 4.1 days, median 8 vs. 4, respectively). The thermotherapy group also had a greater incidence of urinary tract infections, frequently in combination with irritative voiding complaints. When evaluating the changes in urodynamics in the transurethral resection group, according to the Abrams–Griffiths nomogram, 76% of patients in the transurethral resection group and 62% in the thermotherapy group were considered to have obstruction before treatment, while at 6 months 15 and 40%, respectively, were still considered to have obstruction.

In another European study, Dahlstrand and associates[13] compared TURP with TUMT. TURP was performed in 32 patients (mean age 70 years) and TUMT in 37 (mean age 67 years). After both treatments, there was an improvement in symptom score, residual urine volume, and flow rate. Cystometry and pressure flowmetry were repeated after 6 months. During treatment, the urethral temperature was allowed to reach a maximum of 44.5°C and the rectal temperature a maximum of 42.5°C. The treatment was given in a single session as an out-patient procedure. With the exception of intraurethrally applied lidocaine hydrochloride jelly (Xylocaine® 2%, Astra, Sweden) no anesthesia was used. If the patient voided adequately after treatment he was discharged. If not, a Foley urethral catheter was placed and left for 1–7 days. The mean operation time for the TURP was 49 min, and the resection weight 17 g. The mean blood volume lost was 282 mL, but no blood transfusions were given. The mean duration of hospital stay was 3.9 days. Early complications in the TURP group were reoperation due to bleeding or to remove clots (3 patients). In the TUMT group, 5 patients could not void after the treatment and were catheterized for 1–7 days. One patient had transient rectal pain in the perineum. Late complications (>1 week after treatment) in the TURP group were urethral stricture (2 patients) and meatal stenosis (2 patients) requiring internal urethrotomy or meatotomy, respectively.

Study	No. of patients enrolled		Symptom score (% improvement)					Peak flow rate (Q_{max}) (% improvement)				
			Baseline	at 3 months	at 6 months	at 12 months	at 24 months	Baseline (mL s⁻¹)	at 3 months	at 6 months	at 12 months	at 24 months
Dahlstrand et al. 1993	79	39 TUMT	11.2	2.3 (79.5)	3.1 (72.3)	2.7 (76)	–	8.0	12.2 (52.5)	12.0 (50)	12.3 (53.8)	–
		40 TURP	13.3	1.6 (88)	0.9 (93.2)	0.9 (93.2)	–	7.9	18.7 (137)	18.8 (138)	17.7 (124)	–
Dahlstrand et al. 1995	69	37 TUMT	12.1	2.9 (76)	2.6 (78.5)	2.2 (82)	2.3 (81)	8.6	11.6 (35)	11.8 (37.2)	12.6 (46.5)	12.3 (43)
		32 TURP	13.6	1.7 (87.5)	1.1 (92)	0.6 (95.6)	1.2 (91.2)	8.6	18.1 (110)	18.6 (116)	18.9 (120)	17.6 (105)
Ahmed et al. 1997	60	30 TUMT	18.5	–	5.3 (71.4)	–	–	10.1	–	9.1 (–10)	–	–
		30 TURP	18.4	–	5.2 (71.7)	–	–	9.5	–	14.6 (53.7)	–	–
D'Ancona et al. 1998	52	31 TUMT	13.3	5.2 (61)	4.4 (67)	4.2 (68.4)	5.8 (56.4)[a]	9.3	15.5 (67)	17.0 (83)	17.1 (84)	15.1 (62.4)[a]
		21 TURP	13.8	3.6 (74)	2.5 (82)	2.7 (80.4)	3.6 (74)[a]	9.3	19.6 (111)	15.3 (64.5)	19.3 (108)	19.1 (105.4)[a]

[a]at 30 weeks

Table 22.4 Comparison of symptom scores and peak flow rates after TUMT to that of TURP-treated patients

Urinary tract infection occurred in 5 and 4 patients in the TUMT and TURP groups, respectively. After 6 months, 4 patients in the TUMT group were not satisfied and 2 underwent TURP, while the other 2 had a repeat session of TUMT. However, the latter two patients did not improve satisfactorily and underwent TURP after the 1-year follow-up. One patient in the TURP group underwent reoperation after 1 year because of bladder neck sclerosis. In both groups, improvements were noted at 3 weeks and maintained at 24 months. In the TUMT group of 31 patients, 26 of them had a >50% reduction in the symptom score at the 2-year follow-up. In the TURP group of 30 patients, 29 of them had a >50% reduction of symptom score at the 2-year follow-up. There was no significant difference in symptom score at 2 years between the treatments. In the TUMT group, the maximum flow rate was 12.3 mL s^{-1} at the 2-year follow-up period ($P<0.001$). There was no significant difference in residual urine at 2 years between the treatments. When pressure-flow measurement was repeated at the 6-month period, the detrusor pressure at maximum flow rate had decreased from 70 to 67 cmH$_2$O in the TUMT group (NS), and from 75 to 36 ($P<0.001$) in the TURP group. The urethral resistance factor decreased from 1.6–2.1 to 1.1–1.5 ($P<0.01$) in the TUMT group, and from 1.9 to 0.1 ($P<0.001$) in the TURP group. In the TUMT group, 26 of 35 patients had a urethral resistance factor of <1.0 at the 2-year follow-up and in the TURP group, 29 of 30 had a urethral resistance factor <1.0. After treatment, erection was preserved in all patients in both groups; half of the patients who had antegrade ejaculation before TURP developed retrograde ejaculation after the operation, compared with none in the TUMT group. In the TUMT group, the prostate volume decreased from 33.9 to 30.3 at 2 years (NS), and in the TURP group from 36.8 to 22.5 at 2 years ($P<0.001$).

Although it is well established that objective improvement is less pronounced than that resulting from TURP, overall symptomatic improvement does occur in TUMT. In a randomized study comparing TURP with thermotherapy, Dahlstrand[13] showed better improvement in peak urinary flow rate at 24 months for TURP (104% vs. 43%, respectively). However, symptomatic improvement was fairly equal for patients undergoing thermotherapy and those in the TURP group (81% and 91%, respectively) There were no serious complications in the thermotherapy group other than transient urinary retention in 5 of 37 patients, which lasted fewer than 7 days. In the TURP group, 3 of 32 patients required reoperation for bleeding or to remove clots. Two patients developed a urethral stricture, and another 2 patients developed meatal stenosis. No patient had retrograde ejaculation in the thermotherapy group.

In a recent study done by D'Ancona and associates,[11] they examined the long-term results of thermotherapy to the results obtained from TURPs by enrolling 52 patients with BPH who were then randomized and treated with either TURP ($n=21$ patients with a mean prostatic volume of 45 mL) or high-energy TUMT ($n=31$ patients with mean prostatic volume of 43 mL). Each patient underwent a follow-up examination 2 years after the surgical procedure.

Before undergoing the procedure, 67% of the patients in the TUMT group were obstructed and, after surgery, 33% remained obstructed. In the TURP group, 78% of the patients were obstructed prior to surgery, and only 14% were obstructed after surgical treatment. During the follow-up visit, the mean symptomatic improvement stabilized at 56% after TUMT and 74% after TURP. The peak urinary flow rates increased by 62% after TUMT and 105% after TURP. The investigators concluded that both forms of treatment show good symptomatic and objective results when followed-up after 2 years or more. Most re-treatments were performed at 1 year or more after surgical treatment. The authors mentioned that 6 patients (19%) who had originally undergone TUMT had to undergo TURP to achieve satisfactory results; four of them were done after a 1-year duration of having had the TUMT. However, 3 patients were not satisfied with the outcome after the additional TURP.

THERMOTHERAPY VERSUS SHAM-CONTROLLED EXPERIMENTS

In one of the first published reports, de la Rosette and associates[14] compared patients undergoing TUMT with a sham-operated group. At the 6-month follow-up in 17 patients, the mean maximum flow improved by 59%, and the mean symptom score decreased by 76%. Whereas, in the sham-operated group, the peak-flow rates improved by a mean of 4% and the symptom scores improved by 44% at the 6-month follow-up.

In a study by Larson and associates,[15] they examined the effectiveness, safety, and impact on the patient quality of life of the TUMT system in the management of BPH. In this study, 169 patients were enrolled and were then randomized to receive either 1 h of microwave (Urologix Targis) treatment ($n=125$) or sham ($n=44$) procedure. The AUA symptom score 6 months after having the microwave treatment diminished by 50% compared with the baseline values, from 20.8 to 10.5 ($P<0.0005$). The sham-treated group also experienced a decrease in the AUA scores, but not to the magnitude of the microwave-treated group ($P<0.01$). Fifty percent of the patients in the microwave-treated group had an AUA score of less than 9 by 6 months. The peak urinary flow rates in the microwave group also showed an improvement at 6 months; there was a 51% increase in the flow rate from 7.8 mL s^{-1} at baseline to 11.8 mL s^{-1} at 6 months ($P<0.0005$). The magnitude of the post-procedural increase in peak urinary flow rate was significantly greater in the microwave than the sham group ($P<0.05$). Furthermore, 47% of the microwave-treated patients had an increase of 50% or more in the urinary flow rate at a postoperative period of 6 months compared with only 24% of the sham group. The microwave treatment also showed a more positive impact on the patient quality-of-life score than did the sham procedure at 6 months postoperatively; the score decreased by 48% from a baseline score of 4.2 to 2.2 at 6 months in the microwave-treated patients ($P<0.0005$, but $P<0.05$ in microwave vs. sham). Moreover,

98.4% of the microwave-treated patients, compared with 83.3% of the sham group, did not require any additional treatment during their 6-month study.

In a recent study conducted by Roehrborn and associates,[16] 220 patients with BPH were enrolled to examine the efficacy of TUMT in a randomized, double-blind, multicenter sham-controlled protocol and followed for a 6-month period. The AUA symptom score improved by 46% in the TUMT group in comparison with the sham group, which showed only a 25% improvement; these differences were not only significantly different from baseline values ($P<0.05$), but also in-between groups ($P<0.05$). The peak urinary flow rate in the TUMT group showed an improvement of 3.0 mL s^{-1} during the 6-month follow-up period, while the sham group showed a 1.7 mL s^{-1} improvement rate; this is a significant difference between the two groups ($P<0.05$). See Table 22.5 for further details.

HIGH-ENERGY (2.5) AND LOW-ENERGY (2.0) THERMOTHERAPY

Using higher-energy thermotherapy (Prostatron software 2.5), investigators have shown a TURP-like prostatic defect on ultrasonography in 42% of the patients. With the use of higher energy, however, the associated risks and complications also increase. Higher energy results in nearly all patients requiring temporary Foley catheter drainage secondary to postoperative swelling. In protocols using the new high-energy machines, average increases in total energy were 40% greater, achieving temperatures of near 75°C, and creating tissue necrosis and cavity formation or thermoablation. Higher-energy output and treatment of the bladder neck resulted in better long-term objective improvement, but a larger percentage of patients experienced retrograde ejaculation.

de la Rosette and associates[17] have found that the Prostatron 2.5 protocol is best suited for patients with larger prostates (>50 g) and with moderate-to-severe bladder outlet obstruction. Based on a study involving TUMT treatment of 340 patients with BPH, Devonec et al.[18] have concluded that the prostate gland of a young patient requires a higher thermal dose than that of an older patient with the same prostate volume in order to achieve a comparable intraprostatic temperature. The transition zone, the origin of BPH in the majority of cases, is more sensitive to heat than the peripheral zone. Furthermore, the acinar cells in the prostate are more resistant to heat than the smooth muscle cells. From these findings, the Prostatron 2.5 system may be appropriate for only a selected number of patients who fit the above criteria, and maybe this will reduce the overall incidence of adverse events that is evident with the 2.5 version.

In one study comparing the low-energy with high-energy TUMT, the results show that improvement in objective parameters, such as the Madsen symptom scores, are similar, regardless of the energy software used (see Table 22.6).[19] However, there was a significant difference in the improvement seen in peak urinary flow rates of men who had undergone high-energy TUMT in comparison with low-energy TUMT; there was a 53% improvement in comparison with 37% improvement observed at the 6-month postoperative period, respectively. There was also significant difference in the improvement of residual urine volume in the Prostatron 2.5-treated patients in relation to the Prostatron 2.0-treated group. None the less, there is a downside of using the high-energy software program. In this same study, there was a higher rate of morbidity in terms of treatment pain, retrograde ejaculation (2.5 vs. 2.0; 44% vs. 0.1%), and postoperative urinary retention (2.5 vs. 2.0; 49% vs. 22%) with the use of the TUMT 2.5 version.

These similar clinical results were obtained from the study done by Perrin and associates.[20] There was no statistical difference between the two energy groups in terms of symptom score, but a significant difference was observed in favor of the 2.5 version when comparing peak urinary flow rates (Table 22.6).

WHICH DEVICE IS BETTER?

A recent study done by Larson and associates examined the efficacy and safety of two microwave antennae used in TUMT, namely the Prostatron (Technomed Medical Systems, Inc.) and the Targis (Urologix, Inc.) (see Figures 22.1–22.4).[15] Their study showed that the Targis microwave antenna provided more targeted heating pattern than the Prostatron device. The Targis antennae generated a focused, symmetrical heating pattern in the phantom-tissue experiments. In contrast, the Prostatron antennae produced an asymmetrical heating pattern in addition to "back heating" along the catheter, thus causing unwanted heating of structures located outside the prostate gland, such as the external sphincter.[15] The investigators believe that the observed "back-heating" (heat that is gradually moving retrogradely up the catheter) with the use of the Prostatron antennae may account for the high incidence of pain felt by the patient during treatment with the Prostatron TUMT system. Moreover, the Prostatron antennae's inability to target thermal energy exclusively to the prostate may explain the high incidence of retrograde ejaculation and other adverse sexual events that are experienced with TUMT use. This same study was reproduced by Bolmsjo et al.[21] in their study; it was found that the Prostatron and Prostcare devices cause a significant amount of "back-heating", causing heat damage to the region surrounding the targeted area.

In another study, Devonec and associates[18] examined and compared the different versions of Prostasoft TUMT systems. The three protocols deliver increasing thermal doses, Prostasoft T-A>Prostasoft II>Prostasoft I Moreover, the effects of microwave heating on the prostate tissue is shown to be a dose-dependent response; the greater the total power applied, the greater the achieved temperature within the prostate and larger histological lesions observed. Thermocoagulation is observed at temperature greater than 45°C, and thermoablation at temperatures greater than 60°C. The intraprostatic temperatures when using the

Study	Device used	No. of patients enrolled		Symptom score (% improvement)				Peak flow rate, Q_{max} (% improvement)			
				Baseline	at 3 months	at 6 months	at 12 months	Baseline (mL s⁻¹)	at 3 months	at 6 months	at 12 months
de la Rosette et al. 1994	Prostasoft 2.0	50	25 TUMT	13.2	5.9 (55)	3.2 (76)	3.3 (75)	9.6	13.0 (35.4)	15.3 (59.4)	14.0 (45.8)
			25 Sham	12.1	8.2 (32.2)	6.8 (43.8)	9.1 (25)	9.7	9.5 (−2)	10.1 (4)	11.3 (16.5)
Ogden et al. 1993	Prostatron	43	22 TUMT	14.5	3.6 (75.2)	3.6 (75.2)	—	8.5	13.5 (59)	13.5 (59)	—
			22 Sham	14.2	13.7 (3.5)	7.7 (46)	—	8.6	8.9 (3.5)	11.5 (34)	—
Barzell et al. 1998	Dornier UroWave	205	135 TUMT	23.8	—	11.9 (50)	11.2 (53)	7.7	—	10.9 (42)	10.6 (38)
			70 Sham	23.8	—	17.5 (26.5)	—	8.1	—	9.1 (12.3)	—
Blute et al. 1993	Prostatron 2.0	110	75 TUMT	13.9	6.3 (55)	—	—	7.2	11.5 (59.7)	—	—
			35 Sham	14.9	10.8 (27.5)	—	—	7.4	9.4 (27)	—	—
Larson et al. 1998	Urologix Targis (T3)	169	125 TUMT	20.8	9.6 (54)	10.5 (49.5)	—	7.8	11.7 (50)	11.8 (51.3)	—
			44 Sham	21.3	14.5 (32)	14.3 (33)	—	7.8	9.2 (18)	9.8 (25.6)	—
de Wildt et al. 1996	Prostatron	93	47 TUMT	13.7	4.7 (65.7)	—	4.2 (69.3)	9.2	13.4 (45.7)	—	13.4 (45.7)
			46 Sham	12.9	10.4 (19.4)	—	8.2 (36.4)	9.6	9.7 (1)	—	10.5 (9.4)
Francisca et al. 1997	Prostasoft 2.0	50	25 TUMT	13.2	5.9 (55.3)	5.3 (60)	—	9.6	13.0 (35.4)	13.9 (45)	—
			25 Sham	11.9	7.9 (33.6)	9.1 (23.5)	—	9.9	9.6 (−3)	9.6 (−3)	—
Nawrocki et al. 1997	Prostasoft 2.0	78	38 TUMT	19.0	—	9.5 (50)	—	8.8	—	9.94 (13)	—
			40 Sham	17.5	—	9.5 (46)	—	9.44	—	9.49 (.5)	—
Roehrborn et al. 1998	UroWave	220	147 TUMT	23.6	11.7 (50.4)	12.7 (46.2)	—	7.7	11.7 (52)	10.7 (39)	—
			73 Sham	23.9	16.2 (32.2)	18.0 (25)	—	8.1	9.6 (18.5)	9.8 (21)	—

Table 22.5 Comparison of TUMT-treated patients to sham-treated patients

Study	Duration of study	No. of patients enrolled	Device used	Symptom score (% improvement)			Peak flow rate, Q_{max} (% improvement)			Residual urine vol. (mL) (% improvement)		
				Baseline	at 3 months	at 6 months	Baseline (mL s⁻¹)	at 3 months	at 6 months	Baseline (mL)	at 3 months	at 6 months
Höfner et al. 1996	6 months	182	Prostasoft 2.0 (n = 97)	13.9	–	5.3 (62)	8.6	–	11.8 (37.2)	105.5	–	71.7 (32)
			Prostasoft 2.5 (n = 85)	13.9	–	5.9 (57.6)	9.6	–	14.7 (53.1)	83.4	–	29.3 (65)
			P-value	NS		0.374	0.04		0.001	0.029		0.001
Perrin et al. 1995	3 months	235	Prostasoft 2.0 (n = 163)	14.1	6.8 (52)	–	10.5	12.7 (21)	–			
			Prostasoft 2.5 (n = 72)	17.5	6.5 (63)	–	9.2	15.2 (65.2)	–			
			P-value		NS			NS				
				% change is significant, P<0.001			% change is significant, P<0.001					

Table 22.6 Summary of results comparing high-energy TUMT versus low-energy TUMT

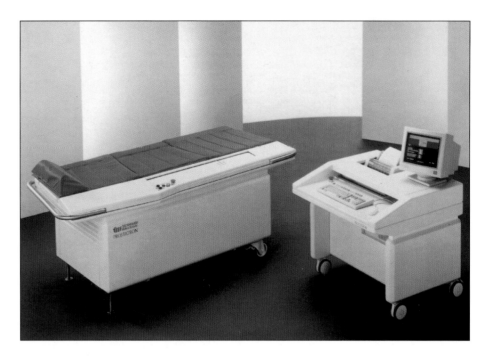

Figure 22.1 Older model of the Prostatron system

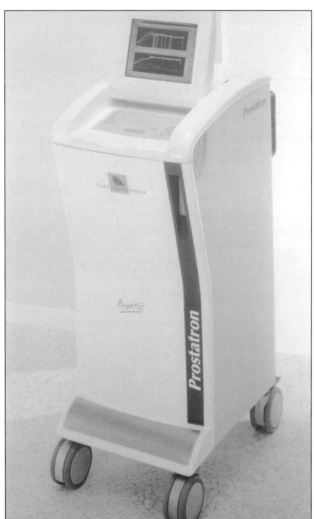

Figure 22.2 Newer model of the Prostatron system

Prostasoft T-A protocol reach >60°C, whereas the Prostasoft II and I protocols reach a temperature of 45–60°C and 45–50°C, respectively. Urodynamic and other studies show that, by increasing power application, there is a significant improvement in the peak flow rate and symptom scores. However, the rate of postoperative urinary retention is also increased with increasing temperature. A large majority of the patients treated with the higher-energy Prostasoft T-A protocol developed edema surrounding the bladder neck region, increasing the outlet urethral resistance. Nonetheless, the authors claim that, despite increasing the temperature to achieve better clinical results, there is no evidence of any damage to non-targeted tissues, such as the rectum, external sphincter, or ureteral orifices.

COMPLICATIONS OF MICROWAVE USE

The most common adverse event after TUMT is urinary retention, noted by Eliasson and associates[4] to be as high as 87% with a mean catheterization time of 16 days. Hallin[7] reported that 34% of patients were unable to void after microwave treatment, and an additional 6% required catheterization within 24 hours after TUMT treatment; in all cases, the catheter was removed within 3 weeks. However, Larson and associates[15] reported that only 8% of their patients required catheterization for urinary retention (Table 22.7). In an interesting study done in Sweden, 30 men with BPH were enrolled to undergo TUMT treatment (Prostasoft 2.5), and half of them were given a Foley catheter while the other half was given a biodegradable stent (SR-PGA) after the procedure, in order to relieve the problems of postoperative urinary retention. The stent was well tolerated by all the patients, and no secondary retention occurred when the stent completely degraded. The investigators stated that the use of the degradable stent

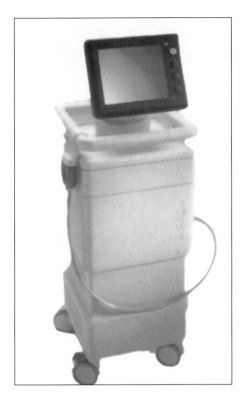

Figure 22.3 The Targis system. Efficient targeted high-energy delivery: high temperatures, necrosis of diseased tissue. Low temperature cooling: preserves urethra, anesthetic-free.

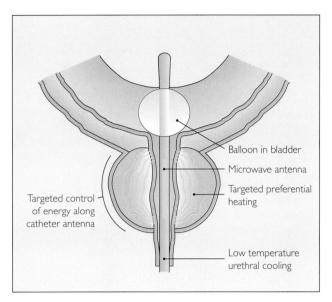

Balloon in bladder

Microwave antenna

Targeted preferential heating

Low temperature urethral cooling

Targeted control of energy along catheter antenna

Figure 22.4 Placement of microwave antenna with targeted energy to the prostate gland. The energy precisely targets preferential and axial microwave heating and preserves the urethra. It delivers energy efficiently and continuously, generating and maintaining peak intraprostatic temperatures >65°C with minimal risk to adjacent structures. Note urethral cooling system and balloon in bladder, which are safety features

solved the problem of post-treatment retention very comfortably for the patient and the drawbacks of the Foley catheter were avoided. This study showed promising results, especially with the use of the higher energy Prostasoft 2.5 protocol, which has been shown to cause a greater incidence of urinary retention.

The second most common complication is hematuria. Stravodimos et al.[5] reported a 49.2% incidence of hematuria, while de la Rosette et al.[17] reported a 76% incidence. de Wildt et al.[1,6] also reported a 76% incidence rate. However, Dahlstrand and co-workers[13] reported no incidence of hematuria.

A significant number of patients also experienced recurrent urinary tract infections (UTI). Some studies revealed that as many as 17.4% of patients presented with a postoperative UTI, and 2% had epididymitis.[15]

Several other studies have shown that sexual dysfunction is evident after microwave treatment. In a clinical trial by Keijzers and associates,[8] there was a reported incidence of 13% with erectile dysfunction and 8% with retrograde ejaculation. De Wildt's[1,6] study reported a 44% incidence of retrograde ejaculation, along with 15% experiencing diminished ejaculatory volume. Stravodimos et al.[5] reported a 9.5% incidence of retrograde ejaculation, while Larson et al.[15] reported a 4% incidence. However, the study done by Eliasson and associates[4] showed a 29% incidence of anejaculation and 28% with impotence after the TUMT procedure. As noted earlier, there is a higher incidence of retrograde

ejaculation, and postoperative urinary retention with the use of high-energy (2.5 version) TUMT in comparison with low-energy (2.0 version) TUMT.

Numerous clinical trials involving microwave treatment for BPH have noted that some patients have experienced urethral stricture postoperatively. In a publication by Sall and Bruskewitz,[22] they reported three cases of prostatic urethral stricture. In a large study using microwave thermotherapy reported by de la Rosette and associates,[17] none of the 116 men who had undergone TUMT had experienced prostatic urethral stricture. In Sall and Bruskewitz's report,[22] 11% had urethral stricture following treatment. Other studies have revealed a low incidence of stricture. The most reasonable explanation of this stricture is probably ischemic or thermal damage by the microwave probe. A combination of coagulation of arteries, with subsequent loss of blood supply (ischemia) to the prostatic urethra, and insufficient cooling from the catheter, resulting in thermal damage to the urethra, might explain the high incidence of prostatic urethral stricture seen in Sall and Bruskewitz's study.[22]

CONCLUSION

The definition of a minimally invasive procedure is one that can be carried out in a single session in an out-patient or office setting with the use of only local anesthetics, not general or regional. This concept is embodied by TUMT. From the results presented in this chapter, TUMT produces a

Complications	% Incidence
Urinary retention	3.3–87
Hematuria	0–76
Urinary tract infections	0–23
Urethral strictures	0–11
Hemospermia	0–2
Epididymitis	0–7
Fistula formation	0–1
Prostatitis	0–6
Sexual dysfunction	
Erectile dysfunction (impotence)	0–28
Retrograde ejaculation	0–44
Anejaculation	0–29
Mean duration of catheterization ≈17 days	

Table 22.7 Complications experienced with TUMT

significant reduction in symptoms related to bladder outlet obstruction secondary to BPH. Unlike TURP, which has debulking ability, TUMT will not attain the peak flow rate improvement that is evident with TURP. High-energy TUMT has demonstrated cavity formation in the prostatic urethra, but the high urinary retention rate and morbidity are the downside of this treatment. One may question whether a marginal improvement in symptom score and peak urinary flow rate is worth the high morbidity of the treatment. This is a justifiable question, but not appropriate. TUMT does not have to have the same effectiveness as TURP in order for it to be considered a successful therapy for BPH. The goal of TUMT is not to debulk the prostatic tissue, which is reserved for invasive surgical procedures like TURP, but to reduce BPH symptoms, with the convenience of out-patient therapy, and without the need for general anesthesia and the high morbidity that is associated with TURP.

REFERENCES

1 de Wildt MJ, D'Ancona FC, Hubregtse M *et al*. Three-year follow-up of patients treated with lower energy microwave thermotherapy. *J Urol* 1996; **156**(6): 159–63.

2 Miyatake R, Park YC, Koike H *et al*. Urodynamic evaluation of alpha-1 blocker tamsulosin on benign prostatic hyperplasia using pressure flow study. *Nippon Hinyokika Gakkai Zasshi* 1996; **87**(8): 1048–55.

3 Tazaki H, Deguchi N, Baba S, Imai Y, Nakashima J. Magnetic resonance imaging following microwave thermotherapy, laser ablation and transurethral resection in patients with BPH. *Urologe A* 1995; **34**(2): 105–9.

4 Eliasson T, Damber JE. Temperature controlled high energy transurethral microwave thermotherapy for benign prostatic hyperplasia using a heat shock strategy. *J Urol* 1998; **160**: 777–82.

5 Stravodimos KG, Goldfischer ER, Klima WJ *et al*. Transurethral microwave thermotherapy for management of benign prostatic hyperplasia: a single-institution experience. *Urology* 1998; **51**: 1008–12.

6 de Wildt MJAM, Hubregtse M, Ogden C *et al*. A 12-month study of the placebo effect in transurethral microwave thermotherapy. *Br J Urol* 1996; **77**: 221–7.

7 Hallin A, Berlin T. Transurethral microwave thermotherapy for benign prostatic hyperplasia: clinical outcome after 4 years. *J Urol* 1998; **159**: 459–64.

8 Keijzers GB, Francisca EA, D'Ancona FC *et al*. Long-term results of lower energy transurethral microwave thermotherapy. *J Urol* 1998; **159**(6): 1966–72 (discussion 1972–3).

9 Walden M, Dahlstrand C, Schafer W, Pettersson S. How to select patients suitable for transurethral microwave thermotherapy: a systematic evaluation of potentially predictive variables. *Br J Urol* 1998; **81** 817–22.

10 Glass JM, Bdesha AS, Witherow RON. Microwave thermotherapy: a long-term follow-up of 67 patients from a single centre. *Br J Urol* 1998; **81**: 377–82.

11 D'Ancona FCH, Francisca EAE, Witjes WPJ *et al*. Transurethral resection of the prostate vs. high-energy thermotherapy of the prostate in patients with benign prostatic hyperplasia: long-term results. *Br J Urol* 1998; **81**: 259–64.

12 D'Ancona FC, Francisca EA, Witjes WP *et al*. High energy thermotherapy versus transurethral resection in the treatment of benign prostatic hyperplasia: results of a prospective randomized study with 1 year of follow-up. *J Urol* 1997; **158**(1): 120–5.

13 Dahlstrand C, Walden M, Geirsson G, Pettersson S. Transurethral microwave thermotherapy versus transurethral resection for symptomatic benign prostatic obstruction: a prospective randomized study with a 2-year follow-up. *Br J Urol* 1995; **76**: 614–18.

14 de la Rosette JJ, Froeling FM, Debruyne FM. Clinical results with microwave thermotherapy of benign prostatic hyperplasia. *Eur Urol* 1993; **23**(Suppl 1): 68–71.

15 Larson TR, Blute ML, Bruskewitz RC *et al*. A high-efficiency microwave thermoablation system for the treatment of benign prostatic hyperplasia: results of a randomized, SHAM-controlled, prospective, double-blind, multicenter clinical trial. *Urology* 1998; **51**: 731–42.

16 Roehrborn CG, Preminger G, Newhall P *et al*. Microwave thermotherapy for benign prostatic hyperplasia with the Dornier urowave: results of a randomized, double-blind, multicenter, sham-controlled trial. *Urology* 1998; **51**(1): 19–28.

17 de la Rosette JJ, de Wildt MJ, Hofner K *et al*. High energy thermotherapy in the treatment of benign prostatic hyperplasia: results of the European Benign Prostatic Hyperplasia Study Group. *J Urol* 1996; **156**(1): 97–101 (discussion 101–2).

18 Devonec M, Ogden C, Perrin P, Carter SStC. Clinical response to transurethral microwave thermotherapy is thermal dose dependent. *Eur Urol* 1993; **23**: 267–74.

19 Höfner K, Jonas U, Miano L *et al*. Low and high energy TUMT: the relation between desobstruction and morbidity. *J Urol* 1996; **155**(5 Suppl): 709A.

20 Perrin P, Devonec M, Houdelette P *et al*. Single-session transurethral microwave thermotherapy: comparision of two therapeutic modes in a multicenter study. In: Marberger M (ed) *Application of Newer Forms of Therapeutic Energy in Urology*. Oxford: Isis Medical Media 1995: 35–9.

21 Bolmsjo M, Wagrell L, Hallin A *et al*. The heat is on – but how? A comparison of TUMT devices. *Br J Urol* 1996; **78**(4): 564–72.

22 Sall M, Bruskewitz RC. Prostatic urethreal strictures after transurethral microwave thermotherapy for benign prostatic hyperplasia. *Urol* 1997; **50**(6): 983–5.

23 Perachino M, Bozzo W, Puppo P *et al*. Does transurethral thermotherapy induce a long-term alpha blockade? An immnohistochemical study. *Eur Urol* 1993; **23**(2): 299–301.

COMMENTARY

Microwaves are transverse electromagnetic waves with frequencies in the range of 30–300 Hz. These travel in a given medium and within the prostatic tissues cause drift, free charge, and polarization of atoms. The initial microwave devices used the transrectal approach but subsequently, the transurethral approach, now called thermotherapy, was utilized to achieve intraprostatic temperatures in excess of 45°C without having to go through heating the rectum. There are several devices in existence now, and some of the more common ones are the Prostatron and the Targis systems. Even the Prostatron device has undergone an evolution from a 2.0 software to a 2.5 software, the latter having the ability to use higher levels of power and higher levels of heating. The TUMT procedure involves placement of the microwave antenna in the urethra, monitoring by ultrasound placed in the rectum, and urethral cooling, which is automated based on temperature elevations set at a certain threshold above body temperature. Treatments using microwave therapy, especially using the 2.0 systems, can be performed in most patients under local anesthesia, although the time taken is close to 1 h. As a result of poor results with the 2.0 system, the 2.5 system was developed and, although this achieves higher intraprostatic temperatures, it requires more anesthesia. While the Prostatron system appears to be satisfactory in relieving symptoms and improving uroflow in 1-year trials, 4-year follow-up trials reveal that more than 50% of patients require additional treatment in the form of TURP or another invasive procedure. In fairness to the microwave therapy results, it must be stated that most other systems such as the interstitial laser and TUNA do not have 5-year follow-up results. In trials where TUMT was compared with TURP, again initial results at 1–2 years appear to be similar in both treatments. As far as symptoms are concerned, reduction is comparative, although uroflow improvement is higher in the TURP group. However, urodynamic studies of patients undergoing microwave have revealed that only 15% of patients in the thermotherapy group are considered to have no obstruction at 6 months, while 40% of patients in the TURP group are considered to have no obstruction. Side effects of the thermotherapy appear to be urinary retention, which occurs in as many as 70–80% of patients and lasts up to 2 weeks. Additionally, hematuria, urinary tract infections, and sexual dysfunction occur in a small percentage of patients.

High-Intensity Focused Ultrasound

S. Madersbacher and M. Marberger

23

INTRODUCTION

The majority of recently developed minimally invasive treatment alternatives for benign prostatic hyperplasia (BPH) make use of the therapeutic effect of heat.[1] There is a close correlation between therapeutic energy and intraprostatic tissue effects and, consequently, clinical efficacy.[1,2] Therapeutic temperatures exceeding 50°C lead to irreversible cell destruction and, above 80–90°C ("thermoablation"), cystic cavities comparable with those after transurethral resection of the prostate (TURP) can be induced.[1,2] Thermoablation can be achieved by microwaves (high-energy transurethral microwave thermotherapy – TUMT 2.5), low-level radiofrequency (transurethral needle ablation – TUNA), or high-intensity focused ultrasound (HIFU).[3–5]

HIFU is based on the emission of a focused high-energy ultrasound wave.[5–7] In non-ideal viscoelastic elements such as biological tissue, the mechanical energy of the ultrasound wave is converted into heat and, within the focal area, temperatures in the range of 80–200°C are generated. This sharp heat impulse leads to an immediate coagulative necrosis of all cellular elements within this focal area.[5–7] As the HIFU beam is focused, thermal damage to intervening tissues as well as areas in the vicinity of the focal zone can be avoided. Hence, HIFU is the only means presently available permitting contact- and irradiation-free in-depth tissue ablation in any solid organ accessible for ultrasound.[5–7] In urology, several organs such as bladder, testis, kidney, and prostate have been subjected to HIFU treatment in experimental and clinical settings.[5–7] By far the widest experience is presently available for the prostate, as several canine and human histological studies as well as data from clinical trials for BPH and localized prostate cancer are available.

The principal aim of this chapter is to provide insights into the physical foundations of this technique, technical requirements, experimental data, and the clinical results so far available. For didactic reasons, we concentrate selectively on prostatic tissue ablation with particular reference to the indication for BPH.

PHYSICAL FOUNDATIONS

ULTRASOUND

Ultrasound is an acoustic mechanical wave consisting of compressions and rarefactions that propagate within a medium.[5–7] The ultrasound wavelength used in medicine is sufficiently short to be brought to a tight focus at depth within the body. This ability to focus means that good resolution may be obtained in diagnostic ultrasound scans (using low output powers) and also that, if sufficient energy is carried within the ultrasound beam, regions of high ultrasonic power are created in which therapeutic effects are generated.[5–7] In general, ultrasound interacts with tissue by thermal and mechanical interactions. The mechanical effects of ultrasound are applied during ultrasonic tissue dissection, contact lithotripsy, and extracorporeal shock-wave lithotripsy and, at least predominantly, for extracorporeal pyrotherapy.[5] Thermal interactions are primarily mediated by acoustic absorption and are the predominant tissue effect during HIFU therapy.[5]

MECHANICAL EFFECTS OF ULTRASOUND

The mechanical tissue effects of ultrasound have recently been reviewed in detail, and some basic aspects and technical terms, which are necessary fully to understand this chapter, are briefly discussed.[8]

Acoustic pressure is exerted on any body immersed in an acoustic field. In a standing wave field, it is greatest at pressure maxima and lowest at velocity maxima.[8] Likewise, **acoustic force** is also exerted on any body immersed in the acoustic field. Non-uniformity of the acoustic field also leads to a time-independent twisting action, which is referred to as **acoustic torque**.[8] **Acoustic streaming** describes the movement of fluid in an ultrasonic pressure field. Where fluid motion encounters boundaries, high-velocity gradients can develop and produce substantial shear stresses. The most prominent mechanical effect of ultrasound on tissue is **acoustic cavitation**, which is defined as the formation and/or activity of gas- or vapor-filled cavities (bubbles) in a medium exposed to an ultrasound field.[8] Generally accepted terms for specific aspects of bubble activity are stable and inertial (collapse) cavitation (also known as transient cavitation). Stable cavitation describes the continuous oscillation of bubbles in response to alternating positive and negative pressure in an acoustic field. The bubble radius varies about an equilibrium value, and the pulsating cavity exists for a considerable number of cycles. Inertial cavitation describes the behavior of bubbles that oscillate about their equilibrium size, grow until the outward excursion of the surface exceeds a limiting value, and collapse violently. Tissue cavitation is a random phenomenon; its occurrence is unpredictable and therefore might lead to uncontrollable tissue destruction.

THERMAL EFFECTS OF ULTRASOUND

As an ultrasound wave propagates through medium, it is progressively absorbed, and the energy is converted to heat in any not-ideally viscoelastic media, such as all biological tissues.[5,8,9] In diagnostic ultrasound systems, the amount of heat generated is extremely small and has not been shown to have any harmful effect. In therapeutic systems, higher intensities are generated, which are capable of inducing thermal damage to cells located within the HIFU-beam focus.[5-9] Thermal effects of ultrasound on tissue are dependent on a number of factors, such as the ultrasonic site intensity throughout the insonified tissues, the absorption coefficient of the insonicated tissue, and the temperature rise throughout the exposed tissues.[5,8,9] For short time intervals (<0.1 s), the temperature rise is proportional to the ultrasonic intensity.[5,8,9] As time increases, temperature rises are modified by thermal conduction and the simple proportionality is no longer valid. In perfused tissues, blood-flow cooling becomes an important additional factor. The damage integral estimates the effects of temperature elevation on tissue structures: tissue changes occur if the heat induction exceeds the threshold level of protein degradation of 45–47°C.

HIGH-INTENSITY FOCUSED ULTRASOUND

A beam of ultrasound can be brought to a tight focus at a selected depth within the body, thus producing a region of high-energy density within which tissue can be destroyed without damage to overlying or intervening structures.[5-7] If the site intensity is set below the tissue cavitation threshold, which is feasible under certain technical settings, the predominant therapeutic effect is the induction of heat.[5-7] This technique is known as ultrasonic ablation, sonablation, focal ultrasound surgery or HIFU; within this chapter, we refer to the latter term. This technique was firmly established in the mid-1950s by the pioneering work of Frank and William Fry and was initially used for ablating brain tissue.[6,10] Subsequent years have seen a steady evolution in understanding the basic physical principles involved in the interaction of this mechanical wave form with biological tissue.[5] In parallel, progress in transducer technology and the advent of new powerful diagnostic tools, such as high-frequency ultrasonography and magnetic resonance imaging (MRI) were the technological basis for recent device designs.[5,11] These developments resulted in the initiation of several human trials, including kidney, bladder, eye, and prostate.

INSTRUMENTATION

The source for HIFU is a piezoceramic transducer, which has the property of changing its thickness in response to an applied voltage.[5-7] This creates an acoustic ultrasound wave with a frequency equal to that of the voltage applied. Frequencies used for HIFU therapy cover a range of 0.5–10 MHz (Table 23.1). The site intensity applied has to be above the temperature threshold, yet below the cavitation threshold to avoid damage to surrounding structures.[5-7] Depending on the ultrasound frequency, the site intensity ranges between 750 and 4500 W cm^{-2} (Table 23.1). The focusing of the HIFU beam is achieved either by placing a lens in front of the transducer or by the transducer itself having a spherical shape.[5] Modern piezoceramics can operate at sufficient power densities with long-term output stability consistent with focal therapy device requirements.[6] Coupling of the transducer to the tissue of interest has to be free of air and usually involves low-loss media, such as degassed water.[5-7] The shape of the focal zone can change significantly, depending on the focal length, exposure time, and site intensity, as was recently demonstrated in vitro and in vivo.[5-7,12-14] Table 23.1 shows presently used HIFU systems with particular reference to urological applications. Regarding prostatic tissue ablation, an extracorporeal or transrectal approach is feasible.[5] For a variety of reasons, such as the vicinity of the HIFU transducer to target tissue and technical and safety considerations, the transrectal approach is clearly superior to the transabdominal approach.[5] In fact, solid animal and human histological data

Manufacturer	Route of application	Frequency (MHz)	Site intensity (W cm^{-2})	Animal data	Human data	References
Sonablate, Focus Surg. Inc., Milpitas, USA	Transrectal	4.0	1200–2200	Prostate, liver, kidney	BPH, prostate cancer, testis, kidney	14–16
Ablatherm, Technomed Int., Lyon, France	Transrectal	2.25	≈2000	Prostate	Prostate cancer	17, 18
Sonacare, Sonacare Inc., New York; USA	Extracorporeal	4.6	?	Eye	Eye (indication: glaucoma)	19, 20
Experimental, Hynynen et al.	Extracorporeal	1.0	?	Muscle	No human data available, soft tissue	11
Toshiba-Research, Tohoku, Japan	Extracorporeal	1.65	4200	Muscle, kidney, prostate	No human data available	21
Experimental	Extracorporeal	1.75	300 W	Muscle, kidney	No human data available	7, 12

Table 23.1 Overview of presently available HIFU systems including principal technical parameters

as well as clinical results are only available for the transrectal system.[5] That is why we concentrate selectively on this approach here.

Transrectal High-Intensity Focused Ultrasound Systems

The transrectal devices were designed to ablate prostatic tissue and incorporate a small imaging and therapy transducer on a single-probe sheath; at present two types of system are available. For air-free coupling of the HIFU beam to tissue (rectal wall), the probe is covered by a condom, which is filled after insertion into the rectum with degassed water. In one device (Sonablate, Focal Surgery Milpitas, USA) the same 4.0-MHz transducer is used for imaging and therapy (Figure 23.1A).[14–16] The focal length is dependent on the crystal used. At present, individual focal lengths of 2.5, 3.0, 3.5, and 4.0 cm are available (Figure 23.1B). The site intensity can be varied from 1260 to 2200 W cm^{-2}. A 4-s interval of therapy (=power on) followed by 12 s power off, is used for obtaining an image update and moving the transducer electronically to the next treatment location. The second transrectal device (Ablatherm, Technomed International, Lyon, France) uses two separate transducers, one for imaging operating at 7.5 MHz, and one for HIFU therapy at 2.25 MHz (focal length 3.5 or 4.0 cm).[17,18] Site intensities in this system have been reported to range between 700 and 2200 W cm^{-2}. Most of the HIFU devices currently being used for clinical trials (including the transrectal ones) damage an ellipsoidal tissue volume approximately 2 mm in diameter and 10 mm long. In order to create a clinically useful tissue volume, a multiplicity of laterally or axially displaced individual lesions are generated by physical movement of the sound head or by electronically sweeping the focused beam.[5,7,14]

Future Technical Developments

The most significant technical innovation for HIFU therapy would be the availability of an annular phased-array transducer with a variable focal length. Such an extracorporeal 10 cm annular phased-array HIFU transducer has been developed recently.[22] This transducer prototype is capable of focusing the HIFU beam between 8 and 12 cm by phasing the array.[22] Once these transducers are at hand, it will be possible simply to mark the respective target area on the computer screen in two dimensions, and the entire area will be precisely ablated. Recently, Ioritani et al. reported on a novel extracorporeal device.[21] The ultrasound source is a spherical piezoceramic transducer (diameter 100 mm; curvature 120 mm) operating at 1.65 MHz. The maximum site intensity at the focal point was 4200 W cm^{-2}. Whether it is possible to miniaturize these phased transducers for transrectal applications, however, remains to be determined.

ANIMAL STUDIES

For human BPH, the best animal model presently available is the canine prostate. Consequently, the histological impact of HIFU on this organ was intensively studied by several groups. Using transrectal instrumentation that is presently

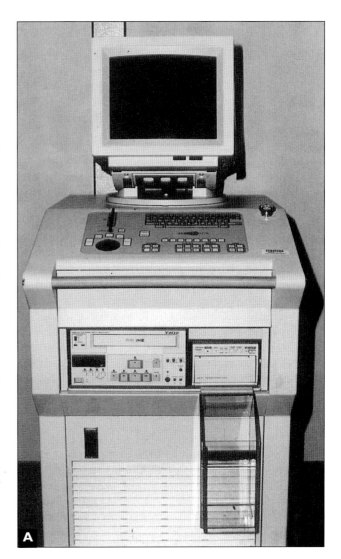

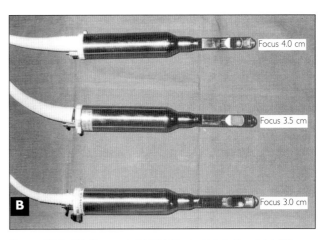

Figure 23.1 (A) Transrectal HIFU-Control Unit (Sonablate®). (B) Transrectal HIFU Probes (Sonablate)

used in human trials for BPH and localized prostate cancer, Foster *et al.*[23] studied the histological impact of HIFU on 26 canine prostates, which were sacrificed in a time interval of 2 hours up to 12 weeks following treatment. Intraprostatic coagulative necrosis was consistently observed. After 14 days, the first cystic cavities were identified, and within 3 months cystic cavities formed in all animals.[23] The surrounding and intervening structures, such as the rectal wall and the prostate capsule, were always intact.[23] A similar study has been conducted by Gelet *et al.*[17] on 37 beagle dogs. Intraprostatic coagulative necrosis was present in the vast majority of animals, and subsequently formed to a cystic cavity after 4 weeks.[17] Two recent canine studies have addressed the issue of increasing the volume of tissue ablated by transrectal HIFU, which is important for enhancing the clinical efficacy in treating BPH and localized prostate cancer.[24,25] With a modified treatment protocol involving several HIFU-treatment zones and different HIFU transducers, Bihrle *et al.*[24] attempted to ablate all prostate tissue except for the extreme anterior aspect of the gland. At histological examination, massive coagulative necrosis comprising approximately 90% of the gland was present. Long-term histological analysis demonstrated only a small rim of prostatic tissue lining a huge intraprostatic cavity.[24] Postoperative recovery in treated animals was uneventful except for a prolonged period of urinary retention. This study demonstrates the possibility of performing subtotal prostatic ablation, with the present technology destroying 90–95% of a canine prostate.[24] An alternative approach to increasing the amount of tissue ablation has been studied by Foster *et al.*[25] using an ultrasound contrast agent. This substance is a suspension of air-filled microspheres, which was introduced into the canine urethra via a transurethral catheter. Canine prostates were subsequently subjected to HIFU therapy with and without the presence of this agent. Histologically, prostates treated in the presence of this agent revealed a significantly enhanced lesion volume. These data demonstrate an enhanced ablative effect when HIFU is used in conjunction with an ultrasound contrast agent.[25] Additional advantages of this approach are the improved imaging of a urethra filled with this agent.[25]

HUMAN HISTOLOGICAL DATA

Despite the encouraging animal data presented above, one has to be aware that the histological impact of heat on the canine and human prostate is not comparable.[5] In addition, there are significant anatomical differences, particularly regarding the route of the urethra. Therefore, it is mandatory to determine the histological impact on the human prostate prior to the initiation of clinical studies.[5] To evaluate this issue in detail, 54 human prostates were treated at the author's institution *in vivo* with transrectal HIFU prior to surgical removal.[14,16,26] All prostates were analyzed histologically following surgery, using whole mount prostatic sections. Mapping of intraprostatic coagulative necrosis was possible in all specimens (Figure 23.2). As early as 1 h after HIFU, intraprostatic necrosis was seen. Epithelial cells exhibited dark staining, pyknotic

nuclei, with the surrounding cytoplasm being narrow and irregularly vacuolized.[14,16,26] The epithelium was detached from the basal membrane and single cells were dissociated. Electron microscopy of fresh lesions (2–3 h after HIFU) revealed severe alterations on the subcellular level. After 7 days, the target area imposed as a classic hemorrhagic necrosis. Within 10 weeks, the coagulative necrosis was resorbed by tissue rich in macrophages and capillary sprouts, and a scar was formed. The border between HIFU-treated and untreated tissue was extremely sharp, comprising only five to seven cell layers.[14,16,26] Thermolesions to intervening tissues were never observed, underlining the safety of the applied system. Using the second transrectal HIFU system presently available, Gelet *et al.*[18] recently reported on the histological impact on the human prostate in a comparable study design. Patients were subjected to prostatectomy 2–48 h after HIFU. While no or only minimal tissue effects were observed in patients with site intensities lower or comparable to those used in canine studies, well-defined coagulative necrosis was consistently present in patients treated with higher site intensities. The respective necroses were rectangular, and their dimensions were equal to, or slightly greater, than the theoretical target volume.[18] Side effects were only minimal.

Hence, transrectal HIFU is capable of inducing precise, well-controllable contact- and irradiation-free intraprostatic ablation in the human prostate. From these studies, it is obvious that transrectal HIFU is highly attractive as a novel minimally invasive therapy for benign tumors, such as BPH, but potentially even more localized prostate cancer.

THE HIFU PROCEDURE

To date, the clinical efficacy of transrectal HIFU for human BPH has been reported only with the device using the same crystal for imaging and therapy.[14,15] Therefore, we describe this procedure in greater detail. HIFU therapy is usually carried out under general or spinal anesthesia, although a subgroup of patients have also been successfully treated under IV sedation.[14,15] Therapy is performed in the classic

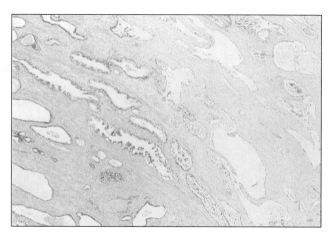

Figure 23.2 Intraprostatic coagulative necrosis following transrectal HIFU

lithotomy position. After a diagnostic cystoscopy, a suprapubic 10-French cystostomy tube is inserted. Subsequently, a 16-French transurethral balloon catheter is introduced to allow exact identification of urethra, bladder neck, and verumonatum during the imaging phase of the procedure. The HIFU transducer is covered by a condom, lubricated with gel, and inserted into the rectum. The condom is inflated with approximately 30 cm³ of degased water for exact air-free coupling of HIFU to tissue. The HIFU transducer is positioned under direct ultrasound guidance using the imaging mode so that the prostatic urethra and bladder neck are located within the target zone. Longitudinally, the treatment zone comprises an area from the bladder neck to the verumontanum. Once the optimal position is obtained, the transducer is immobilized with a locking arm device. HIFU treatment is started after removal of the transurethral catheter. After the initial zone is treated in the 12 o'clock position, the transducer rotates laterally and creates another zone in the far lateral aspect of the transverse plane.[5,14,15] Ultimately seven to nine sectors are subjected to therapy in the transverse plane.[5,14,15] Once HIFU therapy is completed, the condom is deflated and the transducer is removed.

CLINICAL RESULTS

Study Design

To date, worldwide, approximately 250 BPH patients have been treated with transrectal HIFU in an international Phase II clinical trial. Inclusion/exclusion criteria were uniform, i.e. peak flow rate (Q_{max}) $\leq$ 15 mL s^{-1}, American Urological Association (AUA) symptom score of $\geq$ 18, prostate volume of $\leq$ 75 mL, and a prostate-specific antigen (PSA) of less than 10 ng mL^{-1}. Post-HIFU, patients were followed at regular time intervals on an outpatient basis, including assessment of symptom score, uroflow, residual volume, transrectal ultrasonography, and serum PSA.

Symptoms and Uroflowmetry

In the initial US series, Bihrle et al.[15] reported on their experience with 15 patients and a follow-up of 90 days. The maximum flow rate increased from 9.3 mL s^{-1} to 10.3 mL s^{-1} (1 month) and 14.0 mL s^{-1} (3 months; +50.5%), and the postvoid residual volume decreased form 154 mL to 123 mL (3 months). The average AUA score decreased from 31.2 (range 22–38) before treatment to 17.1 (range 8–32) at 30 days, for an average improvement of 45.2%. At 90 days, the average symptom scores improved to 15.9, for an average improvement of 48.4%. We recently reported on our initial series of 50 patients, 20 of whom were followed for 12 months (Figure 23.2).[14] The maximum urinary flow rate (Q_{max}, mL s^{-1}) increased from 8.9±4.1 to 12.4±5.6 (6 months, n=33) and 13.1±6.5 (12 months, n=20). In the same time period the postvoid residual volume (mL) decreased from 131±120, 59±42, and 35±30, and the AUA symptom score declined from 24.5±4.7, 13.4±4.7, and 10.8±2.5. Overall, we observed a 47% improvement in uroflow and a 53% decrease in

urinary symptoms 1 year after treatment.[14] In principle, these data were confirmed in a recent update of more than 100 patients treated at our institution.[5] Nakamura et al.[27] recently reported on the long-term clinical efficacy with this approach in 22 patients, who completed a 2-year follow-up. The Q_{max} increased from 7.6±0.6 mL s^{-1} preoperatively to 9.3±0.7 mL s^{-1} ($P<0.001$) after 24 months. During the same period, the International Prostatic Symptom Score decreased from 23.7±0.4 to 6.9±0.9 ($P<0.001$) and the Quality of Life score from 5.2±0.1 to 2.3±0.3 ($P<0.001$). The overall response at 1 year using these three parameters was as follows: excellent 23%, good 41%, fair 18%, poor 18%.[27] These data demonstrate that HIFU for BPH achieved durability of clinical response up to 2 years in 60% of treated patients.[27]

Intraprostatic cystic cavities, comparable to post-TURP, were demonstrable by transrectal ultrasonography in approximately 25% of patients.[14,15] These lesions appear within the first 6 weeks after therapy and are still present 12–24 months thereafter (Figure 23.4).[14,15]

Pressure-Flow Studies

To obtain further insight into the effect of transrectal HIFU on bladder outflow obstruction, 30 patients underwent multichannel pressure-flow studies before and after transrectal HIFU (mean time interval 4.5 months).[28] Only patients with a urodynamically proven obstruction defined by a linear passive urethral resistance relation (linPURR) of $\geq$ 2 were eligible. Madersbacher et al.[28] observed a reduction in the detrusor opening pressure (cmH$_2$O) from 70±23 (mean±SD) preoperatively to 51±22 ($P<0.005$) postoperatively, and a decline in the detrusor pressure at maximum flow (cmH$_2$O) from 74.2±24 to 57±15 ($P<0.005$).[28] The linPURR dropped from 3.7±1.1 preoperatively to 2.2±1.2 ($P<0.005$) (Figure 23.5). According to the Abrams–Griffiths nomogram, 24 (80%) patients

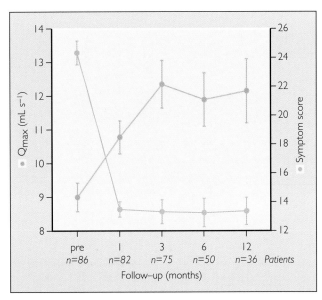

Figure 23.3 AUA-symptom score and Q_{max} before and after transrectal HIFU

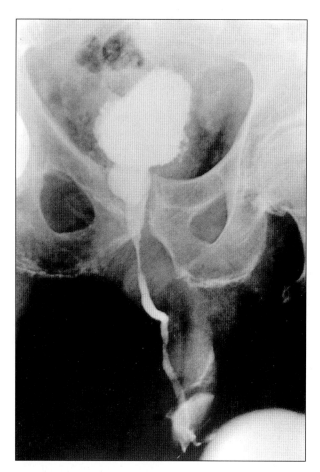

Figure 23.4 Voiding cystourethrogram 12 months following HIFU

were classified preoperatively as obstructed, the remaining 20% as being in equivocal zone.[28] Postoperatively, 13% were unobstructed, 50% in the equivocal zone.[28] However, 37% of patients were still obstructed after HIFU therapy, rated according to this nomogram.[28] These urodynamic data indicate that transrectal HIFU is capable of relieving the infravesical obstruction and of improving objective and subjective BPH parameters.[28] However, the urodynamic changes have to be classified as moderate. Consequently, transrectal HIFU, at least in its present form, should only be considered for moderately, but not severely obstructed, symptomatic BPH patients.

Side Effects

Overall, HIFU treatment is well tolerated.[14,15] Rectoscopy done immediately after the procedure yielded normal results in all but two patients (see below), demonstrating the safety of this approach. The predominant side effect, observed in almost all patients, was a urinary retention. Therefore, we routinely placed a 10-French cystostomy catheter intraoperatively, which was removed on an outpatient basis after a mean of 6 days. The majority of sexually active patients reported on a hematospermia, which disappeared spontaneously after 4–6 weeks. In our series of 102 consecutive patients, we observed two severe complications. In one patient, a perforation of the descending colon approximately 50–60 cm above the treatment zone occurred.[14] This complication was caused by inadvertent overfilling and subsequent rupture of the condom that covered the ultrasound probe to approximately 500 mL. At surgery, remnants of the condom were found at the site of perforation. This complication, which occurred in the early phase of this series (patient 9), led to reconstruction of the filling apparatus and the probe in such a way that the problem can now be reliably avoided.[14] The second severe complication was a thermolesion of the rectum, requiring surgical intervention. This lesion was most likely caused by using an inappropriately high site intensity exceeding 2300 W cm^{-2}. As a consequence, the maximum site intensity is now set at 2000 W cm^{-2}.

Summary – Clinical Data

The clinical data published to date indicate that transrectal HIFU is capable of improving subjective and objective BPH parameters, and that the degree of bladder outflow obstruction can be reduced in the majority of patients.[14,15,28] The greatest advantage of this approach is the capability of inducing contact-free intraprostatic necrosis, thus avoiding urethral manipulation. As a result, postoperative dysuria and urethral discomfort is almost absent, and theoretically, the risk of urethral strictures should be minimal. However, there are also significant disadvantages involved: among these are the expensive equipment, the sophisticated technical OR set-up and the anesthesia requirements. Finally, although these Phase II clinical data have demonstrated the clinical efficacy, it has to be emphasized that the definitive role of this technique can only be determined in a randomized Phase III clinical trial.

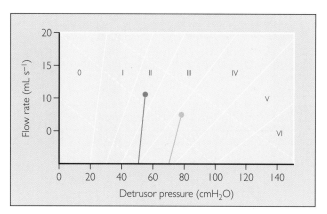

Figure 23.5 Analysis of linear-PURR before and after HIFU

CONCLUSION

Several experimental and clinical studies have proven the feasibility, safety, and efficacy of thermoablation of the prostate by transrectal HIFU. The canine and human histological data confirm that this technique is capable of destroying prostatic tissue while preserving intervening structures such as rectal wall and posterior prostate capsule. The crucial advantage of transrectal HIFU over other currently tested minimally invasive treatment options for BPH, such as TUMT, TUNA, and laser prostatectomy, is that the treatment is contact free.[3,4,29–32] Therefore it is feasible selectively to coagulate periurethral tissue via the transrectal route, avoiding the side effects and risks associated with urethral or intraprostatic manipulation. As the clinical experience with this technique is still limited, it is certainly premature to predict the future role of transrectal HIFU as a minimally invasive treatment option for BPH. However, clinical data of Phase II trials so far available allow some conclusions. HIFU treatment for BPH is associated with very low postoperative morbidity. The therapeutic efficacy of HIFU is comparable to that of high-energy TUMT and TUNA but inferior to laser prostatectomy.[3,4,29–32] Clinical data indicate a lasting (24 months) therapeutic effect of HIFU therapy for BPH.[27]

As the first clinical studies with transrectal HIFU were initiated only 3 years ago, there is considerable room for further improvements. The optimal anesthetic protocol still needs to be defined. The majority of patients have been treated under either general or spinal anesthesia. At the University of Indiana, four out of five patients were successfully treated under IV sedation.[15] Patients were operated on as out-patients with no anesthetic recovery room time. The possibility of a prostatic block as an anesthetic regimen is currently evaluated. In addition, the impact of intraprostatic lesion volume and location on the clinical outcome is currently determined. Probably the most important technical improvement would be the availability of a phased-array HIFU transducer with variable focal length.[22] Once these transducers are at hand, it will be possible simply to mark the target zone identified in two planes on the computer screen and the respective area will be precisely ablated.[22] Furthermore, the availability of varying focal sizes and shorter duty cycles would help to cut down treatment time.

Whether HIFU therapy will gain a place in the armamentarium for 21st century BPH therapy will depend on a variety of factors, such as the durability of the clinical response, the costs of the procedure and of the HIFU machine, the possibility to be performed as day surgery, anesthesia requirements and, finally, the results and costs of competing thermoablation techniques, such as high-energy TUMT or TUNA as well as laser prostatectomy.

In conclusion, HIFU represents an exciting method of minimally invasive surgery without affecting intervening tissue. Although many reports demonstrate its efficacy in the treatment of BPH in a Phase II trial, it is obvious that HIFU will have a major impact in the field of minimally invasive surgery (extracorporeal, transrectal, transvaginal, etc.) for treatment of malignant tumors.[33–38] Theoretically, all organs accessible for ultrasound are potentially suitable for this kind of therapy.[5,38]

REFERENCES

1 Smith PH, Marberger M, Conort P *et al*. Other non-medical therapies (excluding lasers) in the treatment of BPH. In: Cockett ATK, Khoury S, Aso Y *et al*. (eds) *The 2nd International Consultation on Benign Prostatic Hyperplasia (BPH), Paris, France, 1993, June 27–30*. Jersey, Scientific Communications International 1993: 453–507.

2 Devonec M, Ogden C, Perrin P, Carter SSC. Clinical response to transurethral microwave thermotherapy is thermal dose dependent. *Eur Urol* 1993; **23**: 267–74.

3 Devonec M, Carter SSC, Tubaro A *et al*. Microwave therapy. *Curr Opin Urol* 1995; **5**: 3–9.

4 Schulman CC, Zlotta AR. Transurethral needle ablation of the prostate: a new treatment of benign prostatic hyperplasia using interstitial low-level radiofrequency energy. *Curr Opin Urol* 1995; **5**: 35–8.

5 Madersbacher S, Marberger M. Therapeutic applications of ultrasound in urology. In: Marberger M (ed) *Application of Newer Forms of Therapeutic Energy in Urology*. Oxford: ISIS Medical Media 1995: 115–36.

6 Fry FJ. Intense focused ultrasound in medicine. *Eur Urol* 1993; **23** (Suppl 1): 2–7.

7 Ter Haar G. Focused ultrasound therapy. *Curr Opin Urol* 1994; **4**: 89–92.

8 Barnett SB, Ter Haar GR, Ziskin MC *et al*. Current status of research on biophysical effects of ultrasound. *Ultrasound Med Biol* 1994; **20**: 205–18.

9 Driller J, Lizzi FL. Therapeutic applications of ultrasound: a review. *IEEE* 1987; **12**: 33–40.

10 Fry WJ, Barnard JW, Fry FJ *et al*. Ultrasonic lesions in the mamalian central nervous system. *Science* 1955; **122**: 517–18.

11 Hynynen K, Darkazanli A, Damianou CA *et al*. Tissue thermometry during ultrasound exposure. *Eur Urol* 1993; **23**(Suppl 1): 12–16.

12 Ter Haar G, Sinnett D, Rivens I. High intensity focused ultrasound – A surgical technique for the treatment of discrete liver tumors. *Phys Med Biol* 1989; **34**: 1743–50.

13 Madersbacher S, Marberger M. Urological applications of high-intensity focused ultrasound. *Curr Opin Urol* 1995; **5**: 147–9.

14 Madersbacher S, Kratzik C, Susani M, Marberger M. Tissue ablation in benign prostatic hyperplasia with high intensity focused ultrasound. *J Urol* 1994; **152**: 1956–61.

15 Bihrle R, Foster RS, Sanghvi NT, Donohue JP, Hood PJ. High intensity focused ultrasound for the treatment of benign prostatic hyperplasia: Early United States clinical experience. *J Urol* 1994; **151**: 1271–5.

16 Madersbacher S, Pedevilla M, Vingers L *et al*. Effect of high-intensity focused ultrasound on human prostate cancer *in vivo*. *Cancer Res* 1995; **55**: 3346–51.

17 Gelet A, Chapelon JY, Margonari J *et al*. Prostatic tissue destruction by high intensity focused ultrasound: experimentation on canine prostate. *J Endourol* 1993; **7**: 249–53.

18 Gelet A, Chapelon JY, Margonari J *et al*. High-intensity focused

ultrasound experimentation on human benign prostatic hypertrophy. *Eur Urol* 1993; **23** (Suppl 1): 44–7.

19 Lizzi FL. High-precision thermotherapy for small lesions. *Eur Urol* 1993; **23**(Suppl 1): 23–8.

20 Silvermann RH, Vogelsang B, Rondeau MJ, Coleman DJ. Therapeutic ultrasound for the treatment of glaucoma. *Am J Ophthalmol* 1991; **111**: 327–37.

21 Ioritani N, Sirai S, Taguchi K *et al*. Effects of high intensity ultrasound heating on the normal and cancer tissue. *Jpn J Endourol ESWL* 1994; **7**: 299.

22 Zanelli CI, Hennige CW, Sanghvi NT. Design and characterisation of a 10 cm annular array transducer for high intensity focused ultrasound (HIFU) applications. Paper presented at the IEEE Symposium 1994.

23 Foster RS, Bihrle R, Sanghvi NT *et al*. Production of prostatic lesions in canines using transrectally administered high intensity focused ultrasound. *Eur Urol* 1993; **23**: 330–6.

24 Bihrle R, Foster RS, Sanghvi N, Fry F, Donohue JP. Transrectal high intensity focused ultrasound subtotal ablation of the prostate in a canine model. *J Urol* 1995; **153** (Suppl): 435A.

25 Foster RS, Bihrle R, Sanghvi NT, Fry F, Donohue JP. High intensity focused ultrasound treatment of prostatic tissue in the presence of an ultrasound contrast agent. *J Urol* 1995; **153** (Suppl): 398A.

26 Susani M, Madersbacher S, Kratzik C, Vingers L, Marberger M. Morphology of tissue destruction induced by focused ultrasound. *Eur Urol* 1993; **23** (Suppl 1): 34–8.

27 Nakamura K, Baba S, Saito S *et al*. A long term response following high intensity focused ultrasound for prostatic hyperplasia. *J Urol* 1996; **155** (Suppl): 405A.

28 Madersbacher S, Klingler CH, Schatzl G *et al*. The impact of transrectal high intensity focused ultrasound on prostatic obstruction in BPH assessed by pressure flow studies. *Eur Urol* 1996; **30**: 437–45.

29 Kabalin JN, Gill HS, Bite G, Wolfe V. Comparative study of laser versus electrocautery prostatic resection: 18 months follow-up with complex urodynamic assessment. *J Urol* 1995; **153**: 94–8.

30 Ogden CW, Reddy P, Johnson H *et al*. Sham versus transurethral microwave thermotherapy in patients with symptoms of benign prostatic bladder outflow obstruction. *Lancet* 1993; **341**: 14–17.

31 Dixon CM. A comparison of transurethral prostatectomy with visual laser ablation of the prostate using the Urolase right-angle fiber for the treatment of BPH. *World J Urol* 1995; **13**: 126–9.

32 Steele GS, Sleep DJ. Transurethral needle ablation of the prostate: does the pressure flow curve change? *J Urol* 1995; **153** (Suppl): 435A.

33 Yang R, Sanghvi NT, Rescorla FJ *et al*. Extracorporeal liver ablation using sonography-guided high-intensity focused ultrasound. *Invest Radiol* 1992; **27**: 796–803.

34 Fry FJ, Johnson LK. Tumor irradiation with intense ultrasound. *Ultrasound Med Biol* 1978; **4**: 337–41.

35 Yang R, Sanghvi NT, Rescorla FJ *et al*. Liver cancer ablation with extracorporeal high-intensity focused ultrasound. *Eur Urol* 1993; **23** (Suppl 1): 17–22.

36 Madersbacher S, Susani M, Kratzik C *et al*. Transcutaneous tissue ablation of human testes by high intensity focused ultrasound. *Eur Urol* 1998; **33**: 195–201.

37 Yang R, Reilly CR, Rescorla FJ *et al*. Effect of high-intensity focused ultrasound in the treatment of experimental neuroblastoma. *J Pediatr Surg* 1992; **27**: 246–51.

38 Gelet A, Chapelon JY. Effects of high-intensity focused ultrasound on malignant cells and tissues. In: M. Marberger (ed) *Application of Newer Forms of Therapeutic Energy in Urology*. Oxford: ISIS Medical Media 1995; 107–14.

COMMENTARY

HIFU is a method of causing heat-induced prostate destruction using ultrasonic energy. Normally in biologic tissue, mechanical ultrasonic energy is converted to heat. By increasing the intensity of the ultrasonic energy and focusing it on a specific area, temperatures between 80 and 200°C can be achieved. As noted in prior chapters, this level of temperature will produce irreversible coagulation necrosis. Also, focusing the ultrasonic beam means that intervening tissues are not injured.

HIFU has been utilized for therapy of many organ systems. The widest experience is with the prostate. The principles governing the use of HIFU have been eloquently discussed in this chapter by Drs S. Madersbacher and M. Marberger. The instrumentation consists essentially of a piezoceramic transducer, which changes in thickness in response to electric current. This change causes acoustic waves with a frequency of 0.5–10 MHz, which are then focused on target tissues. For a variety of technical and safety reasons, transrectally applied HIFU appears optimal to target the prostatic adenoma. The transrectal devices incorporate both imaging and treatment systems on a single or separate probes, and are available with varying focal lengths to accommodate varying prostate sizes. Phased-array transducers with variable focal lengths have also recently become available.

The pioneering work in this area has been carried out by Madersbacher and Marberger and associates in Vienna, Austria. Their preliminary conclusions are that HIFU is an attractive minimally invasive therapy not only for BPH but also for carcinoma of the prostate. The HIFU procedure can be performed under IV sedation, although mostly it is performed currently under general or spinal anesthesia. The procedure involves initial placement of a 10-French suprapubic tube to drain the bladder. A Foley catheter is placed in the urethra during the imaging phase of the procedure; subsequently, this catheter is removed while the HIFU treatment is performed. The HIFU probe is targeted at the prostate using a transrectal approach and the prostate is treated circumferentially in seven to nine sectors. Lesions of 2×10 mm are created circumferentially during therapy. To date, over 250 patients have been treated worldwide in clinical Phase 2 trials. In Drs Madersbacher and Marberger's experience of over 100 patients, there was a 47% improvement in uroflow and a 53% decrease in symptom scores following 1 year of treatment. These results have essentially been mirrored in worldwide trials. However, pressure-flow studies before and after HIFU conducted in 30 patients revealed only a moderate improvement in objective parameters using the Abrams–Griffith nomogram. The authors, therefore, advise caution and that in its present form HIFU be reserved for patients with moderately but not severely obstructed prostates.

Side effects of the therapy include urinary retention, which is resolved by the presence of a suprapubic catheter for 6 days. Other complications include rectal injury, which is rare at less than 2%. Additionally, their injuries occurred early in the clinical trial and subsequent modifications of the system have resolved them.

In summary, HIFU is a promising though evolving therapy. Experience in the USA is limited. Its major advantage is the capability of inducing contact-free coagulation necrosis without the need for urethral manipulation. As a result, postoperative irritative symptoms and urethral injury are minimal. The disadvantages include only moderate improvement in symptoms, and the need for anesthesia in a significant number of patients, as well as the capital expense of the equipment.

Stents and Spirals in Benign Prostatic Hyperplasia: the European Experience

24

G.M. Lennon and J.M. Fitzpatrick

INTRODUCTION

Benign prostatic hyperplasia (BPH) is the commonest neoplastic growth in men, and prostatic outflow obstruction secondary to BPH constitutes the commonest cause of male urological symptoms. While transurethral resection of the prostate (TURP) remains the gold standard for treating prostatic obstruction, a number of studies in the latter half of the 1980s raised questions regarding the long-term safety and efficacy of TURP.[1,2]

Furthermore, elderly debilitated patients may have several contraindications to surgery for BPH. These patients ultimately end up with a long-term indwelling catheter with the attendant sequalae, i.e. infection, encrustation, stone formation, and discomfort. In the last decade, there has been an explosion of interest in non-surgical and less-invasive surgical alternatives to transurethral resection of the prostate. Of the new modalities, prostatic stents now represent a viable alternative to long-term catheterization in the elderly unfit patient, and, more recently, the indications have been extended for use in elective fit patients as an alternative to TURP.

BACKGROUND

The concept of using a stent for splinting the lobes of the prostate was derived from the original use of stents in the vascular system for preventing arterial restenosis following angioplasty. Fabian was the first to modify this concept, producing the first urethral stent for the treatment of outlet obstruction secondary to BPH.[3] However, it was not until the advent of stenting for urethral stricture disease that the

use of prostatic stents became more widespread. Since then, two types of stents have emerged: the temporary removable stent and the long-term permanent tubular mesh stent. These stents are now available in differing lengths, diameters, materials, and designs, which are listed in Table 24.1.

TEMPORARY STENTS

Temporary prostatic stents are designed for short-term use to relieve bladder outlet obstruction and to serve as an alternative to an indwelling Foley catheter or suprapubic tube in high-risk patients considered unfit for surgery. The stents are designed for short periods of use, usually <6 months and can be inserted and removed easily endoscopically. The Urospiral and Prostakath (Porges, Paris, France; Pharma-Plast Doctors and Engineers, Copenhagen, Denmark) are stainless steel coils, the latter being gold plated to inhibit encrustation. With this design, the proximal tip of the coil extends through the bladder neck and is tightly coiled within the prostatic urethra. A straight segment crosses the external sphincter and membranous urethra and ends in a short coil in the bulbous urethra (Figure 24.1). This design maintains stent position without interference with the sphincter mechanism.[4,5]

In high-risk elderly patients, these temporary stents permit normal micturition with an acceptable side-effect profile compared with Foley catheters. Success rates have been reported in the range of 50–90%. Potential problems include encrustation, migration, and breakage. Stress incontinence has been reported in about 33% of patients and chronic bacteriuria noted in less than 20%. If required, stent replacement can be easily accomplished. Because of the stent design, however, urethral

Name	Manufacturer	Type	Composition	Design	Diameter (French)
Intraurethral catheter	Angiomed	Temp.	Polyurethrane	Malecot	16 (OD)
Urospiral	Porges	Temp.	Stainless steel	Spiral	21 (OD)
Prostakath	Pharma-Plast	Temp.	Stainless steel (gold coated)	Spiral	21 (OD)
UroLume wallstent	American Medical Systems	Perm. mesh	Superalloy	Tubular mesh	42 (ID)
Intraprostatic stent	ASI	Perm.	Titanium	Tubular mesh	35 (ID)

Table 24.1 Prostatic stents

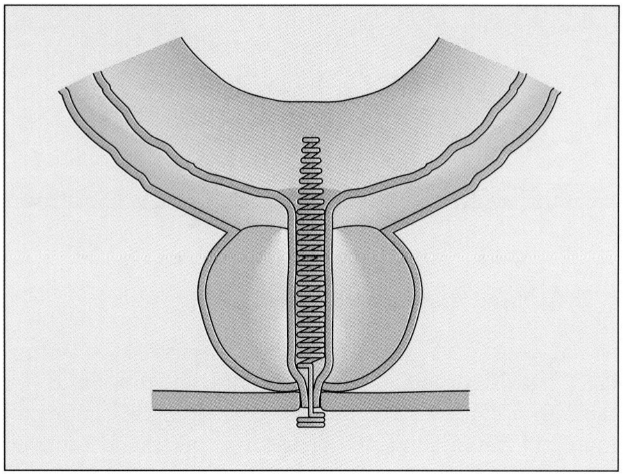

Figure 24.1 Diagrammatic representation of a prostatic stent (the Prostakath) *in situ* in the prostatic urethra

Source: From Prostatic Stents. Kaplan SA, Hoo H. In *Current Surgical Techniques in Urology.* 1990, Vol 3, Issue 4

catheterization and cystoscopy cannot be performed with the prosthesis in place.

One of the earliest and most basic form of these temporary stents was the intraurethral catheter described by Nissenkorn.[6] It has a double Malecot design, which holds the stent in place within the prostate. Nissenkorn reported 3-year follow-up on 94 patients with BPH, unfit for surgery. Seventy-eight had been treated with long-term catheters and 16 had severe symptomatic obstruction.

All stents were inserted under direct vision and local anesthesia and 80.8% of patients had their obstruction relieved. Almost 1 in 5 stents had to be removed earlier than intended because of incorrect positioning or displacement. Irritative symptoms were common in all patients, but these were transient. The author recommended changing the device (which is easily accomplished) 6–12 monthly to minimize the possibility of infection or obstruction.

In 1993, Ozgur *et al.*[7] reported their initial experience with the Urospiral in 31 patients unfit for prostate surgery. All stents were placed under local anesthetic with good results at 4-month follow-up. Guazzoni *et al.*[8] compared 20 patients with the Urospiral and 18 patients in whom a permanent UroLume was inserted. Both groups did well, with somewhat better flow rates and symptom score improvements in the UroLume group at 12-month follow-up. Encrustation was a problem in the Urospiral group, with displacement occurring in 6 patients. However, the temporary stent is easily replaced under local anesthetic and may be a cheaper alternative in patients requiring temporary treatment only.

Anson *et al.*[9] used the Urospiral in 10 patients with advanced carcinoma of the prostate and either urinary retention or severe obstruction. The patients were commenced on antiandrogens following insertion of the stent,

which was removed 3 months later. All patients voided satisfactorily following stent removal, although one patient subsequently required a limited TURP. This limited stent period considerably reduces the risk of displacement, encrustation, and infection, none of which occurred in this series.

Karaoglen *et al.*[10] investigated the Urospiral in 18 similar high-risk patients, all of whom voided successfully post-implantation with satisfactory bladder emptying. Complications in this group included hematuria in 2 patients, migration in 1, and infection in 8.

Thomas *et al.*[11] published their results with the Prostakath in 87 patients considered high risk for conventional surgery. Sixty-four patients presented with acute retention. Fifty-seven (89%) voided successfully, while 7 failed to void. Of 14 patients with chronic retention, 5 voided successfully while 9 failed to void or were incontinent and required an alternative procedure. Complications seen in this series included hematuria resulting in clot retention (5%), stent migration (15%), recurrent urinary tract infections (10%), and encrustation (4%).

Braf *et al.*[12] evaluated the Prostakath (32) and Urospiral (23) in a series of 55 men followed for 12–16 months. There were 10 and 8 failures in the Prostakath and Urospiral group, respectively. Long-term complications in the Prostakath included urinary tract infections 4, failure to void 2, stricture 1, and encrustation 3. Complications in the Urospiral group included urinary infection in 4, migration 1, failure to void 1, and stricture 1. One patient in each group died of urosepsis at about 18 months post-stent insertion.

Temporary stents have the great advantage of ease of insertion under local anesthetic. They produce immediate relief of obstruction and are relatively cheap. They do, however, remain in contact with urine and therefore have a limited life expectancy. Their relatively small lumen precludes endoscopic examination or catheterization without first removing the stent. Nevertheless, in the older unfit patient with a limited life expectancy temporary stents represent a useful alternative to permanent urethral catheterization.

PERMANENT STENTS

Probably the widest experience with permanent prostatic stents has been with the UroLume (American Medical Systems, Minnetonka, MN), and the Intraprostatic stent (Advanced Surgical Intervention, San Clemente, CA) (Figures 24.2–24.4). Both devices consist of a tubular woven mesh made of superalloy and titanium, respectively. The UroLume comes in a range of lengths from 1.5 to 4.0 cm and a diameter of 14 mm. The self-expanding properties of the mesh press it against the lobes of the prostate with a radial force, preventing migration and permitting epithelialization of the wire mesh. The large internal diameter of these stents (Table 24.1), permits easy instrumentation once the lumen has epithelialized. This has usually occurred within about 6 weeks, thus greatly reducing the tendency to encrustation.[13]

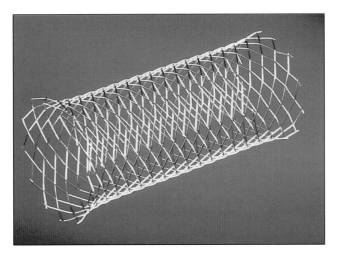

Figure 24.2 The AMS UroLume® prosthesis

Source: UroLume® Endoprosthesis, courtesy of American Medical Systems, Inc., Minnetonka, MN. Illustration by Michael Schenk

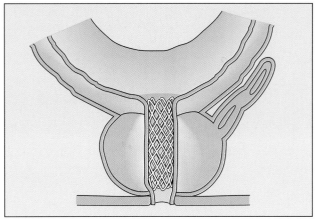

Figure 24.4 Diagrammatic representation of the ASI Intraprostatic stent positioned within the prostatic urethra

Source: From Prostatic Stents. Kaplan SA, Koo H. *Current Surgical Techniques in Urology.* 1990, Vol 3, Issue 4

The ASI Intraprostatic stent differs in several respects to the wallstent. The titanium is neither flexible nor self-expanding and requires a non-compliant balloon catheter to dilate it to its final fixed diameter of 35 French in the prostatic urethra (Figure 24.7). Under caudal or light general anesthesia, cystoscopy is first performed and the prostatic length measured with a special calibrated catheter. The appropriate length stent is then selected, premounted on a balloon catheter, and inserted to lie just distal to the bladder neck and proximal to the external sphincter. The balloon is then inflated to 4 atm. or 120 lb in^{-2} under direct vision using a 0° telescope, expanding the stent to its final 35-French diameter.

Kirby *et al.*[14] inserted the titanium stent in 30 patients with acute urinary retention considered unfit for surgery. Satisfactory voiding was achieved in 25 patients with a mean maximum flow rate of 10.7 mL s^{-1} and a mean residual urine of 50 mL. Five stents required removal, and epithelialization was noted to be incomplete in all cases.[13] Urinary tract infection was noted in 10 individuals, who, however, responded to antibiotic therapy. The authors concluded that the titanium stent was an acceptable alternative to TURP or long-term catheterization in high-risk patients.

TECHNICAL ASPECTS OF STENT PLACEMENT AND REMOVAL

It is generally recommended that prophylactic antibiotic should be administered prior to stent insertion. A cystoscopy is first performed to assess the condition of the urethra/bladder and to measure the length of the prostatic urethra from bladder neck to verumontanum. This can be measured with a calibrated balloon catheter or ureteric catheter.

Alternatively, a flexible cystoscope can be placed at the bladder neck and verumontanum respectively and both positions marked on the shaft of the scope at the

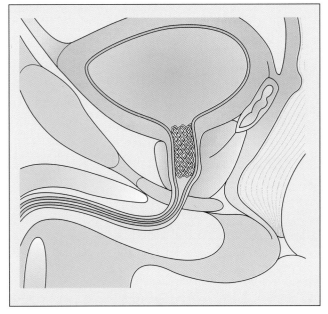

Figure 24.3 Diagrammatic representation of the UroLume® wallstent positioned within the prostatic urethra

Source: UroLume® Endoprosthesis, courtesy of American Medical Systems, Inc., Minnetonka, MN. Original illustration by Michael Schenk

In high-risk patients unsuitable for surgery (usually due to cardiorespiratory disease), these stents may be placed in the prostatic urethra under local/regional anesthesia. The UroLume prosthesis is inserted transurethrally into the prostatic urethra by means of a special delivery instrument shown in Figures 24.5 and 24.6. During insertion, the delivery instrument keeps the stent compressed until its release, when it self-expands, pressing out against the lobes of the prostate from the bladder neck to the verumontanum. The instrument allows direct visualization of the prosthesis throughout the implant procedure, permitting accurate deployment of the stent at the bladder neck and away from the external sphincter mechanism.

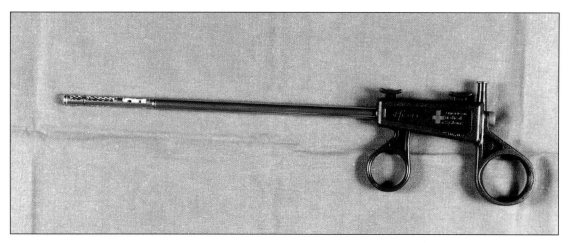

Figure 24.5 The delivery instrument showing the stent covered by the outer retractable sheath

Source: UroLume® Endoprosthesis, courtesy of American Medical Systems, Inc., Minnetonka, MN. Illustration by Michael Schenk

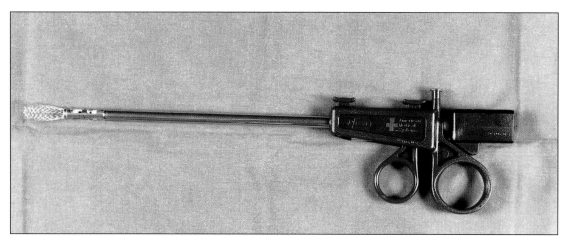

Figure 24.6 The delivery instrument showing the stent partially deployed

Source: UroLume® Endoprosthesis, courtesy of American Medical Systems, Inc., Minnetonka, MN. Illustration by Michael Schenk

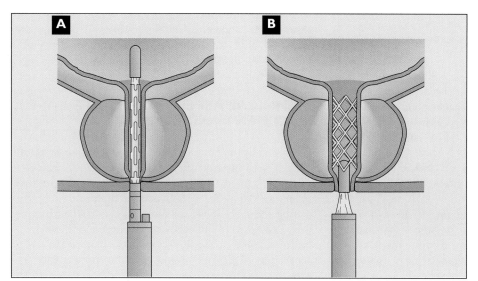

Figure 24.7 The ASI titanium stent mounted on its balloon carrier positioned in the prostatic urethra before (A) and after (B) deployment

Source: From Kirby R, Heard SR, Miller P, *et al.* Use of the ASI titanium stent in the management of bladder outflow obstruction due to benign prostatic hyperplasia. *J Urol* 1992; 148(4): 1195

urethral meatus. The interval between the marks corresponds to the length of the prostatic urethra. However, the calibrated balloon catheter is probably the more accurate method.

The stated length and diameter of the UroLume refers to the unconstrained measurements of the stent. If the stent remains under any compression within the prostate, it may not attain its full 14 mm diameter and so may be slightly longer than the stated length. While prostatic stents usually reach their full diameter, this may take 1–2 days, and so allowance must be made for this at the time of surgery by selecting a stent 0.5 cm shorter than the measured length of the prostatic urethra.

The urethra is next dilated to 28 French. A 0° telescope is inserted into the delivery instrument with or without the optional telescope stabilizer, and the instrument positioned at the bladder neck. The front superior safety button on the instrument is depressed and the trigger-like front finger grip is pulled posteriorly (Figure 24.6). This allows the retractable sheath (which covers the stent) to slide back into the outer shaft. The prosthesis is deployed but not released and can be retracted back into the sheath if the position appears unsatisfactory. Care is taken to ensure the prosthesis does not protrude into the bladder or encroach on the external sphincter by moving the telescope to visualize these structures.

When a satisfactory position is obtained, the prosthesis is released by depressing the rear security button, which detaches the stent from the delivery instrument. The trigger device of the instrument now locks, preventing any attempt to resheath the prosthesis. The delivery instrument is now withdrawn with a slight rotatory motion, while continuing to view the stent to ensure displacement does not occur. The final position can be checked with a 17-French cystoscope, but the scope should not be placed through the prosthesis at this point in order to avoid displacement.

If the prostate is not sufficiently covered, a second stent can be placed overlapping the first prosthesis by at least 5 diamonds. Again, care must be taken not to dislodge the first prosthesis when placing the second prosthesis.

PRECAUTIONS AND COMPLICATIONS OF STENT PLACEMENT

Care should be taken to ensure the prosthesis does not extend into the bladder or encrustation may occur. Similarly, the prosthesis must not extend into the external sphincter or stress incontinence will result (Table 24.2).

A cystoscopy should be performed to check the final position of the prosthesis. Care must be taken not to displace the prosthesis. If the prosthesis is not in satisfactory position, it may be adjusted in a proximal or distal direction by grasping several diamonds with a urological alligator forceps at either end of the stent and pulling or pushing the stent into the required position.

If the patient fails to void, a suprapubic tube must be used. Urethral catheterization is contraindicated until the prosthesis is covered with urothelium (Table 24.2).

- Meatal or urethral strictures, which cannot be dilated to 26 French.
- The presence of active urinary tract infection.
- Patients in whom bleeding may seriously impede visualization of the prosthesis placement.
- Presence of a fistula at the proposed prosthesis location.
- Bladder stones.
- Neurogenic bladder.
- Conditions which may require transurethral manipulations within 1 month of stent placement.
- Patients with known or suspected cancer.
- Large median lobe of the prostate.
- Prostatic urethra less than 2 cm in length.
- Prostatitis.
- Small prostate, i.e. bladder neck obstruction without lateral lobe involvement.

Table 24.2 Contraindications to stent placement

REMOVING A PROSTHESIS

If the position is unsatisfactory and stent removal is necessary the following procedure is recommended.

A guidewire is passed through the working channel of a resectoscope sheath, into the urethra and through the lumen of the prosthesis, allowing it to coil up in the bladder. The sheath is removed and passed alongside the wire. An alligator forceps is used to push the stent into the bladder.

With a grasping forceps, the tip of the wire is withdrawn into the sheath and brought out of the urethra. The sheath is removed and replaced over both ends of the wire and guided back into the bladder. The prosthesis is pulled into the sheath by pulling firmly on both ends of the wire and the sheath removed. If the stent has already epithelialized, it must first be resected using a low setting current, followed by the same steps outlined above.

EXPERIENCE WITH THE UROLUME PROSTHESIS

In 1988 Milroy et al.[15] first described the use of a urethral wallstent (Medinvent, Lausanne, Switzerland), for the treatment of recurring urethral strictures. This stent was made from surgical grade stainless steel and woven in the form of a tubular mesh, which was self-expanding once released from its small-diameter delivery catheter. After first dilating the stricture to 30 French, the UroLume endourethral prosthesis was placed across the strictured area. In this preliminary report, 8 patients were treated. Complete epithelial covering was noted to occur with these stents, with follow-up flow rates approaching those seen following TURP. Since then, over 270 patients have been treated by this group with a newer form of urethral wallstent (the AMS UroLume) with successful outcomes. These stents have subsequently been adapted for use in neuropathic patients with detrusor sphincter dyssynergia[16] and in the prostatic urethra as an alternative to TURP in medically unfit patients.[17]

Williams et al. described the use of the Medinvent stent for use in the prostatic urethra in patients with both acute[22] and chronic urinary retention.[18] All patients were considered high risk for surgery, and all stents were placed under radiological guidance. Twenty patients voided spontaneously, except for one patient with chronic retention. Median flow rates declined from an initial 20 mL s^{-1} at 1 week to 14 mL s^{-1} at 15 months. Although 8 deaths and 2 strokes occurred in the follow-up period, none was procedure-related. Nineteen out of 21 had infected urine prior to stent insertion, but this declined progressively with time to 5 patients at the last follow-up.

In this series 15 patients experienced extreme urgency of micturition for the first 3–4 days, and in 3 patients this persisted for up to 8 weeks. Eight patients experienced urge incontinence lasting from 3 to 21 days, while 4 patients experienced stress incontinence, which was persistent in 2 cases. They found that once epithelialized, the stents were not prone to displacement by instrumentation but urged caution and the use of a suprapubic catheter if a catheter was required.

In 1990, Chapple reported on a series of 12 men with BPH, considered poor risk for surgery, treated with the UroLume Endourethral Prosthesis. Seventy-five percent (9) were in acute retention. Of the 12, 95% were fully satisfied with the outcome and voiding satisfactorily with mean peak flow rates of 13.6±4.7 mL s^{-1}.[17] All patients experienced irritative voiding symptoms immediately after stent placement, which settled over a period of months. One patient with detrusor instability experienced severe frequency and urgency.

This series was later updated to 45 high-risk patients, again with very similar results. Forty-two patients (93%) were satisfied with the outcome following initial problems with frequency, urgency, and urge incontinence. Complete epithelialization was noted at between 4 and 6 months. Hyperplastic tissue growth through the interstices of the stent was seen at 6–9 months but this subsided in 12–18 months and was not deemed clinically significant. Five of 45 stents (11%) were removed without apparent difficulty.[17]

Milroy *et al.*[19] reported on a series of 140 patients from a multicenter European study (94 with BPH and 46 with acute retention). In both groups of patients, voiding was satisfactory post-UroLume placement. In the non-retention group, mean peak flow rates increased from 9.3 mL s^{-1} to 17.3 mL s^{-1} and mean symptom score declined to 7.6. In the retention group, peak flow rates and symptom score were 13.5 mL s^{-1} and 3 post-stent insertion. Eleven stents in the series were removed for malposition and a further three for persistent side effects.[20]

Similar changes in symptom scores, flow rates, and residual urine data were reported by Oesterling *et al.*,[21] who reviewed the multicenter North American experience with prostatic stenting. The UroLume endoprosthesis was placed in 126 healthy men suffering from BPH (95 with BPH and 31 with acute retention). In the non-retention group, mean symptom scores, residual volumes, and peak flow rates went from 14.5±0.5, 85±9 mL, and 9.1±0.5 mL s^{-1} to 5.4±0.5, 47±8 mL, and 13.1±0.7 mL s^{-1} respectively at 24 months. In the retention group, symptom scores and peak flow rates were 4.1±1.4 and 11.4±1.0 mL s^{-1} at 24

months. The majority of stents were covered at 12 months. Explantation was required in 17 patients for migration in 5, recurrent obstruction in 5, encrustation 2, and persistent irritative voiding symptoms and perineal discomfort in 4.

In 1993, Williams *et al.*[22] described their results of treating 140 patients with symptomatic BPH with the UroLume. In this study, 81 men had at least 6 months follow-up, while a further 36 had reached 12 months. The mean symptom scores were 5.3 and 6.5 at 6 and 12 months, respectively. Mean peak urinary flow rates were maintained at 14.9 and 14.7 mL s^{-1} at 6 and 12 months. Explantation was required in 12 patients due principally to stent migration.

Owing to the problem of stent shortening with consequent malpositioning, a modified stent was designed, which demonstrated less shortening following insertion and expansion. Design changes included an increase in diameter of the wire and the crossing angle was changed from 142 to 110°. This modified stent was evaluated in a multicenter European trial.[23] There were 91 patients with symptomatic BPH and 44 with urinary retention. In the non-retention group mean symptom scores improved from 14.1±0.4 to 4.7±5.1 at 18-month follow-up. Mean peak flow rates and residual urines went from 9.3±3.3 mL s^{-1} and 166 mL to 17.1±9.4 mL s^{-1} and 28±50 mL, respectively.

In the retention group, the symptom score, peak flow rates, and residual urine volumes at 18 months were 4.6±2, 13.7±7.3 mL s^{-1} and 37±70 mL, respectively.

While these results were promising, a higher rate of complications (38%) was seen with the modified stent. Explantation was required in 21 patients due to intractable detrusor instability, stent migration, encrustation, persisting obstruction, and severe epithelial hyperplasia.

PROSTATE STENTS AND LONG-TERM WAITING LISTS

In 1994, Schneider *et al.*[24] reported on the impact of the UroLume on their long-term waiting list for prostate surgery. The UroLume was successfully introduced in 60 out of 70 patients chosen from the long-term waiting list. The majority of cases were performed as day-case procedures under a general anesthetic.[23] Short-term results were promising with 72% of patients symptomatically improved, and showing a doubling of mean peak flow rates. Stent displacement required removal in 10 patients. The waiting time for prostatic surgery was reduced from 3 to 2 years, and the authors concluded that the UroLume could offer an expedient solution to this type of public health problem.

MALIGNANT PROSTATIC OBSTRUCTION

Guazzoni *et al.*[25] described the use of the UroLume wall-stent for the treatment of retention secondary to advanced carcinoma of the prostate. The stent was placed in 11 stage-D prostate cancer patients considered high surgical risk, with urinary retention unrelieved by maximal androgen blockade. All patients voided spontaneously with good symptomatic relief. At 1 year, 10 patients were evaluable and 9 of the 10 had non-obstructed flow rates.

The side-effect profile was similar to that seen in benign disease. All patients had marked irritative symptoms and transient hematuria, which resolved over the first 2 months and 2 weeks, respectively. Severe perineal pain was seen in 2 patients, which again resolved spontaneously. Two cases of transient urothelial hyperplasia were seen, which regressed to normal by 6 months. Complete urothelial covering was seen at 12 months and in no case did stent occlusion occur owing to malignant overgrowth. No major complications were seen and no patient required stent explantation. The authors point out that TURP in advanced cancer of the prostate may be associated with a significant rate of intraoperative and postoperative complications, including bleeding and incontinence, and that the UroLume offers a viable alternative to a TURP or long-term catheter in this type of patient with urinary retention.

THE TITAN INTRA-PROSTATIC STENT

The Titan Intra-Prostatic Stent (Boston Scientific Corporation, Watertown, MA) has been reported on by several groups.[14,26–28] The stent is a tubular mesh similar to the UroLume and is composed of titanium, a material known for its tissue biocompatibility, corrosion resistance, and low toxicity. The stent comes in several lengths from 19 to 50 mm at 4-mm increments.

In 1993, Kaplan et al.[27] reported on 68 patients who underwent insertion of the stent, 38 of whom were in acute retention. The stents were inserted under direct vision and expanded to 33 French using a balloon catheter. The mean preoperative symptom score decreased from 16.8 to 3.2 at 18 months. The mean postvoid residual urine decreased from 74 mL to 36 mL and the mean peak urinary flow rate increased from 3.9 mL s^{-1} to 14.4 mL s^{-1} at 18 months. Seventeen stents (25%), were removed, 10 owing to malpositioning of the stent and 7 because of treatment failure. Transient hematuria and urinary infections were noted in 43 (63%) and 6 (9%) patients, respectively.[27]

Miller et al. treated 148 patients deemed unfit for surgery with the Titan Intra-Prostatic Stent.[28] Satisfactory voiding was re-established in 89% of the patients with a mean post-stent peak flow rate of 13.1 mL s^{-1} and postvoid residual urine of 60 mL.

The last few years has seen the introduction of several newer stent materials and designs, including nitinol (the Prostacoil) a flexible thermosensitive product;[29–31] the Memokath, a spiral composed of titanium nickel alloy, with shape memory properties;[32] and the SMA endoprosthesis, another metal alloy with special shape memory properties.[33] Results with these newer designs appear promising in the short term, but, as with the more established stents, will require longer-term evaluation.

PROBLEMS ENCOUNTERED WITH PROSTATE STENTS

In 1995, Parikh and Milroy[34] reviewed some of the problems they had encountered in their first 270 AMS UroLume patients. Choosing the correct size of stent to be used is clearly vital. The length of the prostatic urethra is probably best measured intraoperatively by use of a calibrated balloon catheter alongside a cystoscope. Experience of urethral length measurements with transrectal ultrasound was found to be unreliable owing to prostatic tissue extending beyond the verumontanum. This gave rise to overestimation of the prostatic urethral length and subsequent incorrect stent size placements.

MEASUREMENT OF PROSTATIC URETHRAL LENGTH

The 12-mL balloon on the AMS calibrated balloon catheter fixes the catheter at the bladder neck and enables accurate measurements of the prostatic urethral length. It is important to note that this length is greater if measured along the posterior wall of the prostatic urethra, compared with the anterior wall. The posterior wall curves concave anteriorly and enters the bladder neck obliquely, giving rise to this length discrepancy. This will cause a stent placed level with the posterior wall of the urethra to project into the bladder in relation to the anterior wall of the bladder neck, with the risk of subsequent encrustation. The urethral length should therefore be measured along both the anterior and posterior walls. The stent size required is usually 0.5 cm shorter than the measured length of the posterior wall.

The apparent position of the bladder neck may also change in relation to bladder volume. Thus, a stent placed at the bladder neck with the bladder empty may in fact protrude into the bladder when it is full. Therefore, measurements of prostatic urethral length should also be made with the bladder full.

IMPLANTATION

The stent should first start opening within the bladder and then be slowly withdrawn until the proximal end of the stent lies at the bladder neck at the 12 o'clock position. This should leave the stent just downstream of the bladder neck at the 6 o'clock position. Again, it is important that the bladder be full during the final positioning or the stent may be placed too far proximally and may project into the bladder, as the bladder subsequently fills with subsequent encrustation. If the stent is placed too far distally, it will encroach on the external sphincter mechanism and cause incontinence. Furthermore, if the stent is not placed at the bladder neck, persistence of obstructive symptoms may result.

Suboptimal stent placement may occur if vision is compromised during placement. This is usually caused by bleeding from the surface of a vascular prostate. This may be helped by overfilling the bladder to try and minimize surface bleeding with a high intravesical pressure.

Alternatively, continuous irrigation and a suprapubic catheter can be used to improve visibility.

The UroLume prosthesis usually expands to its full 14 mm diameter after 24–48 h. Incomplete expansion can be detected by the pattern of the diamonds at the time of placement. If the stent is fully expanded, the diamonds are noted to be longer in the transverse axis. Conversely, if not fully expanded the diamonds appear longer from front to back. Allowance must be made when positioning the stent for the gradual complete expansion in the first 24–48 h.

Placement of a second stent to cover a small amount of residual apical tissue is probably best avoided at the time of initial stent insertion. The majority appear to void satisfactorily and can have a second overlapping stent placed subsequently if clinically indicated. This approach will avoid unnecessary additional stent placements and also obviates the risk of displacing the first stent when introducing the second.

HEMATURIA

Occasional intermittent hematuria may occur following stent insertion until epithelialization is complete. This is generally mild and self-limiting. Hematuria can occasionally cause clot retention, and is best managed with a suprapubic tube secured with a suture, as the wires can cause balloon perforation. A urethral catheter is best avoided for at least 1 month post-stent insertion, to avoid displacement. By 4 weeks, epithelial covering is usually well advanced, allowing catheterization or endoscopic instrumentation to be carried out.

RETENTION

Retention of urine may occur due to clot retention as described above or, more commonly, in the setting of patients with chronic urinary retention. A suprapubic catheter is recommended in this group and can be left *in situ* for 4–6 weeks if they fail to void immediately. The majority have a successful outcome. Those with detrusor failure may require a long-term catheter or intermittent self-catheterization. Transrectal ultrasound is useful for checking stent position and detecting obstructing apical tissue, which can be treated with a second stent. This should not, however, be done for at least 48 h for the reasons mentioned above.

INCONTINENCE

Incontinence will clearly occur if the stent is placed overlapping the sphincter. Patients may also develop significant irritative symptoms of frequency, urgency, and urge incontinence, particularly if there is pre-existing detrusor instability. Symptoms tend to resolve gradually over the first 1–2 months, but may require treatment with oxybutynin hydrochloride.

INTRASTENT HYPERPLASIA

Varying degrees of intrastent hyperplasia may be seen with the UroLume prosthesis. This tends to settle spontaneously over a period of 6–12 months, but can in some cases be severe enough to warrant resection. Normal healing has been the experience following resection of the hyperplastic urothelium.

PAIN/EJACULATORY FUNCTION

Perineal/prostatic pain is not uncommon following stent insertion and can on occasion be severe. However, the pain tends to be transient lasting 2–4 weeks and appears to decrease with stent epithelialization. Patients should be warned in advance of this possibility. Standard analgesics plus an α-adrenergic blocker may be of help. Persistent pain may require stent removal on occasion.

Despite the fact that the bladder neck is being splinted open by these devices, the reported incidence of retrograde ejaculation appears to be quite low. In the series by Milroy *et al.*[20] the reported incidence of retrograde ejaculation in those patients who were sexually active was only 20%.

RELATIVE CONTRAINDICATIONS TO PROSTATIC STENTS

The UroLume is not recommended in very small or large prostates and in the presence of a large median lobe. The latter tends to displace the prosthesis anteriorly, resulting in a double-barrel urethra and incomplete epithelialization.

SUMMARY

The past decade has witnessed over 100 studies on the role of prostatic stents in the management of urinary retention and symptomatic BPH. These preliminary studies indicate that prostatic stents are an effective and safe treatment both for those unfit for surgery and also for fit patients with symptomatic bladder outflow obstruction due to BPH. Although the majority of studies have involved the UroLume endoprosthesis, there are a range of alternative products currently being investigated in clinical trials. While the ultimate stent has not as yet been developed, the most recent data suggest that prostatic stents are a safe and effective treatment for BPH in selected patients.

REFERENCES

1 Roos NP, Wennberg JR, Malenka DJ *et al*. Mortality and reoperation after open and transurethral resection of the prostate for benign prostatic hyperplasia. *N Engl J Med* 1989; **320**: 1120–5.

2 Malenka DJ, Roos NP, Fisher ES *et al*. Further study of the increased mortality following transurethral prostatectomy: a chart based analysis. *J Urol* 1990; **144**: 244–50.

3 Fabian KM. Der intraptostatische "Partielle Katheter" (Urologisch Spirale). *Urologe* 1980; **23A**: 236–41.

4 Nordling J, Holm HH, Klarskov P. The intraprostatic spiral: a new device for insertion with the patient under local anaesthesia and with ultrasonic guidance with 3 months follow up. *J Urol* 1989; **142**: 756–62.

5 Parker CJ, Birch BR, Connelly A *et al*. The Porges Urospiral: a reversible endoprostatic prosthetic stent. *World J Urol* 1991; **9**: 22–28.

6 Nissenkorn I. The intraurethral catheter – three years of experience. *Eur Urol* 1993; **24**: 27–30.

7 Ozgur GK, Sivrikaya A, Bilen R, Biberoglu K, Gumele Hr. The use of intraurethral prostatic spiral in high risk patients for surgery with benign prostatic hyperplasia. *Int Urol Nephrol* 1993; **25**: 65–71.

8 Guazzoni G, Bergamaschi F, Montorsi F *et al*. Prostatic UroLume Wallstent for BPH patients at poor operative risk: clinical, uroflowmetric and ultrasonographic patterns. *J Urol* 1993; **150**: 1641–47.

9 Anson KM, Barnes DJ, Briggs TP *et al*. Temporary prostatic stenting and androgen suppression: a new minimally invasive approach to malignant prostatic retention. *J R Soc Med* 1993; **86**: 634–8.

10 Karaoglan U, Alkibay T, Tokucoglu H *et al*. Urospiral in benign prostatic hyperplasia. *J Endourol* 1992; **6**: 455–61.

11 Thomas PJ, Britton JP, Harrison NW. The Prostakath stent: four years experience. *Br J Urol* 1993; **71**: 430–7.

12 Braf Z, Sofer M, Chen J *et al*. Long term experience with two different intraurethral coils in BPH patients. *J Urol* 1994; **151**: 396A.

13 Chapple CR, Milroy EJ, Richards D. Permanently implanted urethral stent for prostatic obstruction in the unfit patient – preliminary report. *Br J Urol* 1990; **66**: 58–64.

14 Kirby R, Heard SR, Miller P *et al*. Use of the ASI titanium stent in the management of bladder outflow obstruction due to benign prostatic hyperplasia. *J Urol* 1992; **148**(4): 1195–7.

15 Milroy EJ, Chapple CR, Cooper JE *et al*. A new treatment for urethral strictures. *Lancet* 1988; **1**: 1424–30.

16 Saurwein D, Gross AJ, Kutzenberger J, Ringert RH. Wallstents in patients with detrusor sphincter dyssynergia. *J Urol* 1995; **154**(92 Pt 1): 495–9.

17 Chapple CR, Milroy EJG, Rickards D. Permanently implanted urethral stent for prostatic obstruction in the unfit patient: Preliminary report. *Br J Urol* 1990; **66**: 58–64.

18 McLoughlin J, Jager J, Abel PD *et al*. The use of prostatic stents in patients with urinary retention who are unfit for surgery. *Br J Urol* 1990; **66**: 66–72.

19 Milroy E. Permanent prostate stents. *J Endourol* 1991; **5**: 75.

20 Milroy E, Coulage C, Pansadora V *et al*. The UroLume permanent prostate stent as an alternative to TURP: long term European results. *J Urol* 1994; **151**: 396A.

21 Oesterling JE, Defalco AJ *et al*. the North American UroLume Study Group. The North American experience with the UroLume endoprosthesis as a treatment for benign prostatic hyperplasia: Long term results. *Urology* 1994; **44**: 353–61.

22 Williams G, Coulage C, Milroy E *et al*. The non operative treatment for bladder outflow obstruction. *J Urol* 1993; **156**: 69–75.

23 Guazzoni G, Pansadoro V, Montorsi F *et al*. A modified prostatic UroLume wallstent for healthy patients with benign prostatic hyperplasia: a European multicenter study. *Urology* 1994; **44**: 364–70.

24 Schneider HJ, De-Souza JV, Palmer JH. The UroLume as a means of treating urinary outflow obstruction and its impact on waiting lists. *Br J Urol* 1994; **74**(3): 393–9.

25 Guazzoni G, Montorsi F, Bergamaschi F *et al*. Prostatic UroLume wallstent for urinary retention due to advanced prostate cancer: a 1 year follow up study. *J Urol* 1994; **152**(5 Pt 1): 1530–6.

26 Perez-Marreo R, Emerson LE. Balloon expanded titanium prostatic urethral stent. *Urology* 1994; **41**(Suppl): 38–44.

27 Kaplan SA, Merril DC, Mosley WG *et al*. The titanium intra-prostatic stent: the United States experience. *J Urol* 1993; **150**: 1624–30.

28 Miller PD, Gillat D, Abrams P. Selection of patients suitable for treatment with the ASI prostatic stent. *J Urol* 1993; **149**: 217A.

29 Yachia D, Beyar M, Aridogan IA. A new large calibre self expanding and self retaining temporary intraprostatic stent (Prostacoil) in the treatment of prostatic obstruction. *Br J Urol* 1994; **74**: 47–52.

30 Gottfried HW, Hautmann RE, Sintermann R *et al*. Memoterm stent for BPH treatment in high risk patients – experience of more than 100 cases. *J Urol* 1994; **151**: 397A.

31 Kiyota H, Machida T, Ohishi Y *et al*. Intraurethral catheter made of Niti-shape memory alloys for benign prostatic hyperplasia. *J Urol* 1994; **151**: 397A.

32 Poulsen AL, Shou J, Oveson H, Nordling J. Memokath: a second generation of intraprostatic spirals. *Br J Urol* 1993; **72**: 331–7.

33 Mori K, Okamoto S, Akimoto M. Placement of the urethral stent made of shape memory alloy (SMA) in the management of benign prostatic hypertrophy for patients contra-indicating other less invasive procedures. *J Urol* 1994; **151**: 398A.

34 Parikh AM, Milroy EJG. Precautions and complications in the use of the UroLume Wallstent. *Eur Urol* 1995; **27**: 1–7.

COMMENTARY

The European experience with stents has been more extensive then the US experience in that more physicians have been willing to use stents for a variety of indications in patients who are at poor risk for surgery. The fact that much of Europe and the UK has a nationalized type of insurance (similar to capitated care in the USA which is still in its infancy) coupled with the fact that, in many of these countries, there are older age groups of patients needing therapy because they have not undergone TURP may be contributing to this occurrence. The collective experience reported and analyzed so expertly by Drs Lennon and Fitzpatrick in this chapter suggest that stents are a viable alternative for patients, especially when combined sequentially with or in addition to other forms of minimally invasive therapy. The biodegradable stents are especially attractive to temporized patients recovering from other procedures, and may indeed be useful as a permanent means of relieving obstruction when they could be exchanged or replaced every 6 months. The stents have certainly undergone evolutionary improvements in materials that are biocompatible, as well as being deployable with more certainty and less complications over the last 10 years. It is the Editor's prediction that, with the improvements in stent technology, the utility of stents will become more common as they will be easy to place under local anesthesia with minimal surgical time. As long as they can be removed without too much operative manipulation, there would be very little disadvantage to their use.

Stents in Benign Prostatic Hyperplasia: the United States Experience

M. Corujo and G.H. Badlani

25

INTRODUCTION

While transurethral resection of the prostate (TURP) is the "gold standard" for the treatment of bladder outlet obstruction (BOO), it is associated with a mortality of 1% and a morbidity of incontinence (2–4%), blood loss, and anesthesia complications (5–10%).[1-4] Urinary stents, however, offer safe and effective alternatives in the poor-surgical-risk patient with BOO or in those patients with obstructive prostatic carcinoma. Stents in the genitourinary tract have been used to maintain patency in the ureter, across uretero- or urethral–intestinal anastomoses, at the bladder neck, and within the prostatic or anterior urethra. It was Chapple *et al.* who initially showed enthusiasm for the use of urinary stents for BOO, over TURP, in the surgically unfit patients.[5] Fabian, in 1980, first introduced the urological spiral (a temporary stainless steel catheter) in the management of BOO in patients who were unfit for surgery.[6] Because of the morbidity and mortality of TURP, less-invasive approaches in the management of BOO have been developed using various forms of thermal ablation such as by lasers, microwaves and rf energy. Unfortunately, these patients often complain of irritative voiding symptoms postoperatively, and about 30% will develop urinary retention from prostatic edema.[7,8] In this population, a temporary stent would be more appropriate than an indwelling catheter with its complications of discomfort and ascending infection.

Permanent stents were initially constructed for use in the vascular system and then adapted for the genitourinary tract.[9] Yachia described several properties that urinary stents should uphold in order to be successful. Stents should be biocompatible, chemically inert, have memory shape after deployment, have adequate tensile strength, and have a low internal–external diameter ratio to allow for optimal flow through the lumen.[10] Initially, stents were constructed in a fixed caliber ("first generation") and would not completely coapt against the urethral wall. These were often complicated by migration. Later self-expanding stents ("second generation") were developed to provide better anchoring within the urethra and thus less risk of migration.

In this chapter, we discuss both temporary and permanent prostatic urethral stents, and the 5-year results of the North American Multicenter clinical trial using the UroLume permanent stent for patients with BOO.

PROSTATE SHAPE

A problem that arises when stenting the prostatic urethra compared with the anterior urethra or ureter is the non-cylindrical shape of the prostate for which a cylindrical stent must be positioned. Furthermore, the bladder neck and prostatic urethra are not at right angles, but rather the prostatic urethra exits the bladder in an oblique fashion. Because the posterior prostatic urethral wall is longer than the anterior prostatic urethral wall, when a stent is placed at the bladder neck, the anterior aspect of the stent will protrude into the bladder and lead to complications of encrustation. To control this, one must position the stent more distally, but this may lead to poor stenting of the bladder neck itself. Proximal migration may also occur after stent placement if the bladder is not full when the stent is initially placed. As the bladder fills, the bladder base stretches, moving the stent proximally into the bladder.[11] Poor apposition of the stent to the urethral wall within the prostatic urethra can also lead to poor epithelialization, more important in permanent stents, which contributes to complications of migration, infection, and encrustation.[12]

TEMPORARY STENTS

Temporary prostatic stents are ideal in those patients with BOO who are either waiting for surgery or who have post-operative urinary retention after heat treatment for BOO (i.e. TUMT). Generally, these stents can be made of metal, polyurethane, or biodegradable materials. Because they are in place for only a short period of time, they are generally constructed into a solid tube made of a tight coil so as to prevent tissue ingrowth and epithelialization, and allow for easy removal. Temporary stents are either removed or changed between 6 and 36 months, unless they are made of bioabsorbable/biodegradable material.

METAL STENTS

There are four designs for temporary metal stents: Uro-spiral (fashioned after the initial design by Fabian), Prostakath, Prostacoil, and the Memokath. The first three stents are similar in that they contain a long prostatic segment followed by a transphincteric space, and then another segment that rests in the bulbar urethra thus anchoring it. The Memokath, on the other hand, is made of one segment.

One disadvantage to some urinary stents is the inability to cystoscope the patient after placement owing to a narrow intraluminal space. Both the Urospiral and the Prostakath are made of stainless steel (the Prostakath is gold plated to resist encrustation), and have external diameters of 21 French, but the internal diameter can only allow a 5- or 6-French catheter. An improvement to this was the Prostacoil, made of nitinol, which is described as self-expanding, and after placement expands to an external diameter of 24–30 French and an internal diameter of 21 French. This can accommodate a rigid 17-French cystoscope. The Memokath is also made of nitinol but has the unique property of expanding in the presence of heat. After the stent is positioned heated water (45–50°C) is placed through the urethra, causing the stent to expand to an internal diameter of 19 French. This stent can accommodate a flexible cystoscope. Adding cold water (10°C) causes the stent to collapse. All the above stents can be removed by using grasping forceps.[13]

POLYURETHANE

There are four designs of polyurethane stents: Nissenkorn, Barnes, Trestle, and ContiCath. The Nissenkorn was introduced in 1989 and is described as a stent (16 French) with two Malecot-like ends, one that rests in the bladder and the other within the prostatic urethra. It has attached to it a nylon string that is used to remove it, by pulling on it.[14] The Barnes is very similar to the above design, differing only in that it lacks the proximal Malecot-like end.[15] The Trestle is made of two tubular stents, connected by a thread with an internal diameter of 22 French. One stent rests in the prostatic urethra while the other is in the bulbar urethra. The ContiCath (Figure 25.1) is the newest design, which is unique because it does not have a lumen. While other

catheters have a lumen that allows urine to drain from the bladder, this stent has deep channels alongside the catheter for urine to pass through. It is anchored in the bladder with a curl, has a prostatic segment of 22 French and a transphincteric segment that ends with a plastic "cage" which prevents proximal migration.[16] We have used this stent as part of a multicenter study in patients with obstructive voiding symptoms waiting for definitive treatment, patients after TUMT, patients after brachytherapy, and patients who developed urinary retention after anesthesia. In these 38 patients with acute urinary retention, 33 (89%) were able to void after the catheter was placed. As part of the study, the catheter was not left in for more than 28 days and, in general, patients tolerated the catheter much better than an indwelling Foley catheter with its cumbersome external drainage bag.

BIOABSORBABLE/BIODEGRADABLE

Generally, the performance of a device placed in the body is determined by two principles: biofunctionality and biocompatibility.[17] Metal stents are made biocompatible by forming a stable oxide layer on their surface, which prevents corrosion of the metal when it is exposed to materials such as urine or blood.

In contrast, bioabsorbable means degradation and metabolism of the material *in vivo*, while biodegradable means the morphological and chemical degradation of the material *in vivo*. Bioabsorbable/biodegradable devices were first used in orthopedics for fracture fixation,[18,19] and their first use in the genitourinary tract was in the anterior urethra. Now they are considered ideal in the management of temporary retention after heat treatment of the prostate. Because they degrade with time, they do not need to be removed. However, one must be sure, as in the case of heat treatment of the prostate, that the prostatic edema has resolved by the time the stent is degraded. One study showed decreased urinary flow rates after 3–4 weeks of VLAP and stent placement due to degradation of the stent and persistent outlet obstruction.[20,21]

The most commonly used compounds are polylactic acid (PLA) and polyglycolic acid (PGA). Both are degraded by hydrolysis.[22–24] These stents can be reinforced with fibrous elements to alter their qualities such that they can self-expand at body temperature after placement, expand quickly, or expand slowly over several weeks.[25] Although ideal in concept, the cost, still undetermined, is likely to be much higher than the temporary polyurethane stents designed for a short period. Since the male urethra is easily accessible for catheter removal, the advantages of a biodegradable stent in relation to its total cost will determine its future use.

PERMANENT STENTS

In contrast to temporary stents, permanent stents are made of metal that is generally woven into a mesh configuration, with wide spaces that allow tissue ingrowth, thus incorporating the stent into the urethral wall. Because these stents

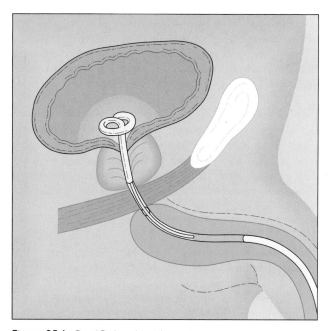

Figure 25.1 ContiCath polyurethane stent

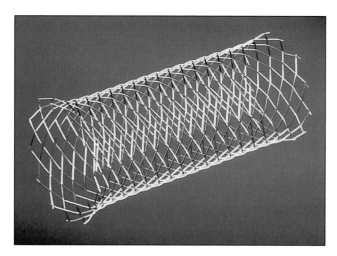

Figure 25.2 UroLume wallstent

are permanent, epithelialization is an important factor that prevents migration, encrustation, and increased tissue response. Currently there are two designs, the expandable ASI titanium stent and the UroLume wallstent (Figure 25.2) a superalloy of stainless steel. The Titan has an expanded diameter of 40 French and is introduced with the aid of a dual lumen catheter and balloon dilation. Biologically more inert than stainless steel, titanium is subject to less corrosion.

Only the UroLume is Food and Drug Administration (FDA) approved for use in BOO, especially in the surgically unfit patient.

In the 5-year review of the North American Multicenter clinical trial, a total of 126 patients with BOO were initially included.[26] Patients were at least 60 years of age and poor surgical risks. Contraindications to placement of the UroLume included: median lobe, active UTI, stricture disease that would warrant immediate catheterization after stent placement, carcinoma of the bladder, prostate or urethra, and prostate length >2.5 cm. (Table 25.1) Prior to placement, the urethra is dilated to 26 French and the prostatic length measured under direct cystoscopic vision, using a measuring guide. With the deployment tool, the stent is partially released and positioned. The stent is placed just distal to the bladder neck and proximal to the verumontanum without occluding the ejaculatory ducts.

Once the position is satisfactory, the stent is completely disengaged and released into the urethra.

Epithelialization begins at placement and by 1 year nearly 90% of the stents is covered. Because of this, patients were not cystoscoped for about 4 weeks, to allow for anchoring of the stents within the urethra. Previously, 2-year data on the UroLume demonstrated a significant decrease in symptom score at 1 month from 14.3 ± 0.5 to 6.4 ± 0.4, which was maintained at 2 years to 5.4 ± 0.5. At 5-year follow-up, symptom score remained low at 8.1 ± 5.1 (Figure 25.3). Mean peak flow rate showed a statistical significance at 1 month with a 57% change from 9.1 ± 3.3 to 16.3 ± 7.3 cm^3 s^{-1}. While significance declined owing to a decrease in the patient numbers at follow-up, flow rates were maintained at 9.1 ± 3.5 to 13.4 ± 5.8 cm^3 s^{-1} at 2 years, and 9.8 ± 3.6 to 11.7 ± 5.9 cm^3 s^{-1} at 5 years (Figure 25.4). In addition, postvoid residual urine showed a statistically significant decrease, with a 72% change from 81.8 ± 77.9 to 24.1 ± 33.6 cc s^{-1} at 1 month. Again, owing to low patient numbers at follow-up, significance was not seen later on, but residuals remained sustained at 66.5 ± 54.3 to 48.0 ± 58.2 cc s^{-1} at 2 years, and 54.6 ± 41.1 to 35.8 ± 43.6 cc s^{-1} at 5 years (Figure 25.5).

Complications of the UroLume such as encrustation, increased tissue response, and migration have generally surrounded poor epithelialization. Owing to the large

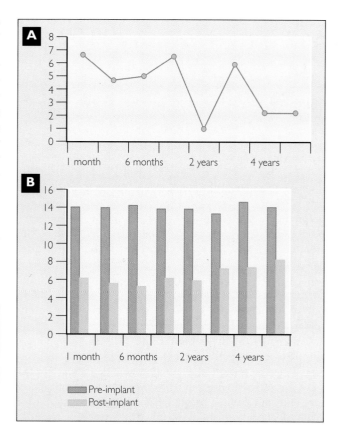

Figure 25.3 (A) Total mean symptom score after UroLume in retention patients. (B) Total mean symptom score before and after UroLume implant in non-retention patients

	Retention patients (n = 31)	Non-retention patients (n = 95)
Prostatic length	3.0 ± 0.8 cm	2.9 ± 0.9 cm
Prostatic volume (% of patients)		
<40 g	78%	55%
40–60 g	20%	32%
>60 g	2%	13%

Table 25.1 Prostatic length and digital rectal examination – estimated prostatic volume in all study patients (n = 126)

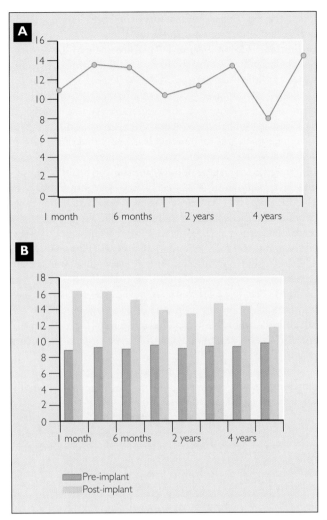

Figure 25.4 (A) Mean peak flow rate (cm³ s⁻¹) after UroLume implant in retention patients. (B) Mean peak flow rate (cm³ s⁻¹) before and after UroLume implant in non-retention patients

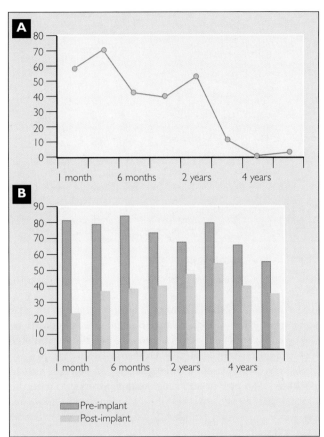

Figure 25.5 (A) Mean residual urine (cm³) after UroLume implant in retention patients. (B) Mean residual urine (cm³) before and after UroLume implant in non-retention patients

internal diameter of the stent, these problems can often be treated endoscopically, either with a TUR loop or with the holmium laser. Generally, encrustation was seen more commonly early on owing to the deployment method of the stents. Stents were generally placed just within the bladder neck, allowing the exposed wire to come in contact with urine and the eventual development of encrustation. In the 5-year review, 30 patients developed encrustation, but in only 5 patients was it severe enough to lead to stent removal. Given the previous discussion on prostatic shape and the stent, at times there could be areas that are not completely compressed against the urethral wall, and this would lead to poor epithelialization with an increase in tissue response. At times, this tissue response can be significant enough to cause obstruction and warrant treatment for removal of this tissue. To date, only 5 patients required removal because of severe tissue response.

Of the 126 patients that had UroLumes placed, at 5 years only 25 have been removed for reasons mentioned

above, in addition to migration, severe irritative symptoms, and difficulties in deployment. Removal is achieved by resecting the newly formed epithelial layer on top of the urethral stent with a TUR loop and then using grasping forceps to either pull it out, or push it into the bladder so that it can be removed through the sheath of the cystoscope.

CONCLUSIONS

While newer ways are developed to treat BOO surgically with a decrease in morbidity and mortality, attention should be given to urinary stents. Stents not only offer a stopgap to definitive therapy but also are a reliable way of treating BOO in patients who are surgically unfit. The ideal stent should be easy to insert and remove, self-expanding, have a large internal diameter (large enough to be able to cystoscope through it), be constructed of material that is biocompatible and the least subject to corrosion. In this chapter, we have reviewed the two classes of prostatic urinary stents – temporary and permanent – including temporary biodegradable stents, discussed the problems associated with prostatic stents because of the shape of the prostate, and reviewed in detail the 5-year data of the North American UroLume Multicenter Trial.

REFERENCES

1 Christensen MM, Bruskewitz RC. Clinical manifestation of benign prostatic hyperplasia and indication for therapeutic intervention. *Urol Clin North Am* 1990; **17**: 509–16.

2 Mebust WK, Holtgrewe HL, Cockett ATK, Peters PC. Transurethral prostatectomy: immediate and postoperative complications: a cooperative study of 13 participating institutions evaluating 3,885 patients. *J Urol* 1989; **141**: 243–7.

3 Nielssen KK, Nordling J. Urethral strictures following transurethral prostatectomy. *Urology* 1990; **35**: 18–24.

4 Fowler FJ, Wemberg JE, Timothy RP *et al.* Symptom status and quality of life following prostatectomy. *JAMA* 1988; **259**: 3018–22.

5 Chapple CR, Milroy EJG, Rickards D. Permanently implanted urethral stent for prostatic obstruction in the unfit patient: preliminary report. *Br J Urol* 1990; **66**: 58–65.

6 Fabian KM. Der intraprostatische "partielle Katheter" (urologische Spirale). *Urologe A* 1980; **19**: 236–8.

7 Barnes DG, Butterworth P, Flynn JT. Combined endoscopic laser ablation of the prostate (ELAP) and temporary prostatic stenting. *Minim Invasive Ther Allied Technol* 1996; **5**: 333–5.

8 Devonec M. Self retaining intra-urethral catheter for prevention of post-operative urinary retention: experience after microwave therapy of the prostate. In: Yachia D (ed) *Stenting the Urinary System.* Oxford, ISIS Medical Media 1998; 329–34.

9 Badlani, GH. Role of permanent stents. *J Endourol* 1997; **11**: 473–5.

10 Yachia D. Overview: role of stents in urology. *J Endourol* 1997; **11**: 379–82.

11 Milroy, EJG, Ng, KJ, Rickards D. Anatomic limitations of prostatic urethra in using cylindrical stents. *J Endourol* 1997; **11**: 455–8.

12 Ng, KJ, Gardener JE, Rickards D, Lees WE Milroy EJG. Three dimensional imaging of the prostatic urethra: an exciting tool. *Br J Urol* 1994; **74**: 604–8.

13 Yachia D. Temporary metal stents in bladder outflow obstruction. *J Endourol* 1997; **11**: 459–65.

14 Nissenkorn I, Slutzker D, Shalev M. Use of an intraurethral catheter instead of a Foley catheter after laser treatment of benign prostatic hyperplasia. *Eur Urol* 1996; **29**: 341–4.

15 Barnes DG, Butterworth P, Flynn JT. Combined endoscopic laser ablation of the prostate (ELAP) and temporary prostatic stenting. *Minim Invasive Ther Allied Technol* 1996; **5**: 333–5.

16 Lightner D, Barrett DM, Schmidt R *et al.* ContiCath: A simple new catheter deigned for continence and volitional voiding past the obstructed urethra. *J Urol* 1998; **159S**: 1171A, 303.

17 Williams DF. Biofunctionality and biocompatibility. In: Williams DF (ed) *Medical and Dental Materials*, Vol. 14 of Cahn RW, Hassen P, Kramer EJ (eds) *Materials Science and Technology.* Weinheim, Germany: VCH 1991: 1–27.

18 Vainionpaa S, Rokkanen P, Tormala P. Surgical applications of biodegradable polymers in huyman tissues. *Prog Polym Sci* 1989; **14**: 679–716.

19 Majola A, Vainiolpaa S, Vihtonen K *et al.* Absorption, biocompatibility and fixation properties of polylactic acid in bone tissue: an experimental study in rats. *Clin Orthop* 1991; **268**: 260–9.

20 Talja M, Tammela T, Petas A *et al.* Biodegradable self-reinforced polyglycolic acid spiral stent in prevention of postoperative urinary retention after visual laser ablation of the prostate-laser prostatectomy. *J Urol* 1995; **154**: 2089–92.

21 Petas A, Talja M, Tammela T *et al.* A randomized study to compare biodegradable self-reinforced polyglycolic acid spiral stent to suprapubic and indwelling catheters after visual laser ablation of the prostate. *J Urol* 1997; **157**: 173–6.

22 Jamshidi K. Synthesis and properties of polylactides. Thesis, Kyoto University 1984.

23 Nakamura T, Hitomi S, Watanabe S *et al.* Bioabsorption of polylactides with different molecular properties. *J Biomed Mater Res* 1989; **23**: 1115–30.

24 Li S, Garreau H, Vert M. Structure poperty relationships in the case of the degradation of massive aliphatic poly-(-hydroxy acids) in aqueous media 1:poly (DL-lactic acid). *J Mater Sci Mater Med* 1990; **1**: 123–30.

25 Talja M, Valimaa T, Tammela T *et al.* Bioabsorbable and biodegradable stents in urology. *J Endourol* 1997; **1**: 391–7.

26 Epstein H, Badlani G, Corujo M, North American UroLume Study Group for BPH. Five year follow-up of the North America UroLume trial in patients with benign prostatic hyperplasia (BPH). *J Urol* 1998; **159S**: 1174A, 304.

COMMENTARY

Urethral stents offer a safe and effective treatment for management of urethral obstruction due to a variety of causes in patients who are poor surgical candidates. Depending on the type and side effects of the stents, they may be used as temporary or permanent devices.

For stents to work, they have to be biocompatible, chemically inert, have memory shape, adequate tensile strength, and low internal–external diameter. Additionally, they need a fixation mechanism to prevent upward or downward migration.

Stents are available in a variety of forms, including permanent self-expanding metallic stents or temporary bioabsorbable/biodegradable ones. Most stents are hollow, allowing urine to pass through. In a more recent concept, solid stents with side channels for urine flow have been constructed. Stents are placed using cystoscopic guidance and special devices, and there are also devices to facilitate removal in case of migration or blockage.

A major side effect of the original metallic stents was encrustation and obstruction. In subsequent models, this has been resolved by having them woven in mesh form, which allows tissue to grow through and epithelialize the internal surface. The bioabsorbable or degradable stents have anchoring devices at the bladder and sphincter ends to prevent upward or downward migration. These may also have either a nylon string attached for removing them, or they are removed by cystoscopic guidance.

A unique use of the polyglycolic acid type of biodegradable stent is to use it temporarily to avoid retention and catheterization in patients undergoing VLAP, TUMT, and other procedures. In a randomized study in Finland, Petas and associates[1] demonstrated that their stents (which gradually degrade over 4–6 weeks) significantly improved time to voiding after surgery as well as patient symptom scores. Furthermore, they were superior to suprapubic tubes, which require an operative procedure and can cause bladder irritative symptoms.

In the USA the only stent that is FDA approved is the UroLume wallstent. This is a stent made of a superalloy of steel in mesh form with an inner diameter of 42 French and inserted using a special cystoscopically guided device. In the multicenter clinical trial of 126 patients, 2-year data revealed a significant decrease in symptom scores, which was maintained in the 35 patients available for follow-up to 5 years. Complications included encrustation, migration, poor deployment, and severe irritative symptoms, necessitating removal of the stent in up to 31.5% of patients at 5 years. The removal can be achieved with specialized instruments that allow the stent to be pushed into the bladder or pulled out. This stent is available for treatment of BPH or urethral strictures. The stent is available in three different lengths (2, 3, 4 cm) to accommodate varying lengths of urethral strictures. Of note, it is contraindicated for use in the anterior urethra and in disruptions due to pelvic fractures.

In summary, it may be stated that urethral stents as currently available can be utilized in a select population to keep the urethra open. The downside appears to be the irritative symptoms and the operative procedure required in removing it in patients when necessary. However, stents appear to be effective treatment in patients who are poor candidates for surgery.

---

1 Petas A, Talja M, Tammela T *et al*. A randomized study to compare biodegradable self-reinforced polyglycolic acid spiral stent to suprapubic and indwelling catheters after visual laser ablation of the prostate. *J Urol* 1997; **157**: 173–6.

Section VI

TRANSURETHRAL AND OPEN SURGERY

Section VI Overview

CONVENTIONAL SURGERY

P. Narayan

Of all the treatments available for the management of BPH, surgery affords the best chance of improving symptoms. In the average patient, transurethral prostatectomy or open prostatectomy results in an 80–85% reduction in symptoms. While complications of surgery are reported to be as high as 18% after TUR, more recent data from Watson and coworkers suggest that the complication rate is closer to nine percent; the most frequent of these are catheter replacement (4%), capsular perforation (2%), and hemorrhage requiring transfusion (1%). Treatment failure at five years is approximately 10% and repeat surgery is only required in about 4% of patients. Incontinence is also rare at 1.2% and is lower, interestingly, compared to an incidence of 2.9% in those who undergo watchful waiting. However, there are other problems with surgery including the need for hospitalization and requirement of anesthesia. Additionally, standard TURP also requires restriction of activities for two to three weeks. Other potential complications include retrograde ejaculation which varies from 30 to 90% depending on the technique. Open prostatectomy also requires an abdominal incision and is associated with potential complications related to open surgery and anesthesia including bleeding, pulmonary problems, blood transfusions, deep vein thrombosis and others.

In this regard, an alternative to TURP is transurethral incision of the prostate (TUIP), a procedure that is equal in efficacy to TURP and has less complications. TURP outcome is well documented and is very comparable to transurethral resection both in short-term as well as long-term studies. It is a relatively easy technique to learn and can be performed under local anesthesia or with IV sedation. The complications of bleeding are low at 1–2% and complications such as TUR syndrome are rare. Antegrade ejaculation is also preserved in 77% of patients after TUIP. Although older series have found a higher incidence of impotence rates, after TUIP, it is lower in more modern series and certainly no higher than that of TURP. Quality-of-life after TUIP has also been found to be very comparable to that of TURP. TUIP is a procedure that is currently under-utilized and in Narayan's opinion deserves more popularity when compared to some of the results of newer minimally invasive techniques, especially for small prostates.

The transurethral vaporization (TVP) technique also has some advantages over standard TURP in that both tissue removal and improved coagulation can be achieved. TVP can achieve results that are very similar to that of TURP and yet allow the procedure to be performed in an ambulatory setting or 23 hour hospital stay. The procedure still, however, requires general or spinal anesthesia in most patients and does have the requirement for use of newer electrocautery machines with higher power output. However, the capital equipment required is still less expensive ($10,000 vs. > $30,000) than that of other minimally invasive therapies and the disposable electrode costs are much lower than that of lasers, TUNA or microwave devices. Using Narayan's technique, antegrade ejaculation can be preserved in over seventy percent of patients after TVP. Irritative symptoms associated with TVP can be avoided by using the combination technique of TURP and TVP and the avoidance of partial burns and inadequate tissue removal. This is facilitated by using newer Force Fx® (ValleyLab®, Denver, Colorado) type of electrocautery machines that have high power output. The technique is also more controlled and easier to learn than standard TURP especially at the apex near the sphincter. The major problems of bleeding and fluid absorption and requirement for hospitalization are nonexistent or very rare with TVP. Currently, the TURP and TVP combination approach is preferred by Narayan for patients who need endoscopic surgery.

Today, for treatment of BPH, if a surgical option is chosen, both patients and physicians need to carefully assess both the need for surgery and the most appropriate surgery. While surgery should not be the last resort for men who fail medical or device therapy, it should not be used as first line therapy in men. If the patient has been fully informed and has chosen to have the option of surgery as his initial treatment, the choice of surgery is determined by a variety of factors including the patients' biases, the surgeon's experience, the availability of equipment in the geographic area and also the medical practices within that area. Certainly there is little controversy to offering surgery as the first choice for patients with recurrent urinary retention, recurrent urinary infections, or other complications such as recurrent hematuria, bladder stones, or renal failure. However, it is not appropriate to recommend surgery for a patient on the grounds that progression is inevitable and that surgical risk will increase with age. It has been shown in many studies that BPH progression is quite variable and that relief of symptoms can be obtained by a variety of techniques including medical management and minimally invasive therapies.

Electrovaporization Principles

A.E. Te and S.A. Kaplan

26

INTRODUCTION

The goal of the surgical therapy of benign prostatic hyperplasia (BPH) is to provide an open anatomic channel for urine to flow easily in the prostatic urethra. Since the advent of electrosurgery in the 1920s and 1930s, the standard use of this technology in transurethral resection of the prostate (TURP) has grown popular and commonplace. Today, TURP remains the mainstay of treating symptoms secondary to BPH, with subjective and objective success rates of 85–90%.[1] Although success rates are excellent, significant morbidity is associated with the procedure. These include bleeding, "TUR syndrome" infection, retrograde ejaculation, impotence, and incontinence.[1,2] In the current drive to develop a surgical alternative to decrease these morbidities, transurethral electrovaporization of the prostate (TUEP), an electrosurgical modification of TURP, has gained attention and popularity owing to its ability to provide near-bloodless tissue ablation or vaporization, with shorter hospital stay and catheterization time than a conventional TURP, with good clinical efficacy.[3–7] The modification reapplies the same electrosurgical principle utilized in the standard TURP to achieve these improved results. The principles of electrosurgery are well known and were described extensively by McLean in 1929.[8] In order to apply electrovaporization effectively, which is a simultaneous application of two major electrosurgical effects, vaporization and desiccation, an understanding of the principles and factors that affect them is essential for a successful surgical outcome.

ELECTROSURGICAL PRINCIPLES

RADIOFREQUENCY CURRENT

Electrosurgery became popular after Bovie, a physicist, and Cushing, a surgeon, collaborated to design a device that was capable of cutting and coagulating tissue. Electrosurgery utilizes a radiofrequency (RF) electric current to cut and fulgurate tissue, and to obtain hemostasis.[9] The frequency selected is important for achieving the desired effects without adverse results. A low frequency such as a 100,000 Hz will stimulate muscles and nerves, and, in effect, electrocute the patient. On the other hand, a high frequency such as 4,000,000 Hz produces a reactive phenomena because it is difficult to confine these high radiofrequency current to wires.[9] For these reasons, electrosurgical tools operate between 400,000 to 1,000,000 Hz, a compromise between two extremes. This frequency varies depending on the generator's manufacturer.

WAVEFORM TYPES

The electrosurgical cutting and fulguration depend on waveform, peak voltage, and the power of the electrical current.

In electrosurgical cutting or vaporization, a characteristic cut waveform is used: a continuously alternating RF sinewave, which delivers a high current capable of delivering high power[9] (Figure 26.1A). This continuous operation generates high heat to create a cutting action with limited hemostasis.

In electrosurgical fulguration, the coagulation waveform is composed of short bursts of high-voltage RF sinewave current with a pause between bursts. The important feature of this waveform is the pause between each burst (Figure 26.1B). Although both waveforms may have the same peak voltage, the average power delivered per unit time is less in the coagulation mode. Because coagulation waveform's power delivery is not a continuous process, it allows for a process of intermittent heat dissipation to occur.

There is also a blend mode, which is a compromise between cutting and coagulation (Figure 26.1C).

GENERATOR POWER

Generator power is equally important. The generator utilized with electrosurgery is responsible for providing a current of sufficient magnitude at the surgical site to create power that is translated into heat to achieve the desired surgical effect. Power that is translated into heat is dependent on the current delivered by the generator and the resistance encountered in the tissue (tissue resistance). Most generators have a power setting on their unit that theoretically reflects the power being generated at the site. However, in this complex interaction, the electrical current is delivered by the generator at variously changing levels to accommodate the different and constantly changing electrical tissue resistance encountered at the surgical site. Optimally, a constant power determined by the generator is delivered to the site. To maintain this constant power, the generator must adjust the current level to the encountered surgical resistance of the tissue. However, older generators did not have this capability. In addition, design limitations and constraints fixed and limited the actual power being delivered at the surgical site. Complicating the interaction

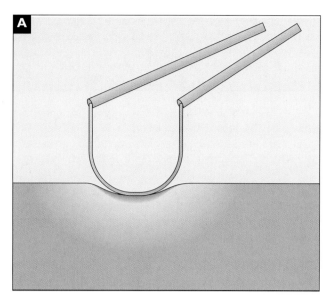

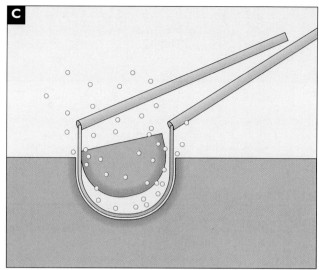

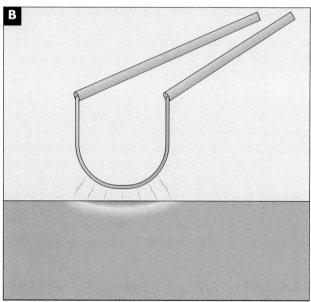

Figure 26.1 The electrosurgical tissue effects produced with the standard resection loop. (A) Desiccation: a low power current generates heat in the tissue that slowly dries it out. (B) Fulguration: a coagulation current with intermittent high voltage sparks is applied with a light touch which fulgurates and chars superficial tissue to a carbon texture and dries it out. (C) Vaporization (cutting): a high energy cutting current rapidly heats cells on contact, causing them to explode into steam. An incision or vaporized space is created in its path

is the fact that electrical tissue resistance can rapidly increase as the tissue dries out. This means that the generator must deliver an increasing voltage level of current to compensate for this increase in resistance to achieve the same power. Thus, during a procedure, power current needs to be adjusted. Each generator has its own power delivery constraints, and determines how efficiently it will deliver actual power at the surgical site to effect the desired surgical result. For example, the Valleylab Force 40 generator is more efficient at vaporization than a Valleylab Force 2 generator. The Force 2 generator's design limits the power to a lower level at higher levels of encountered resistance loads compared with the Force 40 generator.[10,11] The Force 2 was designed for electrosurgical instruments with smaller areas of contact, unlike the electrovaporization electrode with the larger surface area. The Force 2 was designed for small sharp contact area electrodes, whose

power requirements for cutting vaporization is less. The Valleylab FX units are more efficient because they utilize microprocessors that are designed to monitor the resistance changes and adjust the current to deliver the same amount of power over a broader range of encountered tissue resistance. The different power/resistance curves of these generators are compared in Figure 26.2. While we used Valleylab generators as examples, there are many other commercial units with similar efficacy based on these power/resistance curves as well as units with microprocessor-power-controlled technology.

Despite an increasing level of power, high electrical resistance of the tissue can easily negate a generator's efficiency at vaporization by drying tissue out to an insulating quality. In this circumstance, heat required for efficient vaporization of this insulating tissue cannot be attained. Conversely, a high power setting in the coagulation mode can achieve a

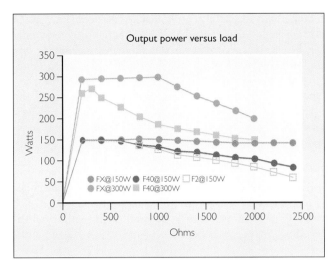

Figure 26.2 Actual power delivered (output power) vs. encountered impedance (load) in various generators. This graph demonstrates the power delivered by specific Valleylab generators, FX, Force 40, and Force 2 at various encountered electrical resistance (load) measured in impedance at the 300 and 150 W setting. At greater impedance, the Force FX delivers the most power while the Force 2 delivers the least at the same impedances. The Force 40 delivers power at a range between the two generators. The impedance area of prostate tissue lies in the 500–1200 ohm range

Source: Adapted from information provided by Valleylab Inc., Boulder, CO

cutting effect if the encountered tissue resistance allows optimal conditions for vaporization.

ELECTROSURGICAL EFFECTS

The three major electrosurgical effects that electrosurgery produces are vaporization, desiccation, and fulguration. Each effect is accomplished with the standard TURP loop in everyday practice.[9]

Electrosurgical desiccation is the simplest to achieve, because a cutting or coagulation current waveform may be applied. An electrode is placed in good contact with the tissue to be desiccated. As current passes through the electrical resistance of the tissue, heat is generated in the water of the contacted tissue. As the tissue gets hot, water is slowly driven out and this tissue becomes desiccated (see Figure 26.1A). Visually, the tissue turns a light brown color, and steams and bubbles as the water is driven out. Persistent electrodesiccation in one area can dry out large areas of tissue, causing coagulation necrosis. A charred or dirty electrode desiccates poorly owing to the insulating effects of dried charred tissue. On persistent desiccation of the same area, the tissue dries out and this increases the electrical resistance of the tissue. When a gradual increase in power is delivered, the increased heat in that area radiates to adjacent areas causing deeper levels of coagulation necrosis.

In electrosurgical fulguration, a superficial charring is created by the coagulation waveform sparking to the tissue surface. The heat is widely dispersed by a combination of the long sparks and the intermittent heating effects. A light touch

is applied with the electrosurgical instrument, and cutting is not the intended effect. As in desiccation, the cells do not vaporize but dry out so as not to be torn apart. This leaves a charred carbon quality surface that forms a seal for hemostasis. Technically, fulguration is a superficial effect that can progress easily to desiccation with persistent application. Thus, coagulation or hemostatic control with electrosurgery involves both desiccation and fulguration (see Figure 26.1B).

In electrosurgical cutting or vaporization, the tissue cells are rapidly heated so that they explode into steam, leaving a space where the cells were present. The rapid heat is generated by delivery of a high current by the contacting surface of the cutting loop. With vaporization, an important factor that directly affects the efficiency of vaporization is the actual surface area of current delivery of the surgical electrode. Current must be applied at a high current density in order to deliver a concentrated focus of power that is translated into instantaneous heat. This high current density of the loop surface is important for achieving a vaporizing effect. In the standard TURP, the loop surface is a thin wire with a high current density, which vaporizes away tissue cells in its path, and thus achieves a cutting effect. Since the effect is instantaneous and fast, the majority of heat is dissipated into the steam and does not conduct into adjacent tissues to dry them out. This heat is carried away by the continuously flowing irrigant fluid. As the electrode moves to fresh tissue, new cells are exploded and either an incision or vaporized space is created. With TUEP, the concept of current density becomes a significant variable factor to understand (see Figure 26.1C).

ELECTROSURGICAL THEORY

With TUEP, two electrosurgical effects are combined to produce the desired effect. Owing to the larger surface area of the roller electrode, more power is required to generate the high current density for vaporizing contacted tissue. As the roller electrode contacts fresh tissue cells, it vaporizes it away at the point of maximum and sufficient current density delivery. As contact is maintained by the rolling effect, the underlying tissue cells start to desiccate instead of vaporizing. This is caused by the increasing resistance of the dried-out tissue as well as the decreasing level of current density at that part of the roller. These factors on the roller electrode combine to lower the power to desiccation level at these trailing edges. Thus, the degree and depth of vaporization and desiccation are governed by the quality of the contact (needs a sufficient level of tactile pressure), power level (set on the generator), and the time spent on that spot by the electrode (determined by resection technique and speed of electrode pass). Since the procedure is performed under water and glycine irrigation, the desiccated tissue is constantly rehydrated. This rehydration makes the tissue available for vaporization on a subsequent pass. Thus, electrovaporization achieves three desired effects: it vaporizes the unwanted tissue, provides hemostasis, and prevents water reabsorption by the development of a zone of desiccation below the vaporized tissue (Figure 26.3).

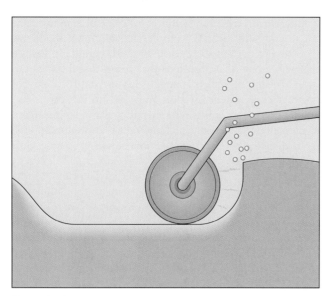

Figure 26.3 Roller electrovaporization: combines vaporization and desiccation

APPLICATION OF PRINCIPLES TO TECHNIQUE

We are currently utilizing a variety of standard transurethral resection equipment, roller electrodes, and electrical current generators to accomplish TUEP. We believe that understanding of the principles is important and allows efficient application of the electrovaporization technique with the variety of equipment utilized.

We currently utilize a Valleylab Force 40, Valleylab FX, and an ERBE generator unit, but have also used the other Valleylab generators such as the SSE2, SSE3, and other Force series generators with the same results. The Force 2 generator has been reported in the community as being less efficient owing to its inherent designed limitation at providing adequate power as tissue resistance increases. This limitation has been discussed previously.

The two features of a generic roller electrode are, first, that its large surface area of contact enables the delivery of a high current density to a large area of tissue to be vaporized, and, second, the subsequent contact rolling effect provides coagulation and desiccation effects. Our widely published experience has been with the VaporTrode, a specially designed grooved roller electrode (Figure 26.4) and a Valleylab Force 40 generator. The electrode developed by ACMI fits standard resectoscope equipment in place of a standard TURP loop electrode. Electrovaporization is generally accomplished at a cutting current of 25–75% higher power than a standard TURP. The average setting was 240 W on a pure cutting waveform current, and up to a 300-W setting can be utilized on the Valleylab Force 40 generator. Occasionally, a 50-W setting on the coagulation waveform current was utilized for pinpoint coagulation.

The procedure is performed under continuous glycine irrigation. Use of the roller electrode element for TUEP requires no specially acquired skills other than that of performing a conventional TURP. Although this technique can be altered according to the surgeon's preference, we preferentially vaporized the middle lobe as needed. Lateral lobe vaporization was then accomplished in overlapping sweeps from the bladder neck to the level of the verumontanum, going clockwise from the 1 o'clock position to the 5 o'clock position, and then counter-clockwise from the 11 o'clock position to the 7 o'clock position, until the desired amount of tissue was removed (Figure 26.5). Sculpting was left until last to complete the vaporization to the desired cavity size. With this technique, vaporization to the crossing white fibers of the surgical capsule was easily accomplished with minimal bleeding. In our experience, small pieces of tissue sufficient for pathology can be collected in the irrigant. However, if larger pieces are required, a sampling resection could easily be performed by just changing to a standard loop electrode during the procedure.

Fulguration is also easily accomplished with the VaporTrode. A standard 22-French, 3-way catheter with saline irrigation or a regular 22-French Foley catheter is placed at the end of the procedure at the surgeon's discretion.

The application of sufficient power to vaporize is important for efficient vaporization. If power is not sufficient, desiccation rather than vaporization will take effect, resulting in more coagulation necrosis.

In addition, contact vaporization is governed by the initial contact current density delivered to the surface tissue to be vaporized. This power level is adjusted on the

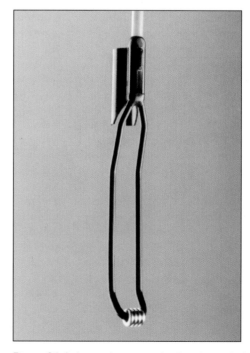

Figure 26.4 A popular grooved roller electrode for electrovaporization: the VaporTrode by Circon-ACMI, Santa Barbara, CA

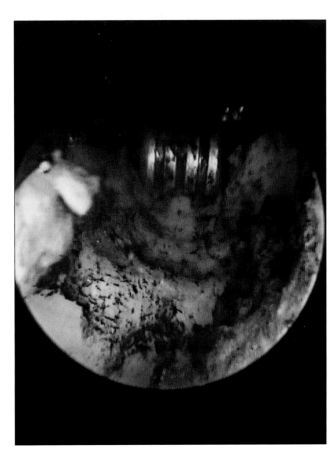

Figure 26.5 An endoscopic view of a roller electrovaporative resection

generator. This power setting can vary among different patients and can increase as the same area is revaporized on subsequent sweeps. In our experience, we determined that leaving the electrode stationary resulted in diminished vaporization, owing to the phenomenon of "electrodesiccation."[12] Electrodesiccation occurs when the electrode is held in one position at a particular spot, causing the tissue to dry out and increasing resistance in the tissue. As resistance increases, the radiating heat created will also desiccate the adjacent tissue. The depth of desiccation was governed by the amount of time spent on that area and the power of the current delivered to overcome electrical tissue resistance. Therefore, the longer the time spent on any particular area and the higher the power applied, the deeper the level of desiccation attained. Electrodesiccation is associated with coagulation necrosis, and significant coagulation necrosis can result in irritative symptoms similar to laser coagulation necrosis. As with all radiating sources of energy, the effect of desiccation diminishes exponentially away from its source. It was noteworthy that fulguration also accomplished desiccation at the coagulation setting.

With the advent of new modified electrovaporative loops, which are basically a thicker wider band than the standard loop, the technique of a standard loop resection is not altered drastically. The same electrosurgical principles apply, and the resectionist has to be aware of the power,

type of current, resection speed, and amount of electrodesiccation produced during each resection pass. These loops have a contact area less than a roller electrode and more than a standard loop. Thus, its general effects of cutting efficiency and hemostatic/desiccative effects fall between the standard loop and the roller electrode.

Finally, a combined loop/roller technique has been utilized to obtain the resection speed of a standard loop TURP and the postoperative advantages of a hemostasis with shortened catheter time and convalescence of a roller electrode resection. This technique involves combining loop resection with a roller resection in the same procedure. However, the perioperative advantage of a hemostatic resection with a roller electrode is not available during the loop portion of the procedure.

OTHER ROLLER ELECTRODES AND DESIGNS

Technically, the first roller electrode available was the standard rollerball used previously to fulgurate bladder tumors. This rollerball can be applied to electrovaporization of the prostate and has been reported by Juma in 20 men with small glands (mean TRUS volume + 31.9 mL) who had lower urinary tract symptoms and a low flow rate.[13] His study reported improvements in American Urological Association (AUA) symptom scores from a preoperative baseline of 22.9±4.2 in 20 men to 5.2±3.2, and in flow rate from a preoperative baseline of 8.9±3.4 mL s^{-1} to 24.3±7 mL s^{-1} in 15 men who completed the 3-month follow-up. Though hospitalization and catheterization were short, the only significant morbidity was a patient who developed bladder neck stenosis at 9 months and another who underwent repeat TURP resection for residual adenoma.

However, the rollerball in our hands, although highly effective for small glands, proved less efficient and effective in vaporizing large glands. This is probably due to the uneven distribution of contact pressure, uneven leading edge, and subsequent variable delivery of current to the tissue. The best vaporative effect with the standard rollerball is the middle portion of the leading edge, where the best contact and current delivery are obtained.

The current ACMI VaporTrode roller electrode design consists of a grooved roller bar that has been in clinical use in BPH for several years (Figure 26.6). The electrode's theoretical advantage, according to the manufacturers, is based on a fundamental electrosurgical principle that current density across an electrode is not uniform but is highest at its edge (Figure 26.6).[14,15] By increasing the number of edges through its grooved design, high current density to tissue is delivered to effect efficient and effective vaporization to a wide contact area. To demonstrate this difference, we compared the volume of human cadaveric prostate tissue vaporized with a standard rollerball with that vaporized with a grooved rollerbar at the same resection speed, tactile pressure, wattage setting, and tissue specimen.[16] The grooved roller

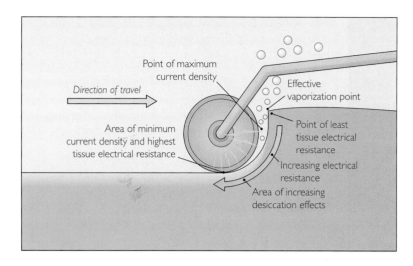

Figure 26.6 Roller electrode electrovaporization. Current travels through the point of least resistance. Current density is highest at the leading edge, where fresh tissue has the least resistance. Current density is lowest at the trailing edge, where desiccated tissue has the highest resistance. The leading edge vaporizes while the trailing edge desiccates and coagulates. Vaporization and desiccation are combined in one motion to remove tissue without bleeding

bar with more edges vaporized more tissue in the same number of passes than the rollerball. Narayan *et al.*[17] has also confirmed this finding in canine prostate. This grooved rollerball design has been the most popular and has been duplicated by several manufacturers.

In addition, several design and material modifications have been aimed at increasing the number and changing the configuration of edges to increase the vaporative effect (Figure 26.7). However, there has been a trade-off in design between vaporization and desiccation. As the roller electrode design became more efficient at vaporization, it became less effective at desiccation and coagulation. To date, the ACMI grooved roller electrode has been the most popular and best-studied device for electrovaporization

of the prostate, and has provided an adequate blend of both effects.

In addition to the grooved roller electrode is the standard 3-mm roller bar, also produced by Storz. Theoretically, owing to its lack of grooved edges, this electrode should be considerably less effective than the ACMI VaporTrode. However, in the authors' hands, it can be effective in vaporizing tissue for BPH in both small and large glands. The explanation of its similar clinical effect lies in the ability to compensate with techniques based on the electrosurgical principles. By increasing power, tactile pressure, and allowing adequate rehydration of vaporized areas, one can compensate for the decreased theoretical efficiency of this roller bar.

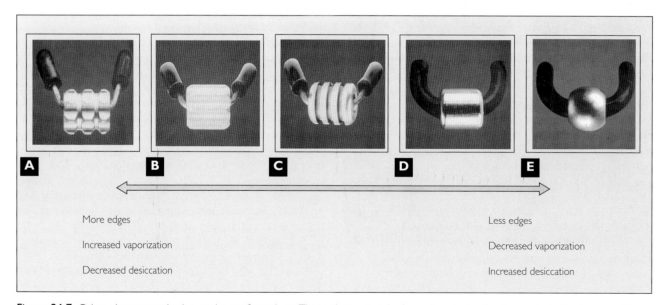

Figure 26.7 Other electrovaporization probe configurations. These electrovaporization roller electrodes demonstrate the incorporation of more edges to increase vaporization efficiency to remove greater amounts of tissue. With increased vaporization efficiency, decreased desiccation effects can occur, since power is delivered more efficiently for a greater vaporization effect: (A) spiked; (B) fluted; (C) grooved; (D) bar; (E) ball

Theoretically, it should be possible to apply the principles and technique of electrovaporization to a resecting loop. Ideally, the loop should combine the desired features of a roller electrode, such as hemostasis, with the ability to resect tissue, like a standard TURP. Several manufacturers have attempted to develop such loops. To date, designs that employ a thin efficiently vaporizing leading edge with a thick desiccating trailing edge seem to be the most logical and safest design. Several loops such as the ACMI VaporTome loop have emerged to achieve this goal (Figure 26.8); however, all have features of compromise between achieving efficient vaporization at the expense of adequate coagulation. They are, as a group, more hemostatic than a standard TURP loop, but less than the grooved roller electrode.

Finally, many "copy-cat" roller electrodes have flooded the market without clinical trials to establish either safety or efficacy. Some roller electrodes are insulated and/or configured differently, and one should not extrapolate the results reported by many with certain electrodes to other products. Our personal experience is that "not all electrodes are built alike." They all confer different vaporization efficiencies, which can be compensated by adjustments in resection technique and generator. How these adjustments

affect coagulation necrosis depth level and irritative symptoms for these "copy-cats" is unknown.

FACTORS AFFECTING VAPORIZATION EFFICIENCY AND COAGULATION EFFICIENCY

Three important issues appear to be recurrent themes in understanding roller electrovaporization: inefficient vaporization, lack of hemostasis, and coagulation necrosis.

When vaporization appears to be inefficient, factors that need to be examined are adequate generator power and the generator's power curve efficiency, tissue resistance, probe current density delivery, and resection technique. Of these factors, the last three are addressed with resection technique. As one takes a vaporative pass over tissue, adequate tactile pressure is required to vaporize the tissue away. Like an electric scalpel, it cuts as deep as one goes. Likewise, a high pressure may run the risk of vaporizing too deeply, while a light pressure serves only to fulgurate and desiccate the tissue without much vaporization. Fulguration is especially evident if the passing tissue and roller electrode look charred. The charring reflects the amount of fulguration effected. Subsequent passes over these areas may prove more difficult to vaporize because the fulgurated and desiccated tissue has a greater tissue resistance. A reused probe, which usually has a charred protein layer, also decreases the effective vaporative surface of the roller electrode. These probes are marketed as a one-time-use tool, because of this effect and the difficulty in cleaning them effectively. In addition, a slow pass may tend to desiccate too much and make subsequent passes less efficient. To compensate for a slow pass, an adequate time of tissue rehydration needs to occur prior to the next vaporative pass. In addition, increased tactile pressure may be utilized. In contrast, a fast pass may not desiccate adequately to obtain hemostasis. If hemostasis is a problem, careful hemostatic slower passes with less power for increased desiccation can be applied. However, a trade-off for increased coagulation necrosis may result.

Like most BPH treatments based on the concept of coagulation necrosis such as visual laser ablation of the prostate (VLAP),[18,19] microwave hyperthermia,[20,21] and transurethral needle ablation of the prostate (TUNA),[22] significant coagulation necrosis from excessive electro-desiccation will result in increased prolonged irritative symptoms, increased tissue sloughing, and a gradual rather than immediate improvement of urinary flow rate postoperatively. However, the documented level of coagulation necrosis remains speculative with TVP in humans. In canine studies presented by Perlmutter et al.[23] electrovaporization with their technique demonstrated a coagulation necrosis zone of 1–3 mm at 3 weeks, which resolved and re-epithelialized after 7 weeks.

Within the last year, modifications to the standard resection loop have been made to incorporate the advanges of an electrovaporative resection while still obtaining a TURP specimen. Many of these loops are available commercially. Preliminary results from a multicenter trial with Circon ACMI's VaporTome demonstrate a more hemostatic

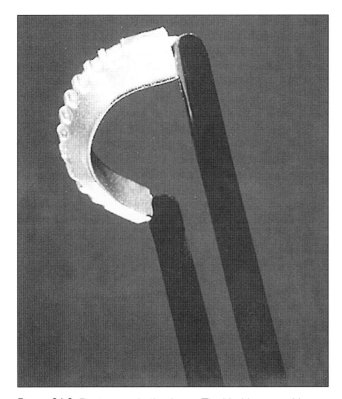

Figure 26.8 Electrovaporization loops. The ideal loop would combine the advantages of roller electrovaporization to resect tissue in a coagulative manner. These loops apply known electrovaporization principles by incorporating an efficiently vaporizing leading cutting edge with a thick coagulating trailing edge. Various loops have been modified to provide a blend of efficient vaporization and desiccation. This loop produced by Circon ACMI is one example

20 Kaplan SA, Shabsigh R, Soldo KA *et al*. Transrectal thermal therapy in the management of men with prostatism. *Br J Urol* 1993; **72**: 195.

21 Blute ML, Tomera KM, Hellerstein DK *et al*. Transurethral microwave thermotherapy for management of benign prostatic hyperplasia. *J Urol* 1993; **150**: 1591–6.

22 Dixon CM. Transurethral needle ablation for the treatment of benign prostatic hyperplasia. *Urol Clin North Am* 1995; **22**(2): 441–4.

23 Perlmutter AP, Muschter R, Razvi HA. Electrosurgical vaporization of the prostate in the canine model. *Urology* 1995; **46**(4): 518–23.

24 Te AE, Laor E, Kaplan SA *et al*. Transurethral resection of the prostate (TURP) vs. vaporization of the prostate utilizing a vaporizing loop (TVLOOP): a multicenter, blinded, prospective comparative study. *J Urol* 1997; **157**(4): 313A (abstract).

25 Kaplan SA, Te AE. Transurethral electroevaporation of the prostate (TVP): A novel method for treating men with benign prostatic hyperplasia. *Urology* 1995; **45**: 566–73.

26 Kaplan SA, Santarosa RP, Te AE. Electrovaporization of the prostate for symptomatic benign prostatic hyperplasia: The 1 year experience. *J Urol* 1996; **155**(5): 405A (abstract).

27 Hamawy KJ, Kim CA, Siroky MB *et al*. Transurethral vaporization of the prostate (TUVP): clinical follow-up at one year. *J Urol* 1996; **155**(5): 404A (abstract).

28 Narayan P, Tewari A, Garzotto M *et al*. Transurethral VaporTrode electrovaporization of the prostate: Physical principles, technique, and results. *Urology* 1996; **47**(4): 505–10.

29 Evans R. TUEVP: initial experience with long-term follow up. (newsletter) *Uro Trends* 1996; **1**(1): 1–5.

30 Kaplan SA, Te AE. A comparative study of transurethral resection of the prostate using a modified electro-vaporizing loop and transurethral laser vaporization of the prostate. *J Urol* 1995; **154**(5): 1785–90.

31 Narayan P, Fournier G, Indudhara R *et al*. Transurethral evaporation of prostate (TUEP) with Nd:YAG laser using a contact free beam technique: Results in 61 patients with benign prostatic hyperplasia. *Urology* 1994; **43**: 813–20.

Electrovaporization of the Prostate: Clinical Results

27

P. Narayan, A. Tewari, and R. Makkenchery

INTRODUCTION

Because of the high cost and morbidity associated with transurethral resection of the prostate (TURP), urologists and researchers have developed several alternative, minimally invasive treatments.[1] Treatments such as thermotherapy, laser ablation, and high-energy focused ultrasound all use heat to destroy prostatic tissue but differ significantly in the degree of heating, the mechanism of delivery, and the latency period necessary for them to be effective. Most of these techniques use sophisticated machinery to deliver a safe and desired amount of heat to the target tissue and are thus expensive and require special equipment and training. Laser prostatectomy has taught us much about simultaneous coagulation and evaporation, leading to renewed interest in electrosurgery, which uses easily available technology for the destruction of prostatic tissue under visual guidance.[2-6] To replace TURP, alternative therapies should have low morbidity and cost, the ability to be performed in an ambulatory setting, achieve a transurethral resection (TUR) defect immediately at the end of procedure (to avoid problems with prolonged catheterization due to swelling and sloughing as occurs in visual laser ablation of the prostate (VLAP) types of procedure), and long-term success with low rates of complications. Electrovaporization, which uses a high current density to destroy tissue, has been used for several years by gynecologists to treat endometriosis.[7]

Modern electrosurgery started when Benjamin Franklin, Mesmer, and John Wesley used static generators for medical applications.[8-13] Several workers are credited with use of high-frequency electrical current in medicine, including Arsenne d'Arsonval, Elihu Thomson, William J Norton, and Nikola Tesla. However, in 1930, WT Bovie (a physicist) and Harvey Cushing (a neurosurgeon) developed the first electrosurgical unit to control troublesome and often fatal bleeding during hypophysectomy. The introduction of solid-state electrosurgical generators in the early 1970s by Valleylab and EMS (now EMS-Darvol) heralded the modern era of isolated outputs, complex waveforms, and exclusive safety features.[8-13]

Electrosurgical applications to treat benign prostatic hyperplasia (BPH) and other urological diseases parallel the development of cystoscopic instruments, optics, and resectoscope design. Existing urological endoscopes and energy sources were initially modified by Beer and Young; Bugbee further modified instruments for electrosurgical

prostatic incision.[8] The predecessor of the modern resectoscope was developed by Stern in 1926, who termed it the "resectotherm".[8] The delivery of cutting current was developed further by Collings in 1932 and the current output was later modified by Sappler, who developed a complex oscillator capable of blending the waveform.[8]

THE SCIENTIFIC BASIS OF ELECTROVAPORIZATION

Electrosurgery uses a radiofrequency, alternating sine-wave electric current between 0.4 and 1.0 MHz for most electrosurgical procedures. Modern solid state electrosurgical units convert a 60 Hz diagonal alternating current into a high-radiofrequency current. By convention, the unaltered uninterrupted sine-wave alternating current is termed cutting current, while interrupted current is coagulating current, and their combination is blended current (Figure 27.1A–C).

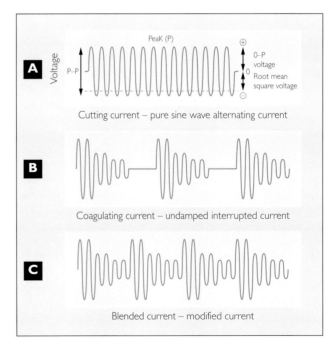

Figure 27.1 Electrosurgical current and waveforms: (A) cutting current – pure sine-wave alternating current; (B) coagulating current – undamped interrupted current; (C) blended current – modified current

Source: With permission from Blackwell Science, *Br J Urol.* **78**: 667–676

The outputs of most electrical appliances are described by power (watts), with voltage and current varying considerably: the work done over time is expressed in joules $(1\ J = 1\ W\ s^{-1})$.[9-12,14-16] Desiccated tissues have a higher resistance (termed impedance in cultured tissue) because there is less saline and blood. The ratio of voltage to current is an important factor responsible for the different effects on the tissue, given a similar electrode size, shape, and tissue exposure time. This is represented by the equation: $W = V \times I$, where W is power, V is voltage, and $I = V/R$ (where R = resistance); thus $V \times V/R = V^2/R$. The "driving force" of increased voltage enables current to arc from the electrode to the tissue more easily; more thermal damage is caused in the tissue as a higher voltage forces more energy into the tissue.[17]

EFFECTS ON TISSUE

The effect of electrosurgical current on living cells is governed by both factors in the tissue and factors related to the electrosurgical current. The latter include frequency, waveform, voltage, power, crest factor, method of delivery (contact vs. non-contact), area of contact (current density), duration of contact, the shape of the electrode, and the presence or absence of arcing. Factors related to the tissue include tissue impedance (which is related to composition), vascularity, mechanical pressure, entrapment of steam (accelerated evaporation phenomenon), and surface cooling.[10-13,17,18] The conversion of electrical to thermal energy is the primary cause of the changes in treated tissue[10-13,17,18] However, a variety of other events also contributes to these changes, including the kinetic energy of steam produced by heat in the interstitium and in the cell, acoustic pressure waves caused by sparking and ionization of the intervening medium, and membrane electrovaporization, which results in the formation of aqueous pores in the lipid bilayer of the cell membrane, which, when large enough, causes cell rupture.[19] Tissue changes are also occasionally caused by faradic effects and capacitance. If the current frequency is >30 kHz, the polarity of the cellular ions alternates so rapidly that depolarization does not occur. Conversely, capacitance is a feature of very high-frequency current, whereby the high electromagnetic field creates an electrical charge in nearby conductors. Capacitance can charge the sheath of an endoscopic instrument and can result in unexpected burns if the charge is released through a small area of contact with the patient's or the surgeon's body.[10-13,17,18]

Living tissue undergoes various temperature-specific changes when alternating current changes into thermal energy (Figure 27.2). Desiccation, coagulation, steaming, and vaporization are all important for electrovaporization (Table 27.1). Desiccation results in cellular dehydration without protein denaturation, and coagulation causes protein bonds to form, creating a homogeneous, gelatinous structure. During coagulation, blood vessels and lymphatics are thrombosed and occluded. Desiccated and coagulated

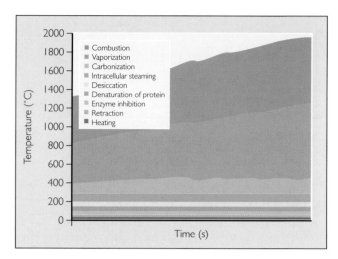

Figure 27.2 The effect of rising temperature on living tissue

Source: Courtesy of Joseph A Smith Jr, MD and Douglas F Milam MD from the book Topics in Clinical Urology: Technique for Ablation of Benign and Malignant Prostate Tissue. New York: Igaku Shoin Medical Publishers 1996.

Temperature (°C)	Effect on tissue
43–45	Tissue retracts
>50	Enzyme activity is reduced
50–60	Protein coagulates
90–100	Desiccation occurs
>100	Water in tissue boils and evaporates
>150	Tissue carbonizes
>300	Tissue vaporizes
>500	Flaming of tissue occurs

Table 27.1 Tissue effects that occur at various temperatures during heat induced treatments of the prostate

tissue are poor conductors of electricity and heat, which results in the accumulation of heat at the tissue surface and, finally, charring and carbonization of tissue. Fulguration spray coagulation (or black coagulation) is the term applied to superficial coagulation and carbonization caused by repeated high-voltage electrosurgical arcs that rapidly increase temperatures to about 200°C.[10-13,17,18]

VAPORIZATION

During vaporization, water changes to steam; to increase the temperature from 37°C to 100°C requires 2.5 kJ of energy/g of tissue. The kinetic energy of the escaping vapor causes microscopic detonations within tissue, further adding to the mechanical rupture of membranes.[4]

FACTORS MODULATING CLINICAL RESULTS

CURRENT-, GENERATOR- AND ELECTRODE-RELATED FACTORS

Unipolar and Bipolar Circuits

In a unipolar circuit, the electrical current flows through the contact electrode, through the body, and finally exits via a ground plate, return plate, or electron sink. Thus, a portion of the patient's body is a part of the electrical circuit. The current affects tissue at the active electrode. Such systems are commonly used for transurethral surgery and electrovaporization. Bipolar systems use miniaturized isolated circuits in which two closely apposed electrodes alternately become active and return electrodes, driven by the alternating current. This system is more precise and less hazardous, but bipolar systems are too weak to be applied to prostate surgery and are used mainly to coagulate delicate tissue, e.g. in neurosurgery.[8–11,16,18]

Frequency and Waveform

Different waveforms of energy affect tissue differently, as seen in Figure 27.1. The pure sine wave and damped continuous sine-wave currents have extensive vaporization properties, whereas modulated undamped and damped waveforms have a predominantly coagulative effect. The blended waveforms have higher peak voltage than pure sine-wave alternating current. However, any one of these waveforms may have multiple effects on tissue depending on other factors.[8–11,16,18]

Electrosurgical Generators

Each make of generator has a different output characteristic and each has varying peak voltage and duty cycles. For prostate electrovaporization, we have obtained the best results with a 300-W setting using a machine that provides a uniform output even with high tissue impedances. Power output is proportional to tissue impedance; most modern machines will automatically adjust the voltage or current as the impedance varies to maintain the desired power output. Additionally, there is a close association between peak voltage and coagulation volume. An increase in power not only results in greater vaporization, but also in a disproportionate increase in the amount of coagulation.[8–11,16,18,20,21] Jennings and associates[22] quantitated the energy transfer during TURP and electrovaporization using a high-frequency microcomputer-controlled Erbe ICC 350 unit in 5 patients. Current, voltage, resistance, and power were similar during resection and electrovaporization, whereas energy transfer was greater during electrovaporization.

Crest Factor

Alternating current varies as a sine wave, and the peak voltage is not maintained evenly throughout the current cycle; the mean voltage is better represented by the crest factor, defined as the ratio of the peak voltage to the root mean square voltage. Changes in the crest factor have the same effect on tissue, as do changes in the voltage.[8–11,16,18,20,21]

Current Density

The thermal effect of the circuit varies inversely with the cross-sectional area of tissue through which current flows at any time, i.e. the current density, given by (power/area)^2.[2] Therefore, the thermal effect can be increased by increasing the current or decreasing the surface area of contact; this relationship further explains why tissue effects vary considerably with the shape and size of the electrovaporization electrode.[8–11,16,18,20,21]

Arcing

When a high-density current is applied to an electrode separated from the target tissue by a medium (gas, steam, or liquid), the intervening medium becomes ionized when the molecules become excited and dissociated. These ions are then accelerated by the strong electrical field and collide with uncharged molecules of the medium. If the electrical field is strong enough (a high current density), the ions will continue ionizing the medium by "avalanche multiplication." As the population of ions approaches a critical density, the equivalent impedance between the electrode and tissue decreases. Current flows and the plasma cloud formed by the excited ionized atoms emit light as some of the ions relax to lower energy states. If the electrical field between the electrodes falls below the minimum required to sustain the plasma cloud, the plasma quickly collapses and the arc is quenched; the arc may be re-established when the field again exceeds the critical current density. The arc may be established on either the positive or negative half-cycle of the sine wave. On the negative half-cycle, the positive ions will be accelerated toward the electrode and the negative charges repelled. The arc is highly localized in both space and time and consists of very short, high current-density discharges capable of intense heating of the target (steaming and vaporization of intra- and extracellular water). Because the arc has a very precise and rapid deposition of energy that dissipates quickly both in time and distance from the point of strike, it is useful for the effective electrovaporization of tissue.[8–11,16,18,20,21]

Shape of the Electrode

The shape of the electrodes can have important implications for contact area, current density, and entrapment of steam in the grooves of the electrode (see Figure 26.7A–E in Chapter 26). The first rollerball type of electrode that was used was made by Circon-American Cystoscope Manufacturers Inc. (Circon ACMI, Stamford, CT, USA) and termed the VaporTrode. The grooved construction of this instrument produces simultaneous coagulation because the area of contact between the grooves is large, and vaporization caused by sparking from the ridges of the instrument causes rapid vaporization. Since several ridges are available on a VaporTrode compared with the single one of the conventional loop, it is theoretically possible to increase the volume of vaporized tissue. Using a combination of vaporization and coagulation, the technique of transurethral electrovaporization of the prostate (TUEP) creates an immediate tissue defect surrounded by a rim of coagulated tissue. As described elegantly by Drs Te and Kaplan there are also temperature differences between the leading and trailing edge of a rollerball electrode (Figure 26.6, Chapter 26). This reduces bleeding and fluid absorption and therefore, TUR syndrome. Currently, several similar electrodes have been made by other manufacturers and are available for TUEP. Most of them use a combination of larger surface area for coagulation, and some modifications for achievement of vaporization. In most instances, there is a trade-off between either higher vaporization or higher coagulation.

Watson and associates[23] performed a study to determine the detailed pattern of prostatic interstitial temperature changes during rollerball electrovaporization and loop electrosurgery in patients with benign hyperplasia. Their studies concluded that the patterns of temperature change during rollerball electrovaporization and loop electrosurgery were similar. Temperatures decreased steeply and significantly with increasing distance from both the rollerball ($P < 0.001$) and loop ($P < 0.001$). Marked mean temperature increases occurred at 1–2 mm from both the rollerball (30.8°C) and loop (34.8°C), and temperatures at this distance were significantly higher than those at greater distances ($P < 0.05$). At 3–5 mm, the mean temperature increase declined by 58% for the rollerball and 68% for the loop. Further declines of 68% and 63%, respectively, were observed at 6–10 mm, and, at distances exceeding 10 mm, the temperature changes were minimal (0.5°C for the rollerball and 0.5°C for the loop). There was no change in temperature at any of the thermosensors near the neurovascular bundles and rectum. The patterns of temperature change with rollerball electrovaporization and loop electrosurgery are closely similar. Interstitial temperature changes during use of the rollerball and loop are transient and highly localized, posing minimal risk of unintended thermal damage to adjacent tissues, including the neurovascular bundles and rectum.

Duration of Contact
Optimal vaporization and coagulation occur when the electrode is tracked across the tissue at 0.5–0.33 mm s^{-1}; the longer the duration of contact, the greater the changes in the tissue.[24] However, if contact is too prolonged, there may be significant peripheral desiccation and coagulation, altering the electrical impedance of the tissue and causing increased charring and carbonization due to a lack of penetration. This was reported in tissue experiments where very slow electrode speeds caused intense heat close to the electrode and damaged it.[24]

Surface Cooling
The irrigant used during electrovaporization needs to be non-ionic and is helpful in washing out the debris and cooling both the electrode and the surface of the tissue.[24]

TISSUE FACTORS
Composition of Tissue and Impedance
Tissues vary considerably in impedance, depending upon their ionic composition and fluid content.[7,10–12,14,16–18] Highly conductive tissues have a high water content and offer little resistance to the current. Tissues such as bone, fat, and any previously desiccated tissue have a high resistance and thus impede the current. This effect is important when low power density is used initially to cause coagulation and desiccation of the prostate, because further attempts to vaporize desiccated tissue results in surface charring, which is preferable towards the end of procedure but is a disadvantage at the beginning. The increased tissue impedance of coagulated tissue causes less vaporization on subsequent passes, leading to an incomplete TUR defect and unsatisfactory results. Therefore, it is preferable to use the higher voltage initially. Once capsule fibers are visible and the adenoma is adequately vaporized, the surgeon should lower the power of the cutting current to increase the coagulation, which will result in more effective hemostasias.

The Heat-Sink Effect
When heat is applied to a vascular tissue for >10 s, some of the energy is transferred to the vascular or lymphatic channels, preventing the accumulation of heat in the peripheral tissues. Because of this heat transfer, lesions made in dead tissue (experiments *in vitro*) are larger than those produced *in vivo*.[4]

EXPERIMENTAL VAPORIZATION AND COAGULATION IN HUMAN AND BOVINE TISSUES

Studies performed in the Editor's laboratory[24] have established several factors that influence the lesions made by vaporization. Lesions made by the VaporTrode instrument were compared with those produced by an Nd:YAG laser fiber.[4] Human and bovine tissues were used and the electrosurgical generator considered a Force 40 S compared with a Force 2. The Force 40 S operates at 90–135 V at 50–60 MHz to insure constant output even with power surges. This instrument delivers a current at 500 kHz and maximum power of 300 W. The maximum peak-to-peak voltage is 3300 V and the crest factor is 2.1 at 100 W at a rate load of 300 ω.

The main findings of the study were (a) an output setting of 300 W produced a significantly greater vaporization lesion and a ring of coagulated tissue around the crater than did a setting of 200 or 250 W ($P < 0.05$); (b) the slower the drag speed of the electrode over the tissue, the greater the vaporization and coagulation volume. The greatest effect was obtained by producing a 10-mm lesion over 20–30 s rather than 5 s: however, drag speeds of <0.33 mm s^{-1} produced excessive carbonization of the floor of the lesion, thus reducing the efficiency of further evaporation of deeper tissues: (c) the Force F40 S, a newer solid-state electrosurgical unit, produced significantly greater volumes of vaporization and coagulation than its previous counterpart, the Force 2 (a 35% greater vaporization volume and 66% greater coagulation volume; $P < 0.05$); (d) a new VaporTrode electrode produced a 50% greater vaporization and 36% greater coagulation volume than an old, used

VaporTrode, ($P<0.05$); (e) the VaporTrode produced more vaporization and 43% greater coagulation than the rollerball, and 711% greater coagulation than the TUR loop; $P<0.05$; (f) the volume of vaporization using the VaporTrode was comparable with a laser lesion produced at high power density (60 W and a drag rate of 0.33 mm s^{-1}); (g) the coagulation volume of the VaporTrode was less than that produced with high- or low-power density lasers (VaporTrode 30 μL; contact laser 40 μL; non-contact 97–109 μL; $P<0.05$).[24]

THE TECHNIQUE OF TRANSURETHRAL ELECTROVAPORIZATION OF THE PROSTATE

TUEP[25–27] begins with a cystoscopic examination of the bladder to detect any associated bladder pathology, i.e. a tumor or stone, and to locate the ureteric orifices. Prostatic size is assessed, and the presence of the median lobe and any extension of apical tissue beyond the verumontanum are noted. Subsequently, a 25.6 French continuous-flow ACMI resectoscope with an attached VaporTrode is introduced into the bladder, with glycine or water used as an irrigant. The electrosurgical unit is set to a pure-cutting current of 300 W. The VaporTrode tip is positioned 1 cm within the bladder but well away from the ureteric orifice. Initial vaporization is carried out on the bladder neck at the 6-o'clock position; subsequently, all tissue between the 5- and 7-o'clock positions on the bladder neck is vaporized. The median lobe, if present, is vaporized by creating successive furrows starting proximally and ending at the prostatic fossa, until all of the median lobe is evaporated. The ureteric orifices are avoided at all times. Gentle pressure and even movements of the electrode from the bladder neck towards the prostate result in a 3–4 mm deep furrow of vaporization as wide as the VaporTrode tip (3 mm). Repeated passes of the VaporTrode result in further deepening of the floor of the furrow. The bladder neck is vaporized only between the 5- and 7-o'clock positions, and passes are repeated until circular bladder neck fibers are visible. The rest of the bladder neck and its mucosa up to 1 cm distal to the bladder neck are preserved to retain antegrade ejaculation. The lateral lobe tissue between the 5- and 11-o'clock positions is next vaporized below the bladder neck. A furrow is initially created from just below the bladder neck to the verumontanum. Repeated passes are made circumferentially from the 5–1-o'clock and 7–11-o'clock positions to achieve complete vaporization of the entire adenoma of both lobes.

On completion of the procedure, the prostatic capsule is visible at several points and any residual tissue is removed by repeated vaporization. After completing the removal of the lateral lobes, the tissue from below the bladder neck to the verumontanum between 5 and 7 o'clock is vaporized. No attempt is made to expose the capsule on the prostatic floor; the tissue of the floor is usually not obstructive and excessive vaporization is unnecessary. Apical tissue is vaporized last, using a combination of mainly retrograde and some antegrade movement of the electrode to achieve smooth vaporization and to avoid "shaggy" tissue at the verumontanum. This preserves anatomical integrity and avoids any inadvertent vaporization of tissue distal to the verumontanum. Excessive pressure on the VaporTrode is avoided at all times to prevent perforation of the capsule and exposure of venous sinuses. The VaporTrode is a powerful instrument and can penetrate deeply.

Bleeding is always minimal and, if observed, can be controlled easily by cauterization. Cutting current is used initially and coagulating current towards the end of the procedure. Using mostly cutting current controls bleeding at the apex. The vaporization between the 11- and 1-o'clock positions on the roof is minimal. Some intact pink mucosa is left at the 12-o'clock position along the entire prostatic fossa to help rapid re-epithelialization of the prostatic fossa. At the end of the procedure, a 20-French three-way Foley catheter is placed in the bladder and connected to a closed drainage system. The irrigation port is left plugged and irrigation is not performed routinely. Bleeding is minimal and occasional, pink-tinged urine clears, usually within 4–5 h. The patients are allowed to go home on the same day with the catheter in place. Patients are taught to remove the catheter themselves, which they do after 12–48 h; a 3-day course of antibiotic prophylaxis is given to all patients.

CLINICAL STUDIES

Kaplan et al.[25] published preliminary results of a study on 25 men (mean age, 63.5 years) with mild-to-moderate symptoms of prostatism who underwent TUEP. The patients were assessed at baseline for both safety and efficacy 1 week, and 1 and 3 months after surgery. These authors evaluated operative duration, change in hematocrit and serum sodium, the postoperative duration of catheterization, the International Prostate Symptom Score (IPSS), peak urinary flow rate (Q_{max}) and postvoid residual urine volume. The symptom score decreased from 17.8 to 5.9 and 4.2 at 1 and 3 months, respectively ($P<0.01$), and the Q_{max} increased from 7.4 to 15.3 and 17.3 mL s^{-1} at 1 and 3 months, respectively ($P<0.02$). The mean operative duration was 40.3 min and the mean interval to catheter removal was 14.6 h. Changes in serum variables included a 0.9% decrease in the hematocrit and a change in sodium of 1.1 mmol L^{-1}. Complications included 3 patients with mild hematuria and 1 with a distal bulbar urethral stricture. There were no associated significant irritative symptoms after the procedure, no patient required recatheterization and none was rendered impotent. The authors highlighted several potential advantages of TUEP, including a significantly lower cost and minimal irritative postoperative symptoms. Te and associates[28] reviewed the records of 93 consecutive patients (mean age 65.2 years) with mild-to-moderate lower urinary tract symptoms who underwent TUEP since August 1994. The patients were assessed at baseline for both safety and efficacy and in follow-up at 1 week ($n=93$) and 1 ($n=87$), 3 ($n=71$), 6 ($n=59$), 9 ($n=44$), and 12 ($n=33$) months. The mean American Urological Association symptom score decreased from 18.6

Study	Device used	No. of patients enrolled	Duration of study (months)	Baseline	Symptom score (% improvement)						
					at ≤2 months	at 3 months	at 6 months	at 1 year	at 2 years	at ≥ 4 years
Porru et al. 1998	Not reported	32	6	26	–	–	8 (69.2)	–	–	–
Gallucci et al. 1996	VaporTrode VE-B	22	1	18	10.5 (42)	–	–	–	–	–
Thomas et al. 1997	Valleylab Force 2	116	4	Not reported	–	67% improvement	–	–	–	–
Matos-Ferreira et al. 1997	Erbe ICC 350E with grooved VaporTrode electrodes	91	12	18.6	–	–	–	5.3 (72)	–	–
Narayan et al. 1996	VaporTrode grooved bar with VE-B Force 405	42	6	24	7.2 (70)	7.7 (68)	7.8 (67.5)	–	–	–
Kaplan et al. 1996	Valleylab Force 40 with Circon ACMI 27F	114	18	16.7	–	7.3 (56.3)	6.5 (61.1)	6.3 (62.3)	5.4[a] (67.7)	–
Kaplan et al. 1995	Circon ACMI 27F with Vallaylab SSE4	25	3	17.8	5.9 (67)	4.2 (76.4)	–	–	–	–
Hamawy et al. 1996	VaporTrode Circon with grooved roller electrode	67	12	21	9 (57.1)	8 (62)	7 (67)	7 (67)	–	–
Perlmutter et al. 1997	VaporTrode Circon w/Valleylab generator	115	6	21.1	–	–	7.1 (66.4)	–	–	–
Desautel et al. 1997	VaporTrode electrode	42	12	20.5	–	7.6 (63)	–	6.7 (67.3)	–	–

[a] at 18 months

Table 27.2 Symptom scores from several published studies using TUEP technique

preoperatively to 8.9, 7.9, 8.1, and 6.3 at 1, 3, 6, and 12 months, respectively ($P<0.01$). The peak uroflow rate (Q_{max}) increased from 7.9 mL s^{-1} to 16.4, 14.1, 14.7, and 17.3 mL s^{-1} at 1, 3, 6, and 12 months, respectively ($P<0.02$). The mean operating time was 47.3 min; 96% of patients had the catheter removed within 24 h and were discharged home on the first postoperative day. There was a mean 1.1 mL dL^{-1} decrease in hematocrit and a 1.4 mEq L^{-1} decline in serum sodium. Complications included mild hematuria (46%), clot retention (5%) (all necessitating transient recatheterization), and distal bulbar urethral stricture ($n=1$). There was an 8% incidence of significant post-procedure irritative symptoms. No previously potent patient reported erectile dysfunction, but there was a 92% rate of retrograde ejaculation. Transurethral vaporization is a potentially useful modification of transurethral resection. There has been significant clinical improvement maintained with minimal morbidity. This early clinical experience highlights several potential advantages of TUEP, including significantly lower cost and minimal postoperative irritative symptoms.

In another report, Kaplan et al.[26] also compared TUEP with high-density laser evaporation and showed that in the 29 patients treated with TUEP the mean symptom score decreased from 15.3 to 4.9 and the Q_{max} increased from 8.2 to 15.6 mL s^{-1} at 3 months. In the 29 patients treated with laser prostatectomy, the mean symptom score decreased from 14.7 to 7.6 and the Q_{max} increased from 9.7 to 14.9 mL s^{-1} at 3 months. There was a significant difference in the incidence of postoperative retention (TUEP, 0; laser, 6), postoperative irritative symptoms (TUEP, 3; laser, 19; $P<0.05$) and the mean duration of catheterization (TUEP, 14.7 h; laser, 79.6 h; $P<0.001$). Since then these authors have published symptomatic improvement in a updated series of 114 patients.[29]

Between November 1994 and May 1996, we treated 60 patients with BPH (mean age 69 years, range 56–83; mean prostatic volume 49.3 mL, range 18–67) using TUEP, who were then followed for a mean of 32.5 weeks (range 15–60). Ten patients were in retention and 8 patients had a well-defined median lobe. The 10 patients in urinary retention were analyzed separately and were not assigned a baseline American Urological Association (AUA) symptom score and Q_{max}. The mean duration of hospitalization was 16.2 h (range 8–24) and the mean duration of catheterization was 22.6 h (range 12–72). There were no statistically significant changes from the baseline in complete blood count, serum electrolytes, and blood gases.[27]

No patient developed clinical or biochemical features of the TUR syndrome. One patient developed hematuria, which lasted for 14 h postoperatively; and he required continuous irrigation of the catheter; his bleeding stopped with no traction or intervention, and the catheter was retained for 3 days. One additional patient developed delayed bleeding, requiring a bladder washout 6 weeks after treatment. This patient had a capsular perforation towards the end of the procedure that was controlled by the insertion of the Foley catheter and by applying traction for 2 h; he needed no irrigation. No patient required a blood transfusion and there were no failures or need for recatheterization at up to 6 months of follow-up.[27] Of the 60 patients, 47 (78%) claimed normal preoperative potency, which was unchanged postoperatively. Of these 47 patients, antegrade ejaculation was maintained in 29 (61%) patients. No patient developed urinary tract infection, urethral stricture, or any other significant morbidity at up to 6 months of follow-up. The results are comparable with others.[25-27]

Several other studies since have shown safety and efficacy of electrovaporization procedure (Tables 27.2 and 27.3). Matos-Ferreira and associates[30] presented their results in 91 patients (median age 65 years) with BPE (median prostate volume 61 mL).[30] Patients were assessed with a general and urological history, the IPSS, urinary tract and prostatic ultrasonography, uroflowmetry, and biopsy of the prostate. An electrosurgical generator (cutting at 200 W and coagulating at 70 W) with grooved electrodes was used to vaporize the prostate. The mean operative duration was 45 min, blood loss was negligible, and the mean duration of catheterization was 24 h. Recatheterization was necessary in 5.5% of patients. The median values before and after treatment were IPSS, 19 and 5; quality of life (QoL) score, 4 and 2; and maximum urinary flow rate 8.3 and 22.1 mL s^{-1} (all $P<0.001$). In nearly all cases, the Siroky nomogram showed that patients became unobstructed.

Few authors including Porru and associates[31] have presented urodynamic outcome following electrovaporization. TUEP was performed in 32 symptomatic patients with BPH. Urodynamic studies with pressure-flow analysis were performed before and 6 months after treatment (see Tables 27.2 and 27.3). All 32 patients showed significant improvement of both subjective and objective obstruction parameters.

COMPARISON OF TUEP AND TURP

In an extensive review of the complications associated with TURP in 3885 patients, Mebust et al. reported significant morbidity in 5.2–30.7% (mean 18%) following the procedure.[1] The risk of mortality within 30–90 days of TURP was 0.53–3.33%, with a mean of 2.01%. In a more recent study comparing TURP with watchful waiting in 249 men undergoing TURP, the overall morbidity rate was 8% in the initial 30 days, with 4% requiring recatheterization, and 1% experiencing hemorrhage requiring transfusion. A mean of 4 days of catheterization was required in 78% of these patients. Postoperative complications included bladder-neck contracture in 3.6%, urethral stricture in 3.6%, and 8.2% for whom the procedure had failed after 3 years of follow-up.[32] A notable feature of this last study was that the mean weight of resected tissue was only 14.4 g and severely obstructed patients and patients in retention were excluded. More recently, Veterans Affairs Cooperative Study (VA Coop) data reveals that morbidity of TURP may be lower but it is still higher than that of TVP.[33]

Study	Device used	No. of patients enrolled	Duration of study (months)	Baseline	Peak urinary flow rate (% improvement) (Q_{max})					
					at ≤2 months	at 3 months	at 6 months	at 1 year	at 2 years	at ≥4 years
Porru et al. 1998	Not reported	32	6	7.4	–	–	18.4 (149)	–	–	–
Gallucci et al. 1996	VaporTrode VE-B	22	1	9.31	20.74 (123)	–	–	–	–	–
Thomas et al. 1997	Valleylab Force 2	116	4	Not reported improvement	–	12.2 mL s^{-1}	–	–	–	–
Matos-Ferreira et al. 1997	Erbe ICC 350 E with grooved VaporTrode electrode	91	12	8.74	–	–	–	21.9 (151)	–	–
Narayan et al. 1996	VaporTrode grooved bar with VE-B Force 40S	42	6	8.8	19.5 (122)	20.1 (128)	20.0 (127)	–	–	–
Kaplan et al. 1996	Valleylab Force 40 with Circon ACMI 27F	114	18	7.9	–	14.8 (87.3)	15.6 (97.5)	16.7 (111.4)	16.5[a] (109)	–
Kaplan et al. 1995	Circon ACMI 27F with Valleylab SSE4	25	3	7.4	15.3 (107)	17.3 (134)	–	–	–	–
Hamawy et al. 1996	VaporTrode Circon with grooved roller electrode	67	12	8.6	18.1 (110.5)	20.7 (141)	19.6 (128)	19.1 (122.1%)	–	–
Perlmutter et al. 1997	VaporTrode Circon w/Valleylab generator	115	6	8.1	–	–	16.1 (99)	–	–	–
Desautel et al. 1997	VaporTrode electrode	42	12	6.2	16.5 (166.1)	–	–	14.4 (132.3)	–	–

[a] at 18 months

Table 27.3 Peak urinary flow rates from several published studies using TUEP procedure

Kaplan and associates compared the safety and efficacy of TURP (Table 27.4).[34] Thirty-two consecutive men (mean age 68.9 years) with lower urinary tract symptoms were treated by TUEP and compared with a cohort of 32 men (mean age 72.8 years) treated by TURP. Parameters of evaluation included AUA symptom score, peak urinary flow rate, adverse events, including serial changes in serum hematocrit and sodium, operative time, postoperative catheterization time, hospitalization time, and days lost from work. A total of 61 patients were available for follow-up at 1 year. None required retreatment. At 1 year symptom score decreased by 12.8 (66%) and 12.2 (67%) and peak urinary flow increased 9.7 ml/s (135%) and 11.3 ml/s (136%) for TURP and TUEP, respectively ($P<0.001$). Operative time was significantly longer with TUEP than with TURP (47.6 ± 17.6 vs 34.6 ± 11.2 min, $P<0.003$). Catheterization time (67.4 ± 13.6 vs. 12.9 ± 4.6 h), hospitalization time (2.6 ± 0.9 vs. 1.3 ± 0.5 days) and days lost from work (18.4 ± 7.6 vs. 6.7 ± 2.1) were significantly greater for resection than electrovaporization, respectively. There were no major complications in the electrovaporization group, while in the resection group 1 patient required transfusion (5 units) and in 1 patient a clinical TURP syndrome developed.

Potency and retrograde ejaculation were normal in 18 of 18 patients (100%) and 13 of 17 (76%) after resection, and 19 of 20 (95%) and 17 of 20 (85%) after TUEP. The results indicated that TURP and TUEP were both effective in reducing lower urinary tract symptoms with similar preservation of sexual function. Both significantly improved peak urinary flow, although resection to a greater degree. Postoperative morbidity, catheterization time, hospitalization time, and days lost from work were significantly less, and operative time was significantly longer with electrovaporization.

Shokeir and associates[35] compared TUEP with TURP in the treatment of 70 men with BPH. Patients with a prostate size of <60 g were prospectively randomized between equal treatment groups; one group underwent standard TURP and the other TUEP. Patients were assessed at baseline and 1, 3, 6, and 12 months after treatment, giving a mean (SD) duration of follow-up of 14.4 (1.9) months (range 12–17). Variables evaluated included the duration of operation, catheterization, and hospital stay, and changes in blood levels of hemoglobin, hematocrit, and sodium 1 h after the operation. The AUA7 symptom score, peak urinary flow rate (Q_{max}), postvoiding residual urine (PVR) volume and sexual function were also evaluated during the follow-up. The mean operative duration of TUEP was 52 min, significantly longer than that of TURP, at 39.7 min ($P<0.001$). One hour after TURP, patients had significantly lower levels of hemoglobin, hematocrit, and Na. The mean duration of catheterization after TURP was 2 days, significantly more than after TUEP, at 1.1 days ($P<0.001$). The mean hospital stay was 2.5 days after TURP and 1.5 days after TUEP ($P<0.001$). Compared with baseline values, the AUA7 symptom score, Q_{max}, and PVR improved significantly in both groups at all intervals of follow-up, and there

were no significant differences between the groups during the follow-up. None of 15 potent men undergoing TURP and two of 18 potent men undergoing TUEP complained of impotence during the follow-up. The authors concluded that TUEP is as effective as TURP in the treatment of BPH in men with a prostate size of <60 g. It also had the advantages of less blood loss, less absorption of irrigant, and a shorter hospital stay, but it had a significantly longer operative duration.

For a summary of symptom scores and peak urinary flow rates from other published reports comparing TUEP with TURP, see Table 27.4.

One disadvantage of TUEP is the lack of tissue for histological analysis. However, if such tissue is needed, the VaporTrode can be exchanged for a routine transurethral resection loop and chips obtained. Lack of bleeding is a major advantage of TUEP, as throughout the procedure the surgeon has a clear field of vision, and the chances of damaging the sphincter or perforating the capsule are thus reduced.

COMPLICATIONS OF TRANSURETHRAL ELECTROVAPORIZATION OF THE PROSTATE

Chow and associates[36] in a retrospective review of 524 consecutive patients who underwent TURP and 302 consecutive patients who underwent TUEP compared the incidence of initial and delayed hemorrhages, the time until a delayed bleed occurred, blood transfusion rates, and the average length of stay in hospital after a bleed. The overall hemorrhage rates for TURP and TUEP were 4.8% and 4.0%, respectively. In the TURP group, there was a 1.1% incidence of acute bleeds and 3.6% incidence of delayed bleeds. For the TUEP group, 0.3% had an acute hemorrhage, and 3.6% were readmitted for clot retention. The average length of time from original discharge to readmission was 12.9 days for the TURP group with a mean repeat stay of 5.7 days. For the TUEP group, the average interval to readmission was 15.4 days with a stay of 3.1 days. The overall rate of hemorrhage for the TUEP group was slightly lower than for the TURP group owing to fewer acute bleeds. However, the incidence of delayed bleeds and clot retention between the two was identical at 3.6%.

Table 27.5 summarizes the side effects reported from several published reports using TUEP procedure for BPH. From this table, it is evident that TUEP is associated with a high incidence of retrograde ejaculation, postoperative irritative symptoms, and hematuria. However, from Table 27.6, which compares the adverse events associated with TUEP with that of TURP, the incidence of hematuria from TUEP is not that high in comparison with TURP. Furthermore, TUEP presents with shorter postoperative catheterization period and hospital stay when compared with TURP. From Table 27.6, it is interesting to note that the incidence of retrograde ejaculation with TUEP or TURP is comparable in all studies, except the one reported by Kaplan and associates[26] in 1995, which stated that the

Study	Device used	No. of patients enrolled		Symptom score (% improvement)				Peak urinary flow rate, Q_{max} (% improvement)			
				Baseline	at 3 months	at 6 months	at 12 months	Baseline (mL s⁻¹)	at 3 months	at 6 months	at 12 months
Cetinkaya et al. 1996	Storz Spike 5 mm 2-system electrode	46	{ 23 TUEP { 23 TURP	Not reported Not reported	Δ = −20.89 Δ = −21.31	— —	— —	Not reported Not reported	Δ = 16.37 mL s⁻¹ Δ = 17.49 mL s⁻¹	— —	— —
Shokeir et al. 1997	Karl Store grooved "spiky" roller electrode	70	{ 35 TUEP { 35 TURP	26.3 25.1	4.5 (83) 4.8 (81)	4.6 (83) 4.5 (82.1)	5.2 (80.2) 4.7 (81.3)	7.8 6.9	19.9 (199) 19.4 (181.2)	19.2 (146) 19.3 (180)	20.1 (158) 18.2 (164)
Kaplan et al. 1998	Valleylab Force 40 with coller fluted electrode	64	{ 32 TUEP { 32 TURP	19.4 18.3	9.2 (526) 8.6 (53)	7.4 (62) 7.9 (57)	6.6 (66) 6.1 (66.7)	7.2 8.3	14.8 (105.6) 16.8 (102.4)	15.6 (117) 18.1 (118.1)	16.9 (135) 19.6 (136.1)
Patel et al. 1997	VaporTrode Spiked Bar with Force FX generator	30	{ 12 TUEP { 18 TURP	21.4 21.6	4.1 (81) 5.2 (76)	— —	— —	7.8 8.1	19.4 (149) 17.7 (119)	— —	— —
Te et al. 1997	Circon grooved VaporTrode	200	{ 100 TUEP { 100 TURP	20.4 21.1		— —	8.0ᵃ (60.8) 9ᵃ (57.3)	9.8 10.2		— —	18.6ᵃ (90) 19.1ᵃ (87.3)
Evans et al. 1997	Not reported	30	{ 15 TUEP { 15 TURP	22 24	10ᵇ (54.5) 12ᵇ (50)	— —	— —	9 9	18ᵇ (100) 14ᵇ (55.6)	— —	— —
Shingleton et al. 1997	Not reported	32	{ 22 TUEP { 10 Laser	22 18	8 (63.6) 6 (67)	5 (77.3) 5 (72.2)	— —	7.7 10.7	17.5 (127.3) 17.6 (64.5)	129 (67.5) 15.3 (43)	— —
Kaplan et al. 1995 (Urology)	VaporTrode	58	{ 29 TUEP { 29 Laser	15.3 14.7	4.9 (68) 7.6 (48.3)	— —	— —	8.2 9.7	15.6 (90.2) 14.9 (53.6)	— —	— —

ᵃ at 9 months
ᵇ at 1 month

Table 27.4 Summary of symptom scores and peak urinary flow rates from studies comparing TUEP with TURP

	Gallucci et al. 1996	Thomas et al. 1997	Matos-Ferreira et al. 1997	Narayan et al. 1996	Kaplan et al. 1996	Kaplan et al. 1995 (Urology)	Perlmutter et al. 1997	Hamawy et al. 1996	Desautel et al. 1997
Hematuria	50%	6.4%	>95%	5%	57%	12%	4%	8%	Present in some
UTI (%)	12.5	10	–	0	2	–	–	–	–
Urinary retention (%)	6.25	–	–	–	0	–	–	–	5
Urinary incontinence (%)	12.5	–	0	0	0	–	2	–	2.4
Postop dysuria and frequency (%)	–	>75	≈50	14	9	–	–	–	–
Duration of post-op catheterization (range: low–high)	48 h	–	24 h (12–36)	23.2 h (12–72)	10.4 h	14.6 h	–	–	–
TUR syndrome (%)	0	–	–	0	0	0	–	–	–
Retrograde ejaculation (%)	100	15	>95	23	84	100	–	–	–
Impotence (%)	–	0	0	0	0	0	–	–	–
Change in Hb or HCT (postop–preop)	1.42 decrease in Hb	–	–	–	1.7% decrease in HCT	0.9 mL dL^{-1} decrease in HCT	–	–	–
Postop hospital stay	2.3 days	–	2.33 days	14.8 h	21.6 h	–	–	≈24 h	–
Bulbar urethral stricture (%)	–	–	1.1	0	2	4	5	1.5	5

N = not reported

Table 27.5 Incidence of TUEP complications

	Cetinkaya et al. 1996		Shokeir et al. 1997		Kaplan et al. 1998		Te et al. 1997		Patel et al. 1997		Kaplan et al. 1995	
	TUEP	TURP	TUEP	TURP	TUEP	TURP	TUEP	TURP	TUEP	TURP	TUEP	Laser
Hematuria (%)	–	–	11.4	5.7	53	60	–	–	–	–	55	72
UTI (%)	–	–	–	–	16	13	–	–	–	–	0	21
Urinary retention (%)	–	–	0	0	0	0	–	–	–	–	0	20.7
Urinary incontinence (%)	–	–	–	–	0	0	–	–	–	–	–	–
Postop dysuria and frequency (%)	–	–	8.6	5.7	16	13	–	–	–	–	7	83
Duration of postop catheterization	1.4 days	1.9 days	1.1 days	2 days	12.9 h	2.8 days	1.1 days	5.5 days	23 h	1.94	13.7 h	3.4
TUR syndrome (%)	0	–	0	0	0	3.1	0	3	0	0	0	0
Blood transfusion (%)	–	8.7	0	0	0	3.1	–	–	0	5.6	0	7
Retrograde ejaculation (%)	–	–	100	100	85	76	–	–	50	–	0	85
Impotence (%)	–	–	11.1	0	5	0	–	–	0	44.4	0	13.3
Urethral stricture (%)	4.3	0	–	–	3.1	3.1	–	–	0	5.6	3.4	0
Change in Hb or HCT	4.14% decrease	6.57% decrease	2.5% decrease	6.3% decrease	2.8 ml dL change in Hb	5.6 ml dL change in Hb	–	–	–	decrease in HCT	1.3 mL dL^{-1} decrease in HCT	3.4 mL dL^{-1}
Post-op hospital stay (days)	–	–	1.5	2.5	1.3	2.6	3.5	7.0	1.2	2.6	–	–

Table 27.6 Summary of adverse events associated with TUEP and TURP

incidence of retrograde ejaculation was 0% in the TUEP-treated group, while 85% experienced it in the TURP-treated group.

USE OF COMBINATION THERAPY

Some patients who have had TUEP have complained postoperatively of significant dysuria and irritative symptoms, which has been noticed by several urologists, including ourselves. The most likely reason for this is that an inadequate TUEP has been performed using the older electrocautery machines (Force 2 Valleylab and similar ones), with sufficient power to handle the larger surface area of roller electrodes. This results in partial burns, ulceration prolonged sloughing of tissue and edema with postoperative irritative symptoms. To avoid these complications and to shorten the operative time of TUEP (which when performed as an isolated procedure does take approximately 150% of the time duration of a standard TURP), we have performed combination therapy in patients who have prostate size >40 grams. We initially start by performing TUEP in a manner similar to that described for the TUEP technique. The only difference is that we avoid evaporating excessive tissue and only make initial single passes from just below the bladder neck to the verumontanum all around the prostate from approximately 11 o'clock to 6 o'clock and from approximately 1 o'clock to 6 o'clock. Once the initial furrows are made, we switch to a regular electrocautery loop. This can be performed using the same resectoscope working element since the electrodes are interchangeable. We then return to resect all the remaining tissue. We subsequently use TUEP again to sculpt the remainder of the prostatic fossa at the end to achieve deep coagulation and remove any residual tissue. This procedure eliminates a portion of the TUEP technique, reducing the time to approximately 30 min, since it is not performed in combination with the TURP technique. Using this technique, we have been able to discharge the patients on the same day of the surgical procedure. Furthermore, these patients have had a reduction in postoperative irritative symptoms, bleeding, and clot-retention problems. Also, the TUEP technique, when performed at the apex of the prostate in a retrograde manner, allows us to avoid inadvertent damage to the sphincter, which cannot be as well controlled during standard TURP. Finally, the combination technique allows some tissue to be recovered, which then can be used for histological detection of cancers if that is a consideration for some clinicians. The main advantage with the use of TUEP, however, is the reduction in bleeding and clot retention because of the large surface area of the electrode, allowing excellent coagulation of venous bleeding. This, thereby, helps to avoid both TUR syndrome and bleeding. The combination therapy may ultimately be the most significant advantage of the availability of rollerball electrodes of various types.

UNRESOLVED ISSUES

Currently, there are certain concerns about TUEP that remain unanswered. The incidence of erectile dysfunction following TURP is 5–34% (mean 13%) and is usually attributed to damage to the cavemosal nerves (which are very close to the prostatic apex) by electrical current.[37–40] TUEP uses a much higher power of cutting current (about double) and may theoretically cause a higher incidence of impotence. Similarly, the use of high-density current on apical tissue may result in electrically induced damage to the external urethral sphincter. The excessive use of coagulating current in these locations should be avoided. The intermittent sine-wave current used for producing low heat and coagulation not only desiccates the tissue but also changes tissue impedance. We have observed none of these complications in the short-term follow-up, but long-term results are not yet reported. The use of electrosurgical current can cause capacitance, which results in high-density current loops between the resectoscope and the urethral mucosa and glands. Urethral strictures after TURP may have been caused by this phenomenon. Muscle twitching and neural stimulation can also occur from such low-frequency currents.[9–11,41] High current density can also result in oxy-hydrogenation of gases in the bladder, due to ionization, and thus can increase the chances of intravesical explosions.[9–11,41] Increased chances of burn injury, pacemaker dysfunction, and corneal damage to the operating surgeon are additional theoretical concerns. Fortunately, modern electrosurgical units are safe, and so far none of these potential hazards has been observed.

CONCLUSIONS

TUEP uses existing electrosurgical principles and equipment and requires no additional technical skills to those already acquired by a urologist. The results of using TUEP to improve symptoms and Q_{max} in patients with symptomatic BPH is promising. The advantages of TUEP over TURP and VLAP include the surgeon's familiarity with the transurethral route, the use of established instruments, the lower cost of the equipment necessary, less training, excellent intra-operative hemostasis and lack of bleeding or fluid absorption, and the ability to produce a complete and predictable TUR-like prostatic defect on completion of the procedure. Additional, randomized studies with more patients will ultimately determine the role of this modality in the management of BPH.

REFERENCES

1 Mebust W, Holtgrewe H, Cocket APC, Peters PC. Transurethral prostatectomy: immediate and post operative complication. A comparative study of 13 participating institutions evaluating 3885 patients. *J Urol* 1989; **141**: 243–7.

2 Leach G, Sirls L, Ganabathi K *et al*. Outpatient visual laser-assisted prostatectomy under local anesthesis. *Urology* 1994; **43**: 149–53.

3 Kabalin J, Gill H, Bite G. Laser prostatectomy performed with a right-angle neodymium:YAG laser fiber at 60 watts power setting. *J Urol* 1995; **153**: 1502–5.

4 Fournier GJ, Narayan P. Factors affecting size and configuration of neodymium:YAG (Nd:YAG) laser lesions in the prostate. *Lasers Surg Med* 1994; **14**: 314–22.

5 Narayan P, Tewari A, Fournier G, Toke A. Impact of prostate size on the outcome of transurethral laser evaporation of the prostate for benign prostatic hyperplasia. *Urology* 1995; **45**: 776–82.

6 Narayan P, Fournier G, Indudhara R *et al*. Transurethral evaporation of prostate (TUEP) with Nd:YAG laser using a contact free beam technique: results in 61 patients with benign prostatic hyperplasia. *Urology* **34**: 1994; 813–20.

7 Sutton C, MacDonald R, Magos A, Broadbent JS. Endometrial resection. In: Lewis BV, Magos AL (eds) *Endometrial Ablation*. New York: Churchill Livingstone 1993; 91–104.

8 Blandy J, Notley RS. The Instruments. In: Blandy JP, Notley RS (eds) *Transurethral Resection*. Oxford: Butterworth-Heinemann 1993; 10–27.

9 Fastenmeier K, Flachenecker GS. High frequency technology: Applications and Hazards. In: Mauermayer W, Fastenmeir K, Flachenecker G, Hartung R, Schütz R (eds) *Transurethral Surgery*. Berlin: Springer 1983; 47–60.

10 Goddard DS. Principles of electrosurgery. In: Glenn JF (ed) *Urologic Surgery*. Philadelphia: JB Lippincott 1983; 879–90.

11 Hulka J, Reich H (eds) *Textbook of Laparoscopy*, 2nd edn. Philadelphia: WB Saunders 1994; 23–46.

12 McCarthy JS. *Physics in Medicine and Biology: Encyclopedia*. New York: Pergamon Press 1986; 319–23.

13 Mitchill J, Lumb G, Dobbie A. *A Handbook of Surgical Diathermy*. Bristol: John Wright 1978: 121.

14 Odell R. Electrosurgery. In: Sutton C, Diamond MP (eds) *Endoscopic Surgery for the Gynaecologist*. Philadelphia: WB Saunders 1959; 303–401.

15 Weyrauch H. Transurethral prostatectomy. In: Weyrauch HM (ed) *Surgery of the Prostate*. Philadelphia: WB Saunders 1959; 303–401.

16 Kramolowsky E, Tucker R. The urological application of electrosurgery. *J Urol* 1991; **146**: 669–74.

17 Munro M. Energy sources for operative laproscopy. In: Gomel V, Taylor PJ (eds) *Diagnostic and Operative Gynaecologic Laproscropy*. New York: Mosby 1995; 26–56.

18 Keckstein J. Tissue effects of different lasers and electrodiathermy. In: Sutton C, Diamond MP (eds) *Endoscopic Surgery for the Gynecologist*. Philadelphia: WB Saunders 1993; 60–70.

19 Lee R, Gaylor D, Bhatt D, Israel D. Role of cell membrane rupture in the pathogenesis of electrical trauma. *J Surg Res* 1988; **44**: 709–19.

20 Valleylab®. *Force 2. Instruction Manual*. Colorado: Valleylab Inc 1985; 7.1–7.11.

21 Valleylab®. *Force 30, Force 40: Instruction Manual*. Colorado: Valleylab Inc 1993; 7.1–7.11.

22 Jennings SB, Karafin LJ, Rukstalis DB. High-frequency electrosurgery using the microcomputer-controlled Erbe ICC 350 unit. *J Endourol* 1998; **12**(1): 67–9.

23 Watson GM, Perlmutter AP, Shah TK *et al*. Heat treatment for severe, symptomatic prostatic outflow obstruction. *World J Urol* 1991; **9**: 7–11.

24 Narayan P, Tewari A, Croker B *et al*. Factors affecting size and configuration of electrovaporization lesions in the prostate. *Urology* 1996; **47**: 679–88.

25 Kaplan S, Te A. Transurethral electrovaporization of the prostate: a novel method for treating men with benign prostatic hyperplasia. *Urology* 1995; **45**: 566–71.

26 Kaplan S, Te A. A comparative study of transurethral resection of the prostate using a modified electro-vaporizing loop and transurethral laser vaporization of the prostate. *J Urol* 1995; **154**: 1785–90.

27 Narayan P, Tewari A, Garzotto M *et al*. Transurethral VaporTrode electrovaporization of the prostate: physical principles, technique and results. *Urology* 1996; **47**: 505–10.

28 Te AE, Santarosa R, Kaplan SA. Electrovaporization of the prostate: electrosurgical modification of standard transurethral resection in 93 patients with benign hyperplasia. *J Endourol* 1997; **11**(1): 71–5.

29 Te AE, Kaplan SA. Transurethral electrovaporization of the prostate. *Mayo Clin Proc* 1998; **73**(7): 691–5.

30 Matos-Ferreira A, Varregoso J. Electrovaporization of the prostate in patients with benign prostatic enlargement. *Br J Urol* 1997; **80**(4): 575–8.

31 Porru D, Scarpa RM, Campus G *et al*. Transurethral electrovaporization of the prostate in benign prostatic hyperplasia. Evaluation of results using different urodynamic parameters. *Scan J Urol Nephrol* 1998; **32**(2): 123–6.

32 Wasson J, Reda D, Bruskewitz R. *et al*. A comparison of transurethral surgery with watchful waiting for moderate symptoms of benign prostatic hyperplasia. The Veterans Affairs Cooperative Study Group on Transurethral Resection of the Prostate. *New Eng J Med* 1995; **332**: 75–9.

33 Bruskewitz RC, Reda DJ, Wasson JH *et al*. Testing to predict outcome after transurethral resection of the prostate. *J Urol* 1997; **157**: 1304–8.

34 Kaplan SA, Te AE. Transurethral resection of the prostate versus transurethral electrovaporization of the prostate: a blinded, prospective comparative study with 1-year follow-up. *J Urol* 1998; **159**(2): 454–8.

35 Shokeir AA, al-Sisi H, Farage YM *et al*. Transurethral prostatectomy: a prospective randomized study of conventional resection and electrovaporization in benign prostatic hyperplasia. *Br J Urol* 1997; **80**(4): 570–4.

36 Chow VD, Sullivan LD, Wright JE *et al*. Transurethral electrovaporization of the prostate versus transurethral prostatic resection: a comparison of postoperative hemorrhage. *Urology* 1998; **51**(2): 251–3.

37 Libman E, Fichten C. Prostatectomy and sexual function. *Urology* 1987; **29**: 467.

38 Lindner A, Golumb J, Korzcak D *et al*. Effects of prostatectomy on sexual function. *Urology* 1991; **38**: 26–8.

39 Gold F, Hotchkiss R. Sexual potency following simple prostatectomy. *NY State J Med* 1969; **69**: 2987–9.

40 Hargreave T, Stephenson T. Potency and prostatectomy. *Br J Urol* 1977; **49**: 683.

41 Boyarsky S. Risk management program in electrosurgery. In: Hinman F Jr (ed) *Benign Prostatic Hypertrophy*. New York: Springer 1983; 855–8.

Transurethral Incision of the Prostate

M. Sall and R.C. Bruskewitz

28

INTRODUCTION

Transurethral incision of the prostate (TUIP) is an old procedure initially described by Guthrie in 1834[1] and Bottini in 1887.[2] However, the first to publish a study of TUIP as a treatment for BPH was Orandi in 1973.[3] Orandi's description was a modification of the technique described earlier by Keitzer *et al.* for incision of bladder neck contractures.[4] Orandi used a combined incision of the bladder neck and the prostate. Initially Orandi[3] did not consider TUIP as an alternative to transurethral resection of the prostate (TURP), but as a new operative treatment option for selected younger patients who had bladder outlet obstruction in spite of smaller prostates, and who were not candidates for resection of the prostate. Since Orandi's first publication, the indications for TUIP have been extended to encompass men of all age groups. The operative technique has been further modified and today TUIP is established as a safe, less invasive procedure with an outcome nearly equal to TURP for men with smaller prostates. It is also a procedure with fewer operative complications and surgical side effects than TURP. Today TUIP is the logical standard for BPH surgical treatment against which new minimally invasive alternatives should be compared.

INDICATIONS

GENERAL

The primary indication for TUIP is bladder outlet obstruction or symptoms believed related to BPH or bladder outlet obstruction in men with smaller prostates. The resectable weight of the prostate should not be more than 30 g (some recommend 20 g), as historically assessed by digital rectal examination and/or cystoscopic measuring of the length from the bladder neck to verumontanum. However, considerable experience with prostate surgery is necessary to estimate the resectable weight with some degree of accuracy. Prostate size is most accurately measured by ultrasonography. The upper limit for prostate size measured by ultrasonography would be 50–60 cm.[3] If TUIP were used in patients with a resectable weight under 30 g about 80% of the patients who undergo TURP in the USA would be potential candidates for incision, based on the study of Mebust *et al.*[5]

The indications for TUIP and TURP are almost equal. TUIP is not indicated in patients with an enlarged median lobe estimated at more than 2 g. Though TUIP is a less invasive operation than TURP, TUIP should not be used in patients who have minimal urinary symptoms and bother, because they will have a reduced chance of noting benefit. Choosing a less morbid approach should not lead to a lessening of the indications for invasive prostatic therapies.

TURP remains the treatment of choice in respect of gross hematuria caused by bleeding from prostatic vessels and prostatitis, where the intention is to remove the prostatic tissue (rare indication). This is also true in cases where pathological examination of the whole prostate is indicated.

TUIP is the preferable surgical treatment in (1) patients with high-risk-associated comorbidity to surgery and anesthesia, because of less blood loss, shorter operative procedure, and because surgery can be performed under local anesthesia;[6] (2) younger and/or sexually active men, because of a better chance of maintaining potency and antegrade ejaculation compared with TURP.[7]

STRONG/ABSOLUTE INDICATIONS FOR SURGERY

(1) Recurrent or persistent urinary tract infection due to bladder outlet obstruction.
(2) Dilatation of upper urinary tract with or without renal insufficiency.
(3) Refractory or recurrent urinary retention which has failed at least one catheter removal with or without additional α-blocker treatment.
(4) Overflow urinary incontinence.
(5) Bladder calculi secondary to bladder outlet obstruction.

MODERATE/RELATIVE INDICATIONS FOR SURGERY

In a patient where the above-mentioned clear-cut indications do not exist, it is necessary to get an overview of the patient's urinary situation by objective as well as subjective measurements and to provide sufficient information to the patient regarding subjective outcomes and complications to assist in his decision-making process. This consists of the following.

(1) Evaluation of urinary symptoms, for example by the American Urological Association (AUA) symptom index. Most often the patient consults his doctor because of increasing urinary symptoms. Symptom score assessment is

of value in quantifying urinary symptoms and later in assessing the patient's subjective treatment outcome. Surgery is normally indicated only for patients with symptoms scores that are either severe (20–35) or moderate (8–19).[7]

(2) Measurement of the patient's degree of bother due to his urinary symptom, for example by using the BPH Impact Index. In patients with similar symptom scores but with a significant different bother scores, studies have shown that patients' bother is one of the better predictors for the treatment outcome.[8]

(3) Uroflowmetry may be performed to give objective evidence of the degree of obstruction and the curve can to some degree be used to differentiate between different causes of obstruction. In the evaluation of BPH, maximal urinary flow rate (Q_{max}) has been found to be the most beneficial flow variable in relation to BPH.[7,9,10] Studies have given good evidence of a relation between treatment success and preoperative Q_{max}.[11] A limitation of uroflowmetry is that flow can be reduced secondary to bladder dysfunction.

(4) Pressure-flow urodynamic investigation is a controversial issue in the diagnosis of obstructing BPH, but should be performed if patients are significantly bothered by urinary symptoms, and uroflowmetry has been inconclusive in the diagnosis of obstruction or if impaired detrusor contractility is suspected.

(5) Postvoid residual urine measured by ultrasonography or by catheterization has not been found to predict the surgical outcome, but patients with a large postvoid residual urine have higher failure rates under watchful waiting.

TRANSURETHRAL INCISION OF THE PROSTATE TECHNIQUE

PREPARATION AND ANESTHESIA

TUIP can be done under general or regional anesthesia or, in selected patients, under local anesthesia eventually as an outpatient procedure.[4,12–15] The patient is placed in the dorsolithotomy position and prepared in aseptic fashion, as for other transurethral procedures. The urethra is anesthetized with lidocaine jelly. A sensory blockade of the prostate, using a 1% lidocaine solution, can be performed with a transperineal infiltration of the lateral prostate lobes or via a resectoscope injection needle at the positions of the incisions. In most patients, parenteral sedation, for example using intramuscular midazolam, can be employed.

OPERATIVE TECHNIQUE

The urethra is calibrated with bougies for a 24-French resectoscope. A resectoscope with a specially designed knife (most often a Colling's knife is used) with cutting current is used to perform the incision. Bilateral 5- and 7-o'clock incisions are most often used (Figure 28.1). As originally described by Orandi,[3] the incisions are started near the ureteral orifice and carried out to the level of verumontanum. The incisions are gradually deepened down to and through the prostatic capsule and bladder neck. Following this maneuver the bladder neck usually springs

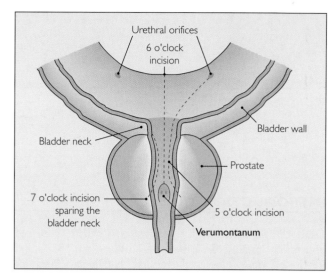

Figure 28.1 Schematic illustration of the dorsal part of the prostate, prostatic urethra, and bladder neck. Incision lines are marked at 5 and 6 o'clock through the bladder neck and prostate. The incision line at 7 o'clock is through the prostate and sparing the bladder neck

apart when the bladder is filled (Figures 28.2 and 28.3). Bleeding is normally easily controlled by coagulation current. However, care must be taken not to cause injury to the rectum, or to cause extravasation following injury to the periprostatic venous plexus. If pathological evaluation is indicated, biopsies can be taken with an endoscopic biopsy needle or loops of tissue can be sampled with resection. After the procedure, a catheter is left in place for about 24 h or until the urine is clear.

Modifications of the original procedure have been developed. Single or bilateral incisions have been performed at a variety of locations. The positions described for a single incision are 5, 6, 7, 8, 10 and 12 o'clock, with 6 o'clock as the most often used. Bilateral incisions, besides the ones described above, have been placed at 4- and 8-, or 3- and 9-o'clock positions. No significant differences have been observed between the different positions or numbers of incisions.

Instruments used for incision include Colling, Orandi and Sachse's knives, and a standard resectoscope. An Nd:YAG laser has also been tried, and has the possible advantage of improved hemostasis.

Complete incision through the bladder neck and the prostatic capsule is often unnecessary in smaller prostates, and sparing of the internal sphincter might reduce the risk for retrograde ejaculation.[16]

Transurethral grooving of the prostate with a standard resectoscope from the urethrovesical junction to verumontanum to the depth of the capsule has shown results similar to TUIP.[17] This has the advantage of reduced risk of extraprostatic injury in larger prostates, where it can be difficult to determine the depth of a simple incision. It also provides tissue for histological examination. The technique of transurethral incision at 4 and 8 o'clock combined with

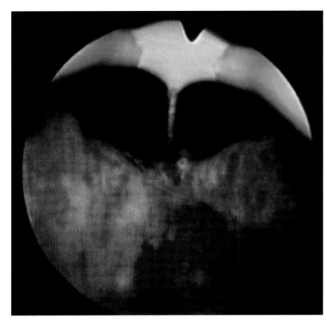

Figure 28.2 Resectoscopic view. Colling's knife in position for incision at 6 o'clock

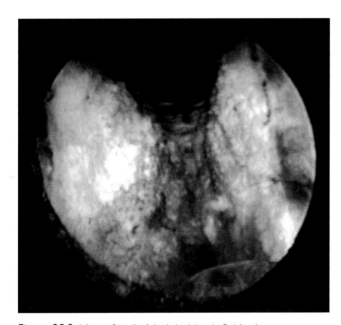

Figure 28.3 View after 6 o'clock incision is finished. Verumontanum at the bottom

posterior resection of the prostate described by Lin has the same advantage.[18] This technique should be particularly preferable in patients with median lobe enlargement, where a normal TUIP is less effective.

COMPARISON OF OPERATIVE FACTORS

Table 28.1 compares TUIP and TURP. TUIP has a reduced procedure time relative to TURP. In randomized studies, the mean time for TUIP has ranged from 15 to 23 min, whereas

for TURP it was found to be between 30 and 59 min. Blood loss, especially if it requires transfusion, is an important issue today because of the increased risk of blood-transmitted diseases after homologous transfusions. Blood loss under TUIP has been about one-third of what was found under TURP, and only two transfusions were required in more than 200 patients evaluated in this respect in randomized studies.[19-24] The TUR-syndrome has never been described after TUIP because of the short operative time and reduced chance of entering the venous plexus. With regard to irrigation fluid, Soonawalla and Pardanani averaged less than 5 L for a TUIP, whereas more than 15 L on average were used for a TURP.[20]

RESULTS

GENERAL

A variety of different measurements have been used to estimate the outcome of TUIP compared with TURP in randomized and matched as well as in non-randomized studies. Different techniques have been used and the maximum size of the prostate has varied from 20 g to more than 50 g, making comparison of different studies difficult. However, when looked at in total, they give a good estimate of the treatment outcome.

SYMPTOMS

In several randomized studies, symptom relief has been measured utilizing symptom scores (Table 28.2). Generally, both operations have been found effective in relieving symptoms. Using a Madsen–Iversen symptom score (with a maximum score of 27) Riehmann et al.[19] found improvement from a mean of 15 preoperatively to a mean of 5 at 3 months postoperatively for TUIP as well as for TURP. Then symptoms increased slightly in both groups over the ensuing 6 years to a level of 10, which was still a statistically significant improvement from the preoperative value.

Patients improved in relation to irritative, as well as obstructive symptoms, and there was no difference in the relief of total irritative and obstructive symptoms between the TURP and TUIP groups.

URODYNAMICS

Peak flow rate has been found to be the most useful urodynamic parameter for evaluating outcome of prostate surgery. TURP, as well as TUIP, has been found effective in improving the peak flow rate in all matched/randomized studies (Table 28.3). However, the improvement has been found to be greater in the TURP groups than in the TUIP groups. Only one randomized study has shown significant difference between TUIP and TURP.[19] This difference was found preoperatively (despite randomization) and at 3–24 months postoperatively, and it continued throughout the entire 72-month period of observation. In one study of 220 patients, mean flow rate has shown more improvement after TUIP than after TURP, in spite of a better peak flow rate in the TURP group.[20] In the same study, the percentage of patients with a high preoperative postvoid residual urine, defined as more than 20% of bladder capacity, was reduced

	n		Prostate size	Incision position (o'clock)	Operating time (min)		Blood loss		Stricture		Retrograde ejaculation (%)		Failure (%)	
	TUIP	TURP	Max	TUIP	TUIP	TURP	TUIP	TURP	TUIP	TURP	TUIP	TURP	TUIP	TURP
Riehmann et al.[19]	61	56	20	6	23	55	54	190	0		35	68	23	16
Dorflinger et al.[22]	29	31	20	7	15	30	10	65	5	1	5	50	27	16
Soonawalla and Pardanam[20]	110	110	30	5 or 7	20	59				3	33	36	6	4
D'Ancona et al.[24]	27	21	30	12					0	2	0	63		
Orandi[21]	66	66	50	5 + 7					2	4	30	41	11	14
Nielsen[23]	24	25	50+	5 or 7	18	45	70	170	0	4			29	20

Table 28.1 Comparison of TUIP and TURP using randomized/matched studies

	Pre-op		Post-op 3 months		1 year		2 years		4 years		6 years	
	TUIP	TURP	TUIP	TURP	TUIP	TURP	TUIP	TURP	TUIP	TURP	TUIP	TURP
Riehmann[19]	15	15	5	5	5.8	5.2	6.5	5	10	9	10	9
Dorflinger[22]	15	16	2.5	1	2	2						

Maximum score = 27

Table 28.2 Comparison of TUIP and TURP using Madsen–Iversen symptom score

	Pre-op		Post-op 3 months		1 year		2 years		4 years		6 years	
	TUIP	TURP	TUIP	TURP	TUIP	TURP	TUIP	TURP	TUIP	TURP	TUIP	TURP
Riehmann et al.[19]	9	11	15	20	16	19	13	19	15	16.5	13	19
Dorflinger et al.[22]	10	8	15	19	15	20	19	20				
Soonawalla and Pardanam[20]	8	8	19	21	19	20						
Orandi[21]	8	8	14	13								
Nielsen[23]	5	5	10	17	9	12						

Table 28.3 Comparison of TUIP and TURP using peak flow rates (mL s^{-1})

from approximately 73% preoperatively to 6% and 7% respectively after TURP and TUIP.

SUBJECTIVE ASSESSMENT OF TREATMENT OUTCOME

Patient-reported subjective outcome has been evaluated in several studies. In one, patients' subjective outcome, weighted on a scale from excellent to worse, was found to be excellent to fair for 95% of the TUIP patients and 90% after TURP.[20] These values were stable over a 2-year observation period. In another trial,[19] using a quality-of-life scale, patients were asked if they were much better to much worse after surgery. The satisfaction rate (better or much better), was about 90% and 85% for TURP and TUIP, respectively, 3 months after surgery. It steadily declined to 55% over a period of 3 years and then stabilized for the TURP group, whereas TUIP declined to the same value over 4 years and then steadily increased to 80% over the next 3 years.

SEXUAL FUNCTION

Evaluation of sexual function has been done in few randomized studies and has been purely subjective, with most attention focused on ejaculation. In all randomized studies comparing TURP and TUIP, retrograde ejaculation has been reported in 35–68% of patients after TURP, while in TUIP patients it was reported to be from 0% to 35%. It has been suggested that one incision results in a smaller risk than two, but in the reviewed studies the highest rate of retrograde ejaculation was found after one incision. Orandi[16] found that a modified technique with sparing of the bladder neck should minimize the problem. However, after performing a single 12-o'clock incision through the bladder neck to verumontanum deepened just to the prostatic surgical capsule, D'Ancona et al.[24] found that all 22 patients still had normal antegrade ejaculation. Dørflinger et al.[22] found that only 1 out of 13 sexually active men had retrograde ejaculation after an incision through the bladder neck and the prostate capsule at a 7-o'clock position.

Generally, new postoperative impotence has been found in a few percent of these few randomized trials where it has been evaluated. Dørflinger et al.[22] found in 43 sexually active men, of whom 19 underwent TUIP, that 15 reported unchanged or better potency and only 1 patient found it to be worse after surgery. Three patients did not report. Of 24 men in the TURP group, 15 reported unchanged or better potency, 4 reported worse potency postoperatively, and 4 were unreported.

TREATMENT FAILURES AND ADDITIONAL SURGERY FOR BLADDER OUTLET OBSTRUCTION

A higher treatment failure has been found after incision than after resection. However, the definition of failure has not been consistent from study to study, and the indication for additional treatment might be a more valid estimation.

In randomized studies, additional surgery after TUIP most often takes place because of continued obstruction due to BPH, and many of the failure patients then undergo a TURP, or some, if due to adhesions between the cut prostate surfaces, a new TUIP.

Bladder neck contractures and strictures are the most common reasons for continued obstruction after TURP. Contractures have especially been a problem after resection of small prostates, whereas they are practically never seen after incision. Riehmann et al.[19] found contracture to occur in 15% of patients after resection of prostates under 20 g, where it was treated with a bladder neck incision or resection.

SUMMARY

TUIP is a cost-effective surgical treatment in relieving urinary outflow obstruction due to BPH in smaller prostates. TUIP is a less-invasive procedure compared with TURP, with shorter operation time, less blood loss, and reduced perioperative morbidity. TUIP is the surgical treatment of choice in high-risk patients where it can be performed under local anesthesia. TUIP is preferable in younger and/or sexually active men because of less risk for retrograde ejaculation. In selected patients, TUIP can be performed as an out-patient procedure under local anesthesia.

REFERENCES

1 Hedlund H, Ek A. Ejaculation and sexual function after endoscopic bladder neck incision. *Br J Urol* 1985; **57**: 164–7.

2 Edwards LE, Bucknall TE, Pittam MR *et al.* Transurethral resection of the prostate and bladder neck incision; a review of 700 cases. *Br J Urol* 1985; **57**: 168–71.

3 Orandi A. Transurethral incision of the prostate. *J Urol* 1973; **110**: 229–31.

4 Keitzer WA, Chervantes L, Demaculang A. Transurethral incision of bladder neck for contracture. *J Urol* 1961; **86**: 242–6.

5 Mebust WK, Holtgreve HC, Cockett ATK, Peters PC. Transurethral prostatectomy: immediate and postoperative complications: a cooperative study of 13 participating institutions evaluating 3885 patients. *J Urol* 1989; **141**: 243–7.

6 Graversen PH, Gasser TC, Larsen EH *et al.* Transurethral incision of the prostate under local anaesthesia in high risk patients: a pilot study. *Scand J Urol* 1987; **106**: 87–90.

7 McConell JD, Barry MJ, Bruskewitz RC *et al. Benign Prostatic Hyperplasia: Diagnosis and Treatment. Clinical Practice Guidelines*, No. 8. AHCPR Publication No. 94–0582. Rockville, MD: Agency for Health Care Policy and Research, Public Health Service, US Department of Health and Human Services 1994.

8 Wasson JH, Reda DJ, Bruskewitz RC *et al.* Comparison of transurethral surgery with watchful waiting for moderate symptoms of benign prostatic hyperplasia. *N Engl J Med* 1995; **332**: 75–9.

9 Jensen KME, Joergensen JB, Mogensen P. Urodynamics in prostatism I. Prognostic value of uroflowmetry. *Scand J Urol Nephrol* 1988; **22**: 109–17.

10 Abrams PH. Prostatism and prostatectomy. The value of urine flow rate measurement in the preoperative assessment for operation. *J Urol* 1977; **117**: 70–1.

11 Jensen KME. Clinical evaluation of routine urodynamic investigation in prostatism. *Neurourol Urodyn* 1989; **8**: 545–78.

12 Orandi A. Urological endoscopic surgery under local anaesthesia: a cost reducing idea. *J Urol* 1984; **132**: 1146–7.

13 Loughlin KR, Yalla SV, Belldegrun A, Bernstein GT. Transurethral incision and resection under local anaesthesia. *Br J Urol* 1987; **60**: 185.

14 Hugosson J, Bergdahl S, Norlen L, Oertengren T. Outpatient transurethral incision of the prostate under local anesthesia: operative results, patient security and cost effectiveness. *Scand J Urol Nephrol* 1993; **27**: 381–5.

15 Birch BRP, Anson KM, Miller RA. Sedoanalgesia in urology: a safe, cost-effective alternative to general anaesthesia. A review of 1020 cases. *Br J Urol* 1990; **66**: 342–50.

16 Orandi A. Transurethral resection versus transurethral incision of the prostate. *Urol Clin North Am* 1990; **17**: 601–12.

17 Simsek F, Türkeri N, Ilker YN, Akdas A. Transurethral grooving of the prostate in the treatment of patients with benign prostatic hyperplasia. An alternative to transurethral incision. *Br J Urol* 1993; **72**: 84–7.

18 Lin C-T. Transurethral incision and posterior resection of prostate for selected patients with benign obstructive prostatic disease. *Urology* 1992; **39**: 508–11.

19 Riehmann M, Knes JM, Heisey D *et al*. Transurethral resection versus incision of the prostate: A randomized, prospective study. *Urology* 1995; **45**: 768–75.

20 Soonawalla PF, Pardanani DS. Transurethral incision versus transurethral resection of the prostate. A subjective and objective analysis. *Br J Urol* 1992; **70**: 174–7.

21 Orandi A. Transurethral incision of prostate compared with transurethral resection of prostate in 132 matching cases. *J Urol* 1987; **138**: 810–15.

22 Dørflinger T, Jensen FS, Krarup T, Walter S. Transurethral prostatectomy compared with incision of the prostate in treatment of prostatism caused by small benign prostate glands. *Scand J Urol Nephrol* 1992; **26**: 333–8.

23 Nielsen HO. Transurethral prostatomy versus transurethral prostatectomy in benign prostatic hypertrophy. A prospective randomized study. *Br J Urol* 1988; **61**: 435–8.

24 D'Ancona CAL, Netto NRJ, Care AM, Ikari O. Internal urethrotomy of the prostatic urethra or transurethral resection in benign prostatic hyperplasia. *J Urol* 1990; **144**: 918–20.

Transurethral Resection of the Prostate for Benign Prostatic Hyperplasia

29

J.P. Blandy

THE INDICATIONS FOR TRANSURETHRAL RESECTION

Half a century ago, when the writer started out in urology, prostatectomy was so dangerous and carried such a high mortality that it was performed only for repeated attacks of acute retention, or when chronic retention of urine became complicated by infection or uremia. As the years went by, and transurethral resection became progressively more safe, the threshold for advising the operation was lowered, and the operation began to be offered on the basis of symptoms, and long before there were any objective signs of damage to the detrusor or the kidneys. At the same time, there came in a new fashion, where, instead of the doctor sitting down and taking a history, the patient was made to complete a questionnaire – from which was calculated a symptom score.[1] Symptom scores are in common use, and it seems to matter little that their results are the same whether the respondent is a man or a woman[2] or that none of them has anything to do with objective urodynamic evidence of out-flow obstruction.[3] It is a pity that symptom scores should now dominate any discussion about the treatment of benign enlargement of the prostate, for this particular Emperor appears to have no clothes on at all.[4]

In fact the purpose of transurethral resection is not so much to relieve symptoms but to prevent the patient suffering unnecessary damage to his bladder or kidneys. Many of the more bothersome symptoms are common to either gender,[2] and reflect changes that are normal with age, including the failure of the antidiuretic hormone to act during the night and the tendency for inferior vena cava to produce more natriuretic hormone.[5] What really matters is that the patient should not be allowed to slide through neglect into renal failure caused by back-pressure, and that his detrusor should not be allowed to become so altered by obstruction that, thanks to the progression of trabeculation, sacculation, and diverticula, it will never work effectively again.

The difficulty here is that most of our current methods of investigation are not able to detect outflow obstruction at a stage before it has begun to do harm. In the current state of knowledge, it is necessary to carry out quite invasive and unpleasant urodynamic tests to detect obstruction to the bladder outflow before there is a significant amount of residual urine or evidence of back-pressure damage to renal function.[6-8] To meet the requirements of the urodynamic purists, every patient must submit to having a suprapubic tube placed in the bladder and another in the rectum, and then pass urine into an unfamiliar flowmeter, in extreme cases in the X-ray room in front of a young lady radiographer. To believe that these measurements are physiological strains ordinary credulity: they are certainly not ordinary practice.

In real life, most urologists compromise, and seek a happy mean – somewhere between operating merely for symptoms that might or might not signify outflow obstruction, and waiting for the bladder to become grossly sacculated and unable to empty itself completely. Today, with the advent of α_1-blockers and 5α-hydrogenase inhibitors, a man with minimal symptoms, a fair flow rate, and negligible residual urine, whatever his imagined symptoms, should probably be left alone, or, if he insists on treatment, be offered one or other of these drugs which appear to confer symptomatic benefit and probably do little harm.[9,10]

INFORMED CONSENT

RETROGRADE EJACULATION
Men who are being advised to undergo transurethral resection of the prostate (TURP) need to understand that afterwards, when they ejaculate, the semen will probably ooze back into the bladder, and be voided in the urine. This does not occur in every case (for it is quite unpredictable) and for most men it is not important. But it must be clearly explained, for when the phenomenon comes as a surprise it generates shame, disappointment, and resentment out of all measure, and litigation is sure to follow.

ERECTILE IMPOTENCE
Even more important, it is necessary to point out that there is also a risk of erectile impotence after transurethral resection. For many years this was thought to be uncommon, but more recent surveys suggest that impotence occurs in about 10% of men and, despite their age, these men mind about it very much.[11,12] Provided the issue has been clearly discussed with the patient, there ought to be no misunderstanding, but when it comes as a surprise, resentment quickly hurries the patient to his lawyer. The prudent surgeon will point out the facts and obtain the patient's written consent.

CONTRAINDICATIONS TO TRANSURETHRAL RESECTION

Most urologists admit that there is an upper limit to the size of prostate that they will treat by transurethral resection, and that for very big glands they get a better result by an open operation, which, in the UK, is invariably the retropubic operation. The difficulty is that few urologists agree how big is too big. This is because the decision has to be subjective. It must be based on the surgeon's awareness of his own limitations, and these are in practice determined not so much by the size of the gland, but by whether the resectoscope lies comfortably in the prostatic urethra, and the landmarks can be safely identified. Sometimes the landmarks are difficult to identify even in a small gland, or the resectoscope is so firmly gripped that it cannot be maneuvered with safety. Sometimes a deformity of the spine or hips prevents insertion of the resectoscope. It is not size alone that determines the method of operation.

PREPARATION

Known urinary infection should always be treated before proceeding to transurethral resection, but whether every patient with sterile urine needs prophylactic antibiotics to cover the operation is still an issue for debate. My practice is to give antibiotics if the patient has been catheterized before the operation, but otherwise to withhold them, hoping that this will avoid breeding multiresistant organisms. With such a policy, however, it is necessary that every member of the urological team is aware of the possibility of sudden unexpected bacteremia and knows what to do.[13,14]

Bleeding can be equally unpredictable, and although it is no longer essential to have blood cross-matched for every transurethral resection, the patient should be grouped and the laboratory should have his serum in case blood is needed in a hurry. When preoperative investigations have shown that the prostate is unusually large, then it is wise to have at least 2 units cross-matched.

POSITION ON THE OPERATING TABLE

Probably dating from the days of perineal lithotomy, patients undergoing cystoscopy or transurethral surgery were customarily put up in a position where the hips and lumbar spine were acutely flexed. In practice, this made it difficult to see the prostate properly during the resection. A position in which the legs are almost horizontal is far more comfortable for surgeon and patient alike and is said to put less strain on the heart (Figure 29.1). Of more practical importance, since many of the men undergoing this operation are elderly and arthritic, the less exaggerated "cystoscopy" position avoids postoperative backache.

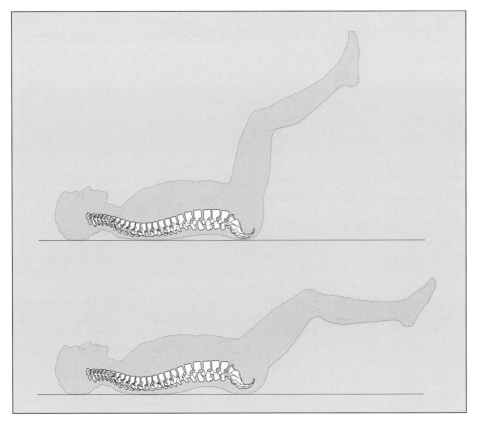

Figure 29.1 Top: incorrect position for transurethral resection – the hips and lumbar spine are needlessly flexed. Bottom: correct position – the legs are almost horizontal

An appropriate drape is applied with a finger-cot to allow the surgeon to monitor the resection with a finger in the rectum. Some kind of sieve to catch the chips of prostate may be incorporated in the drape.

EQUIPMENT

Today there is a wide choice of resectoscopes on the market, all of which have Storz–Hopkins rod lens systems, fiber light, and excellent mechanics. A continuous irrigating sheath may be preferred, or the conventional system: these are matters for personal preference. For teaching purposes, a closed circuit television will be needed.[15,16]

Newcomers to transurethral resection will probably find it easier to use a 0° or direct viewing telescope, instead of the traditional 30° lens, which is a vestige from the days of filament lamp-lit instruments.

There are two other considerations, which are both more important than the type or even the make of endoscopic equipment that are used. First, there must always be enough spare parts: sheaths wear out, loops break, telescopes turn misty. Adequate back-up must be ensured. Secondly, on purchase of endoscopic equipment, it should be ensured that the supplier offers a rapid and reliable repair service, preferably providing a replacement telescope if one goes wrong.

IRRIGATING FLUID
Today there is no question but that a non-electrolytic irrigating fluid should be used, which will not cause hemolysis when it enters the bloodstream.[17–19] There is little to choose between 2.5% glucose, sorbitol–mannitol, or glycine solutions. The really important thing is the fluid must be non-hemolytic and perfectly sterile.

DIATHERMY
Thanks to the development of solid-state circuitry, the diathermy equipment of today is light-years away from the quaint apparatus with which the pioneers of transurethral resection had to contend. Nevertheless, there are two guiding principles which do not change, even if one need not understand the arcane mysteries of electronics.

(1) There must be more than one diathermy machine in the hospital: even the best of them sometimes go wrong, and a resection should never be started without there being a spare one to call upon.

(2) The surgeon must check the diathermy system himself in every case. A diathermy burn is a terrible complication, which can nearly always be avoided by making sure (a) that the earth pad is correctly sited, where it can be seen and adjusted, i.e. *not* under the patient's sacrum; (b) that there is no contact between the patient and any metal object through which a diathermy current might find its way to earth.

AVOIDING DEEP VENOUS THROMBOSIS
The legs should rest on suitable supports, which avoid compression of the calf. Supportive stockings probably help to avoid thrombosis as do pneumatic boots that intermittently squeeze the feet: neither can do any harm. Whether every patient should be given heparin is a different issue: many surgeons feel that the risk of bleeding is bad enough during transurethral resection without making it worse. On the other hand, when there is some important indication for anticoagulants, it has been my experience that one can control the bleeding perfectly well even when subcutaneous heparin has been given, although unhappy experiences with patients on small daily doses of aspirin, makes me advise them to leave off this medication for a week prior to surgery.[20,21]

ANESTHESIA
My advice over many years to my younger colleagues has been to take care in choosing the anesthetist they wish to work with, but not to tell him how to do his job. Surgeons share a widespread misconception that spinal or epidural anesthesia is more safe in the elderly man. Anesthetists know that this is not so. The anesthetist can get more oxygen into the patient's brain (which is the overriding safety factor) with an inhalation technique. All anesthetic techniques, if expertly performed, can give good operating conditions: it is up to the surgeon to make clear what he needs.

(1) There should be no undue congestion of the pelvic veins: CO_2 retention can be a potent cause of this, and a skilled anesthetist can take appropriate steps even in the most blue-nosed old smoker.

(2) The patient must not cough – or at least, if he is going to cough, you need warning of it, or the resectoscope may be jerked through the capsule.

(3) He must not develop an erection. Almost the single most dangerous intraoperative complication is for the patient to develop an erection. It can occur insidiously. First the bleeding increases. Next the surgeon becomes aware that the resectoscope is being gripped in the penis, which has become turgid. The third and most dangerous stage is when the elongated penis pushes the resectoscope down the urethra. By now bleeding has already made the vision worse, and it is all too easy to mistake the sphincter for the prostate, and with one misguided stroke of the resectoscope loop to render the patient permanently incontinent (Figure 29.2).[22]

TECHNIQUE OF TRANSURETHRAL RESECTION

Transurethral resection has to be learned in the operating room, and the following description is intended only to highlight some of the points which may be of help to others.

PRELIMINARY CYSTOURETHROSCOPY
Begin the operation by passing a cystoscope along the urethra using the 0° telescope under vision. Note any narrow parts in the urethra for which a preliminary internal urethrotomy may be required. Identify the external sphincter, the verumontanum, and the top of the middle lobe, which will give you a good idea of the size of the prostate. Then

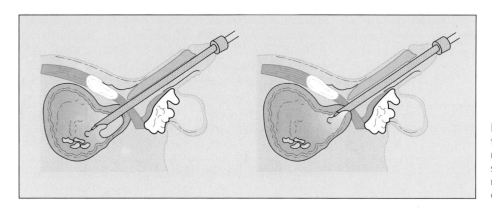

Figure 29.2 An erection elongates the penis and may push the resectoscope out past the sphincter: it is probably the single most dangerous intraoperative complication

exchange the 0° telescope for the 70° and carry out a careful cystoscopy, looking for unexpected tumors, stones, and diverticula. If you find a diverticulum make sure you have looked all round inside it, especially if it has a swollen or inflamed mouth – a sinister sign of cancer inside. Identify the ureteric orifices. Empty the bladder, and then carry out a rectal examination.

INTERNAL URETHROTOMY

To prevent the formation of urethral stricture many urologists slit the urethra on every occasion using the blind urethrotome of Otis or the visual one of Sachse. It is not necessary in every case. If a 24 F sheath is used, and urethrotomy is performed only if it is gripped by the urethra, urethrotomy will be needed in only 10% of cases.

PRELIMINARY DIATHERMY OF PROSTATIC ARTERIES

The main vessels of the prostate enter at 10, 2, 5, and 7 o'clock (Figure 29.3). When the prostate is bulky, it is helpful to begin by coagulating these vessels before beginning the resection. Apply the roller ball and coagulation current

to the four quadrants until the prostatic tissue is whitened. This prevents much of the bleeding that would otherwise be encountered during the rest of the resection.

FIRST STEP: FINDING THE LANDMARKS

The verumontanum is the inferior landmark and the key to safety in transurethral resection of the prostate: it should be in your mind's eye at every stage of the operation, and you should not hesitate to return to it again and again to verify your position (Figure 29.4).

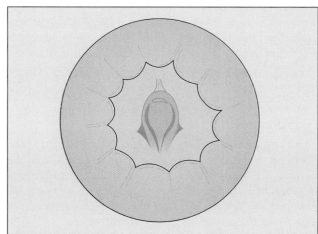

Figure 29.4 The inferior landmark – the verumontanum is the key to safety in prostatectomy

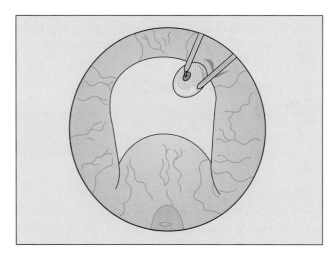

Figure 29.3 Preliminary coagulation of the sites of entry of the main arteries of the prostate makes for a relatively bloodless operation

The superior landmark is the circular muscle of the bladder, which is hidden under the middle lobe. As middle lobes vary so much, one needs to resect more or less tissue to uncover these fibers (Figure 29.5). When the middle lobe is small, it takes only one or two chips to reveal the bladder neck fibers (Figure 29.6). With a bulky middle lobe, on the other hand, it may take some time to uncover these fibers, during which it is necessary to keep the bites of the resectoscope loop regular and even (Figure 29.7) or else the middle lobe will be divided into two lumps, which make the rest of the operation very confusing (Figure 29.8).

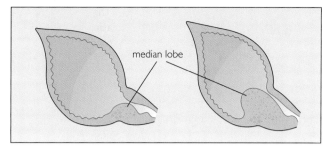

Figure 29.5 The upper landmark – the transverse fibers of the bladder neck – is hidden under the adenoma of the middle lobe

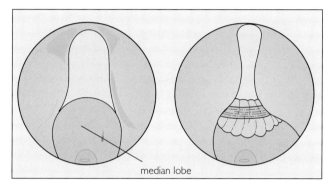

Figure 29.6 When the middle lobe is small it only takes one or two chips to reveal the bladder neck fibers

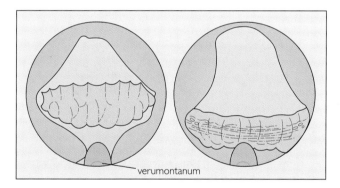

Figure 29.7 When the middle lobe is big it must all be removed to display the bladder neck fibers. The dome of the middle lobe must be taken away evenly

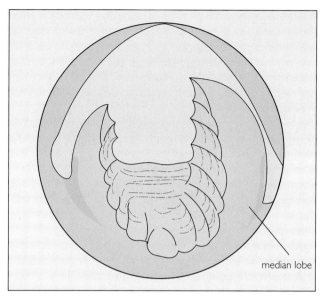

Figure 29.8 If by mistake the middle lobe is bisected two very awkward lumps are formed which can be needlessly confusing

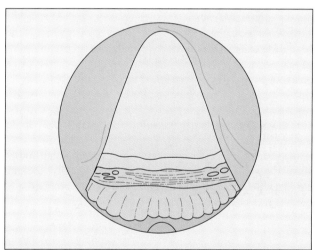

Figure 29.9 The rest of the middle lobe is taken away down to within a few millimeters of the verumontanum, and out to the edge of each lateral lobe

When the middle lobe is quite large, the resection should be continued with a second series of evenly placed bites of the loop within a few millimeters of the verumontanum, and on either side laterally to the junction of middle and lateral lobes (Figure 29.9). When this is done cleanly and neatly, there is a clear edge of bladder neck fibers stretching from one lateral lobe to the other. A few large vessels are constantly present in the 7 o'clock and 5 o'clock corners and, although the preliminary coagulation will have controlled most of these, it is worth spending a few moments making sure that every one has been sealed off, because when you return to it later in the operation a thin layer of blood clot will often conceal the openings of the vessels.

At this stage, the upper limit of your resection has been established, and sometimes one finds that there is really no more prostate to be removed – the bulk having been made up by the middle lobe.

RESECTING THE LEFT LATERAL LOBE
Now rotate the resectoscope round so that the anterior midline comes into view. There is almost no adenoma in the midline at 12 o'clock, so that the loop should be directed upwards and laterally at about 1 o'clock to begin

to find the edge of the left lateral lobe and separate it from the "capsule" (Figure 29.10). As you make your trench, if the preliminary coagulation has sealed the anterior prostatic arteries, there will be very little bleeding, but time spent controlling any that occurs is time well spent, and will result in the rest of the resection of the lateral lobe being almost bloodless.

Once the 1 o'clock trench has been carried round to about 3 o'clock, the lateral lobe begins to fall backwards and medially into the gap formerly occupied by the middle lobe. It is now possible to cut it away in a series of bites, which keeps the top more or less flat (Figure 29.11). It is a mistake to hollow out the lateral lobe, for then a tiresome flap falls down to hide the verumontanum and confuse everything (Figure 29.12).

Once the main part of the lateral lobe has been cut away, it is helpful to work with one finger in the rectum to lift the lateral lobe upwards and inwards (Figure 29.13).

If you have been fortunate with your preliminary coagulation, the resection of the lateral lobe will be almost bloodless, but in any event, once you have resected one lateral lobe completely, i.e. down to the "capsule", take your time to go over the whole of the interior surface of the exposed "capsule" to make sure that all the bleeding has been stopped.

THE CAPSULE

In TURP, surgeons have come to refer to a certain endoscopic appearance as "the capsule," i.e. where criss-cross bands of fibrous tissue, separated by pale gray areas, have a different appearance from that of the adenoma, which resembles white bread (Figure 29.14). In fact, Page showed very clearly[23] that when you see this "capsule" you are looking at a very thin layer made up partly of compressed adenoma, and partly of fibrous tissue, the whole being thinner than the resectoscope loop. You are actually looking through this tissue at the fat surrounding the prostate, i.e.

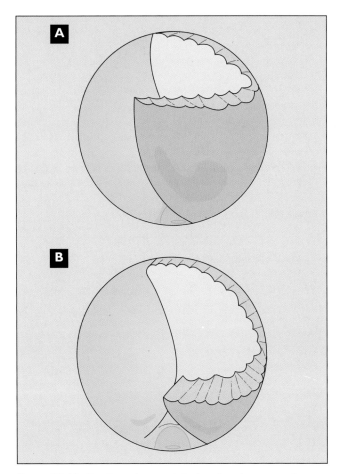

Figure 29.11 Continue the trench in the plane between adenoma and capsule (A): this allows the lateral lobe to fall back (B). Keep the resection flat and even

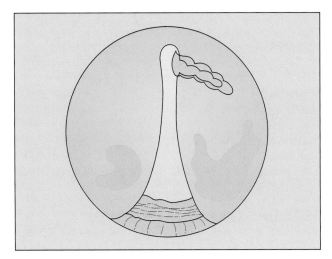

Figure 29.10 Resecting the left lateral lobe: begin by making a trench at 1 o'clock

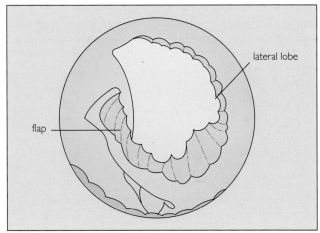

Figure 29.12 Do not hollow-out the lateral lobe, otherwise a flap will fall down and hide the verumontanum

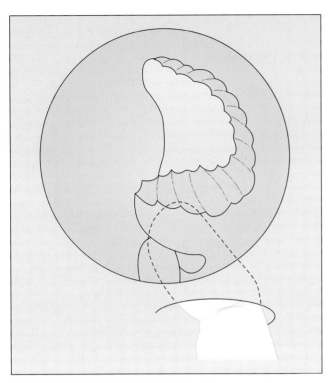

Figure 29.13 Once the main mass of the lateral lobe has been removed, a finger in the rectum to lift the rest of it towards the lumen makes the resection easier

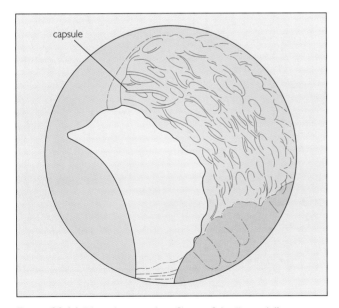

Figure 29.14 The criss-cross lacy fibers of the "capsule" represent a very thin layer of tissue

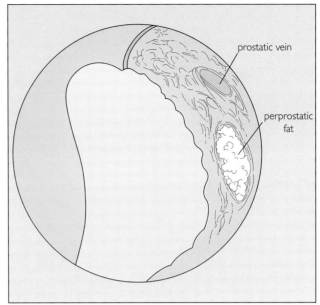

Figure 29.15 A black hole in the "capsule" is probably the inside of a prostatic vein: if you can see fat you are outside it

HEMOSTASIS

Throughout the resection, small bleeding vessels are sealed with the loop using the coagulating current. When there is a larger vessel, and when you are doing your final round of hemostasis after removing the lateral lobe, it is more efficient to use the roller ball electrode, taking great care not to use it in the vicinity of the verumontanum for fear of injuring the sphincter, which lies just below it.

A number of crafty tricks help with achieving hemostasis.

(1) When a bleeding artery is pumping straight at you, confusing you with a red mist, advance the resectoscope above the vessel, angulate the beak against the wall of the prostate, and then creep up on the bleeder from behind as you slowly withdraw the resectoscope (Figure 29.16).

(2) At the end of the resection, when you are satisfied that you have controlled all the spurting arteries, empty the bladder and go all over the area again while, with one finger, restricting the inflow of irrigant: this will allow you to detect bleeding from small veins and allow them to be coagulated (Figure 29.17).

(3) Sometimes you can be confused by what seems to be furious bleeding. Search as you may, you cannot find the artery. This may be "bounce bleeding" from the opposite side of the cavity (Figure 29.18), and it is worth looking at the diametrically opposite wall for the source.

THE SECOND LATERAL LOBE

When all the bleeding has been controlled from the first lateral lobe, turn your resectoscope again to the anterior midline at 12 o'clock. You will probably find that it has shifted over to the untouched side. Start a second trench at 10

you have almost gone too far. It is small wonder then that when you examine the interior of the capsule after you have removed the lateral lobe, you often see glistening globules of fat, and occasionally the lumen of a vein (Figure 29.15).

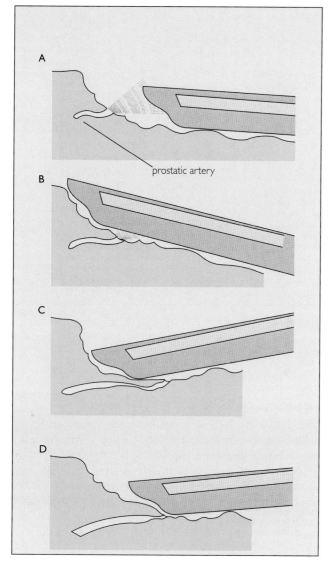

Figure 29.16 When an artery is pumping straight at you (A), advance the resectoscope beyond it (B), angulate it to squeeze the vessel (C), and then slowly remove it to show where the artery is situated (D)

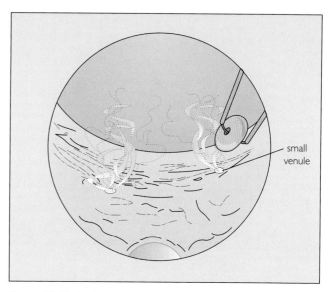

Figure 29.17 At the end of the resection, empty the bladder and cut down the flow of irrigant to show the little puffs of blood coming from small veins

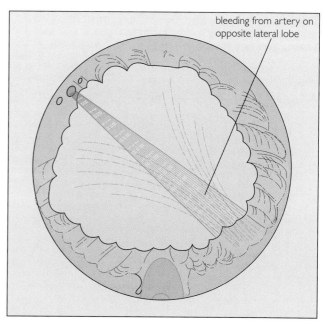

Figure 29.18 Bounce bleeding: if in doubt look at the opposite wall of the cavity

o'clock (Figure 29.19) and proceed exactly as with the first side: free the lateral lobe, allow it to drop back, and cut it away evenly with an even series of strokes that keep the ridges and furrows more or less level (Figure 29.20). Finish by going all over the inner surface of the capsule to stop the bleeding.

THIRD STAGE: TIDYING UP
When the second lateral lobe is finished, evacuate all the chips, go over the inner surface of the capsule once again to control residual bleeding, and then withdraw the resectoscope just downstream of the verumontanum. Now you will often see a tiny shoulder of apical tissue on either side of the verumontanum (Figure 29.21). This can safely be left alone: it will not cause obstruction, and excessive zeal to resect

this little remaining gram or two of adenoma may damage the sphincter.

Sometimes the residual shoulder of apical adenoma is larger, and obviously projecting into the lumen. In such a case you may see Nesbit's "white line" at the lower end. Lift up the apex with a finger in the rectum, and trim away the remaining tissue down to the white line: a cautious back cut is permissible here (Figure 29.22). One last look round to check hemostasis, one last evacuation of remaining chips of prostate, and the operation is done.

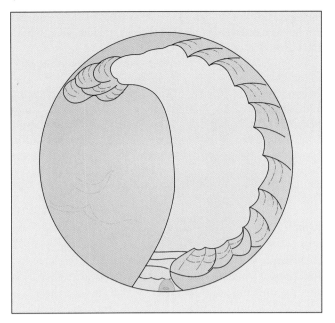

Figure 29.19 Starting to resect the right lateral lobe: the "midline" has shifted over

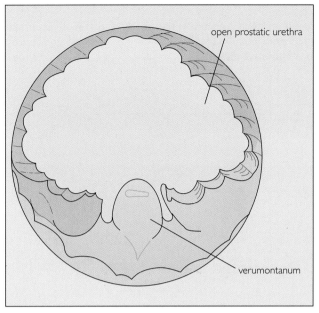

Figure 29.21 The view at the end of the operation from just below the verumontanum. Small lumps of apical tissue cause no trouble, but removing them might

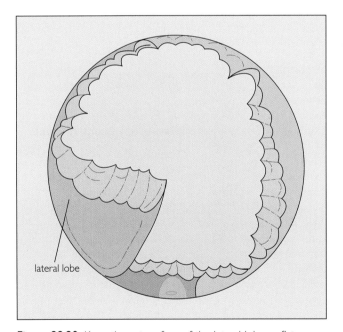

Figure 29.20 Keep the cut surface of the lateral lobe as flat as possible: avoid hollowing it

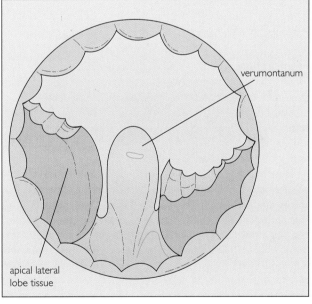

Figure 29.22 A large lump of apical tissue might cause obstruction. Note Nesbit's white line – never resect below this. A finger in the rectum helps to offer up the apical adenoma to the loop

CATHETER

Several systems of postoperative irrigation are in use. Many urologists rely on the patient's own diuresis to keep the urine clear of clots, encouraging this with intravenous fluids and frusemide. Others, who use a suprapubic cannula for continuous flow resection, leave a catheter in the suprapubic track. My preference is to use a 22 French 3-way latex Foley catheter. The irrigation is started on the table, finishing off the glycine used for the resection, and thereafter continued with physiological saline. If the irrigant is not crystal clear at the end of the operation, inject 40 mL of water into the balloon, and apply traction to compress the remaining small veins around the bladder neck (Figure

29.23). The irrigation can usually be slowed down after about an hour, depending on the color of the effluent, and stopped after 6–12 h. The catheter is removed on the 2nd postoperative day.

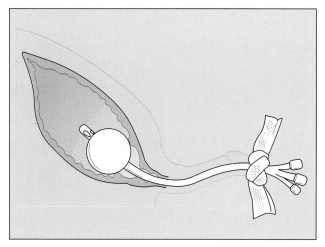

Figure 29.23 Traction on the balloon squeezes the veins at the neck of the bladder

COMPLICATIONS DURING THE OPERATION

Hemorrhage

Hemorrhage on the table is the most important complication, and cannot always be avoided. It can usually be controlled by careful application of the roller ball diathermy, but when it is uncontrollable, it may be necessary to evacuate the clot, stop the operation, insert a Foley catheter, and apply traction, as described above.

Much more rarely, the bleeding, usually from a large atheromatous prostatic artery, is so furious that one can see nothing through the sea of blood, and traction with the catheter fails to stop it. Under these circumstances, the only mistake is to dither and delay. Open the retropubic space: incise the capsule, enucleate any remaining adenoma, suture ligate the bleeding vessels and, if necessary, insert a pack. It is better to explain an unexpected abdominal incision to the patient, than an avoidable death to his widow.

Perforation

Modern understanding of the anatomical nature of the transurethral resectionist's "capsule"[23] makes it obvious that there must be a few small perforations of the "capsule" in every operation, and it is equally obvious that they usually cause no harm. However, when a large vein is laid open, or a large expanse of fat has been exposed, then the operation should be terminated, and the bleeding controlled, if necessary by traction on the catheter. Such perforations are usually recognized after completing the resection of one lateral

lobe, and it is gratifying to know that most of these patients are relieved of their symptoms and never come back to have the other lobe removed.

Erection

As explained above, this is a very dangerous complication and should be dealt with the moment it is noticed. Complaining to the anesthetist and changing the anesthetic agent are equally futile. Inject the penis with Aramine or 0.001% epinephrine, while asking the anesthetist to monitor the blood pressure. The erection will subside immediately, and the operation can then proceed.[22] If these measures fail, stop the operation.

POSTOPERATIVE COMPLICATIONS

Reactionary Hemorrhage

Reactionary bleeding may occur in the recovery room. Usually the nursing staff will report that the catheter has become blocked with clot. Sucking out the clot and changing the catheter are usually the only necessary measures, but from time to time they do not work, and the catheter quickly blocks again. In these cases, the sooner the patient is returned to the theater and anesthetized again the better. Remove the catheter. Pass the resectoscope. Wash out all the clots with an Ellik evacuator and then search carefully for the offending vessel. Sometimes merely evacuating the clot is enough to stop the bleeding.

Secondary Hemorrhage

This occurs 7–10 days after the operation. It is more common when there is infection, but may occur even when the urine is sterile. Patients should be warned that there may be a little bleeding, and understand if you explain this in terms of the bleeding that is familiar when a scab comes away from a wound in the skin. Occasionally, secondary hemorrhage leads to clot retention, when it may be necessary to catheterize the patient and wash out the bladder.

The Transurethral Resection Syndrome

Intravasation of irrigating fluid may give rise to dilutional hyponatremia: the altered membrane potential of nerves and muscles gives rise to malfunction of muscles and nerves producing bradycardia and other more bizarre signs and symptoms, while intracellular edema causes fits and coma.

A number of factors may contribute to the transurethral resection (TUR) syndrome: opening periprostatic veins, allowing pressure to build up in the bladder, an excess of intravenous fluids, and inappropriate secretion of the antidiuretic hormone, which occurs in as many as 25% of these elderly patients.[24,25] Its onset is very variable: usually there is loss of consciousness, sometimes fits or hemiparesis suggest a cerebrovascular accident, and occasionally there is transient blindness. Most men recover spontaneously thanks to a good diuresis, but when there are uncontrollable fits it may be safer to give the patient 50 mL of 29.5% (hypertonic) saline slowly, through a central venous catheter.[26,27]

The TUR syndrome is uncommon, and not always associated with prolonged resection of very large glands. There are a number of preventive measures.

(1) A weighing machine may be attached to the operating table, which will give warning of loss of the irrigating fluid into the systemic circulation. In practice, so many gadgets and monitors are attached to the patient during the operation that it is difficult to get a true measurement of the weight of the patient alone.

(2) Another system is even more elegant: a minute amount of alcohol is added to the irrigating fluid, and the anesthetist regularly samples the expired air with a Breathalyzer.[28,29]

(3) The Iglesias continuous irrigating resectoscope was designed to prevent an excessive rise of pressure within the bladder:[30] others prefer to perform transurethral resection with a suprapubic cannula *in situ* to allow a continuous escape of the irrigant.

In the early days of transurethral resection, when distilled water was used as the irrigating fluid, hemodilution was sometimes accompanied by hemolysis. The liberated hemoglobin was filtered into the glomeruli, concentrated in the tubules, and there allowed to block them, with resulting uremia which, in the days before hemodialysis, was usually fatal.

Incontinence

Three types of incontinence are seen after transurethral resection.[31]

Genuine Stress Incontinence

Genuine stress incontinence, lasting for a few weeks, is not uncommon after an otherwise successful transurethral resection. The patient experiences a little loss of urine when he coughs or strains, possibly because the supramembranous intrinsic part of the external sphincter complex has become slack over the years. This improves spontaneously, and the improvement may be hastened by perineal floor exercises. Only a complete urodynamic investigation can distinguish this from detrusor instability.

Detrusor Instability

If detrusor instability has been detected prior to the operation by the presence of inappropriate and involuntary detrusor contractions during urodynamic studies, then the patient should be warned that after the operation coughing or straining may precipitate a detrusor contraction with resulting loss of urine. Since most of these examples of detrusor instability are secondary to outflow obstruction, the condition usually improves rapidly without treatment. Only urodynamic studies can distinguish this from the genuine stress incontinence referred to above and, as both types of incontinence are self-limiting, it is seldom necessary to put patients through these investigations.

Damaged Sphincter

Endoscopy shows a sphincter that does not close completely or has a segment missing from its ring (Figure

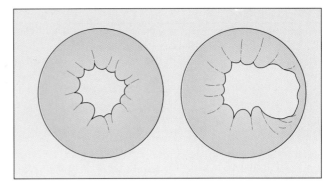

Figure 29.24 The urologists nightmare: a segment has been cut out of the supramembranous intrinsic sphincter

29.24). Urodynamic investigations will show a stable detrusor and a urethral pressure profile with a greatly impaired urethral closing pressure. This does not improve spontaneously. The patient is condemned to use either an external compression device such as a Cunningham clamp, wear a urinal, or undergo the implantation of a Brantley–Scott type of artificial sphincter.[32]

Unhappy Outcomes after Transurethral Resection

When careful follow-up studies are carried out on large numbers of patients who have undergone transurethral resection, there is a surprising proportion who are not happy with the result – somewhere between 25 and 35%.[33,34] No doubt some of these inferior results arise from poor case selection, especially when the operation has been advised for "irritative" symptoms, e.g. frequency and nocturia, for which there are many causes other than prostatic outflow obstruction. Others are the obvious consequences of complications such as a urethral stricture, retrograde ejaculation, or impotence, which were either not expected or not explained. The plain fact is that the operation is still far from perfect.

The Need for a Repeat Transurethral Resection

In the pioneering days of transurethral resection, it was often said that the operation was in some way "incomplete," and that if only an open enucleation had been done the patient would not have come back. Today it is accepted that the residual prostatic tissue in the compressed periphery of the prostate can give rise to new formation of benign hypertrophy and occasionally to new obstruction. The incidence is variously estimated to be from 3 to 13%.[35,36]

Long-term Aftermath of Cardiac Disease

In 1989 a retrospective study of men who had undergone transurethral resection in three different countries and were then followed up, suggested that there was an unexpectedly high incidence of cardiac disease during the years after the operation.[37,38] There was a flurry in the dovecotes, and the findings were hotly disputed.[39–41] However, the suspicion had been raised, and the argument will, no doubt, long continue.

EPILOGUE

To those who can remember the crude, old-fashioned, transvesical operations with so much danger and discomfort for the patient, transurethral resection came as nothing short of a benign revolution. Perhaps today it may be being done too often. Undoubtedly, it is still not perfect. But no operation can be expected to succeed if it is done badly, or for the wrong reasons, and, of all urological procedures, there is no other which is so well worth doing well.

REFERENCES

1 Ko DSC, Fenster HN, Chambers K et al. The correlation of multichannel urodynamic pressure-flow studies and American Urological Association symptom index in the evaluation of benign prostatic hyperplasia. J Urol 1995; 154: 396–8.

2 Lepor H, Machi G. Comparison of AUA symptom index in unselected males and females between 55 and 79 years of age. Urology 1993; 42: 36–41.

3 Hines JEW. Symptom indices in bladder outlet obstruction. Br J Urol 1966; 77: 494–501.

4 Abrams P. Managing lower urinary tract symptoms in older men. Br Med J 1995; 310: 1113–7.

5 Kikuchi Y. Participation of atrial natriuretic peptide (hANP) levels and arginine vasopressin (AVP) in aged persons with nocturia. JPH J Urol 1995; 86: 165–9.

6 McGuire EJ. The role of urodynamic investigation in assessment of benign prostatic hypertrophy. J Urol 1992; 148: 1133–6.

7 Hofner K, Jonas U. Urodynamics in benign prostatic hyperplasia. Curr Opin Urol 1996; 6: 184–8.

8 Rollema H. Clinical significance of symptoms, signs, and urodynamic parameters in benign prostatic hypertrophy. In: Krane RJ, Siroky MB, Fitzpatrick JM (eds) Clinical Urology. Philadelphia: JB Lippincott, 1994: 847–79.

9 Caine M, Perlberg S, Meretyk S. A placebo-controlled double blind study of the effect of phenoxybenzamine in benign prostatic obstruction. Br J Urol 1978; 50: 551–4.

10 Andersen JT, Ekman P, Wolf H et al. Can Finasteride reverse the progress of benign prostatic hyperplasia? A two year placebo-controlled study. Urology 1995; 46: 631–7.

11 Hanbury DC, Sethia KK. Erectile function following transurethral prostatectomy. Br J Urol 1995; 75: 12–13.

12 Thorpe AC, Cleary R, Coles J et al. Written consent about sexual function in men undergoing transurethral prostatectomy. Br J Urol 1994; 74: 479–84.

13 Hall JC, Christiansen KJ, England P et al. Antibiotic prophylaxis for patients undergoing transurethral resection of the prostate. Urology 1996; 47: 852–6.

14 Hargreave TB, Botto H, Rikken GH et al. European collaborative study of antibiotic prophylaxis for transurethral resection of the prostate. Eur Urol 1993; 23: 437–43.

15 O'Boyle PJ. Video-endoscopy: the remote operating technique. Br J Urol 1990; 65: 557–9.

16 Notley RG. Closed circuit television for the urologist. In: Blandy JP, Notley RG (eds) Transurethral Resection, 4th edn. Oxford: Isis Medical Media 1998.

17 Creevy CD. Hemolytic reactions during transurethral prostatic resection. J Urol 1947; 58: 125–31.

18 Bunge RC, Barker AP. Hemolysis during transurethral prostatic resection. J Urol 1948; 60: 122–23.

19 Beirne GJ, Madsen PO, Burns RO. Serum electrolyte and osmolarity changes following transurethral resection of the prostate. J Urol 1954; 93: 83–6.

20 Hedlund PO. Post-operative venous thrombosis in benign prostatic disease: a study of 316 patients using the I¹²⁵ fibrinogen uptake test. Scand J Urol Nephrol 1976; Suppl 27.

21 Wilson RG, Smith D, Paton G et al. Prophylactic subcutaneous heparin does not increase operative blood loss in transurethral resection of the prostate. Br J Urol 1988; 62: 246–8.

22 McNicholas TA, Thomson K, Rogers HS, Blandy JP. Pharmacological management of erections during transurethral surgery. Br J Urol 1989; 64: 435–7.

23 Page BH. The pathological anatomy of digital enucleation for benign prostatic hyperplasia and its application to endoscopic resection. Br J Urol 1980; 52: 111–26.

24 Goel CM, Badenoch DF, Fowler CG et al. Transurethral Resection Syndrome: a prospective study. Eur Urol 1992; 21: 15–17.

25 Norris HT, Aasheim GM, Sherrard DJ, Tremann JA. Symptomatology, pathophysiology and treatment of the transurethral resection of the prostate syndrome. Br J Urol 1973; 45: 420–7.

26 Worthley LIG, Thomas PD. Treatment of hyponatraemic seizures with intravenous 29.2% saline. Br Med J 1986; 292: 168–70.

27 Arieff AI. Management of hyponatraemia. Br Med J 1993; 307: 305–8.

28 Ekengren J, Hahn RG. Continuous versus intermittent flow irrigation in transurethral resection of the prostate. Urology 1994; 43: 328–32.

29 Hahn RG, Stalberg HP, Gustafsson SA. Intravenous infusion of irrigating fluids containing glycine or mannitol with or without ethanol. J Urol 1989; 142: 1102–5.

30 Iglesias JJ, Stams UK. How to prevent the TUR syndrome. Urologe 1975; 14: 287–98.

31 Krane RJ, Fitzpatrick JM. Postprostatectomy incontinence. In: Fitzpatrick JM, Krane RJ (eds) The Prostate. London: Churchill Livingstone 1989; 191–5.

32 Scott FB. The artificial sphincter in the management of incontinence in the male. In: Kaufman JJ, Raz S (eds) Urologic Clinics of North America, Symposium on Urinary Incontinence. Philadelphia, WB Saunders 1978; 375–91.

33 Thorpe AC, Cleary R, Coles J et al. Deaths and complications following prostatectomy in 1400 men in the Northern Region of England. Br J Urol 1994; 74: 559–65.

34 Doll HA, Black NA, McPherson K et al. Differences in outcome of transurethral resection of the prostate for benign prostatic hypertrophy between three diagnostic categories. Br J Urol 1993; 72: 322–3.

35 Chilton CP, Morgan RJ, England HR et al. A critical evaluation of the results of transurethral resection of the prostate. Br J Urol 1978; 50: 542–6.

36 Neal DE. Prostatectomy – an open or closed case. Br J Urol 1990; 66: 449–54.

37 Roos NP, Wennberg J, Malenka DJ et al. Mortality and reoperation after open and transurethral resection of the prostate for benign prostatic hyperplasia. N Engl J Med 1989; 320(17): 1120–4.

38 Malenka DJ, Roos N, Fisher ES et al. Further study of the increased mortality following transurethral prostatectomy: a chart-based analysis. J Urol 1990; 144: 224–7.

39 Mebust WK, Holtgrewe HL, Cockett ATK et al. Transurethral prostatectomy: immediate and post-operative complications. A

cooperative study of 13 participating institutions evaluating 3885 patients. *J Urol* 1989; **141**: 243–7.

40 Jenkins BJ, Sharma P, Badenoch DF *et al*. Ethics, logistics and a trial of transurethral versus open prostatectomy. *Br J Urol* 1992; **69**: 372–4.

41 Hargreave TB, Heynes CF, Kendrick SW *et al*. Mortality after transurethral and open prostatectomy in Scotland. *Br J Urol* 1996; **77**: 547–53.

Open Prostatectomy in Benign Prostatic Hypertrophy

30

C. Cascione, M. Patel, and P. Narayan

INTRODUCTION

There are no other surgical procedures that better exemplify the daring and ingenuity of early physicians beyond those performed by pioneering urologic surgeons. Eugene Fuller[1] of New York is credited with reporting the first successful series of six patients who underwent complete suprapubic prostatic enucleation in 1895. In the early 1900s, Sir Peter Freyer of London refined the procedure and popularized it with his report on a series of 1600 cases.[2,3] Remarkably only a 5% mortality rate was reported. The proportion of this achievement is even more striking when one considers the hazards of operating without an aseptic environment, in the absence of modern instrumentation, anesthetics, and antimicrobial medications. This procedure was performed by blind enucleation through a 2–3-in. suprapubic midline incision, usually within 15 min.

A low vertical (vesical) incision with visualization of the bladder neck and placement of hemostatic sutures was reported by O'Conor and Nanninga in 1963 and 1972.[4,5,6,7] They reported no mortalities in a series of more than 300 patients in 1982. Transcapsular (retropubic) prostatectomy was first reported by Von Stochum in 1909, but gained popularity after a report of 20 successful procedures performed by Terrence Millin in 1945.[8]

Simple prostatectomy (open enucleation) is an efficient, highly effective, and safe surgical treatment for benign obstructive prostatic disease. Successful surgical outcomes remain reliant on proper patient selection and adherence to proven surgical principles.

The technical complexities of this procedure have diminished proportionately in relation to the surgical skills, which the majority of urologists have mastered through radical prostatectomy. The frequency of this procedure decreased with the advent of improved endoscopic instrumentation, pharmacologic therapy, minimally invasive procedures, together with early detection and treatment of incipient benign obstructive prostatic disease. Pharmacologic therapy, specifically, selective α-1A-adrenergic blockade, could conceivably portend an increase in the need for open prostatic surgery, as continued prostatic growth may overwhelm the efficacy of this therapy and exceed the limits of safe endoscopic treatment.

PATIENT ASSESSMENT

Indications for an open prostatectomy are grouped into two categories, as absolute and relative. In the latter category, the patient's treatment preference and his financial status (such as medical insurance), and previously failed pharmacologic therapy are the indications. As for the compelling indications, prostatic adenomatous growth of greater than 60 g, associated intravesical disorders (such as massive vesical calculus, functionally significant bladder diverticula, etc.), and ankylosis of the hips are the indications that necessitate the use of open prostatectomy for benign prostatic hyperplasia (BPH).

Many of these patients are elderly, and often present with some chronic system disease; evaluation of these patients must be carefully done, remembering that the open prostatectomy is usually an elective procedure. This includes a detailed patient history and physical examination. A complete medical and urological history should be obtained. A standard medical history and review of the systems is necessary with specific references made to current medication usage. Past history of diabetes, polyuric states and neurologic illnesses as well as of surgery in the pelvis or urogenital system is mandated. The urologic history should include voiding function characterizations and AUA symptom score. In addition, any history of urinary tract infections, hematuria, urolithiasis, and sexual dysfunction should be obtained.

During physical exam, the abdominal, pelvic, inguinal, and genital regions should be focussed; a thorough examination of these areas is essential in obtaining the overall clinical picture. In addition, an evaluation of the musculoskeletal system is required, with specific references made to the range of hip motion and the presence of any spinal deformities (lordosis, kyphosis, scoliosis, herniations, etc.). To conclude, a digital rectal exam (DRE) must be performed to evaluate the strength of the anal sphincter tone and to examine the contour of the posterior surface of the prostate gland. An elevation in serum prostatic specific antigen requires transrectal ultrasonography (TRUS) with possible biopsy. A guaiac test is included as part of the DRE to rule out presence of microscopic/occult blood in the rectum; this test may also unmask any hidden coagulopathies, which would be a contraindication for open prostatectomy.

At the time of the pre-admission testing, a blood and

urine sample is obtained from the patient for CBC, PT/PTT, TT, serum PSA level, SMA-7 (for an estimation of renal function via measuring serum creatinine and BUN levels), and urinalysis with urine culture and sensitivity. Pre-operative type and cross-match of two units of blood is usual. If possible, consider the use of cell saver or normovolemic hemodilution and type and screen of blood, in lieu of cross-match.

Traditionally, the role of radiologic imaging studies in the evaluation and management of BPH has been to (1) assess the volume of adenomatous prostate; (2) determine the degree of bladder dysfunction and volume of residual urine; and (3) rule out the presence of other pathology either related or unrelated to BPH. An ultrasound of the bladder is a useful test in patients planned to be subjected to open prostatectomy. The test can detect high residual urine (which may necessitate postoperative intermittent catheterisation) and also alert the clinician to other pathologies such as bladder diverticula or calculi. While a large prostate size can be documented by DRE, it should be confirmed by a TRUS which would also assess presence of median lobe and any asymmetry of prostatic lobes.

It is recommended that a chest X-ray should be done, preferably within 3 months of the scheduled surgery. Other radiologic imaging studies for the routine evaluation of the upper urinary tract in BPH patients are not recommended; they are neither cost effective nor do they have any impact on the clinical outcome. The Clinical Practice Guidelines (CPG) do not recommend upper urinary tract studies for BPH evaluation except under special circumstances (i.e. cases of protracted, complete obstruction of the prostatic urethra). The major indication for upper tract radiologic evaluation is hematuria.

In addition to radiologic and imaging studies, the patient should be scheduled for flexible urethrocystoscopy. Even though it is not recommended by the CPG as a test for determining the need for therapy, cystoscopy is indicated in men with a history of hematuria, stricture disease, urethral injury, or prior lower urinary tract surgery/instrumentation. Additionally, when the need for surgical therapy has been finalized, cystoscopy should be done for several important reasons, all of which will provide more insight into the patient's anatomy and help determine a strategic surgical approach. Cystoscopy should be done to (1) document the presence of ureteral peristalsis and to determine the position of the urethral orifices in order to prevent any inadvertent injury; (2) assess the configuration of the prostatic urethra; (3) assess the bladder capacity and presence of bladder trabeculation and diverticula (this information provides an idea of expected postoperative recovery); and (4) identify any BPH-associated intravesical disease (such as cystolithiasis, bladder calculi, small (less than 5 mm) bladder neoplasms) that is not visible by preoperative imaging studies.

PREOPERATIVE MANAGEMENT

The patient should be admitted the morning of the surgery date. Preadmission testing (PAT) includes a CBC, SMA-7, urinalysis with urine culture/sensitivity, and blood type and cross-match. The patient should be instructed to self-administer a Fleets enema during the evening prior to surgery. In addition, the patient should be informed to withdraw from taking any liquids or solid foods (NPO) after 12 a.m. (midnight), the evening before surgery. Finally, but most importantly, the patient must be instructed to cease taking aspirin, non-steroidal anti-inflammatory medication and all other potential blood thinners 1 week prior to surgery.

The use of antibiotics as prophylaxis treatment prior to surgery should strongly be considered, especially if the patient has a history of prostatitis or prostatolithiasis, even in the absence of pyuria or urine-cultured bacterial growth. If the cultured urine is positive for bacterial growth, infection is treated with perioperative ampicillin or cefazolin, limited to three doses. Antibiotic coverage should be restarted again when the urinary catheter is removed; this time, ciprofloxacin or trimethoprim–sulfamethoxazole is the preferred choice.

During the office visit in which surgical intervention to treat the BPH was decided, an informed consent should be obtained from the patient. The informed surgical consent document should include reference to potential intra-operative and postoperative complications, and the risks of potential blood transfusion. There should also be documentation of the patient's understanding of alternative forms of medical and surgical therapy. It is no longer prudent to obtain informed consent for "cytoscopy, possible transurethral resection of prostate, possible open prostatectomy." Preoperative assessment should allow reasonable certainty and agreement by the patient of the planned surgical procedure. In addition to the above, the patient must have the intraoperative risks and postoperative complications explained in lay terms (Table 30.1). The patient should also be informed of the possible poor outcomes after an open prostatectomy, such as urinary incontinence and retention.

SELECTION OF OPEN PROSTATECTOMY PROCEDURES

For simple prostatectomy, the suprapubic approach is the easiest to learn, but it lacks the control that is found in the retropubic enucleation. Suprapubic resection is indicated for prostate glands that have a large median lobe or where there is a need for additional procedures such as cystolithotomy or diverticulum excision. The retropubic approach avoids a bladder incision and is also better for hemostatasis. Table 30.2 summarizes the advantages of each type of prostatectomy.

TRANSVESICAL (SUPRAPUBIC) PROSTATECTOMY[9,10,11]

As mentioned before, this procedure is standardized for the removal of large adenomas (>60 g). After the preliminary work-up is completed, the patient should be prepared for

Intraoperative risks	Postoperative complications	Poor outcome
1. Severe bleeding 2. Injury to ureters	1. Bleeding 2. Infection 3. Pulmonary embolus 4. Urethral stricture 5. Prolonged cystostomy site drainage 6. Sexual dysfunction	1. Incontinence 2. Urinary retention

Table 30.1 Risks, complications, and outcomes of open prostatectomy

Transvesical (suprapubic)	Transcapsular (retropubic)
1. Associated intravesical procedures: (a) Diverticulectomy (b) Cystolithotomy 2. Predominance of intravesical prostatic component 3. Limited retropubic scarring (theoretical advantage for potential future radical retropubic prostatectomy)	1. Improved hemostasis (intracapsular bleeding) 2. Predominance of intraurethral prostatic component 3. Reduction of bladder spasms associated with cystotomy

Table 30.2 Selection of open prostatectomy procedures

surgery. It is recommended that the patient be given a spinal anesthesia as opposed to general anesthesia, unless contraindicated or technically impossible. This spinal anesthetic not only yields excellent intraoperative analgesia and muscle relaxation, but also reduces postoperative urethral irritation (due to Foley catheter), pelvic pain, and bleeding. Awakening from general anesthesia is often associated with disorientation and an attempt by the patient to pull out his urinary catheter or expel it with a forceful Valsalva maneuver because of irritation; thus, general anesthesia should be avoided when possible.

The operating room should be supplied with a prostatectomy set, in addition to lobe forceps, 3 Deaver retractors, a Balfour retractor with a flexible blade or a Jacobson (3-bladed bladder) retractor, several Allis clamps and several 2-in. vaginal packs (Table 30.3) The suprapubic prostatectomy should commence via the following sequence.

(1) The patient should be placed in the supine position, with the sacrum elevated in a kidney rest or folded sheet. The operating table is broken slightly, while the suprapubic area is elevated by approximately 20° of Trendelenburg tilt. Note that if manually elevating the prostate from the rectum during enucleation is anticipated, the patient's left leg should not be strapped to the table but allowed to drape freely. The operative area, penis, and scrotum are prepared with Betadine (iodine) solution and draped in a sterile fashion from the mid-thighs to approximately 6 cm above the umbilicus. A Foley catheter is inserted and the bladder is filled with approximately 250 cm^3 of sterile saline. The catheter is then removed (Figure 30.1).

	Transcapsular		Transvesical
Retractors Self-retaining Handheld	Millin	Bookwalter Deavers, thin Malleable, medium	Balfour with deep blades and bladder blade
Catheters	24 French Foley with 30-cm^3 balloon	CBI tubing – saline irrigant	24 French 3-way Foley catheter, 30-cm^3 balloon 26 French Malecot catheter
Clamps		Allis, Babcock, ring forceps	
Suction catheters		Yankauer Tip (two)	
Miscellaneous		Vaginal packing 2 in., bulb syringe, pneumatic leg compression devices	
Suture		0 Dexon or Vicryl, 2-0; 0-chromic catgut (5/8 in. needle)	
Optional		Cell Saver (autotransfusion) Lighted Yankauer suction tip	

Table 30.3 Instrumentation

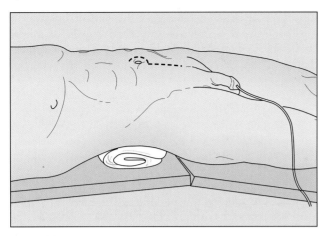

Figure 30.1 Patient is placed supine with a roll under sacrum to elevate it

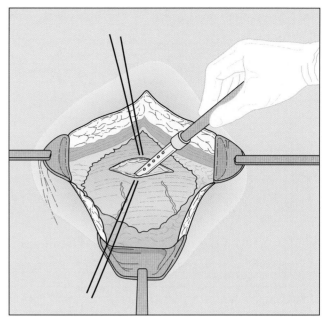

Figure 30.2 A midline incision is made, a transverse cystotomy is used to open the bladder

(2) Midline or Pfannenstiel incision is made from the anterior surface of the symphysis pubis to the left side of the umbilicus. The linea alba and rectus muscles are separated in the midline and gently retracted laterally, as the transversalis fascia is grasped with forceps and sharply incised with scissors. The peritoneum is gently swept cephalad from under the surface of the rectus muscles and the dome of the bladder with a sponge stick to expose the bladder in the space of Retzius. Precautions should be taken to avoid injury to the inferior epigastric vessels. Retractor blades are then positioned for maximal exposure; Bookwalter or Balfour self-retaining retractors can be utilized (Figure 30.2).

(3) A transverse cystotomy is made approximately 2 cm above the bladder neck and 0-chromic stay sutures are placed above and below the intended site of incision of the vesical neck. However, one should be cautious not to place the sutures into the prostatic capsule. Serosal vasculature is fulgurated with cautery, while the bladder is opened with cutting current between stay sutures. Bladder contents are aspirated with pool suction tip, and the bladder is inspected, while expanding the incision with two index fingers. The bladder dome is retracted with thin Deavers, over open wet sponges. After inspection and palpation of the vesical neck and the bladder interior to remove any debris, such as calculi, the ureteral orifices are identified.

The trigone is then depressed with a sponge stick and the traction suture is tensed. The bladder neck mucosa is incised circumferentially around the protruding prostatic adenoma with blended current, superficially cutting into the adenoma. The plane of dissection between the prostatic capsule and adenoma is developed by using Metzenbaum scissors; this is done by gently spreading the blades of the curved scissor (which is facing anteriorly, with tips pointed downward).

(4) To start the enucleation, an index finger is inserted into the anterior plane of dissection and all bladder retractors and sponges are removed. The patient, at this time, should be maneuvered into the Trendelenburg position. The index finger is then placed into the distal prostatic urethra between the two lobes, forcing the fingertip anteriorly and in the midline plane through the urothelium. The dissecting finger is then swept in an arc from 10 to 2 o'clock to the apex of the bladder (Figure 30.3). The arc of dissection is broadened until the urethral mucosa at the apex can be divided by pressure between the thumbnail and the pad of the index finger (Figure 30.4). In an obese patient, a finger in the rectum to elevate the prostate may help enucleate the adenoma. The anterior commissure is then ruptured and dissection is carried out laterally until the apical urethra can be completely divided. Metzenbaum scissors may be digitally guided to sharply divide apical urethral mucosa or adhesions between the adenoma and surgical capsule; one must be cautious not to hook into the prostatic capsule with the edge of the scissors. The digital dissection is then conducted posteriorly and behind the middle lobe to remove the specimen, making sure both lobes are free before proceeding to free either one completely. It is commonly practiced and (at times) necessary to remove large lateral lobes separately. Gentle traction may be placed on the adenoma with a Babcock clamp to facilitate dissection; however, early separation of apical mucosa is necessary to avoid traction injury to the striated sphincter (Figure 30.5). After completely enucleating the adenoma, the

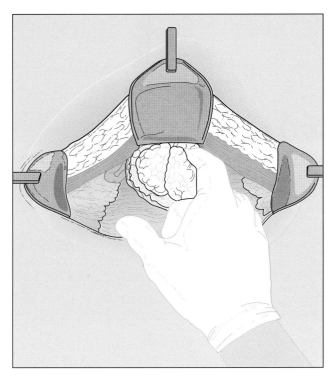

Figure 30.3 An index finger or 'Kittner' (clamp with a small gauze) is used to enucleate the prostate

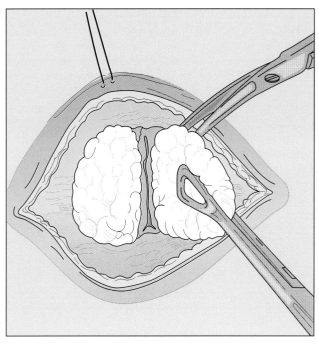

Figure 30.5 Scissors are used to sharply divide apical urethral mucosa

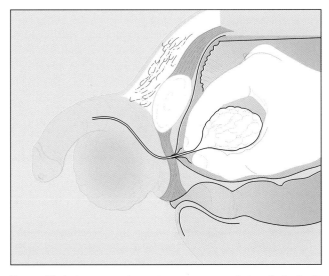

Figure 30.4 The apex of the adenoma can usually be pinched off using the index finger and thumb

bladder epithelium is pinched off or sharply incised. Finally, the prostatic fossa is examined for any remaining adenoma tissue.

(5) To establish hemostasis, a 2-in. wet vaginal packing is compressed into the prostatic fossa with a thin Deaver and pressure is maintained for 5 min to allow the fossa to contract (which aids in hemostasis of the venous blood).

The bladder neck is then grasped with an Allis clamp at the 6-o'clock position, and 2–0 chromic (figure-of-eight) suture ligatures are passed at the 5-o'clock and 7-o'clock positions, while avoiding the ureteral orifice. The first suture should be placed deep in order to get a bite of the prostatic capsule along with the main prostatic arteries, and a superficial layer of the bladder epithelium. This is of great importance, because the main arterial blood supply feeding the adenoma is from the urethral branches of the prostatic arteries, which enter the capsule, distal to the bladder neck at the 5-o'clock and 7-o'clock positions. Thus, excessive bright-red bleeding most likely originates from these arteries, and they must be ligated with the 5-o'clock and 7-o'clock positioned sutures.

After placing the first suture, it is retracted to elevate the bladder neck for the placement of the next set of sutures. Two additional sutures are then placed, one each at the 11-o'clock and 1-o'clock positions in order to catch the anterior arterial branches. None of the four sutures should be cut, because they can be used later to inspect the fossa for any bleeding sites. Further sutures of 3–0 are then placed as needed. If the neck is small or fibrous, a wedge is excised from the posterior lip. The vesical epithelium over the rim of the fossa is then tacked with fine plain catgut (PCG) sutures to prevent vesical neck contracture. The packing is then slowly removed and the fossa is inspected for bleeding with a Deaver retractor or ring forceps. (A lighted suction tip may be very helpful.)

Bleeding from the prostatic fossa may be brisk and may require the following special hemostatic procedures.

(a) *Catheter traction*: To control venous oozing, the balloon of the Foley catheter is pulled to the bladder neck and inflated to 100 cm^3 (approximately 5 lb of pressure), making sure the balloon is not in the fossa. A hemostatic substance, such as Surgicel, may be first inserted into the prostatic fossa. This traction should be released within 12–24 h (see below).

(b) *Plication sutures*: This procedure should be utilized when there is persistent bleeding without an obvious identifiable source. To accomplish this, the capsule is first folded lengthwise like a fan, and several rows of transverse 0-chromic catgut sutures on 5/8 curved needles are placed in the posterior capsule, running from one side of the fossa to the other to bring the capsule together.[5]

(c) *Purse-string bladder neck*: A #1 nylon suture is woven with a free needle around the bladder neck through the mucosa and passed through the bladder wall anteriorly, in a purse-string fashion. The sutures should then be wrapped around, crossing the midline anteriorly and exiting through the entire thickness of the anterior bladder wall. A 24-French Foley catheter with a balloon should now be placed through the bladder neck. The bladder neck is then tightened down over the Foley catheter, which is placed to traction via inflating the balloon. Once inflated, the sutures are drawn around the catheter to close the vesical neck. These sutures are also then passed through the anterior abdominal wall, just superior to the symphysis; the sutures should be pulled, so enough tension is present to close the bladder neck around the catheter, separating the fossa from the bladder. The suture is then anchored over a button on the lower abdominal wall. The purse-string suture may be removed within 24–48 h, and the balloon catheter is removed on the second postoperative day (Figure 30.6).[12]

If the latter two procedures are performed, a cystostomy tube must be inserted to allow for irrigation. This is done by making a stab wound in the anterior abdominal wall, and introducing a Mayo clamp through the wall of the abdomen and bladder. A 30-gauge Malecot catheter, the tip cut obliquely at a

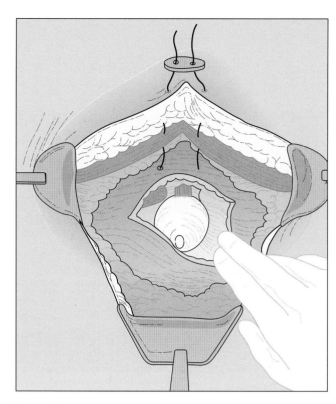

Figure 30.6 A purse string suture around the bladder neck may be occasionally necessary to achieve hemostasis

30° angle, is placed between the tongues of the clamp, and is pulled through the tract introduced by the Mayo clamp. The catheter should be placed against the bladder wall, but away from the trigone by using a purse-string suture at the site where the catheter exits through the bladder wall.

(6) *Closure*: A 24-gauge French two-way Foley urethral catheter with 30 cm^3 balloon is brought out along with a 26 French Malecot cystostomy tube through a separate stab wound. If bleeding is a problem, a three-way catheter is placed to allow for postoperative irrigation. Catheter traction should be placed if persistent venous oozing is evident. The bladder is closed in layers with running 0-chromic catgut suture. The field is drained with a Jackson–Pratt bulb suction catheter through a separate stab wound. The catheters are irrigated to test for any leakage of fluid and bleeding. The incision site should be covered with iodine ointment, abdominal pads, and Montgomery straps. The suprapubic tube should be secured to the abdomen with tape, while the urethral catheter is secured to the penis.

(7) *Postoperative care*: Continuous bladder irrigation may be maintained with sterile saline infusion through either of the two catheters. If there is persistent and uncontrollable bleeding in clots, the patient must be immediately taken to the operating room for clot

evacuation via the use of a resectoscope, with the placement of a suprapubic tube for continuous irrigation.

The urethral catheter is removed within 48 h, if urine is clear. The suprapubic cystostomy tube is clamped on the fifth day and removed if postvoid residual volume is small. However, if drainage persists, a 22-gauge catheter with a 30 cm^3 balloon is inserted for a few days. If a purse-string suture was used, it is removed on postoperative day 1. In the absence of a purse-string suture and bleeding, the balloon can be deflated and the catheter subsequently can be removed as early as postoperative day 2. The Jackson–Pratt drainage tube should be removed after all other catheters have been removed.

Ambulation is achieved on the first postoperative day; however, lower extremity pneumatic compression devices are maintained while in bed for 3–4 days, postoperatively. Oral intake can begin as soon as anesthesia has worn off. The patient also should be adequately hydrated, either orally or through IV. Not withstanding any complications, the patient can be discharged on postoperative day 4 or 5.

TRANSCAPSULAR (RETROPUBIC) PROSTATECTOMY[9,10,11]

Prior to the surgical procedure, the patient should be advised to evacuate his bowel. Any pre-existing urinary infection or prostatitis should be treated as mentioned in the suprapubic prostatectomy section. Several surgeons have suggested that the patients should wear veno-occlusive stockings intraoperatively also.

In the operating room, the patient should be given an epidural anesthetic or general anesthesia. The operating room should be supplied with a prostatectomy set, in addition to Deaver, Balfour, and Millin retractors; small, medium, and large-sized lobe forceps (two of each needed); a curette; a T-clamp; a bladder-neck spreader; several curved sponge sticks; Mayo scissors; Metzenbaum scissors (curved and straight); bipolar coagulating forceps; and several 2-in. vaginal packs. See Table 30.3 for a detailed summary of necessary equipment needed for surgery.

The retropubic proctectomy should commence via the following sequence:

(1) *Position*: The patient should be placed supine on the table with the sacrum elevated on a kidney rest or folded sheet (see Figure 30.1). The table is broken slightly to elevate the suprapubic area; the table is tilted to a 20° angle in the Trendelenburg position. The patient is prepped and draped in a sterile fashion from the mid-thighs to approximately 6 cm above the umbilicus. the bladder is emptied of urine with sterile Foley catheter insertion. A cystoscopy should be performed at this time, if not done previously.

(2) *Incision*: A midline from the symphysis pubis to the left side of the umbilicus or Pfannenstiel incision is made.

The recuts muscles are separated in the midline and gently retracted laterally, as the transversalis fascia is grasped with forceps and sharply incised with scissors. The peritoneum is gently swept cephalad from under the surface of the rectus muscles with a moist sponge stick, avoiding injury to the inferior epigastric vessels. Superficial connective tissue beneath the pubic bones may be gently retracted with a moist laparotomy pad and scored with Bovie coagulation current to enter the space of Retzius. Self-retaining retractor blades are placed to expose the bladder neck and anterior surface of the prostate. A malleable retractor, padded with a moist laparotomy pad, will help to depress the bladder and to retract the prostate into the surgical field (see Figure 30.2).

(3) Loose areolar connective tissue is swept laterally off the bladder neck and prostatic surface with a sponge stick or Kittner dissector. A right-angle clamp or packing forceps held with a double-gloved hand grasp is used gently to retract fat and small superficial vessels from the prostatic capsule surface, as coagulation current of 60 W passes through the instrument. Three opened wet 4×4 sponges are then packed on each side of the prostate to assist exposure of the gland (Figure 30.7).

(4) Palpation of the Foley catheter balloon facilitates bladder neck location. Two rows of hemostatic, interrupted sutures of 2–0 Vicryl or Dexon on a 5/8 in. needle are passed at 1 and 2 cm distal to the bladder neck. These sutures are passed through a full thickness of the prostatic capsule, superficially into the prostatic adenoma, and tied down tightly. Twelve-o'clock sutures are placed on slight traction to define tissue planes, as the capsule is opened between suture lines with Bovie cutting current. Remove the Foley catheter, and spread Metzenbaum scissor blades in the plane between the adenoma and surgical capsule (one may cut superficially into the adenoma with the Bovie instrument if the proper plane is not readily distinguishable) (Figures 30.8 and 30.9).

(5) *Enucleation*: The index finger is inserted into the anterior plane of dissection, sweeping in an arc between 10 and 2 o'clock, toward the apex of the gland. The arc of dissection is broadened until the urethral mucosa at the apex can be sharply divided with Metzenbaum scissors or pinched apart between thumbnail and pad of index finger. Digital dissection is performed laterally and posteriorly toward the bladder neck. It may be necessary to sharply incise areas of capsular adhesions or thickened mucosa at the bladder neck. The adenoma is delivered through the capsulotomy with Babcock clamps. A very large adenoma must frequently be divided for enucleation pushing the index finger through the anterior commissure into the urethra (Figures 30.10 and 30.11).

(6) *Hemostasis*: The fossa is packed with 2-in. wet vaginal packing and compressed with pressure exerted with a Yankauer suction tip or thin Deaver retractor. The

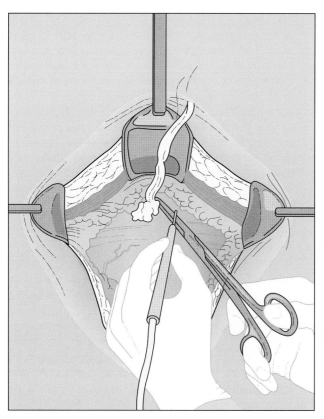

Figure 30.7 Loose areolar tissue over the bladder neck is removed using a forceps, Kittner, and electrocautery

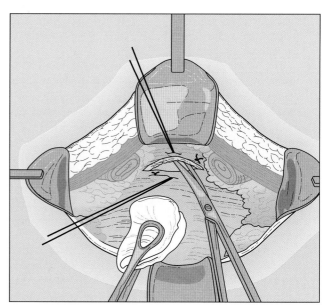

Figure 30.9 The capsule is opened using electrocautery and scissors

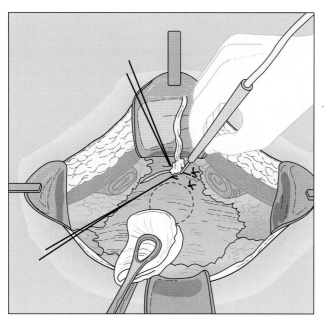

Figure 30.8 Two rows of hemostatic sutures are placed on the prostatic capsule

bladder neck is grasped at 6 o'clock with an Allis clamp and a figure-of-eight 2–0 chromic hemostatic sutures are placed through the prostatic capsule and bladder neck at 5 and 7 o'clock (Figure 30.1). Additional sutures may be required at 11 and 1 o'clock. Any redundant posterior lip of bladder neck is resected and the mucosa is sutured down to the prostatic capsule, posteriorly, with running 2–0 chromic catgut. (Five cubic centimeters of Indigo Carmine, given intravenously, will help verify ureteral orifice peristalsis.) The packing is removed and any bleeding sites are cauterized (Figure 30.12).

Hemostatic measures discussed in the section transvesical prostatectomy would also be applicable here; however, transcapsular access generally allows point fulguration of arterial bleeding sites. Walsh and Oesterling described achieving complete hemostasis with ligation of the dorsal vein complex and lateral prostatic pedicles, prior to capsulotomy.[11]

(7) A 24-gauge French 3-way Foley catheter with 30 cm^3 balloon is passed into the bladder. Place the catheter to slight traction and irrigate the bladder with a bulb syringe until clear. A cystostomy is generally not necessary, but may be inserted at this point if there is concern of continued bleeding and necessity for brisk continuous bladder irrigation. Close the capsulotomy with running sutures of 0-Dexon or Vicryl, beginning at the lateral extremes. Test the closure with irrigation and oversew any leaks. A Jackson–Pratt drain is placed in the space of Retzius and brought out through a separate abdominal stab wound.

(8) *Postoperative care*: Maintain continuous bladder irrigation with sterile saline, as required. Remove the

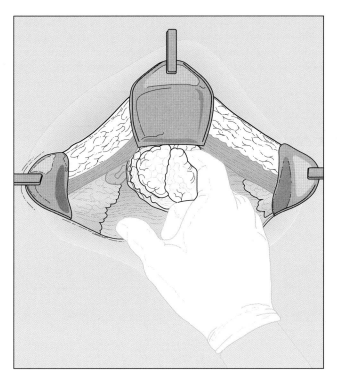

Figure 30.10 The index finger or Kittner dissector is used to enucleate the adenoma

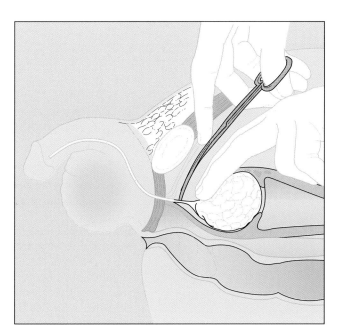

Figure 30.11 The apex of the adenoma is sharply divided using scissors

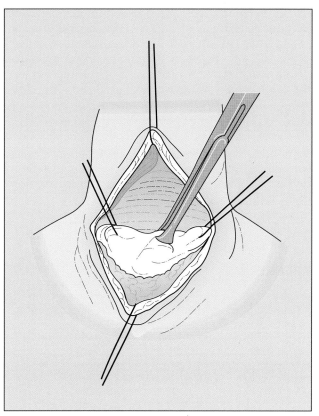

Figure 30.12 Hemostasis is secured initially by pressure and subsequently by 20 chromic catgut sutures

COMPLICATIONS OF OPEN PROSTATECTOMY

The most frequently encountered and potentially dangerous complication of open prostatectomy is that of intraoperative hemorrhage. Other complications are rare (see Table 30.4). If bleeding is persistent, it may require endoscopic cauterization, assuming attempted tamponade has failed. While setting the patient up in the OR for the endoscopic procedure, several laboratory exams should be ordered in an attempt to find any kind of clotting disorders. The following tests are recommended: CBC, PT/PTT, TT,

Foley catheter within 5–7 days. Ambulation is achieved on the first postoperative day; however, lower extremity pneumatic compression devices are maintained while the patient is in bed for 3–4 days, postoperatively.

Complication	%
Hemorrhage (requiring transfusion)	15
Urethral stricture or bladder neck contracture	2–8
Wound infection	4
Epididymitis	2–3
Stress urinary incontinence	1–2
Pulmonary embolus	<1
Impotence	<1
Osteitis pubis	<1
Mortality	<1

Table 30.4 Complications of open prostatectomy

clotting factor VIII levels, fibrinogen level, and fibrin-split products. In addition, protamine activity should be monitored for an estimation of clot degradation. Note that a chronic alcoholic may have decreased amounts of clotting factors (specifically, 2,7,9,10) due to extensive liver damage and malabsorption. However, this should be evident when preoperative PT/PTT tests were ordered. If severe bleeding is present, the incision site should be reopened, packed with 2-in. gauze pads, and traction with a balloon should be applied. Postoperative disseminated intravascular coagulation (DIC) is of great concern, especially pulmonary emboli; this should be carefully watched for by examining PT/PTT, TT, and fibrin-split products.

Another concern during every surgical procedure is wound infection; however, this is rare. If an infection is evi-dent from the presence of an elevated WBC count, fever, chills, erythema of the incision site, and (possibly) UTI, the patient should immediately be placed on IV antibiotics. Postoperatively, the release of chronic obstruction may lead to postobstructive diuresis. This should be carefully monitored. Management of and different types of diureses are well explained in Chapter 10.

CONCLUSION

Open prostatectomy is a procedure which is required in approximately 3–5% of patients with obstructive BPH. It is a procedure that must be held within the armamentarium of all urologists, as a highly effective, efficient, and safe form of therapy.

REFERENCES

1 Fuller E. Six successful and successive cases of prostatectomy. *J Cutan Genitourin. Dis* 1895; **13**: 229.
2 Freyer PJ. A new method of performing prostatectomy. *Lancet* 1900; **1**: 774.
3 Freyer PJ. One thousand cases of total enuceation of the prostate for radical cure of enlargement of that organ. *Br Med J* 1912; **2**: 868.
4 O'Conor VJ Jr, Nanninga JB. Low suprapubic prostatectomy: a continuing report. *J Urol* 1972; **108**: 453.
5 O'Conor VJ Jr. An aid for hemostasis in open prostatectomy: capsular plication. *J Urol* 1982; **127**: 448.
6 Nanninga JB. Suprapubic and retropubic prostatectomy. *AUA Update Series* 1984; **V**: 111.
7 O'Conor VJ Jr, Bulkley GJ, Sokol JK. Low suprapubic prostatectomy: comparison of results with the standard operation in two comparable groups of 142 patients. *J Urol* 1963; **90**: 301.
8 Millin T. Retropubic prostatectomy: new extravesical technique; report on 20 cases. *Lancet* 1945; **2**: 693.
9 Shah P Jr, Abrams PH, Fineley RCL *et al.* The influence of prostatic anatomy and the different results of prostatectomy according to the surgical approach. *Br J Urol* 1979; **51**: 549–51.
10 Stutzman RE, Walsh PC. Suprapubic and retropubic prostatectomy. In Walsh PC, Retik AB, Stamey TA *et al.* (eds) *Campbell's Urology*, 6th edn. Philadelphia: WB Saunders 1992.
11 Walsh PC, Oesterling JE. Improved hemostasis during simple retropubic prostatectomy. *J Urol* 1990; **143**: 1203–4.
12 Malament M. Maximal hemostasis in suprapubic prostatectomy. *Surg Gynecol Obstet* 1975; **120**: 1307.

COMMENTARY

The suprapubic or transvesical prostatectomy was the first really preferred method for removal of adenoma. Currently, the procedure is done with good visualization under direct vision allowing control of bleeding and meticulous repair of bladder neck to prevent contractures. The advantages of the suprapubic technique are the ability to treat bladder pathology such as diverticula and calculi. The disadvantages, which are minor, include a bladder neck incision and cystotomy, which can be avoided in the retropubic technique. The retropubic technique, which is preferred by the Editor, requires an incision over the prostatic capsule but has the advantage of better visualization of the prostate, and allows precise excision of the adenoma at the apex of the prostatic urethra. The prostatic blood vessels need to be meticulously secured in both techniques and is more easily done with a capsular incision. The experience of most surgeons with radical prostatectomy allows for several modifications to the original retropubic technique including use of sutures at the 5- and 7-o'clock positions at the prostatic pedicles prophylactically. One can ligate the Santorini plexus if required. On several occasions, the Editor has also used a combined approach in which a retropubic vertical capsular incision is used to begin the operation and, subsequently, a small added "T" extension is made into the bladder neck to release the median lobe.

To prevent bladder neck contractures it is important to suture the posterior mucosa of the bladder neck on to the prostatic capsule.[1] This allows rapid and smooth epithelialization. The use of a suprapubic catheter is conventional, although more recently some surgeons avoid this.[2] With current availability of ultrasound and other options for endoscopic management, a blocked Foley catheter can be reinserted if necessary. Most surgeons, however, still leave a suprapubic tube for several days postoperatively.

The open prostatectomy techniques, however, all have surgical morbidity associated with an abdominal incision, requirement of anesthesia (including pulmonary and cardiac and cerebrovascular complications, deep venous thrombosis, etc.), possible blood transfusions, and wound-related problems. Other complications have been associated with open prostatectomy such as postoperative urinary incontinence. There is 1.9% probability of having stress urinary incontinence and a 0.5% probability of having total urinary incontinence following open enucleation. The suprapubic technique is associated with a higher probability of stress urinary incontinence (2.6%) than the retropubic method (1.6%).[3] Interestingly enough, the probability of stress urinary incontinence and total urinary incontinence is much higher when patients are treated with TURP in comparison to open prostatectomy; the percent probabilities are 2.2 and 1.0, respectively. Two more complications resulting from surgical intervention for BPH are urethral stricture and bladder neck contracture. In an analysis by Roehrborn, open prostatectomy presented with a probability of urethral stricture and bladder neck contracture of 2.6% and 1.8%, respectively, with a combined probability of 4.3%.[3] It should be noted that the probability of urethral stricture and bladder neck contracture was much more during the suprapubic technique compared with the retropubic method: 5.1% vs. 1.0% for urethral stricture, and 2.9% vs. 1.0% for bladder neck contracture. In comparison to suprapubic prostatectomy, TURP shows a much lower probability of urethral stricture (3.1%) and bladder neck contracture (1.7%).

Maintaining or restoring sexual function is of increasing importance to patients suffering from BPH. Various surgical procedures cause varying incidence of sexually related complications such as impotence and retrograde ejaculation. Roehrborn analyzed data from several studies using surgical intervention for BPH management.[3] From his analysis, it was determined that the incidence of retrograde ejaculation was considerably higher in patients undergoing suprapubic prostatectomy (80.8%) than in those undergoing TURP (70.4%) and retropubic prostatectomy (65.0%). Further-

more, 16.4% of the patients who had undergone suprapubic prostatectomy and who were previously potent were impotent after the surgical procedure. In comparison, 15.6% and 13.6% of the previously potent patients were impotent after retropubic prostatectomy and TURP, respectively. In order to avoid impotence and retrograde ejaculation, the Editor prefers the use of TUNA or staged TURP/TUVP in all large glands. TURP morbidity has diminished considerably over the last several decades.

In 1962, Holtgrewe and Valk reported the morbidity and mortality of TURP in 2015 cases.[4] They found a mortality rate of 2.5% and a morbidity rate of 18%. The leading cause of death was myocardial infarction, and the most common morbidity problem was epididymitis (6%) followed by pneumonia (1.3%). In 1974, using data allocated from 2223 patients, Melchior and associates[5] reported a mortality rate of 1.3%, with the leading cause being myocardial infraction. In a recent report by Mebust and associates, of the 3885 patients reviewed, the mortality rate for TURP was 0.2%, with only one patient dying of a myocardial infarction.[6] The postoperative morbidity rate was 18%; this mostly consisted of patients with greater than 90 minutes resection time, prostate size >45 g, history of acute urinary retention, and patient age greater than 80 years (see Figure 30.11). Most recently, morbidity of TURP in the VA Cooperative trial was 9%.[7] In the Editor's recently reported results with TUNA in large glands (average 45 g; range up to 160 g) the overall morbidity from TUNA was quite reasonable at less than 8.8% percent.[8] However, the disadvantage of TUNA over TURP is that it may only be about two-thirds as efficacious and in large glands the procedure may take 1.5–2 h involving 12–18 treatment sites.

1 Malamet M. Maximal hemostasis in suprapubic prostatectomy. *Surg Gynecol Obstet* 1965; **120**: 1307.

2 Walsh PC, Oesterling JE. Improved hemostasis during simple retropubic prostatectomy. *J Urol* 1990; **143**: 1203.

3 Kirby R, McConnell JD, Fitzpatrick JM *et al*. Standard surgical interventions: TUIP, TURP, OPSU. In: *Textbook of Benign Prostatic Hyperplasia*, 1st edn. Oxford: Isis Medical Media 1996; 342–78.

4 Holtgrewe HL, Valk WL. Factors influencing the mortality and morbidity of transurethral prostatectomy: a study of 2015 cases. *J Urol* 1968; **87**: 450.

5 Melchior J, Valk WL, Foret JD, Mebust WK. Transurethral prostatectomy: computerized analysis of 2223 consecutive cases. *J Urol* 1974; **112**: 634.

6 Mebust WK, Holtgrewe HL, Cockett ATK, Peters PC. Transurethral prostatectomy: immediate and postoperative complications. A cooperative study of 13 participating institutions evaluating 3885 patients. *J Urol* 1989; **141**: 243–7.

7 Flanigan RC, Reda DJ, Wasson JH, Anderson RJ, Abdellatif M, Bruskewitz RC. 5-Year outcome of surgical resection and watchful waiting for men with moderately symptomatic benign prostatic hyperplasia: a Department of Veterans Affairs Cooperative Study. *J Urol* 1998; **60**: 12–17.

8 Kahn S, Alphonse P, Tewari A, Narayan P. An open study on the efficacy and safety of transurethral needle ablation of the prostate in treating symptomatic benign prostatic hyperplasia: the University of Florida experience. *J Urol* 1998; **160**: 1695–1700.

FUTURE TRENDS

P. Narayan

The management of BPH has undergone a tremendous change in the last decade. It is clear that symptoms are what bother patients and relief of symptoms is currently the ultimate goal of the therapy. Documentation of obstruction by pressure-flow studies is not necessary in most patients undergoing BPH therapy. In studies where TUR was performed without prior invasive urodynamic studies, 80% of patients had relief of symptoms while in those with documented obstruction on pressure flow TUR produced relief in 90% of patients. This 10% difference is not cost effective, nor a logical reason, to perform invasive pressure-flow studies routinely in 90% of patients who may not benefit from it. Pressure-flow studies are indicated in special circumstances where the question of obstruction is in doubt and the patient may have bladder dysfunction. With the advent of minimally invasive therapies, patients are willing to accept therapy failure provided irreversible side effects are avoided. Many of the patients in the Editor's practice come in seeking a one-time surgical alternative to perhaps partially beneficial or intolerable medical therapy. Patients are willing to pay $5000–$10,000 for a laser, TUNA, or microwave provided they have no irreversible side effects. This patient-driven therapy has resulted in the recent popularity of minimally invasive treatments, despite the fact that none of them is as efficacious as standard TURP. In the future, I anticipate that we will see more such minimally invasive treatments available with lower side effects, improved efficacy, and lower costs.

The use of various instruments to assess health-related quality of life (HRQOL) has also focused physicians' attention on the fact that patients do perceive a decrease in sense of well-being secondary to urinary symptoms and that therapy of most types (medical or surgical) improves patients' perception of HRQOL and health status. Primary care physicians are aware of this fact, and currently prescribe pharmaceutical agents routinely for BPH. This is a paradigm shift from a decade ago when urologists were the primary care givers for patients with BPH. The aging of the world's population especially in the western hemisphere will increase the need and use of medical therapies in BPH.

With regard to epidemiology and natural history, the data suggest that progression of BPH is highly variable and dependent not only on patient age, family history, and perception of symptoms, but also lifestyle and availability of various therapeutic options. Treatment should not be offered simply because of inevitability of progression or because surgical risk increases with age. The BPH guidelines in various countries are beginning to consolidate these findings into their recommendations on BPH management guidelines. It is important that urologists do not embrace new tests and treatments without proper peer review and scientific data.

With reference to etiopathogenesis, there is considerable interest and several new advances in understanding of BPH at a cellular and molecular level. It is clear that normal androgenic function is required to establish but not maintain BPH. Once established, BPH cells can be maintained by growth factors and other cytokines released from themselves and nearby cells. While testicular testosterone is important, adrenal androgens can sustain BPH. The use of the Type II 5α-reductase inhibitor finasteride has demonstrated that prostate size decreases only 30% with 90–95% suppression of DHT. Other mechanisms maintaining BPH growth include Type I 5α-reductase inhibitors in liver, skin, and genital tissues, adrenal androgens, as well as growth factors and other molecules. Orchiectomy also does not result in total ablation of the prostate since adrenal androgens converted by peripheral 5α-reductase can maintain prostatic cell growth. Another factor of emerging importance is that stromal cells are the initial targets of DHT and that stromal cells influence epithelial cell growth probably by influencing basal epithelial cells (which also contain 5α-reductase) to regenerate and form luminal epithelial cells. The communication systems between these cells are complex and include cytokines, growth factors, cell adhesion molecules, and other factors. These reactions are also modulated by neuroendocrine cells which are influenced by both hormones and neurotransmitters. A majority of this work has come from studies on prostatic cancer, and it appears that some of the growth factors involved in growth and differentiation of normal prostatic cells may also function as oncogenes in malignancy. It has also been discovered that in malignancy the androgen receptor in prostatic cells can be abnormal. The clinical implication of this finding is that, while some agents such as flutamide, an anti-androgenic agent, can suppress growth initially in prostate cancer cells, mutations can result in anti-androgens causing cell proliferation, which may explain why PSA rises in some patients who are on anti-androgens. Additionally, there are recent data that the estrogen receptor has two subtypes α and β, with the β-receptors present on prostatic cells. This fact has several implications, since it is known that estrogen can suppress prostatic epithelial cells but may have a stimulatory effect on stromal cells.

The clinical implications of these findings include the possibility that newer agents, such as growth factor inhibitors and combined Type I and II 5α-reductase inhibitors, may have a role in suppressing established BPH. Phase II trials using the new Type I and II 5α-reductase inhibitors are currently in progress. The molecular data also provide insight into the mechanisms of action of some phytoestrogenic agents such as genistin and biochanin, which are active ingredients in soy extract and other herbal medications commonly used for BPH therapy.

Work by Steers, DeGroat and others has focused on the role of the irritable bladder and detrusor instability (DI) as a major contributor to symptoms in patients with BPH. DI due to obstruction is seen in 50–80% of men with BPH and may be a major factor in etiology of BPH symptoms. The neural innervation of the prostate comes from sympathetic, parasympathetic, and somatic sources, but at a cellular level there is tremendous cross-talk between the various types of nerves and neurotransmitters.

It is increasingly obvious that, apart from acetylcholine and norepinephrine, there are a number of other neurotransmitters involved in nerve-to-cell communication between bladder, urethra, and the prostate. These include non-cholinergic, non-adrenergic transmission via ATP mechanisms, direct effects via nitric oxide mechanisms, and also neurotransmitters associated with a variety of muscarinic- and adrenergic-receptor subtypes at the muscle, spinal, and pelvic ganglia. The net result of their interactions is that there is a bladder response to obstruction, that bladder behavior is modified by obstruction at the outlet, and that this response is variable based on the degree and duration of obstruction.

At a molecular level, there is also evidence that obstruction results in enhanced sensitivity of the bladder to non-specific stimulation, including shift of depolarization

Drug	Mechanism of action
Propantheline Br	An anticholinergic/antimuscarinic that also inhibits the action of acetylcholine at the postganglionic nerve endings of the parasympathetic nervous system.
Methantheline Br	Anticholinergic
Emepronium Br	Anticholinergic
Terbutaline	Sympathomimetic; a β-adrenergic receptor agonist which activates adenyl cyclase which converts ATP to cAMP for the activation of secondary messenger system, such as protein kinase.
Clenbuterol	Sympathomimetic
Terodiline HCl	An anticholinergic drug with calcium blocking action with calcium antagonist properties; it was effective in reducing urge incontinence, but was withdrawn from the market because of serious side effects, such as prolonged QT interval and ventricular arrhythmias.
Tolterodine	A Ca^{2+} channel blocker with muscarinic receptor antagonistic properties; it is indicated for treatment of patients with an overactive bladder with symptoms of urinary frequency, urgency, or urge incontinence.
Levcromakalim	ATP-sensitive K^+ channel opener/activator, causing smooth muscle relaxation inducing a glibenclamide-sensitive hyperpolarization of the membrane potential
Zeneca ZD6169	ATP-sensitive K^+ channel opener/activator with in-vivo selectivity for smooth muscle of the urinary bladder; it significantly reduces or prevents PGE₂-induced bladder activity by causing hyperpolarization of the smooth muscle membrane and a reduction in calcium activity; optimal for inhibition of bladder detrusor instability (hyperreflexia) with minimal, if any, cardiovascular adverse events.
Darfenicillin	Mu-3 antagonist
Duloxetine inhibitor	Norepinephrine and serotonin re-uptake
Resiniferatoxin	An ultra-potent (quinone) vanilloid agonist with high affinity for vanilloid receptor; inhibits the NADH-plasma membrane electron transport system and induces apoptosis in transformed cells.
Capsaicin	An ultra-potent (quinone) vanilloid agonist with high affinity for vanilloid receptor and is responsible for the pungent taste of hot peppers. It initially stimulates polysynaptic nociceptors and subsequently inhibits them, causing the NADH-plasma membrane electron transport system to be inhibited and inducing apoptosis in transformed cells.
Genistin	A plant isoflavonoid contained in a methanol extract of Radix puerariae. Currently its mechanism of action is controversial: while some studies have shown that it has tyrosine kinase antagonist activity, others have not.

Table 31.1   Medical agents with potential for management of lower urinary tract symptoms

potentials of bladder muscle cells. Clinical implications of this data are that medications to treat BPH will include combinations of α-blockers with perhaps bladder muscle relaxants such as Ca^{2+} channel blockers (see Table 31.1), K^+ channel openers, non-specific anesthetics of bladder muscle, as well as other agents.

With regard to medical therapy, α-blockers are clearly the first choice for patients and doctors in most countries today. The availability of superselective α-blockers such as tamsulosin has made it possible to prescribe medication and provide some relief even for elderly patients and nursing home residents who might otherwise be condemned to a catheter for life. The uroselective α-blockers also have additional advantages in that the incidence of clinically significant postural hypotension and syncope is rare. The elderly have a 10–15% incidence of spontaneous postural hypotension based on decreased sensitivity of baroreceptors, also created by aging; this is further exacerbated in patients who have volume depletion. These states include patients with cardiac disease, those on diuretics, those with diabetes, and those who are sedentary. The standard α-blockers are not recommended in such patients even for treatment of hypertension because of the fear of postural hypotension. In the future, we anticipate more superselective agents on the market with low side effects and improved tolerance. The availability of agents that are used once a day and avoid titration are an added benefit

and future agents have to compete on these grounds also. Even with these advantages, there is now a trend towards intermittent rather than daily therapy with medical agents. A recent study noted that alternative day (every other day) α-blockers were just as effective as daily use of their medications. In older patients, especially where the average number of pills per day is over six, there is very little desire to continue one more pill on a chronic basis. I have used α-blockers in my practice in many patients on an intermittent basis when symptoms appear to worsen as during travel, conferences, stress, and other situations. In these instances, patients use the medication only for a week or two.

With reference to surgery and minimally invasive therapies, it is now evident that patients prefer minimally invasive therapies that protect quality of life (i.e. low side effects) even if therapies are not immediately effective (few weeks as in TUR) and of unknown long-term durability (provided that at least durability data of 2–3 years is available).

The future challenge is for therapies to be more office based, short in duration, urologist friendly, and reasonable in cost. The availability of injectable therapies and improvements in biodegradable stents suggest that this form of treatment may have a role in BPH management, since these treatments are easy to perform and theoretically have low side effects.

Future Trends in Benign Prostatic Hyperplasia

31

G. Janetschek

For several decades the treatment of patients with benign prostatic hyperplasia (BPH) was relatively simple; there was only the choice of transurethral resection of the prostate (TURP), open surgery, or treatment with plant extracts. Over the past decade, however, the number of methods available for the management of BPH has been rapidly increasing. This goes for both medical and surgical therapy. Even for the specialist, it has become difficult to understand the true impact of each of these modalities, and it is still more difficult to anticipate their potential use in the future. Looking back, we have to concede that time and again we pursued elusive goals, and in many instances researchers have burdened themselves with an enormous workload without achieving the expected success. On the other hand, the progress which has actually been made would not have been possible without this research. However, we are currently not at the end but rather at the beginning of a long road. The different medical therapies available have to be evaluated for their effects and side effects, and the new technologies have to be optimized before they can be compared with each other in controlled studies, and, after some years, several of these modalities will probably be of historical interest only.

Despite the progress made in the management of BPH, its etiology remains unclear; therefore the prospects for prevention are still poor. There is an urgent need for analytic studies on BPH in order to identify the risk factors and thus improve the prospects for prevention. Age is definitely a risk factor, since males under 30 years of age do not develop BPH. About half the male population has developed BPH by age 50, and the incidence rises to 88% in the eighth decade of life. To date, however, no definite correlation has been established for other risk factors such as food, smoking, or sexual activity. The findings that white Europeans and Americans develop BPH more frequently than native Asians and Africans, while African and Asian immigrants to the USA develop BPH at similar rates to their Caucasian counterparts are suggestive of environmental or dietary factors. Yet, these observations, intriguing though they may be, cannot settle the issue.

INVESTIGATIONS

PRESSURE-FLOW STUDIES

It has been known for a long time that there is no direct correlation between the size of the prostate, the severity of symptoms, and the degree of bladder outlet obstruction. The pathophysiology of prostatism is most likely to be multifactorial. On account of the multitude of treatment modalities available today, it is essential to differentiate carefully between irritative symptoms and true obstruction in order to be able to select the most suitable therapy. Even though there is a general consensus that pressure-flow studies are the best tool for diagnosing true bladder outlet obstruction, they are rarely part of the preoperative work-up in BPH patients and are included only in an insignificant number of current publications.[1] Even sophisticated single-blind and double-blind prospective randomized studies do not include pressure-flow studies and, therefore, do not provide the necessary data.[2,3] In our comparative study on TURP and various laser techniques, the American Urological Association (AUA) symptom scores, peak flow rates, and postvoid residual volumes of the various cohorts did not reveal any significant differences, whereas pressure-flow cystometry clearly demonstrated that objectively assessable relief of obstruction was achieved only in the patients undergoing TURP.[4] Today we are, in fact, confronted with innumerable studies that lack urodynamic data and are therefore unsuitable for deciding on the most appropriate therapeutic modality; they only contribute to the widespread confusion that can be observed in this matter today. It may well be that in the foreseeable future urodynamics will be an indispensable part of the preoperative work-up in every BPH patient.

Furthermore, urodynamic studies can be expected to contribute to a better understanding of the underlying disease by differentiating between bladder outlet obstruction, poor detrusor contractility, and irritative symptoms. Improved preoperative work-up resulting in a more appropriate selection of the treatment modality would, in itself, be a great step forward in terms of therapeutic outcome. Retrospective studies have shown that about 30% of patients undergoing TURP did not actually suffer from urinary obstruction.[5] Not only could these patients have been spared an operation, but they might also have benefited from less invasive and more promising alternative methods. Currently, urodynamic studies are far from being used as a routine investigation; nevertheless, they represent the only way of obtaining objective preoperative diagnostic data. Yet, the choice of the most suitable treatment modality must be based on objective data, and it may well be that initiating therapy without preceding urodynamic assessment, even though not considered necessary at present, will be regarded as malpractice in the near future.

ULTRASONOGRAPHY

Currently, several techniques employing electric current, laser light, ultrasound, radiofrequency, and microwaves, as well as other forms of energy are used for the resection of prostatic tissue. Yet only rarely are their effects on the prostate documented. This may not be essential for routine therapeutic modalities, but if the efficacy of a treatment modality is to be evaluated in a controlled study, exact morphologic evaluation that should provide more data than just the size of the prostate is a must. This morphologic investigation has to be reliable, easy to perform for the physician, and not uncomfortable for the patient; it has to be documented in a reproducible form and should be repeated prior to treatment and several times during the follow-up period. While computed tomography (CT) scans are rather expensive and yield only little morphologic data, magnetic resonance imaging (MRI) is capable of providing more detailed information on the prostate, yet it is even more expensive and also troublesome for the patient.

In the 1960s, ultrasonography was introduced as a new imaging technique in urology; since then it has become a valuable diagnostic tool in the assessment of disorders of the genitourinary tract. With the advent of instruments for performing transrectal ultrasound, the indications for ultrasonography have been extended to include the prostate. Three-dimensional (3-D) transrectal ultrasonography (TRUS) is the first imaging technique capable of simultaneously demonstrating relevant structures in three planes; apart from the sagittal and horizontal planes, the region of interest can be assessed in the coronal plane as well (Figure 31.1). The structural differences of the prostatic zones in normal prostates and in BPH can be clearly identified.[6] The coronal plane provides important additional information; above all, the central zone and the enlarged transition zone can best be identified in this plane. The ultrasound equipment used in our department consists of a Combison 330 and a Voluson 3D multiplanar endorectal transducer (7.5 and 10 MHz) produced by Kretztechnik (Austria). This special transducer has two focusing ranges (short- and long-range). The investigation is performed with the patient in the right lateral position. Initially the relevant region is targeted with normal real-time imaging. Subsequently, a volume scan of this region is performed, which takes approximately 3–4 minutes. All ultrasonographic data obtained are collected in a volume image store. On the monitor of the system, three sections of the prostate can be displayed simultaneously in the horizontal, sagittal, and coronal planes. The coronal plane represents a calculated artificial section, which cannot be obtained by conventional ultrasonography. Since it is no longer necessary for the patient to be present once the volume scan has been obtained, the sonographer can take his/her time to evaluate the recorded ultrasound images later on. With the

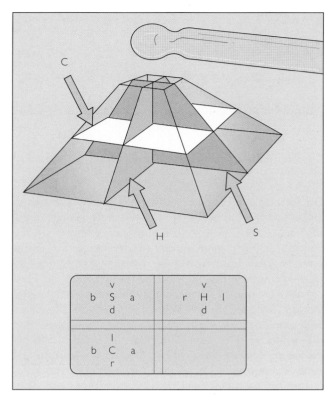

Figure 31.1 Three-dimensional TRUS. On the monitor (bottom) three sections of the prostate are displayed simultaneously: S=sagittal plane; H=horizontal plane; C=coronal plane; a=apical; b=basal; v=ventral; d=dorsal; l=left; r=right

Source: From H. Strasser *et al. Urology* 1996; **47**: 485–490, with permission from Elsevier Science

Combison 530, the data of the volume scan can be permanently stored on a floppy disk so that the pre- and postoperative status of the prostate can be compared at any time in real-time quality. This means that any targeted area within the prostate can be investigated for changes resulting from the treatment. This novel method of follow-up is unique and opens up new, as yet unknown, perspectives.

The effects of any type of treatment on prostatic tissue can be documented in relation to the zones of the prostate, and changes within the tissue occurring over a longer period of time can be demonstrated in a kind of "time-lapse photography."

Several ultrasonographic studies have shown that, compared with other ultrasonographic techniques, planimetric volume measurement of the prostate has the lowest variability (5% volume variation). The Kretz ultrasound equipment also contains a special program for planimetric volume measurement. But it is 3-D ultrasonography that has paved the way for volumetric assessment of the transition zone; it is a simple, easy, and quick method of determining not only the volume of the prostate as a whole, but also the volumes of its zones. Planimetric volume measurement is undoubtedly the most precise method of determining the volume of the prostate. Volumetry of the different prostatic zones before and after therapy and a correlation of these data with pressure-flow studies would provide reliable and objective data for determining which tissue is to be removed and to what extent in order to obtain optimum relief of obstruction. Since it is obviously an abnormal growth of the transition zone that is responsible for bladder outlet obstruction, therapeutic efforts should be focused on the removal of precisely this prostatic zone. The efficacy of therapy in this respect can be monitored by means of 3-D TRUS while pressure-flow urodynamics can demonstrate improvement in function (Figure 31.2). Pre-operative volumetry revealed a prostatic volume of 26.7 mL, while the volume of the transition zone in the same patient was 9.8 mL. Following thermotherapy using the T3 device (Urologix, USA), the prostatic volume decreased to 17.5 mL, which corresponds to a reduction in size by 9.2 mL (35%). The transition zone – the true target of therapy – decreased from 9.8 mL to 1.1 mL. The reduction in volume, which amounts to 8.7 mL (89%), demonstrates the efficacy of therapy. Urinary flow increased by 130%, and a pressure-flow study revealed complete relief of obstruction. Such studies should be undertaken to investigate, for example, why a 20–30% decrease in prostatic volume after treatment with finasteride results in an increase in the maximum flow rate by only 1.5 mL. It can be assumed that all zones of the prostate decrease in volume to about the same extent so that finally the degree of obstruction does not change significantly.

The technology described above is now on the market. The next step in this development will be a 3-D ultrasonographic system including 3-D color Doppler ultrasonography. With such a system, it will be possible intra- and immediately postoperatively to visualize with utmost precision the degree and exact localization of prostatic tissue damage produced by any kind of energy and to follow closely the post-therapeutic course and monitor any inflammation, absorption, scar formation, or cystic transformation that may occur. Conventional transrectal probes for performing color Doppler ultrasonography are available already, and the development of a 3-D color Doppler system can be expected in the near future.

MEDICAL THERAPY

FINASTERIDE

For many years, plant extracts were the only kind of medical therapy available; although they were used in a great number of patients, these drugs failed to show significant effects over placebo. The trend among a considerable number of patients toward non-surgical treatment has now led to the development of various new pharmacologic treatment options. All endocrine therapies known to reduce the size of the prostate, such as GnRH antagonists, cyproterone acetate, and flutamide, act on the male hypothalamic–pituitary–gonadal axis. Yet, they are only rarely used for the treatment of symptomatic BPH because of their severe side effects.

The 5α-reductase inhibitor finasteride is a new endocrine treatment option that has no severe side effects.

It has been safely used in symptomatic BPH patients who are not yet candidates for surgery but for several reasons, the overall success rate has not come up to expectations.[7] In a double-blind, placebo-controlled multicenter study including 707 patients treated for 7 months, a mean decrease in prostatic volume of 19% was observed for the finasteride group, whereas in the placebo group the prostatic volume increased by 12%. Surprisingly, the increase in flow rate did not correlate with this decrease in volume, and the mean peak flow rate increased by only 1.5 mL s^{-1}. Urodynamic studies were not performed, therefore the true degree of obstruction before therapy and relief of obstruction after finasteride administration could not be assessed.[8] By comparison, an 8–15% reduction in prostatic volume following laser therapy was found to result in a more pronounced increase in the mean peak flow rate (8–9 mL s^{-1}).[4] These inconclusive data indicate that the mechanism of obstruction is still poorly understood.

As already mentioned above, it may be speculated that finasteride administration results in uniform shrinkage of all prostatic zones, and does not affect the periurethral adenoma to a greater extent than the normal prostatic tissue. A decrease in total prostatic volume does not necessarily mean that the obstruction has been relieved. In this context, one has to keep in mind that the size of the prostate does not correlate with the degree of obstruction at all. Laser treatment, by contrast, obviously targets the periurethral tissue that has to be removed. In view of the small amount of tissue that is removed, relatively good relief of obstruction can be achieved with this technique.[4] An exact evaluation of the different zones of the prostate before and after treatment by means of 3-D ultrasonography might be expected to provide valuable data, but such a study has not been performed as yet.[6]

Finasteride does not act by instantly relieving the obstruction, as erroneously believed by many, but by halting the progressive enlargement of the gland. Therefore, patients with mild or moderate BPH are candidates for finasteride therapy, whereas those with advanced disease still require surgery. In other words, these two treatment modalities do not compete, but supplement each other.[9] It has been shown that finasteride can produce a sustained decrease in prostatic size for up to 5 years, and the same is true for its effects on clinical symptoms and maximum flow rate.[10] Future studies and the results of long-term follow-up will show whether the disease indeed does not progress in the long run, whether there is a group of patients in which prostatic growth continues despite finasteride administration, and whether there are clinical parameters capable of identifying such a group in advance. Moreover, the efficacy of the drug may be enhanced by developing 5α-reductase inhibitors that block Type 1 and Type 2 isoenzymes, the latter obviously being the more important one. The major disadvantage of finasteride administration is that it has to be continued indefinitely to maintain a therapeutic response. Consequently, cost-effectiveness is a concern, and the question arises as to whether in the long run surgical therapy will not be superior in this respect. On the other

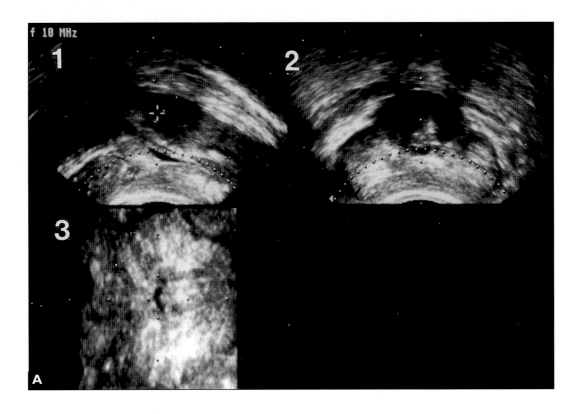

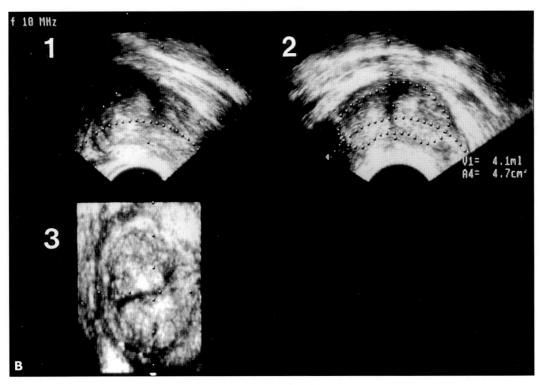

Figure 31.2 (A) Three-dimensional ultrasound of the prostate. The prostatic volume is 26.7 mL. The central and transition zones are best displayed in the coronal plane (3). The volume of the transition zone is 9.8 mL. (B) Three-dimensional ultrasound after transurethral microwave therapy (TUMT). The volumes of the prostate and transition zone are reduced to 17.5 and 1.1 mL, respectively

hand, it should be up to the patient to decide whether he prefers lifelong medical therapy or surgery, which, hopefully, has to be performed only once.

ALPHA₁-ADRENOCEPTOR ANTAGONISTS

There are two ways in which BPH causes bladder outlet obstruction. The first is by a static component, which is primarily related to the enlargement of the gland; most therapeutic concepts, including hormonal treatment, therefore, are aimed at a reduction in prostatic size. The second factor contributing to obstruction is a fluctuating dynamic component, which is related to the tone of prostatic smooth muscle and is regulated by neural activity.[11] The tone of prostatic smooth muscle is mediated by α_1-adrenoceptors.[12] Selective α_1-adrenoceptor antagonists act on smooth muscle by relaxing the tone, which results in a decrease in urethral resistance. Phenoxybenzamine, a non-selective α-blocker, was the first to be used for the treatment of BPH.[13] It proved to be effective, but did not gain widespread acceptance on account of its serious adverse side effects. In 1977, it was reported that prostatic smooth muscle tone is mediated by the α_1-subtype of the α-adrenoceptor.[14] Prazosin was one of the first α_1-adrenoceptor subtype antagonists available on the market. The main problem with α_1-selective agents is their effect on the smooth muscle portion in the walls of blood vessels, which in susceptible individuals, particularly diabetics, may give rise to postural hypotension. Recently, three subtypes of the α_1-adrenoceptor have been identified. They were initially described as α_{1a}, α_{1b}, and α_{1c}, but the classification has been changed, and the subtypes are now termed the α_{1d}, α_{1b}, and α_{1a} adrenoceptor. It is the α_{1a}-adrenoceptor subtype that mediates prostatic smooth muscle tone. The pharmaceutical industry is now actively engaged in the development of α_{1a}-adrenoceptor subtype antagonists, which are expected to be highly efficient without causing hypotension and other adverse reactions. However, it is also conceivable that the therapeutic effect of α_1-blockers is mediated by factors other than prostatic smooth muscle.[12]

At the 1995 AUA meeting in Las Vegas, two studies were presented investigating the effect of tamsulosin, an α_{1a}-blocker (old classification: α_{1c}).[15,16] Tamsulosin has been shown to be effective, safe, and well tolerated without the usual cardiovascular adverse events. These promising preliminary results have been confirmed by a double-blind study on its long-term efficacy.[17] Recently, the incidence of untoward reactions to tamsulosin has been demonstrated to be essentially the same in both young and old patients and not significantly different from that in placebo controls and the general population. In addition, tamsulosin did not reveal statistically significant differences compared with placebo with regard to pulse rate as well as supine and standing blood pressure.[18] These preliminary data need to be confirmed by others; at the same time, new substances are being investigated as the search for prostate-specific α_{1a} antagonists continues.[19]

In terms of clinical impact, α_1-blockers and finasteride differ significantly. On the one hand, α_1-blockers provide a more immediate response, but on the other hand, they have more severe side effects, the most serious being hypotension. This may change once more specific α_{1a} antagonists have proved efficient. Alpha₁-adrenoceptor antagonists do not influence the growth of the prostate at all. Therefore, they cannot substitute for or postpone surgery, but can only be employed to relieve symptoms in the interval between their onset and final therapy.

Alpha₁-blockers are the only therapeutic option targeting the dynamic component of bladder outlet obstruction, whereas all other treatment modalities are directed at the static component, which means that they reduce the size of the prostate. One exception might be microwave thermotherapy, which by some authors is supposed to destroy the α-receptors in the bladder neck and prostate. However, a study investigating these receptors before and after treatment has not been undertaken so far. On account of their different mode of action, α-blockers can – at least in theory – be combined with any other form of therapy to achieve a synergistic effect. The most promising concept appears to be the combination of α_1-blockers and finasteride. However, this approach cannot be recommended until prospective studies providing sufficient data on both efficacy and side effects have been performed.

SURGICAL MANAGEMENT

TRANSURETHRAL RESECTION OF THE PROSTATE

For several decades, open surgery and transurethral resection were the only surgical approaches available for the treatment of BPH. Great technical progress has been made in the past 30 years, and the morbidity associated with transurethral resection has been dramatically decreased. The overall complication rate, however, has remained virtually unchanged, ranging between 15 and 18%.[20] Therefore, great efforts have been made to develop possible alternatives which, ideally speaking, can match transurethral prostatectomy in efficacy but entail fewer complications. As a by-product of the advances achieved with the help of modern technology, the technique of TURP has been significantly improved, and further developments are currently under investigation.

Videoprostatectomy was introduced by O'Boyle et al. in 1984.[21] Though the introduction of a video camera has not enhanced the efficacy or decreased the morbidity of TURP, it makes it easier and more comfortable for the surgeon to perform the procedure, reduces the risk of contact with blood or urine, and greatly facilitates the teaching of TURP.

Wickham and coworkers have developed a prototype robot to enable the surgeon to perform TUR of the prostate more accurately, efficiently, and rapidly. An industrial robot, the Puma Unimate 6-axis robot arm, was modified to perform precision prostatectomy in vitro. A support and safety frame is positioned over the patient's perineum. The surgeon then manually introduces a conventional resectoscope into the urethra and attaches it to the robotic frame. The anatomic parameters of the prostate assessed by TRUS are loaded into the computer, which drives three electrical motors and the resectoscope that automatically resects the predetermined area of prostatic tissue. In initial trials, 30 patients were treated by manually moving the frame, and in the second phase only 3 patients have so far undergone fully automated resection.[22]

Several problems were encountered, which have not been fully overcome. In the early phase, the maximum volume that could be resected was only 18 mL, but this problem was solved by several modifications. Two of the initial 30 patients presented with residual median lobe tissue requiring additional manual resection. Furthermore, setting up the robot proved to be rather time consuming. The major disadvantage of the original robot, though, was that it could not be used for achieving hemostasis. Hence, after the resection had been performed by the robot, the surgeon had to coagulate all bleeding vessels manually, which proved quite tedious and time consuming, since heavy bleeding was encountered in many cases. In summary, there was no benefit in terms of operative time, and the procedure was much more complicated than a simple TURP; therefore automated TURP was abandoned. More recently, Wickham has started to use the robot again. Instead of a resectoscope, he now uses a VaporTrode in an attempt to solve the problem of hemostasis, but no results have been published as yet.

The morbidity of TURP is essentially related to hemorrhage; bleeding requiring one or more units of blood was seen in 4.2% of 1211 patients undergoing TURP at our department.[20] It must be added, though, that the risk of hemorrhage almost exclusively depends on the size of the prostate. Among our patients the average prostate was no larger than 37 g, and with this prostatic size blood transfusions are rarely needed. Nevertheless, great efforts are being made to reduce blood loss. A new electrosurgical loop with a wedge-shaped design has been developed for TURP. It is wider than the standard loop and thickens from front to back. With this design, it is possible to coagulate the resection bed as the chips are carved out, thereby minimizing blood loss. Pure cutting power simultaneously of 27 W was found to allow easy resection as well as optimum hemostasis, thus combining the benefits of both TURP and electrovaporization.[23]

In order to compare the safety of TURP by means of the wedge device (275 W) vs. the standard loop at a power setting of 150 W, the tissue changes in the prostate have been assessed in the canine model by recording the temperatures in and near the prostate as well as by means of gross and microscopic pathology. Gross pathology revealed that either technique created a cavity in the canine prostate without capsular perforation or damage to adjacent tissues or organs. Microscopic pathology yielded a 2-mm zone of superficial coagulation in the tissue following wedge resection. Real-time thermometry demonstrated a minimal rise in temperature in the prostatic capsule and rectum with both standard loop and wedge resection. On account of these favorable results, similarly shaped loops have been developed by several companies (Figure 31.3).[24]

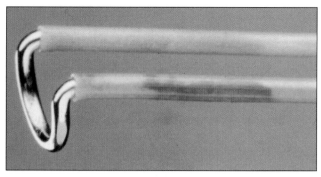

Figure 31.3 Special loop design for combined vaporization and resection (Wolf, Germany)

Modulation of the high-frequency generator may also contribute to reduced blood loss. In this instrument, the cutting and coagulating currents alternate and are switched automatically by an electronic device, depending on the resistance of the tissue. The initial results obtained with this prototype generator are very promising.[25]

Several innovative techniques of tissue ablation have been developed on the basis of TURP. Prostatic tissue can be vaporized with a rollerball electrode, the so-called VaporTrode, using existing endoscopic instrumentation and high-frequency generators. The great advantage of this method is that it is associated with minimal blood loss.[26] Different new designs of the electrode, which are expected to improve its efficacy, are currently being tested.

Since the application of high-frequency electrical power involves a number of hazards to the patient such as burns, nerve and muscle stimulation, or urethral stricture, the electrical parameters to which patients are exposed during tissue vaporization have been assessed in a clinical study. In vaporization, a 10-fold increase in input power was measured within identical application times compared with TURP. This means that in vaporization the power and the current density applied to the patient are as unfavorable as the properties of unregulated generators used in the past. Therefore, long-term follow-up of patients undergoing tissue vaporization is necessary to exclude urethral stricture.[27]

ROTORESECT

The Rotoresect, a completely new device for tissue ablation, has been developed with the aim of reducing the morbidity of TURP.[28] The Rotoresect device utilizes the coagulating high-frequency current to reduce bleeding and at the same time facilitates constant mechanical tissue ablation by means of a rotating ablator electrode fitted with semi-sharp resection wings (Figure 31.4). The ablation rate is regulated by the rotation speed. The Rotoresect, which is introduced into the urethra under visual control, first coagulates the prostatic tissue, which then increases in consistency and is subsequently shaved off by the ablator electrode. In the porcine model, the tissue ablation rate and blood loss were quantified *ex vivo* using blood-perfused kidneys ($n=30$) and then compared with loop resection and

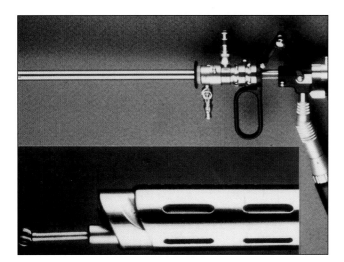

Figure 31.4 Rotoresect with coagulating ablator electrode (Storz, Germany)

electrovaporization (grooved roller/rollerball). Furthermore, transurethral rotoresection of the prostate and open partial resection of the liver were carried out in five dogs (*in vivo*). The animal study *ex vivo* demonstrated that the rate of tissue ablation increases with the frequency of the coagulation current and the rotation speed of the ablator electrode. The tissue ablation rate achieved by means of the Rotoresect was shown to be comparable to that of loop resection (5.5–6.0 g min⁻¹) which was more than double the rate of electrovaporization (1.7–2.0 g min⁻¹). In standard loop resection, blood loss was several times higher (16.5–18.0 g min⁻¹) than in rotoresection and electrovaporization (<2.3 g min⁻¹). The canine trials *in vivo* demonstrated that, with this new surgical tool, TURP and open segmental liver resection can be performed with minimal bleeding. The Rotoresect is a promising new instrument for tissue ablation in parenchymal organs, which is of great help in transurethral, laparoscopic, as well as open surgery. Currently, clinical trials are under way to evaluate the long-term efficacy and safety of transurethral rotoresection of the prostate for BPH.

LASER

In the past few years several techniques using laser technology have been developed for tissue ablation in the prostate. We have performed a prospective study comparing TURP with contact laser, interstitial laser, and TULIP.[4] All patients underwent detailed preoperative evaluation, including assessment of the AUA symptom score, uroflowmetry, determination of postvoid residual volume, TRUS to assess the prostatic volume, and pressure-flow studies. These investigations were repeated over a follow-up period of up to 1 year after surgery.

For contact laser treatment, a wide-angle zero-degree telescope has been developed in collaboration with Storz (Germany) to accommodate the semirigid fiber of the neodymium:yttrium–aluminum–garnet (Nd:YAG) laser on

which the contact tips are mounted.[29] By working the handle of the mechanism, the contact tip can be protruded forward up to 3 cm. The contact tips, which are available in many shapes, are produced by SLT and permit cutting, coagulation, or ablation. Recently, a right-angle probe has been developed to facilitate treatment of the lateral aspects of the prostate near the apex. Contact tips 4.0 and 5.0 mm in diameter have been developed, since the speed and efficacy of tissue ablation are very much dependent on the size of the contact tip.[29]

Nevertheless, laser vaporization has proved to be slow and time consuming, hence the technique has been limited to small prostates. In our experience, intraoperative bleeding was minimal, only few postoperative complications were encountered, and the results were slightly better than those of the laser techniques mentioned above. Good micturition was achieved immediately after removal of the indwelling catheter on the first or second postoperative day, which seems to be the greatest advantage of the contact laser technique. However, the overall results were clearly better for TURP. Consequently, we have abandoned Nd:YAG contact laser vaporization following the aforementioned study, mainly because of the slow speed and the small amount of tissue ablation. Possibly, future advances in fiber technology will permit higher energy densities to be delivered to the prostate so that vaporization becomes efficient enough to provide a valid alternative to TURP once again. Several groups are currently investigating the efficacy of the holmium laser, which appears to show great promise.

The Nd:YAG laser was also used for interstitial laser therapy. Precise positioning of the laser fiber was achieved with the help of a specific 3-D ultrasound guidance system, which was adapted for this purpose in collaboration with Kretz (Austria).[30] With this guidance system, the laser fibers can be positioned at any desired site in the prostate. This helps to preclude overlapping areas of tissue coagulation. Furthermore, precise placement of the laser fibers permits relatively large volumes of prostatic tissue to be coagulated with minimal bleeding and under no pressure of time (no TUR syndrome). In patients presenting with large prostates, interstitial laser therapy is certainly a good therapeutic option, which is associated with low morbidity. It is, therefore, particularly suitable for patients with advanced BPH who are in poor general health, as for these patients the lack of immediacy of the therapeutic effect does not present a significant drawback. We continued to use interstitial laser therapy for this group of patients after the results of our comparative study were in. However, more recently the technique has been abandoned in favor of thermotherapy. New diode laser systems specifically suited for interstitial laser therapy have been developed in the past few years. They are much smaller than Nd:YAG lasers, and in addition, they are far less expensive.

The well-known TULIP system has yielded the poorest results of the therapeutic modalities studied; in addition, it turned out to be associated with a high rate of complications and the highest rate of reoperations. This is why it is no longer used in clinical practice.

To understand the potential of the holmium laser compared with the widely used Nd:YAG laser, we have to go back to the physics of laser. The considerable differences in clinical effect between the large variety of surgical lasers are attributable to the great diversity of their wavelengths and of the resulting absorption characteristics of prostatic tissue. Absorption of laser energy produces heat in the tissue, which in turn results in a combination of ablation – vaporization and cutting – and coagulation.

The depth of penetration of laser energy into tissue largely depends on the absorption coefficient. The CO_2 laser, for example, with a wavelength in the mid-infrared portion of the spectrum is highly absorbable in water, which is the largest constituent of soft tissue. Therefore, the CO_2 laser has a very short absorption length, which means that it does not provide deep tissue penetration. Once laser light is absorbed by tissue, it is immediately converted to heat. These physical properties result in a "what you see is what you get" effect of the CO_2 laser on human tissue. Its endoscopic application is limited, since its light does not pass through flexible fibers. The Nd:YAG laser, by comparison, has the lowest absorption coefficient with regard to water, melanin, and hemoglobin. Hence the Nd:YAG laser has the greatest absorption length, which means that it has a deeper penetration than any other laser. Clinically, the Nd:YAG laser produces deep coagulation necrosis. When high energy is delivered during contact laser application, the tissue is vaporized on the surface so that deep penetration does not occur any longer. Owing to its physical properties, the Nd:YAG laser is better suited to produce deep necrosis than surface vaporization. The holmium:YAG (Ho:YAG) laser with a wavelength of 2.140 nm and an absorption length of 0.5 mm is somewhere between the CO_2 laser and the Nd:YAG laser. Its clinical applications are identical to those of the carbon dioxide wavelength, but the Ho:YAG laser has the benefit of a more pronounced coagulative effect. Since it can be delivered through flexible fibers, it can be expected to be very valuable for endoscopic tissue vaporization.

Both the feasibility and efficiency of endoscopic prostatic tissue ablation by means of the high-energy, free-beam Ho:YAG laser were demonstrated in the canine model. Significant tissue loss and sizable prostatectomy defects were produced acutely with adequate hemostasis.[31] Over the past 2 years, three different techniques employing the Ho:YAG laser for prostatectomy have evolved in clinical practice.[31] Holmium was used in combination with Nd:YAG in a procedure termed combination endoscopic laser ablation of the prostate (CELAP). Holmium laser ablation of the prostate (HoLAP) employs the Ho:YAG laser primarily to vaporize obstructing tissue, whereas holmium laser resection of the prostate (HoLRP) uses the holmium wavelength for resecting tissue in a mode similar to standard TURP. In a comparative study on these three different modalities, HoLRP proved to be superior. It produces a cavity identical in appearance to that achieved in TURP, is a relatively bloodless procedure, results in immediate improvement in flow rates and voiding symptoms, and is associated with low recatheterization rates and minimal morbidity.[32,33] A randomized, prospective clinical trial based on urodynamic studies demonstrated that HoLRP results in earlier improvement of voiding symptoms, fewer problems with dysuria, and better relief of obstruction than Nd:YAG laser prostatectomy.[34]

TRANSURETHRAL MICROWAVE THERAPY

The application of very high energy produces high surface temperatures resulting in tissue vaporization. Lower energy applied over a longer period of time, by comparison, heats a larger volume of tissue and results in coagulation necrosis. Relief of obstruction is achieved only after the necrotic tissue has been absorbed, which may take several weeks. Different sources of energy other than laser (sidefire, interstitial) such as microwaves, radiofrequency, and high-intensity focused ultrasound are alternative novel techniques used to produce coagulation necrosis. These technologies, however, vary greatly in their modes of application (transrectal vs. transurethral; catheter vs. needle), energy applied, temperature achieved within the prostate, the size, form and localization of the lesion achieved, and, last but not least, in the degree of invasiveness. The disadvantages of these methods compared with techniques that immediately remove the tissue are the postoperative irritative symptoms and the delayed relief of obstruction. On the other hand, they offer the advantage of reduced operative invasiveness, which is the decisive parameter when selecting the most suitable technique from among the modalities resulting in coagulation necrosis, provided, of course, their efficiency is adequate. Currently, none of these techniques can be considered preferable, since data from prospective randomized studies including pressure-flow measurements and exact ultrasonographic evaluation are still lacking. The ideal would be a method that does not require anesthesia, can be performed on an outpatient basis, is cost effective and easy to apply, involves minimal morbidity, results in relief of obstruction and symptoms in a high percentage of patients, and has a low retreatment rate. The final objective is a machine for the resection of the prostate similar to ESWL for stones. At present, however, there is no such method, and probably never will be, which meets all demands; at the moment it seems that thermotherapy has the potential to come closest. This technique has one advantage over all other methods that produce coagulation necrosis, namely the uniformity of hyperthermia in the transition zone. By comparison, all other techniques produce several "hot spots" with the tissue in between remaining at a low temperature. Over the past few years, we have used interstitial Nd:YAG laser therapy in patients with large prostates who were unfit for TURP. This method worked well and the outcome was good; however, anesthesia was required, and the procedure was time consuming and quite complicated.[4] In this highly selected risk group, we have recently abandoned interstitial laser therapy in favor of the

T3, a third generation thermotherapy device.[35] This device is currently under investigation in our department. The early results have been so encouraging that we intend to use it as an alternative to TURP (Figure 31.5). No anesthesia is required for this treatment, which takes but 1 hour and can be performed on an outpatient basis.

Heat treatment of tissue was first performed in a cancer patient by Busch in 1866.[36] Tumor cells are more sensitive to heat than normal cells, and temperatures between 42°C and 44°C may suffice to produce irreversible damage. The development of tissue heating by means of microwaves facilitates the application of thermal energy deep within the lateral lobes of the prostate. The first clinical devices employed a shielded antenna within the rectum, with simultaneous cooling of the rectal wall. These so-called hyperthermia devices created temperatures of up to 45°C within the prostate. Though the clinical results did show subjective improvement, the objective response was poor, and the widespread skepticism about microwave therapy stems from these early controversial data.[37-39]

Advances in microwave engineering have led to the development of flexible antennas that can be introduced into the urethra to permit direct application of heat to the obstructing tissue. The Prostatron, the first thermotherapy device, generated temperatures in excess of 45°C, but the results obtained were unsatisfactory.[40] It has been demonstrated that the outcome of thermotherapy improves with increased energy delivery and increased intraprostatic temperatures.[41] Currently available devices have difficulty maintaining high temperatures, as they shut off upon rectal heating. Owing to the design of its microwave antenna, the T3 device directs the energy preferentially to the lateral and anterior portions of the prostate, where temperatures as high as 80°C can be achieved (Figure 31.6).

The mean temperature reaches a maximum of 54°C at a radial distance of approximately 0.5 cm from the urethra and does not decrease below 45°C up to a distance of 1.6 cm. By means of the T3 device, uniform thermoablation of a broad zone of obstructing tissue that is demonstrable on histopathology can be achieved. On account of two factors, namely the antenna's capability of focusing thermal energy mainly on the anterolateral prostatic portion on the one hand, and the exponential reduction in temperature with decreasing distance from the microwave antenna on the other, significantly higher intraprostatic temperatures can be maintained without inducing potentially treatment-limiting rectal heating.[42,43] Depending on the design of the microwave antenna, the temperature profiles relative to the distance from the urethra may vary significantly among the different microwave thermal treatment systems. This must be taken into account when comparing these systems. The initial clinical results with the T3 device are excellent, and there is a high degree of patient satisfaction; however, follow-up data that include pressure-flow studies and ultrasonography of the prostate are still lacking.[35,44]

The vasculature and composition of the prostate are known to vary considerably among different individuals and the blood flow has been shown essentially to influence intraprostatic heating.[45] Consequently, we are now using a transrectal color Doppler probe before and after transurethral microwave therapy (TUMT) to investigate this issue.

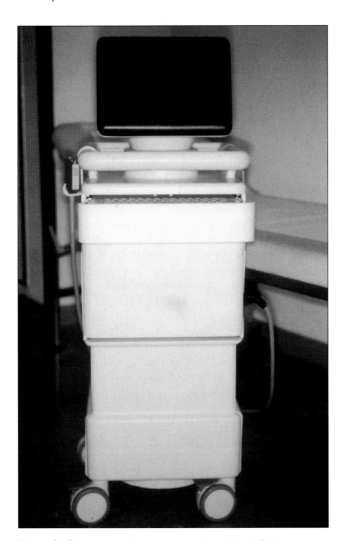

Figure 31.5 T3 thermotherapy system (Urologix, USA)

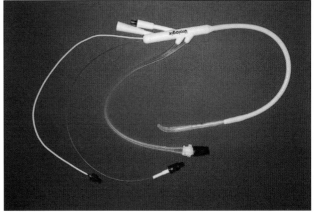

Figure 31.6 The microwave antenna of the T3 system (Urologix, USA) is placed within a transurethral catheter. Owing to the design of the antenna, preferential heating of the anterolateral portion of the prostate is achieved

It has been speculated that to some extent the effect of thermotherapy may be due to lesions of α-receptors, but no data are available as yet to support this hypothesis.

POSTOPERATIVE STENTING

The major drawback of minimally invasive treatment modalities resulting in coagulation necrosis is the delayed therapeutic effect. In order to avoid post-treatment catheterization, postoperative insertion of a prostatic stent of absorbable material (polyglycolic acid (PGA) stent, Bioscience Inc., Tampere, Finland) appears to be a very attractive option.[46]

A recent study has demonstrated that following high-energy thermotherapy for large, severely obstructing BPH, it was possible in all patients to preclude postoperative retention and catheterization by inserting a biodegradable PGA stent. Only minimal irritative symptoms were observed.[47] However, following laser prostatectomy PGA stenting resulted in severe irritative symptoms, so that the stents had to be removed in a great number of patients.[48] Obviously, the concept of postoperative stenting is not valid after laser prostatectomy, since this technique destroys the urethral epithelium, whereas in thermotherapy it remains intact.

EXPERIMENTAL MODEL FOR TISSUE ABLATION

It is difficult to compare directly the effectiveness of the various techniques of tissue ablation. Therefore, a standardized model permitting the assessment of tissue ablation and the related blood loss has been developed.[49] For this purpose freshly slaughtered porcine kidneys perfused with Tyrodes solution are utilized *ex vivo*. During ablation the kidneys are perfused with completely heparinized porcine blood at a pressure of 120–140 cmH$_2$O, so that the speed of tissue ablation and amount of blood lost can be quantified. The resection loop and vaporization electrodes have been compared using this model.[50] Electrovaporization techniques (ball, roller) were found to have a markedly reduced hemorrhagic tendency. However, compared with loop resection the ablation speed was slower.

CONCLUSIONS

A tremendous amount of research into the management of BPH has been performed so far, which has brought about a dramatic increase in therapeutic options. Nevertheless, a great number of questions remain to be solved, and only the future will show which of the methods presented in this book will stand the test of time. A number of studies on the early experience with minimally invasive methods have reported the therapeutic benefit of the novel techniques to equal that of TURP, which, however, could not be confirmed in subsequent randomized, double-blind studies. TURP still has an important role in the management of BPH, but medical treatment and minimally invasive techniques have to be given due consideration, and patients can be expected to benefit from all these efforts to improve therapy.

Yet there is an inherent danger in the diversification of therapeutic modalities. Just imagine a patient running through all treatment options available, beginning with some form of medical therapy, perhaps an α-blocker. After a while, because of side effects, for example, the drug might be replaced by finasteride for several years. Next, some form of minimally invasive therapy may have to be undertaken, which is not unlikely to require revision surgery. Finally, TURP is performed, and hopefully our patient is then free of symptoms and still continent. Such a patient history must not become the order of the day.

This cascade of therapeutic modalities is also responsible for the dramatic increase in total cost for the treatment of BPH. Since financial resources are rapidly decreasing, cost-effectiveness has become a major concern. The social security system may not be able and willing to afford therapeutic options of limited efficacy and a high likelihood of retreatment, when there is a more efficient alternative. The most costly aspect of any BPH treatment regimen is obviously its failure rate. As cost-effectiveness is going to be an important issue, the question will arise as to whether expensive medical treatment over many years should not be replaced by an efficient but less costly operation. An interesting study states that the cost of finasteride therapy for 10 years equals the cost of a single TURP.[10] Obviously, as soon as new medical therapies become available, there is an increasing patient demand for these treatment options. Of course, extremes have to be avoided, and the best road to take will lie somewhere in the middle. An operation that may seem expensive in an elderly patient might be very cost effective in a young patient compared with the non-surgical alternative. Still, the final decision for any type of treatment will always be up to the patient and the physician, and the information presented in this book is intended to help them to make the right choice.

REFERENCES

1 Höfner K. Urodynamic evaluation of lower urinary tract dysfunction. *Curr Opin Urol* 1992; **2**: 257–62.

2 Oesterling JE, Issa MM, Roehrborn CG *et al*. A single blind prospective randomized clinical trial comparing transurethral needle ablation (TUNA™) to transurethral resection of the prostate (TURP) for the treatment of benign prostatic hyperplasia (BPH). *J Urol* 1996; **155**: Abstract 372.

3 Keoghane S, Lawrence K, Doll H *et al*. One year data from the Oxford Laser Prostate Trial: a double blind, randomised controlled trial of TURP and contact laser prostatectomy. *J Urol* 1996; **155**: abstract 28.

4 Horninger W, Janetschek G, Watson G *et al*. Are contact laser, interstitial laser and TULIP superior to transurethral prostatectomy? *Prostate* 1997; **31**: 255–63.

5 Schäfer W, Rübben H, Noppeney R, Deutz FJ. Obstructed and unobstructed "prostatic obstruction." A plea for objectivation of bladder outflow obstruction by urodynamics. *World J Urol* 1989; **6**: 198–203.

6 Strasser H, Janetschek G, Reissigl A, Bartsch G. Prostate zones in three-dimensional transrectal ultrasound. *Urology* 1996; **47**: 485–90.

7 Glazier DB, Lee G, Weiss RE *et al*. Urodynamic assessment of the efficacy of finasteride. *J Urol* 1995; **153**: abstract 361.

8 Andersen JT, Ekman P, Wolf H *et al*. Can finasteride reverse the progress of benign prostatic hyperplasia? A two-year placebo-controlled study. *Urology* 1995; **46**: 631–7.

9 Moore E, Bracken B, Bremner W *et al*. Proscar®: five-year experience. *Eur Urol* 1995; **28**: 304–9.

10 Geller J, Kirschenbaum A, Lepor H, Levine AC. Therapeutic controversies: clinical treatment of benign prostatic hyperplasia. *J Clin Endocrinol Metab* 1995; **80**: 745–7.

11 Caine M, Pfau A, Perlberg S. The use of alpha-adrenergic blockers in benign prostatic obstruction. *Br J Urol* 1976; **48**: 253–63.

12 Lepor H. Role of long-acting selective alpha-1 blockers in the treatment of benign prostatic hyperplasia. *Urol Clin North Am* 1990; **17**: 651–9.

13 Caine M, Perlberg S, Meretyk S. A placebo-controlled double-blind study of the effect of phenoxybenzamine in benign prostatic obstruction. *Br J Urol* 1978; **50**: 551–4.

14 Berthelson S, Pettinger WA. A functional basis for the classification of alpha adrenergic receptor. *Life Sci* 1977; **21**: 595–606.

15 Lepor H. Clinical evaluation of tamsulosin, a prostate selective alpha 1c antagonist. *J Urol* 1995; **153**: abstract 182.

16 Abrams P, Schulman CC, Vaage S. The efficacy and safety of 0.4 mg tamsulosin once daily in symptomatic BPH. *J Urol* 1995; **153**: abstract 184.

17 Lepor H. Long-term evaluation of tamsulosin, a prostate selective alpha 1 antagonist. *J Urol* 1996; **155**: abstract 1099.

18 Chapple C. Tamsulosin: tolerability in older and younger symptomatic BPH patients. *J Urol* 1996; **155**: abstract 1057.

19 Noble AJ, Chess-Williams R, Couldwell CJ, Chapple CR. The affinity of a new prostate selective α1 adrenoceptor antagonist at functional α1-adrenoceptors. *J Urol* 1996; **155**: abstract 1108.

20 Horninger W, Unterlechner H, Strasser H, Bartsch G. Transurethral prostatectomy: mortality and morbidity. *Prostate* 1996; **28**: 195–200.

21 O'Boyle PJ, Lumb GN, Appleton GVN. Videoprostatectomy. In: *Endourology, Third Congress Issue*. Karlruhe Verlag 1984; 323–4.

22 Timoney AG, Eng M, Hibberd RD, Wickham JEA. Use of robots in surgery: development of a frame for prostatectomy. *J Endourol* 1991; **5**: 165–8.

23 Perlmutter AP. "The Wedge": a new resection loop for transurethral prostatectomy. *J Urol* 1996; **155**: abstract 1101.

24 Perlmutter AP, Vallancien G. Thick loop transurethral resection of the prostate. *Eur Urol* 1999; **35**: 161–5.

25 Hartung R, Barba M, Leyh H, Fastenmeier K. Verbesserung der Hochfrequenz-Chirurgie bei der TURP: Koagulierendes Schneiden. *Urologe A* 1995; **74**: abstract V9.1.

26 Kaplan SA, Te AE. Transurethral electrovaporization of the prostate: a novel method for treating men with benign prostatic hyperplasia. *Urology* 1995; **45**: 566–73.

27 Leyh H, Fastenmeier K, Barba M, Hartung R. Electrical current and power applied to the patient during transurethral vaporisation of the prostate. *J Urol* 1996; **155**: abstract 1047.

28 Michel MS, Köhrmann KU, Weber A *et al*. Rotoresect: a new technique for resection of the prostate: experimental phase. *J Endourol* 1996; **10**: 473–8.

29 Bartsch G, Janetschek G. The development of an endoscope and of contact probes for transurethral laser surgery of the prostate. *J Urol* 1994; **151**: abstract 424.

30 Strasser H, Janetschek G, Horninger W, Bartsch G. 3-D sonographic guidance for interstitial laser therapy in benign prostatic hyperplasia. *J Endourol* 1995; **9**: 497–501.

31 Kabalin JN. Holmium:YAG laser prostatectomy canine feasibility study. *Lasers Surg Med* 1996; **18**: 221–4.

32 Fraundorfer MR, Gilling PJ. The holmium laser in the treatment of benign prostatic hyperplasia. *J Urol* 1996; **155**: abstract 29.

33 Gilling PJ, Cass CB, Cresswell MD, Fraundorfer MR. Holmium laser resection of the prostate: preliminary results of a new method for the treatment of benign prostatic hyperplasia. *Urology* 1996; **47**: 48–51.

34 Gilling PJ, Fraundorfer MR. Holmium laser resection of the prostate versus Nd:YAG coagulation prostatectomy: a randomised prospective, urodynamics-based trial. *J Urol* 1996; **155**: abstract 30.

35 Ramsey EW, Miller PD, Parsons K. Preferential heating using transurethral microwave thermoablation (T3) improves clinical results. *J Urol* 1996; **155**: abstract 368.

36 Busch W. Uber den Einflusse welchen heltigere Erysipeln zuweilen auf organisierte neubildungen. *Verh Naturheil Preuss* 1866; **23**: 28–30.

37 Lindner A, Braf Z, Lev A. Local hyperthermia of the prostate gland for the treatment of benign prostatic hypertrophy and urinary retention. *Br J Urol* 1990; **65**: 201–3.

38 Strohmaier WL, Bichler KH, Flüchter SH, Wilbert DM. Local microwave hyperthermia of benign prostatic hyperplasia. *J Urol* 1990; **144**: 913–17.

39 Yerushalmi A, Fishelovitz Y, Singer D *et al*. Localized deep microwave hyperthermia in the treatment of poor operative risk patients with benign prostatic hyperplasia. *J Urol* 1985; **133**: 873–6.

40 Devonec M, Berger N, Perrin B. Transurethral microwave heating of the prostate or from hyperthermia to thermotherapy. *J Endourol* 1991; **5**: 129–36.

41 Perrin P, Devonec M, Houdelette P *et al*. Transurethral microwave thermotherapy: higher energy protocol improves clinical results. *J Urol* 1995; **153**: abstract 821.

42 Larson TR, Collins JM. An accurate technique for detailed prostatic interstitial temperature-mapping in patients receiving microwave thermal treatment. *J Endourol* 1995; **9**(4): 339–47.

43 Larson TR, Bostwick DG, Corica A. Temperature correlated histopathologic changes following microwave thermoablation of obstructive tissue in patients with benign prostatic hyperplasia. *Urology* 1996; **47**: 463–9.

44 Blute M, Bruskewitz R, Lason TR, Mayer R, Utz W. U.S. wide multi-center study results of a new high temperature office based microwave system (T3) for the treatment of BPH. *J Urol* 1996; **155**: abstract 1590.

45 Larson TR, Collins JM. Increased prostatic blood flow in response to microwave thermal treatment: preliminary findings in two patients with benign prostatic hyperplasia. *Urology* 1995; **46**: 584–90.

46 Kemppainen E, Talja M, Riihelä M *et al*. A bioresorbable urethral stent. *Urol Res* 1993; **21**: 235–8.

47 Dahlstrand C, Pettersson S. Resorbable stents can prevent retention after high energy TUMT for large symptomatic benign prostatic hyperplasia. *J Urol* 1996; **155**: abstract 384.

48 Costello AJ, Crowe HR, Asopa R. Long term results of randomized laser prostatectomy versus TURP: modification of laser prostatectomy technique with biodegradable stent insertion. *J Urol* 1996; **155**: abstract 22.

49 Michel MS, Niedergethmann M, Henkel TO *et al*. A new standardised ex vivo model for the evaluation of alternative tissue ablation methods. *J Endourol* 1995; **9**: abstract O3–30.

50 Köhrmann KU, Michel MS, Alken P. Loop, rollerball or vaportrode: an experimental comparison. *J Endourol* 1995; **9**: abstract O3–31.

Index

Note: Page references in *italics* refer to Figures; those in **bold** refer to Tables